MOSBY'S
NEUROLOGY
PSYCHIATRY
ACCESS SERIES

Washington University

Adult Psychiatry

OTHER BOOKS IN MOSBY'S NEUROLOGY PSYCHIATRY ACCESS SERIES

Parmelee, Child and Adolescent Psychiatry

David, Child and Adolescent Neurology

Corey-Bloom, Adult Neurology

MOSBY'S
NEUROLOGY
PSYCHIATRY
ACCESS SERIES

Washington University
Adult Psychiatry

Samuel B. Guze, MD
Editor

Spencer T. Olin Professor of Psychiatry
Head of the Department
Washington University School of Medicine
Saint Louis, Missouri

Ronald B. David, MD
Series Editor

Children's Neurological Services
Associate Clinical Professor of Pediatrics
Medical College of Virginia
Virginia Commonwealth University
Richmond, Virginia

Mosby

St. Louis Baltimore Boston Carlsbad Chicago Naples New York Philadelphia Portland
London Madrid Mexico City Singapore Sydney Tokyo Toronto Wiesbaden

Mosby
Dedicated to Publishing Excellence

A Times Mirror Company

Vice President and Publisher: Anne S. Patterson
Editors: Laura DeYoung and Michael Brown
Developmental Editor: Rebecca Gruliow
Associate Developmental Editor: Jennifer Byington Geistler
Editorial Assistant: Marla Sussman
Project Manager: Deborah L. Vogel
Production Editor: Karen L. Allman
Designer: Pati Pye
Manufacturing Manager: Theresa Fuchs
Cover Art: Bob Cass

Printed in the United States of America
Composition by Clarinda Company
Printing/binding by Maple-Vail Book Mfg Group

Mosby-Year Book, Inc.
11830 Westline Industrial Drive
St. Louis, Missouri 63146

Library of Congress Cataloging in Publication Data
Adult psychiatry / [edited by] Samuel B. Guze. — 1st ed.
p. cm. — (Mosby's neurology psychiatry access series)
Includes bibliographical references and index.
ISBN 0-8151-3993-4
1. Psychiatry. I. Guze, Samuel B., 1923- . II. Series.
[DNLM: 1. Mental Disorders—diagnosis. 2. Mental Disorders--therapy. WM 140 A244 1996]
RC454.A319 1996
616.89—dc20
DNLM/DLC
for Library of Congress 96-15338
CIP

96 97 98 99 00 / 9 8 7 6 5 4 3 2 1

Contributors

Carmen Bayon, MD
Visiting Fellow,
Department of Psychiatry,
Washington University School of Medicine

Laura Jean Bierut, MD
Instructor in Psychiatry,
Washington University School of Medicine

Kevin John Black, MD
Instructor in Psychiatry,
Washington University School of Medicine

Kelly Botteron, MD
Assistant Professor of Psychiatry,
Washington University School of Medicine;
Assistant Professor of Radiology,
Mallinkrodt Institute of Radiology,
Saint Louis, Missouri

C. Robert Cloninger, MD
Wallace Renard Professor of Psychiatry,
Washington University School of Medicine

Wilson M. Compton, MD
Assistant Professor of Psychiatry,
Washington University School of Medicine

John N. Constantino, MD
Instructor in Psychiatry and Pediatrics,
Washington University School of Medicine

John G. Csernansky, MD
Gregory B. Couch Professor of Psychiatry,
Washington University School of Medicine

Stephen H. Dinwiddie, MD
Associate Professor of Psychiatry,
Washington University School of Medicine

Wayne C. Drevets, MD
Associate Professor of Psychiatry,
Associate Professor of Radiology,
Assistant Professor of Anatomy and Neurobiology,
Washington University School of Medicine

Nuri B. Farber, MD
Assistant Professor of Psychiatry,
Washington University School of Medicine

Samuel B. Guze, MD
Spencer T. Olin Professor of Psychiatry
and Head of the Department,
Washington University School of Medicine

Barry A. Hong, PhD
Associate Professor of Medical Psychology
in Psychiatry,
Washington University School of Medicine

Richard W. Hudgens, MD
Professor of Psychiatry,
Washington University School of Medicine

Keith Eugene Isenberg, MD
Associate Professor of Psychiatry,
Washington University School of Medicine

Barbara A. Koppe, MSW, LCSW
Supervisor, Psychiatric Social Work,
Barnes Hospital,
Saint Louis, Missouri

Richard E. Mattison, MD
Associate Professor of Child Psychiatry,
Washington University School of Medicine

Steven O. Moldin, PhD
Formerly:
Assistant Professor of Medical Psychology
in Psychiatry,
Washington University School of Medicine,
Saint Louis, Missouri;
Currently:
Chief, Genetics Research Program,
Schizophrenia Research Branch,
Division of Clinical and Treatment Research,
National Institute of Mental Health,
National Institutes of Health;
Rockville, Maryland

George E. Murphy, MD
Professor Emeritus of Psychiatry,
Washington University School of Medicine

Elliot C. Nelson, MD
Assistant Professor of Psychiatry,
Washington University School of Medicine

John W. Newcomer, MD
Assistant Professor of Psychiatry,
Washington University School of Medicine

Carol S. North, MD
Assistant Professor of Psychiatry,
Washington University School of Medicine

Thomas R. Przybeck, PhD
Research Assistant Professor of Anthropology in Psychiatry,
Washington University School of Medicine

Daniel D. Pugh, MD
Associate Professor of Psychiatry,
Washington University School of Medicine

Devna Rastogi-Cruz, MD
Instructor in Psychiatry,
Washington University School of Medicine

Eugene H. Rubin, MD, PhD
Professor of Psychiatry,
Washington University School of Medicine

Dragan M. Svrakic, MD, PhD
Assistant Professor of Psychiatry,
Washington University School of Medicine

Richard D. Todd, PhD, MD
Ittleson Professor of Child Psychiatry,
Professor of Genetics,
Washington University School of Medicine

Richard D. Wetzel, PhD
Professor of Medical Psychology in Psychiatry,
Professor of Neurology and Neurological Surgery,
Washington University School of Medicine

Sean H. Yutzy, MD
Assistant Professor of Psychiatry,
Director of Forensic Services,
Washington University School of Medicine

Charles F. Zorumski, MD
Professor of Psychiatry and Neurobiology,
Washington University School of Medicine

To our many students, residents, and fellow faculty members, past and present, who, over the many years, helped shape our thinking and practice with regard to the care of psychiatric patients.

Foreword

Each book in this series is built on a structural framework that was well received by critics and readers alike in David, *Pediatric Neurology for the Clinician.* Each volume is divided into three sections:

- Tools for diagnosis
- Diseases and disorders
- Common problems

Also included to facilitate a physician's use of this book are:

- Diagnostic tables
- "Pearls and Perils" boxes
- "Consider Consultation When . . ." boxes
- Selected annotated bibliographies
- A complete bibliography

Diagnostic tables are based on a discriminator model to promote clearer understanding and are superior to a criterion-based model and others that lack similar specificity. Classification systems induce an orderliness in thinking and enhance our ability to communicate effectively. A review of the most enduring hierarchial classification systems, particularly that of Linnaeus (that is, phyla, genera, species), makes clear the value of grouping according to discriminating features, as well as the value of simplicity, expandability, and dynamism.

The goal, whatever the classification system, is to seek the most powerful discriminating features that produce the greatest diagnostic clarity. Much of the confusion that arises in diagnosis may be the result of the clinician who unwittingly crosses the anatomic, pathologic, pathophysiologic, phenomenologic, and etiologic classification domains used in medicine (for example, the inclusion of anatomically-oriented "temporal lobe seizures" in a phenomenologically based classification system that includes complex partial seizures). Some conditions, such as brain tumors, are classified according to their histopathology and lend themselves well to this classification system. Others, such as headaches and movement disorders, are classified phenomenologically and are therefore much less easily classified. In other cases, discriminators must encompass inclusionary as well as exclusionary features. At times, we can only use a criterion-based system or construct tables to compare features. Discriminating features should avoid crossing domains. Arbitrarily, we label as consistent features those that occur more than 75% of the time; features are considered variable when they occur less than 75% of the time. The diagnostic tables should be viewed, therefore, only as a beginning in the extremely difficult effort to make diagnosis more precise and biologically based. How well this book accomplishes the goals of identifying the most powerful discriminating features for maximum diagnostic clarity is limited by the current state-of-the-art in child and adolescent psychiatry. In some areas, several features, when clustered together, serve to discriminate.

> Whoever having undertaken to speak or write hath first laid for themselves some [basis] to their argument such as hot or cold or moist or dry or whatever else they choose, thus reducing their subject within a narrow compass.
>
> Hippocrates

As Hippocrates has suggested, structure is the key to learning. Unless there is a structure onto which knowledge can be built, confusion and disorganization are the inevitable consequences. Although each text in this series reflects appropriate stylistic differences among content editors, each is built on the same structural framework; hence the value of these texts to the users. It is therefore my fondest wish that these texts be on your desk rather than on your bookshelf.

As a part of this foreword, I would like to acknowledge some of the people who have made key contributions to this effort. They include Craig Percy, who initially saw the potential of this effort; the National Institute of Neurological Disease and Stroke (NINDS)* for their support in nosologic research and to the investigators who were involved with this NINDS project; Dr. Katherine Bick, whose help was invaluable in the final review of the manuscript; Dr. Grover Robinson, a long-time friend (who suggested the "Consider Consultation When . . ." boxes for the present series); Ms. Laura DeYoung, Mr. Michael Brown, and all of the Mosby team who made this vision a reality; and Dr. Samuel Guze, with whom I share a passion for biologically based diagnostic specificity.

Ronald B. David, MD

*NINDS 1PO1NS20489-01A1

Preface

This book has certain distinctive attributes. First, it is directed to generalists or primary care practitioners, physicians who nearly always need to know a good deal concerning psychiatric conditions and how to think about and manage them. For the same reason, it is also directed to medical students and residents. We of course hope that it will, at the same time, be of use to psychiatrists and other mental health professionals. For all such potential readers, we have tried to make clear that psychiatric disorders are very common, widespread, and often disabling; have great impact on the victim's life and family; and often carry risk of premature death. *No illnesses cause more widespread suffering and devastation to the victims and their relatives.*

We have tried to make clear that the most appropriate approach for dealing with psychiatric conditions is to use the concepts and strategies from general medicine: emphasizing diagnosis and differential diagnosis, course, outcome, complications, treatment, etiology, pathogenesis, and epidemiology. This approach is what is meant by the term *Medical Model,* which encapsulates the above concepts and strategies.

Because this Department of Psychiatry has played a central role in the application of the Medical Model to psychiatry and in its gradual acceptance by the field, we concluded that drawing our authors from the Department's faculty would maximize the likelihood of a consistent and useful book.

Our readers will not be surprised by our conviction that the future of psychiatry will increasingly depend on research in the neurosciences (including of course neuropharmacology), genetics, and neuroimaging, as well as continued improvements in clinical skills, epidemiology, and the organization of medical care (including psychiatry) generally.

Finally, but of great importance, we have tried to make clear that psychiatric conditions are the most characteristically human of medical problems, dealing as they do with temperament, personality, thinking, emotion, learning perception, motivation, sexuality, interpersonal relationships, and character. No medical conditions require more sensitivity and compassion from the physician. These attributes in turn depend on significant knowledge and training because physicians must understand, recognize, and accept the validity of psychiatric disorders to reflect to the patient and family the understanding and sympathy that are essential for good medical care. If our book helps achieve these goals, we shall be truly gratified.

Samuel B. Guze, MD
Richard W. Hudgens, MD
Eugene H. Rubin, MD, PhD
Charles F. Zorumski, MD

Contents

section one

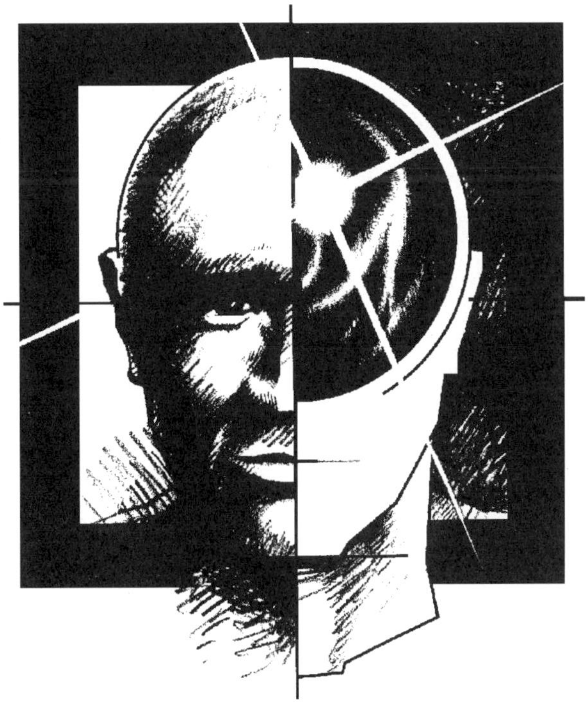

Assessment and Evaluation

Richard W. Hudgens, MD

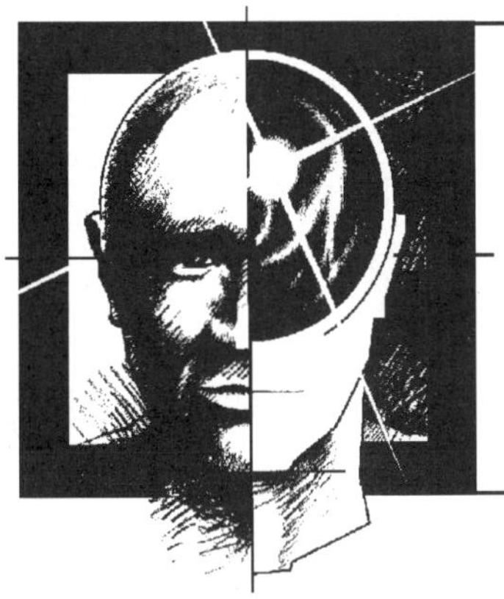

chapter 1

Psychiatry and the Medical Model

Kevin John Black, MD and Samuel B. Guze, MD

Psychiatry is a medical specialty concerned with disturbances of thought, emotions, and behavior. This definition may seem simple and obvious, but it is a product of a long and contentious history. Over the years, mental illnesses have been assessed, explained, and treated in different ways. This book teaches an approach to mental illness that has been called the *medical model of psychiatry.* This is simply the consistent application, in psychiatry, of modern medical thinking and methods. In this chapter, we briefly review the history that led up to this conceptual approach to mental illness and discuss some alternative views. After describing several practical benefits of the medical model, we attempt to debunk some common myths about psychiatry.

Psychiatry Defined

In the previous paragraph, psychiatry was defined as a medical specialty concerned with disturbances of thought, emotions, and behavior. Notice what this definition does not say. There is no reference to what causes the disturbed thinking, mood, or behavior. Psychiatry is not concerned only with illnesses that have psychological causes. One reason for this is that many different illnesses can cause the same symptoms, and treatment and prognosis are often quite different. For instance, depressed mood can be caused by manic-depressive illness, personality disorder, alcoholism, hypothyroidism, stroke, bereavement, or everyday disappointments. When patients seek help, they rarely wear labels indicating the cause of their symptoms; diagnosis is an essential part of the physician's duty. The differential diagnosis of these mental symptoms is a medical question for which psychiatrists are best suited by nature of their education and training. A second reason for not limiting psychiatry to illnesses with psychological causes is that treatment for psychiatric syndromes can be similar no matter what the etiology, and psychiatrists have expertise in these symptomatic treatments. For instance, the manic syndrome can be effectively treated with hospitalization, medication, or electroconvulsive therapy (ECT), whether it is the result of bipolar disorder or encephalitis. A third reason is that there are few, if any, illnesses known to have purely psychosocial etiologies. For most major mental illnesses, etiological knowledge remains incomplete, but there is strong evidence for genetic and biochemical components.

In other words, psychiatry is best defined by the clinical manifestations of its patients and not by what causes these manifestations (see the Pearls & Perils box to the right). Thus hallucinations are psychiatric symptoms whether they are caused by drug use, brain tumors, or schizophrenia, and major depression is a psychiatric syndrome whether it is the result of reserpine, stroke, or bipolar disorder.

Another medical specialty, neurology, is also concerned with disturbances of thought, emotions, and behavior. Naturally there is a considerable overlap of interests. For instance, there are conditions for which expertise is shared by the two specialties (such as Tourette's disorder, Alzheimer's disease, and sleep disorders). There are illnesses in each specialty without clear pathology (such as torticollis and panic disorder) and illnesses in either specialty with clear pathology (for example, stroke and Wilson's disease psychosis). There are several conditions that were treated by psychiatrists a century ago but are now treated by neurologists (such as epilepsy and neurosyphilis). Most commonly, there are illnesses that take patients to both neurologists and psychiatrists (such as depression and somatization disorder). Obviously there are differences: neurologists do not commonly treat mania or personality disorder, and psychiatrists do not commonly treat epilepsy or multiple sclerosis. However, there is enough overlap between the two specialties to discredit the simplistic notion that pathology and etiology reliably distinguish them.

PEARLS & PERILS

WHAT IS PSYCHIATRY?

- Psychiatry is a medical specialty concerned with disturbances of thought, emotions, and behavior.
- Psychiatric practice still includes "organic" disorders of cognition and mood.
- Psychiatric illnesses can be reliably diagnosed.
- Most psychiatric illnesses can be effectively treated but often go untreated.
- Psychiatric illnesses are real, common, and serious, yet they remain stigmatized.
- People with mental illnesses deserve a physician's care as much as people with other equally severe illnesses.

Models of Mental Illness

As Western civilization has changed and science has progressed, theories of illness have changed. Mental illness is no exception. The history of these changes explains a great deal of current popular opinion about mental illness. A brief and selective synopsis of this history follows.

Pre-1800s

Hippocrates wrote:

> From the brain, and from the brain only, arise our pleasures, joys, laughter and jests, as well as our sorrows, pains, griefs and tears. . . . It is the same thing which makes us mad or delirious, inspires us with dread or fear. . . . and [produces] acts that are contrary to habit. These things that we suffer all come from the brain when it is not healthy, but becomes abnormally hot, cold, moist, or dry.

In other words, psychological symptoms, like physical symptoms, were ascribed to alterations in bodily elements or humors. The term *melancholia* (literally *black bile*) reflects this conception. Other ancient cultures also attributed emotions and thought, like sensation or movement, to bodily dysfunction. The brain was sometimes implicated, but so were the heart, bowels, and uterus. However, bodily disease was not always presumed. Mental illness in several cultures was ascribed to mystical or supernatural influence. However, these same influences were often believed to cause somatic illnesses as well. In other words, mental and physical illnesses have often been thought to have similar causes.

However, a competing idea over time has been that mental illnesses are by their nature different from other illnesses. In this view, the causes, treatments, and study of mental illnesses are assumed to be different from those of physical illnesses. This concept derives in part from a philosophical view, represented and solidified by René Descartes, that mind and body are of two different genera, neither knowable by the methods used to study the other. This concept of mind-body duality has been prominent for the last several centuries and underlies much of the debate mentioned in succeeding paragraphs.

Origins of the Medical Model

The late nineteenth century was a time of great strides in medicine. Among others who could be named, Koch and Pasteur elucidated the role of bacterial pathogens in infectious disease. Virchow developed modern pathology, and with clinical-pathological correlation, he laid the foundations of a new specialty, internal medicine, which relied on the application of biology to everyday clinical medicine. The English surgeon Hunter tested the safety of new treatments before they were applied to patients. These and other advances in basic medical science in the nineteenth century led to the dramatic and well-known medical discoveries of the twentieth century.

Perhaps more important than the scientific discoveries themselves, however, was a new approach to illness. Many specific discoveries or treatments have come and gone over the last century. However, the empirical approach to medical research has remained more constant. This approach to illness had roots in the late 1600s, when Sydenham championed the ideas that symptoms with a given cause fell into natural groupings, or syndromes, and that study of such syndromes was the best approach to uncovering the causes of the presenting symptoms. Koch, Pasteur, Virchow, Hunter, and others contributed specific important discoveries to medical science, but they changed medicine in a broader way by beginning to use controlled studies that tested a hypothesis. This method of discovery, the scientific method, soon spread to clinical medicine. This change was solidified in the early twentieth century when Fisher laid the foundations of modern biostatistics. Case studies, personal experience, and authority were no longer the unquestioned basis of medical epistemology. Instead a reliance on the scientific method has come to generally characterize modern medical training. In other words, at the core of modern medicine is thinking about patients scientifically.

Even before modern research methods had matured, psychiatry shared in these advances. Philippe Pinel, considered by his contemporaries to be the leading French authority in general medicine, is often credited with founding psychiatry as a medical discipline with his 1801 textbook on insanity, which discussed psychosis as properly falling within the purview of medicine. He felt that mental illness should be classified by a "deep study of the symptoms" rather than by presumed etiology. Antoine Bayle linked general paralysis of the insane to the pathological lesions of neurosyphilis and later suggested that other forms of insanity should also be studied with clinical-pathological correlation. Karl Friedrich Kahlbaum contributed the careful, longitudinal study of psychiatric symptoms and sought to find commonalities among a group of patients with similar course and outcome. Emil Kraepelin used this longitudinal approach, motivated by Sydenham's assumption that etiology could best be discovered by studying syndromes, to divide schizophrenia from manic-depressive illness. As chair of an influential department of psychiatry, Kraepelin also brought together a number of renowned psychiatric scientists, including Alois Alzheimer, to study mental illness with scientific methods. Julius Wagner-Juaregg not only developed fever therapy for neurosyphilis, which won him the Nobel Prize, but also made fundamental contributions to the treatment of endemic cretinism. Hans Berger invented the electroencephalograph, which had tremendous implications for the diagnosis and treatment of epilepsy. Not surprisingly, these discoveries led to great hope for further advances for the treatment of other forms of psychosis through continued biological investigations. Leading physicians such as Griesinger, Maudsley, Schneider, and Wernicke believed that insanity was a disease of the brain and best studied by the methods of neuropathology.

Again, the specific discoveries of this period of psychiatry are not the focus of this chapter. Rather, they are important as instances of applying the philosophy and techniques of general medicine to psychiatry. This medical model of psychiatry was based on a few key assumptions. First was the notion that the same approach should be used for mental illnesses as for other illnesses. One corollary of this assumption was that there exist different psychiatric illnesses with different causes, courses, and optimal treatments. Second was an increasing insistence that empirical proof after open hypothesizing and skeptical inquiry was the best way to test a medical theory. In other words, the scientific method should be medicine's approach to knowledge. This belief gradually spread from basic research into the clinical domain. Thus the quintessential attribute of medical psychiatry is thinking about patients scientifically. A third assumption was the hope that an increased understanding of the physiology of the brain would eventually improve the care of patients with mental illness. Different psychiatrists of this time accepted these assumptions to greater and lesser degrees. However, it is hard to resist the impression that this medical model of psychiatry was responsible for the intellectual climate in which the important psychiatric discoveries of the late nineteenth century could be made.

The Psychoanalytic School

However, increasing knowledge of neuroanatomy confirmed that some patients had signs of neurological dysfunction that did not correspond to anatomical pathways—*conversion symptoms* in current terms (see Chapter 16). The neurologist Sigmund Freud (a contemporary of Wagner-Juaregg) had a special interest in these cases. He eventually developed an extensive theory of human behavior that did not depend on altered brain function to explain abnormal behavior. In the early and mid-twentieth century, American psychiatry turned almost wholly to the psychoanalytic theory of Freud and his followers. Psychiatry's former interest in "organic" illnesses such as pellagra, epilepsy, and neurosyphilis all but disappeared.

The extent of psychiatry's loss of interest in the brain was shown by the encephalitis lethargica epidemic of 1917. Most physicians felt that the unusual psychological and motor signs of encephalitis reflected abnormal brain functioning. As a result, they learned a great deal about basal ganglia physiology. However, similar signs had long been described in patients with schizophrenia. Thus psychodynamic explanations of these unusual postures and movements were readily available, and psychiatrists of the day largely ignored these valuable clues to abnormal brain function.

Psychodynamic theory has a voluminous literature and has changed over time, including division into several schismatic viewpoints. It cannot be thoroughly covered in the space available. Briefly, psychodynamic theory presupposes that some record of past experiences is maintained by the individual but is inaccessible to ordinary recall. These unconscious parts of the mind are thought to greatly affect a person's day-to-day actions. These effects can be noted through properly interpreting slips of the tongue, the content of recurrent dreams, free association, and symptoms, and they are also thought to be reflected in several aspects of culture. According to this theory, the unconscious not only influences daily life but also produces pathological behavior, especially if difficult early life conflicts involving powerful emotions have not been correctly resolved. Unconscious motives are perhaps most evident in certain situations that either obviously or symbolically recapitulate important situations from early life. One such situation is the special relationship between a doctor and a patient; this develops strongly in the course of psychoanalysis. Often a patient's actions toward the therapist appear to be reenactments of relationships with powerful figures of the patient's past rather than truly appropriate responses to the present situation. Interpretation of this transference—that is, explaining the symbolism of these actions to the patient—is thought to have powerful therapeutic potential.

It is more relevant to this discussion that "above all, psychodynamic psychiatry is a *way of thinking*" (Gabbard, 1990). This way of thinking is what characterized American psychiatry for much of this century. For the purposes of this book, it is worth noting the following concepts of traditional psychodynamic thought: (1) emotions and behavior are thought to have similar causes in both health and illness; (2) most psychiatric symptoms can be explained within the constructs of psychodynamic theory without reference to neuroanatomy or physiology; (3) the form of a symptom, such as a hallucination vs. a dream, is not considered as important as the specific content or meaning attributed to the symptom by the patient or the therapist; (4) there is a relative emphasis on individual precipitants to an illness rather than common features among groups of patients; (5) the optimal mode of treatment is thought to be similar for many different psychiatric symptoms; and (6) knowledge is acquired by special training and is heavily influenced by personal experience, single case studies, expert opinion, and tradition. The empirical methods of scientific inquiry are generally considered unnecessary or inappropriate.

The reader may note that these beliefs differ radically from the assumptions of the medical model and that they drastically lessen the urgency of diagnosis, biological investigation, and controlled studies of causation and interventions. The consequences for day-to-day clinical management of patients are significant, compared with the medical model view that accurate diagnosis, recognition of clinical uncertainty, and reliance on treatments with proven efficacy are essential to good patient care.

Psychology

Whereas psychoanalysis dominated American psychiatry for much of the twentieth century and was essentially limited to physicians, others continued to study behavior from other perspectives. Experimental psychology began to make substantive contributions to scientific knowledge about cognition, especially about normal learning of narrowly defined tasks. Theories derived from investigations of animal learning were extrapolated to human learning, and methods were devised for the reproducible testing of certain aspects of mental function. Importantly, these roots inspired an underlying philosophical model that abnormality consisted primarily of quantitative variation from normal, rather than categorical difference.

Naturally the observations of experimental psychology were extrapolated to abnormal human behavior and emotional states. Neuropsychology developed as the application of experimental testing methods to humans, especially to neurology patients. Several clinical tests originated as elaborations of the bedside neurological and mental status examinations. These methods proved clinically useful in helping localize abnormalities of brain structure or function. A field with related interests is behavioral neurology, which examines alterations in cognition and behavior in patients with known pathologic conditions of the brain. Behavioral theory discusses mental illnesses in terms of experimental psychology, drawing attention to observable undesired behaviors and the observable antecedents and consequences of such behavior. Clinical efforts based on this theory tend to eschew discussion of syndromes, focusing instead on eliminating specific unwanted behaviors by environmental manipulation. For instance, attention might be given to diminishing the frequency of a patient's excessive hand washing rather than to diagnosing obsessive-compulsive disorder (OCD) vs. schizophrenia. A more recent clinical offshoot, cognitive behavior therapy (CBT), extends these techniques from strictly externally observable phenomena to also include patients' self-reported thought content. Thus errors of logic are considered to be treatable causes of depression, anxiety, personality disorder and perhaps even psychosis. Cognitive psychology is a newer science that attempts to dissect actions, including inferred mental activities, into clearly defined, reproducible atoms of mental function that can hopefully be studied free of extraneous variables. With this approach, specific steps in mental processing can be examined in healthy subjects or hypothesized to underlie the symptoms of patients.

These approaches, when applied to mental illness, tend to share certain features with the medical model, including an emphasis on consistent application of the scientific method. However, there are important differences. Historically, psychology has assumed that mental processing is generally similar in health and in psychiatric illness and that symptoms arise from inappropriate learning rather than from brain dysfunction. Another difference has been psychology's focus on specific, single aspects of mental processing rather than on syndromes, which have characterized the medical approach to illness.

Psychosocial and Cultural Models

Some have held that mental illness is but the expected, or normal, response to living in an increasingly abnormal world. Advocates of this view have attributed the excess of depression in women to intolerable role demands or oppression in society. Similarly, the fact that schizophrenia is more common in inner cities has been interpreted as evidence that schizophrenia is produced by poverty, crowding, and other conditions of urban life. These explanations are intuitively appealing, but empirical support is less clear. "That psychiatric disturbances arise from the social and psychological environment appears to be so plausible that hypotheses often are not critically examined" (Guze, 1992). Even when these questions are subjected to research, several methodological issues make meaningful studies more difficult than is often recognized. However, careful epidemiological research can be done and has addressed some of these issues. For instance, the balance of evidence concludes that schizophrenia is more common in the inner city not because it is born there but because it migrates there. That is, people who develop schizophrenia come from approximately equivalent social environments as those who do not, but as the illness progresses they often move into less privileged settings. Perhaps the main difficulty with the psychosocial model of mental illness is that it fails to explain why some individuals become ill in certain environments but most do not.

More extreme versions of the psychosocial model of mental illness include claims that there is no such thing as mental illness but merely an intolerant society. Eccentricity, in this view, is interpreted as pathological solely because society tends to ethnocentric bigotry. According to this argument, people intentionally choose to report hallucinations, delusions of persecution, or depression, and hence they should not be forced to conform. Some advocates of this position claim that there is no justification for reifying schizophrenia as an illness when there are no clearly consistent chemical or anatomical abnormalities.

One argument against this position is that many people affected by mental illness suffer greatly. To view these illnesses as voluntarily chosen lifestyles seems incomprehensible to physicians who work daily with such suffering. A second objection is that the major mental illnesses are quite similar in their clinical features and prevalence across a wide range of cultures that are more and less accepting of eccentricity. More importantly, it is hard to reconcile this view of mental illness with the fact that bipolar disorder, for instance, is largely a genetic illness. Regarding the complaint that these are not illnesses because their causes remain unknown, a little historical reflection may persuade the reader that a century ago, the causes of general paresis or pellagra were equally unknown. To imagine that they suddenly became illnesses when their causes were discovered is hard to accept. Equally untenable is the supposition that we have already discovered the causes of all illnesses affecting the brain. Migraine, torticollis, and other neurological illnesses remain equally baffling.

The psychosocial view of mental illness more often surfaces in a milder form. When discussing major depression in a patient with a stroke, for instance, it is common to hear medical personnel state, "I'd be depressed too." This sympathetic view unfortunately falls short of the facts, since the majority of stroke victims never experience the syndrome of major depression. The specific factors that lead to major depression in some but not all stroke patients might never be elucidated if the cause is assumed to be obvious. This example also highlights the common confusion of *understandable* and *normal*. It is entirely understandable when an elderly smoker with diabetes and a strong family history of coronary disease suffers angina after shoveling his walk in the cold. However, concluding that this makes angina normal is only a more obvious, not a more egregious, error than calling secondary depression normal.

Resurgence of the Medical Model of Psychiatry

In the last 25 years, there has been a dramatic change in American psychiatry. The psychodynamic way of thinking about mental illness is gradually being replaced by a more empirical approach to validation of diagnosis and treatment. To a large extent, this can be attributed to four practical benefits derived from applications of the medical model to psychiatry. The first impetus for change was perhaps the discovery of *dramatically effective somatic treatments* for mental illness. One of the criticisms of psychoanalysis from Abraham Myerson, a leading neurologist of 50 years ago, was that its methods would have been embraced nearly universally by physicians if it had provided clearly superior therapeutic results. In contrast, many psychiatric hospitals were virtually emptied with the discoveries of ECT in 1938, lithium salts for mania in 1949, and chlorpromazine in 1952. These somatic treatments had clear, significant efficacy. These therapeutic discoveries coincided with several *clinical discoveries that reminded psychiatrists that the brain was involved in mental illness*. For instance, reserpine, which depletes the brain of monoamines, was found to precipitate melancholia, and drugs that inhibited degradation of monoamines were found to treat melancholia. As another example, when computed tomography (CT) became available the cerebral ventricles were shown to be enlarged in people with schizophrenia compared with those of control subjects. The possibility that some mental illnesses might arise from brain dysfunction offered an alternative etiological view to psychodynamic theories, and the strict methods used to test biological hypotheses suggested that psychological theories should be subjected to equal rigor.

Another advance that helped reform psychiatry was the development of *reliable diagnostic criteria* that followed the outline of diagnostic rules in general medicine. The Washington University criteria for research diagnosis, published in 1972, rapidly became the most commonly cited of all psychiatric publications. These criteria had demonstrably high reliability, paving the way (as intended) for meaningful etiological research. On the clinical front, physicians were hungry for a reliable way of communicating about their patients. When the American Psychiatric Association introduced the third revision of its *Diagnostic and Statistical Manual* (DSM-III) (1980), derived from the Washington University criteria, it rapidly became a bestseller (for more information on diagnosis, see Chapter 2). Finally, psychiatry was the beneficiary of (and often the originating force behind) powerful *new research tools*. These included modern epidemiological methods for teasing out psychosocial and biological causes of illness, mathematical tools for the genetic study of common diseases and quantitative traits, and imaging techniques that allowed the structure and function of the brain to be examined during life. These research tools further boosted hopes that the causes of mental illness might eventually be uncovered.

What the Medical Model of Psychiatry Is and Is Not

These four major advances are well known, but the medical model of psychiatry, as taught at Washington University, has not spread as widely. Perhaps because of this, some have erroneously concluded that the medical model is synonymous with an openness to biological causes of mental illness, or even with "an exclusive focus on body chemistry and the prescribing of psychoactive drugs. Nothing could be more incorrect" (Guze, 1992). In fact, the essential defining point of the medical model is a way of thinking about patients.

We believe this way of thinking to be critically important. Physicians swear an oath to "first, do no harm," but unscientific thinking on their part can harm patients. When physicians uncritically accept hypotheses about a patient's illness, they tend to believe that the cause of the symptoms is obvious. This comforting fallacy can lead to major—even fatal—errors in treatment. "We can make this error whether we favor a biological, dynamic, cognitive or biopsychosocial etiology, and can avoid it only by recognizing that clinical hypotheses must be treated as critically as research hypotheses" (Black, 1994). Thus skepticism about etiology and treatment is as crucial for the clinician as it is for the researcher.

Specifically, the medical model of psychiatry does not assume that all mental illnesses will turn out to have biological causes. Rather, psychiatrists who use the medical model examine critically the evidence for any proposed etiology. Theoretical speculation can be useful "if it produces testable hypotheses" (Goodwin and Guze, 1989). However, experience has taught us that many theories have been plausible but wrong, and many more theories remain altogether untested. In the words of one critical physician, "one good experiment is worth a dozen subtle theories piled dubiously and uncertainly" (Myerson, [1944] 1994). In other words, for a theory to be attractive or plausible "is not enough; systematic and controlled data are necessary" (Guze, 1992). Thus the medical model of psychiatry makes no specific assumptions about etiology. It does share the assumptions of general medicine that there are different causes for different illnesses and that careful study of patients and of normal physiology may help elucidate those causes, just as it has in the past.

Similarly, the medical model does not condone uncritical acceptance of pharmacological treatments or uncritical rejection of psychotherapy (see the Pearls & Perils box below). On the contrary, specific psychotherapeutic techniques have demonstrated efficacy for many patients, and somatic treatments have shown little or no efficacy for some conditions. The emphasis is not on choosing a treatment congruent with the illness's presumed etiology but on a demand for empirical demonstration of safety and efficacy. Beyond specific treatments, an ongoing compassionate, supportive, educational dialogue with the patient is certainly part of the physician's role for all patients (see Chapter 20). We could hardly recommend any clinical practice in which patients had "to demand that they be listened to rather than simply medicated" (Gabbard, 1990).

Some have characterized the empiric approach to psychiatry as superficial. This charge of superficiality seems to come in three flavors. First, some have interpreted the research focus on objective signs of illness as synonymous with a lack of curiosity about the inner workings of the mind. This hardly fits our experience with psychiatrists who use the medical model. A fascination with the varieties of mental experience is nearly ubiquitous among such physicians. Instead medical model psychiatrists tend not to be satisfied with explanations of symptoms at the superficial psychological level. Rather, they wish to understand the underlying pathophysiology responsible for the psychological manifestations. Furthermore, psychiatrists who use the medical model tend to be frustrated with superficially plausible explanations of causality, preferring instead provable hypotheses that may lead to firm etiological knowledge.

The misconception that medical model psychiatry is not interested in the subjective psychological experience of the patient may result from the medical model's reliance on objective findings as a basis for diagnosis. Somatization disorder (Briquet's syndrome), for instance, was defined by a pattern of lifelong unfounded physical complaints largely because this produced reliability of diagnosis. Yet the overall clinical presentation of such patients, including their psychological and interpersonal difficulties, was a central motivation for the study. It is after all the subjective experience of symptoms that commonly motivates patients to seek treatment; thus the subjective perceptions of patients are the common working material of the psychiatrist and the basis for her empathy. The difficulty is that rarely have such perceptions been made precise enough to have any solidly demonstrated value in guiding treatment. Our contention is that to base treatment decisions for patients on any unproven theory, no matter how plausible, is risky and rarely likely to be in the patients' best interest. It is comforting to believe that one knows how to approach nearly every patient, but there are enough clinical situations without proven treatment options that such knowledge is but a placation of the physician's wishes to avoid ambivalence—possibly at the patient's expense.

A second sense of superficiality with which medical model psychiatry has been charged is a narrowness of scope. This scientific approach to patient care, it is said, does not fully appreciate the human condition. Clearly a medical approach to psychiatry does not explain all of human behavior! But this was never its intent. The medical model's hope, though considerably less grand, is no less worthwhile: namely, that over the long run an empirical approach to psychiatric diagnosis and treatment will prove to be in the patient's best interest. Besides, there are risks to any model of mental illness which attempts to also explain all of normal mental and social life. Although psychiatrists naturally benefit from broad interests in these directions, "if our claims for special knowledge and expertise are too broad, we run the risk of diluting our credibility" (Black, 1994). It is sheer hubris to expect that psychiatrists have discovered not only the best approach to mental illness but also the best view of normal mental life and the answers to many serious philosophical and religious questions.

PEARLS & PERILS

WHAT IS THE MEDICAL MODEL OF PSYCHIATRY?

- The medical model is the consistent application, in psychiatry, of modern medical thinking and methods.
- The medical model of psychiatry is a way of thinking about mental illness.
- The medical model relies on the scientific method rather than theory to guide clinical practice.
- Successful approaches to "physical" illnesses can be applied to mental illnesses.
- Optimal knowledge of psychiatric disorders requires continued study of brain physiology.
- The medical model does not assume that all psychiatric illnesses have genetic or biochemical causes.
- Psychotherapy is an important part of psychiatric practice.
- The medical model of psychiatry does not pretend to explain all of human experience.

Finally, medical model psychiatry has been accused of fostering a superficial understanding of patients. But this is a misunderstanding. Black (1994) wrote:

> Reliance on diagnosis and data does not mean one should know one's patients shallowly. Diagnosis, after all, is "the careful examination and description of the patient's condition" (Guze, 1992). Both our ability to provide good care and our enjoyment of psychiatric practice depend on how well we know our patients. So much of compliance, motivation, and therapeutic success hinge on the doctor-patient relationship, rather than on knowledge of a particular piece of data. In fact, thinking scientifically about one's patients obliges one to know more, not less, about them because so many questions of diagnosis and management remain unanswered by controlled studies.

Knowing patients well is crucial in psychiatry but may be equally important in general medicine. This is because "a mental disease is a disorder of the person following the laws of general pathology like any other disease" (Meyer, [1897] 1994).

The most serious charge against the medical model is that a scientific approach to patient care somehow precludes empathy. Our belief is that nothing could be farther from the truth. "Scientific skepticism is in no way incompatible with compassion for the sick or disabled. In fact, it is the desire to help patients that causes one to be frustrated by the lack of definite knowledge about what really helps and what does not. There are few things more humanitarian than the effective use of knowledge to relieve suffering" (Guze, 1970).

Practical Benefits of the Medical Model

We have taken a good bit of space to discuss philosophical issues relating to psychiatry. The primary justification is our belief that a consistent application of the scientific method to clinical psychiatry will help patients over the long run. Thus we feel that this medical model should underlie all subsequent chapters in this volume. However, this approach to psychiatry also has a number of practical benefits for psychiatrists, neurologists, and other physicians at all levels of training. A description of some of these benefits follows (see the Pearls and Perils box to the right.).

A Common, Accessible Language for Education and Collaboration

Implicit in the medical model is an insistence on reliable diagnostic methods. One practical benefit is that the experience of senior physicians can be more easily shared with students and residents. Obviously, students must still gain clinical experience to identify signs of illness, such as tangential speech or an Argyll Robertson pupil. However, with clear diagnostic criteria they can already have some idea of what is meant by paranoid schizophrenia or secondary mania.

If this benefit were limited to medical novices, reliable diagnostic methods could serve as a temporary nursemaid and then be abandoned. However, modern diagnostic criteria also improve a physician's continuing medical education. Before widespread acceptance of research diagnostic criteria, it was difficult to know if treatment studies reported in the literature had any relevance for one's own patients, since different investigators meant different things by even such common terms as *schizophrenia*. On the other hand, it is now possible to read a study of a new treatment for schizophrenia and know whether a patient shares important features with the patients studied. Finally, using specific diagnostic criteria, physicians can discuss patients with colleagues and have some hope of communicating clearly.

A Hope for Discovery of Etiology and Treatment

The hope for successful research into the causes and treatment of mental illness is a significant *raison d'être* for the medical model of psychiatry. It shares the power of empiricism that has propelled all successful branches of science. We have discussed some historical support for the success of this approach, but

PEARLS & PERILS

PRACTICAL BENEFITS OF THE MEDICAL MODEL OF PSYCHIATRY

- Reliable diagnosis allows better patient care.
- Patients are more likely to receive treatments based on scientific evidence of efficacy.
- The medical model allows a unified approach to all patients, without unreasonable illness boundaries.
- It encourages early recognition of psychiatric illness by nonpsychiatric physicians.
- The medical model of psychiatry promotes careful differential diagnosis of psychological symptoms.
- Diagnosis is a common, accessible language for education and collaboration.
- The medical model of psychiatry provides the tools and motivation for discovery of etiology and treatment.
- This model has a proven track record in psychiatric science.
- Applying the medical model of psychiatry may help medical practice be enjoyable for a lifetime.
- This model has important implications for public policy.

it bears repetition that the major discoveries of psychiatry and medicine in general can be attributed largely to the assumptions of the medical model.

A Unified General Approach to All Patients

Internists, neurologists, and other physicians spend years in training, learning among other things a tried and true approach to their patients. This approach includes gathering careful historical information from the patient, conducting a general or focused examination, matching the patient's symptoms and signs with those of a known syndrome if possible, and turning to controlled studies to support diagnostic and therapeutic actions. Special techniques have developed in each specialty appropriate to its needs, but this underlying approach is nearly universal in medicine. Patients with psychiatric illnesses constitute a large share of the practice of physicians in other specialties. If a completely different approach were required for psychologic as opposed to bodily complaints, then physicians of other specialties would understandably feel at a loss when faced with these patients. However, if physicians adopt a medical model approach to mental illness, then their general medical skills—careful history and examination, identification of a syndrome, and reference to the diagnosis and treatment of similar illnesses in the literature—serve equally well for psychiatric patients and for all other patients.

A medical approach to all patients helps not only physicians but patients. For instance, important psychiatric syndromes such as dementia or major depression are often overlooked by nonpsychiatrist physicians. When evaluation is not limited to physical complaints, patients receive better care. Similarly, many idiopathic psychiatric illnesses include physical signs (such as the motor retardation of major depression) that are prone to be overlooked if the illness is assumed to be psychological.

No Need for Unreasonable Illness Boundaries

Many common clinical situations defy the dualistic supposition that mental and physical illnesses should be separated. For instance, there is good evidence that obsessive-compulsive symptoms are an integral part of Tourette's disorder as mental equivalents of motor tics. Similarly, depressive symptoms can be the earliest manifestations of Parkinson's disease, and psychosis is a common side effect of antiparkinsonian medication. Depression, dementia, and psychosis are as much a part of Huntington's disease as is chorea (see Chapter 26). It seems arbitrary and wasteful for a physician to need to "change gears" mentally when assessing affective or cognitive signs compared with motor signs of the same illness. Many physicians have also shared the frustration of dealing with separate insurance rules for the same patient, depending on whether psychiatric or neurological symptoms are more prominent at the moment.

The Enjoyment of Medical Practice

Among the many factors that can make medical practice an enjoyable vocation for a lifetime is the excitement of evaluating a new patient. Considering that a large fraction of patients seen in primary care practices have psychiatric illness, a physician's approach to these patients becomes important. If symptoms and signs of depression, somatization disorder, or anxiety are approached with the medical model, the nonpsychiatric physician may be more likely to view these complaints as part of the challenge of medical science and part of the healing art of helping those who are suffering. If patients with psychological complaints are instead seen as an extraneous distraction from "real illness," much of medicine, especially primary care medicine, may become frustrating.

Saving Lives

Schizophrenia, major depression, panic disorder, and mania are diseases with high morbidity and mortality. They are also among the most treatable of medical conditions. With treatment, their remission rates are easily comparable to those of hypertension, angina, and other common general medical disorders. If these conditions are viewed as separate from other medical conditions, the physician may miss an opportunity for sharing in rewarding clinical results. If the primary care physician does not see these diseases as part of her duty, the physician may even unintentionally contribute to a death (see Chapter 27).

Differential Diagnosis

Almost all major mental illnesses have a broad medical differential diagnosis. Although they are not the most common causes of psychological symptoms, secondary psychiatric illnesses are far from rare. For instance, the schizophrenic syndrome can be caused by Wilson's disease, adult metachromatic leukodystrophy, or habitual intoxication with phencyclidine or amphetamine. Fatigue and depression are sensitive indicators of hypothyroidism and other endocrine disorders. In fact, for most psychiatric presentations one can generalize the words of Gelenberg (1976) regarding catatonia: "Like hypertension . . . catatonia discovered on physical examination should spur a medical investigation to uncover the probable cause."

Aside from the fact that differential diagnostic considerations provide much of the enjoyment of medical practice, psychological symptoms can be significant clues to general medical illnesses. However, these symptoms are nonspecific enough that a good working knowledge of psychiatry is required to sort out their likely cause. If psychological complaints are simply assumed to be the result of life stressors or intrapsychic conflict rather than as symptoms whose differential diagnosis should be pursued as warranted by the rest of the history and examination, many patients will not receive optimal treatment.

Societal Considerations

There are many practical repercussions of the way physicians view mental illness. Among these are effects on psychiatric research and on insurance for mental illness. Research funding for mental illness has rarely received the public financial support that it would merit on a basis of societal cost, extent of disability, or even prevalence. To some extent this may be attributed to a public perception that cancer or stroke are real and dreadful diseases that strike indiscriminately, whereas mental illnesses are not illnesses but weaknesses that can be avoided by personal effort. When physicians support this dichotomous view of illness, research for its prevention and cure is slowed.

On another front, the nearly ubiquitous discriminatory policies that underinsure mental illnesses as compared with other illnesses, if not entirely the result of greed and exploitation of ignorance on the part of insurers, must be largely the result of a view that mental illnesses are not real. To the extent that physicians (who should be patients' best advocates) support such discriminatory policies, they share in the responsibility for the pain and suffering the policies cause. Instead, physicians can spread the knowledge that treating serious psychiatric illnesses actually saves money. "We may have to control the growing costs of health care, but we should not do it by discriminating against a particular category of illness that can be as painful, disabling, and life-threatening as most other serious medical conditions and that is often long-lasting and broadly pervasive in its manifestations" (Guze, 1992).

Myths About Psychiatry

Considering the difficulties psychiatry has faced in defining itself over the last century, it is perhaps no surprise that there are a number of common misconceptions about the field. The following paragraphs address a few of the more prevalent myths.

Myth: Psychiatric Illnesses Aren't Real

This assertion is hard to rebut in a few sentences, and the serious reader is referred to the discussions by Kendell or Guze mentioned in the annotated bibliography. However, a few points answer many arguments commonly given to support this assertion. If real illnesses always have identifiable pathologies, then several general medical problems today (such as hypertension or migraine) are not diseases, and "most of the great scourges of mankind have only become diseases during the last hundred and fifty years" (Kendell, 1975). Furthermore, to require known pathology implies the bold assumptions that current methods for finding pathology are already perfect, and that physicians already know exactly where to apply which tools. In fact, "the availability of more powerful research tools has shown that whether or not one associates a given illness with pathology depends largely on the [power] of one's research methods" (Csernansky, Black, and Faustman, in press). Additionally, if only serious illnesses are real, then the major mental illnesses certainly qualify. They are associated with a great deal of suffering, and they cause death and disability to a greater extent than many nonpsychiatric illnesses. Another way of judging the seriousness of an illness is to consider its effect on the biological fitness of the individuals affected. Judged in this way, schizophrenia (for instance) is clearly a serious illness.

The fact that this issue is raised in psychiatry much more often than in general medicine largely reflects the tacit assumption of mind-body duality. Kendell (1975) wrote:

> Most doctors never give a moment's thought to the precise meaning of terms like illness and disease, nor do they need to. They simply treat the patients who consult them as best they can, diagnose individual diseases whenever they can, and try to relieve their patients' suffering even if they can't. At times they are well aware that they are dealing with matters other than illness [e.g., childbirth], but rarely do they pause to consider what is the essential difference between the two. The practical nature of medicine is not conducive to theorizing.

Myth: Psychiatry is an Inexact Science

Of course psychiatry is an inexact science, just like all of clinical medicine. The only myth here is the implicit idea that other medical specialties somehow escape this charge. In fact, medicine itself is an inexact science.

Myth: Even Psychiatrists Can't Agree on Diagnosis

This is a special case of the previous myth. The best brief answer is perhaps that diagnostic dilemmas are not limited to psychiatry but are part of the reality of all of clinical medicine. In diagnostic studies of many general medical conditions, it is apparent that perfect diagnostic concordance is nearly impossible (see Table 2-2, p. 20). Research on the major psychiatric illnesses, for which specific laboratory tests are generally unavailable, has had to face this difficulty head on. As a result, recent studies of psychiatric diagnosis show high diagnostic reliability. The methods developed by psychiatric researchers to improve clinical judgments and quantify diagnostic concordance have since been recognized and adopted by other specialties for illnesses in which laboratory tests play a minor role. Chapter 2 further addresses the reliability of psychiatric diagnosis.

Myth: Psychiatric Illnesses Are Diagnoses of Exclusion Only

This unfortunate idea seems to come from three prevalent fallacies: (1) *psychiatric* means *unexplained;* (2) psychiatric disorders are not treatable; and (3) psychiatric disorders are not medically serious. Two facts replace these fallacies. First, undiagnosed illness does not imply psychiatric illness. For instance, follow-up studies of single conversion symptoms show an alarmingly high rate of neurologic and systemic disease. Conversely, diagnosing a valid syndrome, even if its cause is not completely known, provides a degree of certainty about prognosis including response to treatment. Sometimes the psychiatric diagnosis provides much more information than the less well-validated physical disorder being assessed (for example, major depression vs. irritable bowel disease). Additionally, the psychiatric disorder under consideration is often at least as treatable as the physical disorder (such as panic disorder vs. coronary artery disease). Often, treatment of the psychiatric disorder is more important than treatment of the "rule-outs" for preventing disability or even death. In short, psychiatric illnesses should be considered early in the medical evaluation, not as a last resort.

Consider the common clinical situation of a middle-aged woman with atypical chest pain. An abnormal stress test has about the same positive predictive value as a coin flip, whereas a clinically definite diagnosis of Briquet's syndrome (somatization disorder) has a 94% chance of still explaining her chest pain on follow-up years later. If this disorder is identified, the physician now has diagnosed a condition known to cause complaints of chest pain, which can explain the presentation. If instead of a careful record review, history, and psychiatric examination, there were a laboratory test with this success rate, no doubt the test would be used much earlier in the evaluation than is commonly done for psychiatric referral.

Myth: People with Mental Illnesses Don't Need a Physician

The usual answer to this invidious myth is: who else is properly trained in differential diagnosis, triage, and both psychological and somatic treatments? This is a crucial point, and for many observers it settles the question.

However, another part of the answer lies in society's expectations for medical care. The current extensive training of physicians arose in the early years of this century. At that time, physicians had few if any effective treatments, and little was known about the pathophysiology of disease. Doctors generally had brief courses of practical study and informal apprenticeships. However, the influential Flexner report revolutionized medical training by its radical suggestions that medical schools require a 4-year degree, including training in chemistry and other sciences, before matriculation and then teach a 4-year curriculum, including additional basic science work, before graduation. Formalized internships were required even after this extensive education. The underlying reason for these changes was the hope that training in the biological sciences would make for better doctors. Not only would they be better situated to find causes and treatments of disease, but they could better analyze new research findings of others and think scientifically about their patients' problems. This hope is arguably more important now than ever, given the vast body of scientific facts available to support the modern practice of medicine and the overwhelming rate at which new biomedical knowledge is being acquired.

The exigencies of wartime, and later the rising costs of medical care, have led to a number of other professionals taking roles traditionally filled by physicians. Psychologists and social workers are not alone in seeking a more direct role in providing patient care; they are joined by nurses, physician's assistants, physical therapists, optometrists, and others. Society now has an important question to answer. Without a doubt these professionals have a role to play in the efficient delivery of medical care, but should they supplant the physician? Put another way, is extensive scientific and medical training no longer the best way to train for providing psychiatric and general medical care? Our contention is that this is still the approach most likely to produce competent practitioners and that society may get what it is willing to pay for.

Finally, to say that people with mental illness don't need a physician is really simply a form of discrimination against a minority. People with mental illnesses already face enough stigma and discrimination. Denying them access to a physician when no such denial is made for other illnesses is only adding injury to insult.

Conclusion

Mental illnesses are real. They are common. They cause a very human form of suffering. They can cause disability and even death. Yet they remain undertreated, stigmatized, and widely misunderstood.

However, applying the methods of modern medicine to psychiatry has led to exciting advances. Several major mental illnesses of a century ago, such as endemic cretinism, neurosyphilis, and pellagra, have been largely eliminated. Psychiatric illnesses can now be reliably diagnosed. The safety and efficacy of many psychiatric treatments have been clearly established, and treatment outcomes in psychiatry are among the most rewarding in all of medicine. And there are almost daily advances in our understanding of how the brain functions in health and disease. The medical model approach to psychiatry, which is largely responsible for many of these advances, offers a proven approach for continuing to help those affected by mental illness.

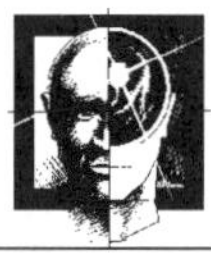

Annotated Bibliography

Guze SB: *Why psychiatry is a branch of medicine,* New York, 1992, Oxford.

This short book offers an introduction to the medical model of psychiatry, explaining its advantages and discussing its implications.

Kendell RE: The concept of disease and its implications for psychiatry, *Br J Psychiatry* 127:305-315, 1975.

This article provides a clear, brief discussion of what defines a disease.

Pichot P: Nosological models in psychiatry, *Br J Psychiatry* 164:232-240, 1994.

A brief history of psychiatric classification is given in this article.

Rogers D: *Motor disorder in psychiatry: towards a neurological psychiatry,* New York, 1992, John Wiley & Sons.

This book challenges the simplistic idea that neurology treats the brain and psychiatry treats the mind (see especially pp. 1-10 and 113-114).

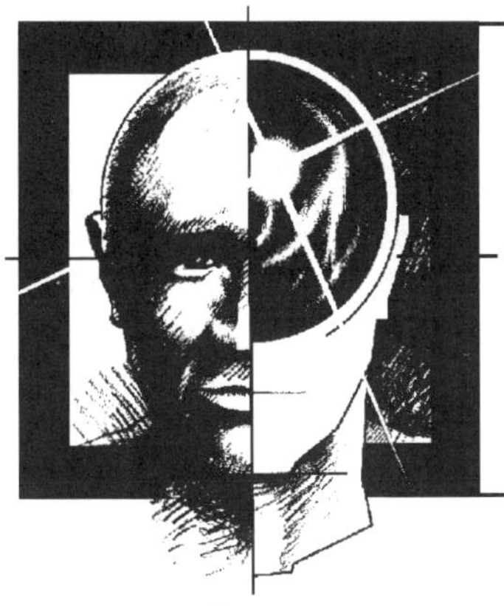

chapter 2

Diagnosis

Kevin John Black, MD and Samuel B. Guze, MD

In Chapter 1, we summarized the origins and features of the medical model of psychiatry—the application of modern medical thinking and methods to disorders of emotion, cognition, and behavior. We also discussed a number of practical benefits of this approach to mental illness. What may not be obvious is that the process of diagnosis is the foundation of modern medicine. In this chapter, we turn our attention to diagnosis and address the questions of why psychological symptoms should be categorized into diagnoses, whether diagnostic criteria for psychiatric illness are useful, and how psychiatric diagnoses are made.

Why Make Diagnoses for Psychological Symptoms?

Background

Among the core goals of medicine are treating illnesses successfully, predicting their outcome, and finding their causes. The process of diagnosis has become fundamental to meeting all three of these goals. From early times, physicians have observed that afflictions tend to fall into syndromes, or patterns of signs and symptoms that are fairly stable across patients. Those with similar signs and symptoms often have a similar prognosis. Additionally, the cause of an illness can often be found by comparing similarities in the backgrounds of different patients with the same syndrome. Treatments that help one patient with a given syndrome often help others with the same syndrome. The process of carefully listening to the patient, examining him, and classifying his symptoms and signs into recognized syndromes is called *diagnosis.*

Diagnosis began with clinical observations alone. However, the advent of modern pathology in the nineteenth century had two significant effects on diagnosis. First, many existing diagnoses made by purely clinical criteria (such as pneumonia) were validated by laboratory findings and autopsy. Second, new diagnostic subcategories arose when different laboratory findings in the same clinical syndrome tended to help predict outcome (for example, streptococcal pneumonia). These new diagnoses based on pathology enjoyed great popularity for a simple reason. They were generally superior to purely clinical diagnoses in the three previously mentioned functions of diagnosis: explaining illness, suggesting treatment, and predicting outcome.

Unfortunately, this change in paradigm helped change the concept of disease from a clinical syndrome to an illness marked by a specific pathological or laboratory abnormality. The effects of this change were felt most in psychiatry, because psychiatrists of the early and mid-1900's largely abandoned illnesses with pathological or laboratory findings (such as neurosyphilis). These psychiatrists also lost interest in diagnosis because they emphasized factors unique to an individual rather than syndromal commonalities among patients and because they assumed that mental processes were similar in health and illness (see Chapter 1). As a result of these changes in psychiatric and general medical thinking, two widespread misconceptions have arisen. One is that meaningful diagnoses are always associated with laboratory or postmortem abnormalities. The other is that diagnosis for physical illness is meaningful, whereas diagnosis for mental illness is nothing but an arbitrary label. These fallacies are common even among physicians. For instance, the problem list for patients seen in other specialties may include the entry "psych problem," even though this label is nearly useless given the wide variety of causes, outcomes, and appropriate treatments for different psychiatric illnesses.

The truth is that diagnosis has invaluable benefits in psychiatry. In Chapter 1, we discussed several practical benefits of using the medical model in psychiatry. Since diagnosis is central to the medical model, many of these benefits are the result of diagnosis. Psychiatric diagnosis has advantages for medical education, research, and clinical care.

Education

Medical education consists largely of gaining access to the medical knowledge of others. This communication of knowledge requires a common language. The general concepts expressed by standardized diagnostic criteria can be made accessible to medical students early, so they have a framework on which to build new knowledge about mental illness. However, medical school is only the beginning of medical education. Standardized diagnostic criteria allow the physician to continue to learn from the experience of colleagues and from medical literature, since the experience of other physicians with their patients is only relevant for patients with similar characteristics. A related clinical benefit of diagnosis is that a common language of diagnosis allows physicians to understand each other and hence collaborate meaningfully in patient care.

Research and Its Long-Term Benefits

A major benefit of diagnosis is that it increases the power of etiological studies. Some opponents of diagnosis suggest that psychiatrists should instead focus on the unique predispositions to illness of each patient. However, if "causal factors are different for each individual case of a given illness," then since "it is primarily through the recognition of common denominators that the study of cause is possible, . . . an emphasis upon the uniqueness of each causal pattern must result in a completely sterile approach" (Guze, 1970). It is no exaggeration to say that without diagnosis, etiological research is nearly useless. The long-term benefits of such research are apparent when one considers the dramatic advances in treatment that have been possible because there is a better understanding of the causes of many medical illnesses.

Clinical Care

The most practical justification for diagnosis is that it allows physicians to meet patients' needs. Patients ask physicians, "What do I have?" "What can you do for me?" and "Will it go away or get worse?" Diagnosis is designed to answer these questions by making the experiences of other patients relevant. These questions also provide a standard for assessing the usefulness of a given diagnosis. Diagnoses are useful to the extent that they help answer these three questions.

All Diagnoses Are Not Created Equal

Validity

Diagnosis is a form of classification intended to help the physician meet a patient's needs. In diagnostic classification, it is presumed that there is an underlying cause for each disease. Under this premise, the job of the classifier is to find the natural classification in which each diagnostic syndrome reflects a single disease entity. However, the classification is needed before there is perfect knowledge about all relevant illnesses. Fortunately, there are certain illness features that tend to identify natural syndromes. Diagnostic systems tend to be most useful when they are based on the careful study of these illness features. If diseases are invented arbitrarily, then the whole procedure is pointless. To make an analogy to a different kind of classification, one could group all red flowers together and call this group "the species *red.*" Although this classification may seem unnatural, it at least has two minimum virtues. There is no argument over whether red flowers exist, and most observers can reliably tell whether a given flower is red or not red. However, there are two serious problems with this classification by color. First, it is not likely to be useful in predicting other features of the flower, such as root structure, preferred climate, and so on. It may not even predict whether the flower will still be red next week! Second, the species *red* is not likely to survive the acquisition of new knowledge about flowers. For instance, phylogeny as defined by gene homology probably differs as much among red flowers as between red flowers and those of other colors. Linnaeus's classification of plants, on the other hand, was based on a careful attempt to discover natural classes. Accordingly, it has not only remained useful for centuries, but it has also been supported by new knowledge, such as that gained through biochemical and genetic studies.

When applied to medical diagnoses, these virtues—present usefulness and stability in the face of new information—reflect diagnostic validity. Physicians can think of validity as the extent to which patients with the same clinical diagnosis turn out to have the same underlying disease. When there is a clear gold standard for diagnosis (such as pathognomonic laboratory or postmortem findings), then judging the validity of clinical diagnosis is relatively straightforward. However, validity is also needed for diagnoses that describe idiopathic illnesses. A valid diagnostic category should be useful in the ways doctors need it to be; it should accurately predict course and treatment response and it should add meaningful information to other valid diagnoses. Furthermore, a valid diagnosis should still be useful after new research. This new research may reveal more precise clinical descriptions, new laboratory findings, and eventually knowledge of etiology and pathophysiology. In other words, validity reflects how reasonable it is to speak of a diagnosis before final information about etiology and pathophysiology is obtained. Box 2-1 describes a method for validating clinical diagnosis in the numerous diseases for which a gold standard has not yet been found.

Some psychiatric diagnoses have met these tests. Schizophrenia, affective illness, and somatization disorder are examples of psychiatric diagnoses that are supported by numerous validity studies (Table 2-1). On the other hand, the validity of many other psychiatric diagnoses has not been adequately studied. A popular example is multiple personality disorder (MPD). Although there is no question that there are patients who consistently report multiple personalities, it is also true that such patients nearly universally meet criteria for one or more well-validated conditions such as antisocial personality disorder, somatization disorder, or substance abuse. It is not clear how much additional information is gained by adding the diagnosis of MPD to these more established diagnoses. Thus this diagnosis has not been clearly delimited from other disorders (Box 2-1). Other steps to validation, such as follow-up and family studies, are also inadequate for MPD.

Unfortunately, MPD is not the only psychiatric diagnosis with questionable validity. Many of the diagnoses listed in DSM-IV still lack clear validation. In fact, Cloninger lamented in 1989 that in the 20 years since development of the Washington University criteria (which describe about a dozen psychiatric illnesses), not one further diagnosis had been adequately validated. Fortunately, increasing attention is being paid to diagnostic validity, and there are now numerous research studies that address the points in Box 2-1.

BOX 2-1

STEPS TO ESTABLISHING DIAGNOSTIC VALIDITY

- Clinical description
- Laboratory studies
- Delimitation from other disorders
- Follow-up study (including response to treatment)
- Family study

From Robins E, Guze SB: Establishment of diagnostic validity in psychiatric illness: its application to schizophrenia, *Am J Psychiatry* 126:983-987, 1970.

TABLE 2-1

SELECTED PSYCHIATRIC DIAGNOSES WITH MORE AND LESS WELL-ESTABLISHED VALIDITY

Validity well established	Validity partially established	Validity poorly established
Alcoholism	Bipolar II disorder	Dysthymia
Schizophrenia	Recurrent brief depression	Hypochondriasis
Panic disorder	Psychotic subtype of major depression	Primary insomnia
Bipolar disorder	Rapid cycling subtype of bipolar disorder	Generalized anxiety disorder
Major depression		Multiple personality disorder
Anorexia nervosa		Reactive psychosis (DSM-III)*
Alzheimer's disease		Borderline personality disorder
Somatization disorder		Seasonal affective disorder
Antisocial personality disorder		Psychophysiological insomnia (ICSD)
Obsessive-compulsive disorder		Psychological factors affecting physical condition

*Defining criteria, when not DSM-IV, are given in parentheses.

Reliability

In one scene from the novel *Twenty Thousand Leagues Under the Sea,* the main characters watch the ocean fish from inside the *Nautilus.* The professor's servant, Conseil, classifies the fish by class, order, family, and genus. But Ned, the whaler, has his own classification. Fish, says Ned, come in two species: good-to-eat and not-good-to-eat (Verne, [1869] 1966). This classification is potentially useful, but it has a much more basic flaw than the red species of flower. Although there is no argument that there exist fish that taste good and fish that taste bad, it is unlikely that any two men on the *Nautilus* would agree completely about which fish belonged in which category. Ned himself may have changed his tastes with time.

This problem, when it occurs in medical diagnosis, is called *poor diagnostic reliability.* Reliability includes both agreement among different examiners and stability of diagnosis by the same examiner on reexamination. Reliable diagnosis is crucial for both the researcher and the clinician. Research on less-valid diagnoses may be pointless, but research without diagnostic reliability is nearly impossible. For clinical purposes, a diagnosis is hardly worth making if it fails to consistently describe the patient, and a diagnosis that means different things to different colleagues can hardly aid communication between physicians.

Studies of diagnosis have uncovered several features that tend to improve reliability (Box 2-2). Some of these features pertain to the diagnosis itself, others pertain to the examiner or type of assessment used to make the diagnosis, and still others pertain to the patient.

BOX 2-2

FACTORS THAT INCREASE DIAGNOSTIC RELIABILITY

Assessment

- Longitudinal vs. cross-sectional data
- Several informants vs. history from patient alone
- Standardized assessment
- Experience of examiner
- Signs and symptoms (vs. symptoms alone)

Diagnosis

- Criterion-based diagnosis
- Greater severity of illness
- "Lumped" vs. split diagnostic categories
- Based on objective vs. subjective criteria

Patient/informant

- Reliability of informant
- Length of acquaintance of informant with patient
- Absence of concurrent substance abuse (minor effect on reliability)

Obviously reliability is improved if each examiner elicits the same symptoms or signs from a given patient. Two main strategies that can be employed for this purpose are using thorough clinical assessments and standardizing the assessment strategy.

A thorough clinical assessment need not involve the use of complicated research tools. The reliability of the psychiatric evaluation can be improved by obtaining a careful longitudinal history from the patient, observing the patient over time, seeking signs of illness as well as symptoms, and obtaining a psychiatric history from other sources (such as friends, relatives, and medical records). In research studies, this approach has been called the Longitudinal, Expert, All Data (LEAD) standard. Thorough clinical assessment is crucial because even when raters use the same diagnostic criteria or definitions, their final diagnoses vary substantially based on which information is available for diagnostic decisions. These techniques are simply good medical practice and at least as important for psychiatric illness as for other medical complaints, yet they are sometimes neglected in psychiatric evaluations. Improving the clinical database in these practical ways often resolves confusion about diagnosis.

For research purposes, diagnostic reliability has also been improved by standardizing the examination technique. Standardized assessment of psychomotor retardation and standardized neurological examinations are examples of obtaining signs of illness in a reproducible way. Well-studied rating scales (such as the Hamilton Depression Rating Scale or Brief Psychiatric Rating Scale) help anchor clinical descriptions to a standard rating of severity. Turning to symptoms, standardized interviews are designed to elicit primarily historical information in a reproducible way. Diagnoses based on these interviews tend to show high reliability. Self-report questionnaires (such as the Beck Depression Inventory, Michigan Alcoholism Screening Test, or Minnesota Multiphasic Personality Inventory) also tend to be reliable. Additionally, some problems, such as substance abuse, are often missed in clinical situations but detected by these techniques. However, some illnesses are known to be poorly diagnosed by standardized interviews or self-report questionnaires. This happens because some conditions usually require longitudinal information from several sources for diagnosis (for example, somatization disorder), other conditions are better defined by physical signs than by symptoms (such as melancholia), and others are poorly remembered or described by patients after recovery (such as hypomania).

Reliability of diagnosis is affected not only by what information is obtained from the patient, but also by how information from the patient is interpreted; in other words, reliability is affected by features of the diagnostic classification itself. Several features of a diagnosis improve reliability. More severe illnesses tend to be more reliably diagnosed than subtle cases or *formes frustes,* so a past episode of major depression is more likely to be recalled by a patient than a past episode of hypomania. It is also easier for physicians to agree on more broadly defined diagnostic categories (for example, schizophrenia vs. affective illness) than on more finely divided subtypes (for example, paranoid vs. undifferentiated schizophrenia). On the whole, more valid diagnoses may also be made more reliably. Thus there is more diagnostic agreement among examiners and over time for schizophrenia than for borderline personality disorder. On the other hand (like the species *red*), some diagnoses have high reliability but unproven validity (such as dysthymia).

However, perhaps the most important characteristic of a diagnosis for reliability has been the clarity of the rules used for diagnosis. It was largely because of poor diagnostic reliability with older, more vague descriptions of psychiatric diagnoses that operationalized criteria were developed for diagnosis in psychiatry.

Operationalized Diagnostic Criteria, Including DSM-IV

Background

Over the past 20 years, several sets of psychiatric diagnostic criteria have been used widely. The most important of these have been the Washington University (Feighner) criteria (1972), the Research Diagnostic Criteria (RDC) (1975), and the third and subsequent editions of the American Psychiatric Association's DSM (DSM-III [1980], DSM-III-R [1987], and DSM-IV [1994]). All have had a dramatic effect on both research and clinical practice. With the advent of these operationalized diagnostic rules, physicians could meaningfully communicate about a patient by saying (for example) that he met RDC criteria for mania. Treatment or follow-up studies done at other institutions suddenly became relevant to a physician's own patients. Etiological studies became feasible.

Although the DSM manuals grew largely from the previous research criteria, there are some important differences. The DSM works are explicitly intended for routine clinical purposes rather than for research purposes, and criteria were largely decided by committees of experts rather than by formal evaluation of diagnostic studies. They describe hundreds of diagnoses rather than a few well-validated ones.

The current standard is the fourth edition of the DSM (DSM-IV). The DSM-IV has been described as the most thoroughly documented set of psychiatric diagnostic criteria in existence. The DSM-IV committee widely publicized draft versions, solicited commentaries from hundreds of organizations and individuals, sponsored extensive literature reviews, supervised field trials of current and proposed diagnoses, and published the results. An effort was also made to unify DSM-IV criteria with the corresponding sections of the tenth edition of the *International Classification of Diseases,* (ICD-10 [1993]). However, pragmatism and committee consensus still had powerful effects on the final document.

DSM-IV: How Good Is It?

The reliability of DSM-III, DSM-III-R, and ICD-10 diagnoses have been extensively studied in samples from all over the world. Since DSM-IV criteria were used in prepublication field trials for several disorders, and since the DSM-IV criteria for many disorders are identical to the DSM-III-R criteria, there is also some information on the reliability and validity of DSM-IV diagnoses. For most diagnoses, modern psychiatric research studies, using operationalized diagnostic criteria and standardized assessments, demonstrate reliability in a range at least comparable to that for other medical diagnoses made by clinical criteria (Table 2-2). Diagnostic reliability tends to be higher for broader diagnostic categories (anxiety disorders vs. panic disorder with agoraphobia), more severe illnesses (mania vs. hypomania), and perhaps for better-validated diagnoses (schizophrenia vs. schizoaffective disorder), but reliability is still acceptable for nearly all diagnoses. In other words, most DSM-IV diagnoses can be reliably assessed.*

Validity is a separate question. DSM-IV–based studies confirm the validity of previously well-validated diagnoses such as schizophrenia. However, although validation studies have now been carried out for some additional diagnoses, the results did not support their validity in many cases (see Table 2-1).

DSM-IV: The Final Episode?

A strong argument could be made that physicians should use one of the published sets of standardized diagnostic criteria until the etiology and pathophysiology are clearly known for more illnesses. Each nosological revision before that time creates difficulties. For instance, to what extent do research findings on Briquet's syndrome (by Washington University criteria)

*The John D. and Catherine T. MacArthur Foundation has sponsored a General Reliability Field Trial to further assess accuracy of DSM-IV diagnoses. Results are not yet published.

TABLE 2-2

RELIABILITY OF SELECTED DIAGNOSES

Diagnosis	Diagnostic criteria/means of assessment	Chance-corrected reliability (κ)*
Alcohol abuse or dependence	DSM-III-R, SCID†	0.96
Substance use disorders (average)	DSM-III, usual clinical interview	0.95
Schizophrenia	DSM-III-R, SCID	0.94
Major depressive disorder	DSM-III-R, SCID	0.93
Migraine	IHS, review of clinical records	0.88
Any personality disorder	DSM-III-R, Dutch version of SCID-II	0.80
Atopic dermatitis	U.K. Working Party criteria, focused clinical examination	0.78
Acute myocardial infarction	Clinical judgment, serial serum enzyme concentrations	0.56-0.92
Erosive esophagitis	Grades 2-4 severity, endoscopy	0.68-0.79
Pneumonia	Chest radiograph	0.71-0.72
Transient ischemic attack	Standardized protocol	0.65-0.77
Dysthymia	DSM-III-R, modified SCID	0.59-0.82
Dysplastic nevus	Skin biopsy pathology	0.55-0.84
Substance use disorders (average)	DSM-III, written case summary	0.69
Lewy body dementia	Newcastle criteria, usual clinical examination	0.50-0.87
Major depression (lifetime)	DSM-III-R, modified SCID	0.52-0.77
Alzheimer's disease (probable or possible)	Modified NINCDS-ADRDA, clinical examination with ADRS scale	0.63
Broken ankle or foot	Original Ottawa ankle rules, semistandardized clinical examination	0.56-0.69
Any personality disorder	DSM-III-R, MDCL-P	0.62
Any ICD-10 mental disorder	ICD-10, written case summary	0.59
Vascular dementia	NINDS-AIREN, case summary plus magnetic resonance imaging	0.46-0.72
Any DSM-III-R diagnosis	DSM-III-R, written case summary	0.53
Suspicion of breast cancer	Mammography	0.47
DSM-IV sleep disorders	DSM-IV, clinical interview	0.26-0.80
Alzheimer's disease (probable or possible)	NINCDS-ADRDA, case summary only	0.51
Obsessive-compulsive disorder	DSM-III-R, SCID	0.40
Prostate cancer	Clinical judgment, digital rectal examination	0.22
Psychotic disorders NOS (average)	DSM-III, written case summary	0.05

*A κ (kappa) value of zero indicates that any diagnostic agreement is purely the result of chance, whereas κ = 1 means that diagnostic agreement is perfect. Generally, κ > 0.75 is interpreted as excellent reliability and κ = 0.60-0.74 is understood to be good reliability. The κ statistic is not an ideal measure of diagnostic concordance, but it is probably the most commonly reported.

†*SCID,* Structured Clinical Interview for DSM-III-R; *IHS,* International Headache Society; *NINCDS-ADRDA,* National Institute of Neurological and Communicative Diseases and Stroke—Alzheimer's Disease and Related Disorders Association; *ADRS,* Alzheimer's Disease Rating Scale; *MDCL-P,* Munich Diagnostic Checklist for the Assessment of DSM-III-R Personality Disorders; *NINDS-AIREN,* National Institute of Neurological Disorders and Stroke—Association Internationale pour la Recherche et l'Enseignement en Neurosciences.

pertain to patients diagnosed with DSM-IV somatization disorder? Since some patients meet criteria for one but not the other, this question has real clinical importance.

Regardless of how long physicians should optimally wait for another revision of the DSM, hopefully DSM-IV will not be the last iteration. The nosology will certainly be improved as knowledge accrues, just as it has in the past. For instance, clinical definitions of general paresis of the insane were largely replaced by a combination of clinical and laboratory information when tests for syphilitic infection became available. Therefore when the causes of bipolar disorder are more completely known, specific laboratory tests or different clinical criteria will be added to the diagnostic definition.

This admission of imperfection in the current diagnostic system leads some to throw up their hands and deny its utility. However, imperfection is far from uselessness. There are at least two good reasons for using a standardized diagnostic system even though it is not the ultimate iteration. First, widely available, reliable standardized diagnostic criteria (even if imperfect) allow physicians to take better care of their patients. The abilities to communicate effectively with colleagues, teach others, and apply studies from other populations are all crucial to good patient care. "True" or final validity is perhaps secondary in importance to these essential benefits of criteria-based diagnosis. Second, the new knowledge that can someday advance psychiatric diagnosis can only be obtained when investigators first agree on the condition under study.

How Are Psychiatric Diagnoses Made?

Clinically-Defined Syndromes with Several Causes

Some medical diagnoses are made primarily by a given laboratory test in the appropriate clinical setting. Others are usually made by clinical judgment alone, either because antemortem laboratory studies have not been useful (as in Parkinson's disease) or because there is no consistent pathology (as in migraine). Most psychiatric diagnoses are made by clinical criteria alone. Just as in other areas of medicine, psychiatric diagnoses are based not on a single feature but on a pattern of symptoms, signs, and course. Chest pain, for example, has numerous causes and outcomes, depending largely on whether the pain syndrome is angina, heartburn, pleuritic pain, or something else. Similarly, most psychiatric symptoms, taken singly, are nonspecific. For instance, the symptom of sadness is a nonspecific symptom that has many causes and vastly different prognoses and treatments, depending on the cause. On the other hand, well-defined syndromes (like primary melancholic depression) are more likely to arise from a single illness, so when a complete syndrome is present, one has greater certainty in treatment decisions.

As discussed, each clinical syndrome of a natural nosology would have a single cause. However, in medicine many syndromes seem to represent final common pathways of clinical expression, and even though recognition of a syndrome narrows the etiological considerations considerably, there often remain several known causes for the syndrome. In psychiatry, this is most obvious with the syndromes known traditionally as organic, such as dementia or delirium. For example, Meyer ([1897] 1994) wrote:

> The most common mental disorders are those of intoxication and fever delirium. In these we see plainly that the mental disease is purely symptomatic, so much so that fever delirium and acute intoxication, with alcohol or other poisons, is not usually looked upon as a mental disease. We look quite correctly on the cause of the fever and on the process of poisoning as the principal pathological feature. The same probably holds for a great number of mental diseases.

However, most other psychiatric syndromes also have a broad differential diagnosis, with several known "organic" causes in addition to the idiopathic (primary) disorders. Autism, mania, major depression, and catatonia are examples of psychiatric syndromes with many medical causes. This does not mean that every patient needs dozens of diagnostic procedures. When the physician has a good knowledge of which conditions cause secondary psychiatric illness, then diagnosis often requires only a prudent consideration of the clinical setting, the medical history, and the psychiatric and neurological examinations. When laboratory testing is indicated, a few well-chosen studies are often adequate.

When an underlying general medical condition is discovered (for instance, hyperthyroidism), other specialists are often involved in treating the primary illness. However, the secondary syndrome (such as mania resulting from hyperthyroidism) remains a psychiatric illness, just as kidney disease is still relevant to nephrologists when it is the result of a rheumatologic process, or cranial nerve abnormalities are still a neurological concern when they are caused by an infectious disease.

Throughout this discussion, we have assumed that diagnosis is made according to the medical model of assigning patients to categories based on syndromes. This is in accord with the goals of medicine to find the cause and optimal treatment of similar illnesses in different patients. As one physician has pointed out, "The treatment of pneumonia by sulpha drugs cannot depend on the fact that *individuals* of *markedly dif-*

ferent background have acquired an infection; it depends on the *sameness of that infection*" (Myerson, [1944] 1994). However, as discussed in Chapter 1, many other models have been proposed for classifying mental illness. One of these is to describe patients by quantifying traits on several dimensions rather than assigning a categorical diagnosis. This alternative form of classification may meet some of the goals of diagnosis, such as improved communication between physicians. It might even be useful for etiological research, although different experimental designs and statistical techniques are required. However, it is doubtful that physicians will entirely turn to a dimensional classification system.

One significant problem with this dimensional approach is its presumption that illness consists largely of quantitative variation from normal. In the past, this presumption has impeded etiological research: if schizophrenia is seen as only an exaggeration of normal idiosyncrasy, why look for a pathogen? In fact, most of the more valid psychiatric diagnoses occur in a bimodal distribution of severity (consistent with well vs. ill), rather than smoothly grading into normalcy. For instance, epidemiological evidence shows that we are not all "a little schizophrenic" any more than we are all "a little parkinsonian." Of course, there is a spectrum of severity within each syndrome, and at times the severity of an illness may be of overriding importance to the patient or treating physician. However, this does not conflict with the validity or utility of categorical diagnosis.

Applying Specific Diagnostic Criteria to Daily Clinical Practice

Most physicians agree that criteria-based psychiatric diagnoses have clear advantages. However, many are uncomfortable with bringing research criteria into day-to-day practice. Some of their concerns can be summarized in two questions, which are discussed in the following paragraphs.

Do I Have to Look Up (or Memorize) the Criteria?

We have discussed how using accepted diagnostic criteria can improve patient care and research. But this presumes the criteria are used correctly. Unfortunately, this is far from universal. One common misconception is that a DSM-IV diagnosis is simply a new name for an old concept; in other words, it is a label to be applied to a patient not by clear rules but based on a gestalt impression of the patient's presentation. When this mistake is made, the benefits of communicating accurately with other physicians or of applying research from the literature to the patient are lost. An example from another specialty may make this more clear. Compare the difference between the two statements, "I think this patient's joint inflammation is probably caused by rheumatoid arthritis," and, "This patient meets research criteria for classic rheumatoid arthritis." Both statements have their place, but they are not at all identical. If physicians commonly confused the two, diagnosing classic rheumatoid arthritis based solely on pattern recognition or a vague clinical impression, then the research diagnosis would lose much of its meaning.

Some physicians feel that the use of written diagnostic criteria is too time consuming. Of course, this is sometimes true. Occasionally the treatment plan does not hinge on the complete accuracy of a diagnosis. Just as with rheumatoid arthritis, if there is a typical clinical picture with good treatment response, the physician may not need to turn to research criteria for diagnosis. However, substantiating a diagnosis is often critical, and the extra time it may take to gather additional history and consult the written criteria can be well spent. Another reason for referring to the diagnostic criteria is that even when physicians believe they are following certain rules for diagnosis, they often actually base their clinical diagnoses on information outside those rules.

Obviously it is not necessary to page through the entire DSM-IV manual for each patient. Common clinical sense can usually eliminate all but a few important differential diagnoses. Additionally, focusing on more valid diagnoses narrows the search to those that are most useful. Finally, the decision trees in Appendix A of the DSM-IV can help the physician narrow the differential diagnosis.

What About Cases That Do Not Seem to Fit the Criteria for Anything?

Although research studies often limit enrollment to classic or typical cases of an illness, physicians in practice take care of a number of patients whose presentations are atypical. These atypical presentations are part of the excitement of clinical medicine, but they can also present the physician with difficult diagnostic dilemmas. Sometimes unusual presentations are the result of comorbid conditions. General medical illnesses, intoxication or withdrawal from psychoactive substances, and mental retardation commonly alter the usual signs and symptoms of psychiatric illness. Furthermore, some conditions manifest differently at different ages or at different times during the course of an illness. Finally, an incomplete clinical database often gives the impression that the patient's presentation is atypical, when in fact further inquiry reveals characteristic "missing" features. However, many cases remain atypical after thorough evaluation. Specific strategies for dealing with comorbid illness and age effects are discussed in the relevant chapters later in this volume. Here we offer two general considerations for dealing with diagnostic uncertainty.

The first consideration is that definite diagnosis should be deferred for many patients. Using conservative diagnostic criteria, about 20% of psychiatric patients remain undiagnosed after adequate investigation. Although it is human nature for physicians to feel uncomfortable with uncertainty, it is usually in the patient's best interest to avoid premature insistence on a diagnosis when features are atypical or information is lacking. Referring to an atypical patient as undiagnosed is more defensible and modest than the alternative, and it avoids the automatic repetition of an unjustified diagnosis by those who review the medical record in the future. Additionally, there is often little point in making a poorly validated diagnosis, no matter how definitely it can be substantiated, since less valid diagnoses tend to offer scanty information about prognosis or treatment. Since some diagnosis is often needed for insurance purposes, DSM-IV allows for a number of "not otherwise specified" (NOS) categories, which we feel should be used liberally in these situations. The label *provisional* can be appended to a diagnosis, or the phrase *rule out* can be prefixed to it when a physician is somewhat more confident. In mild cases, a diagnostic decision can often be deferred altogether until the illness declares its presence (or until it is clear there is no illness).

The second general consideration arises from the need to do *something* in medical practice in the face of diagnostic uncertainty. For instance, patients who are acutely psychotic usually need some form of intervention before there is enough information to make a definite diagnosis. Two techniques can be helpful here. The first is to explicitly decide when a hunch is being expressed and when a diagnosis is based on standard criteria and supported by clear evidence. It may be helpful for a physician to record both types of diagnosis in the medical record to support therapeutic decisions in the face of insufficient data. For instance, the physician may suspect that a patient has major depression, even though it may not be clear whether the symptoms are persistent, related to alcohol use, or the result of a general medical condition such as hypothyroidism. In some cases it may be prudent to start psychotherapy, prescribe an antidepressant, or hospitalize the patient before such information can be obtained. In this case the physician might have the following thoughts: "From currently available history, I believe this patient probably has mild recurrent major depression. However, tests of thyroid function, clinical follow-up, and further history from family members regarding his mood symptoms and alcohol use will be important in firming up the diagnosis. The DSM-IV diagnosis at present is depressive disorder not otherwise specified (NOS)."

There is a second, more formal technique that can help the physician choose a course of action in the face of diagnostic uncertainty. This involves the field of decision analysis. In its more elaborate incarnations, this can involve lengthy analyses of alternative choices and numerical probabilities. These analyses can help greatly in research and teaching, but most physicians find them too time consuming for routine clinical use. However, in its simplest form, decision analysis harks back to the well-known medical aphorism, "When you hear hoofbeats, think horses, not zebras." For instance, since delirium is much more common in the hospital than in the office, it should be carefully ruled out in hospital patients with psychiatric symptoms but screened for quickly in outpatients. Although these vague statements of likelihood often suffice for day-to-day clinical practice, more information can be gained when a physician is willing to invest a little effort in learning simple decision analytic techniques. For instance, learning a few relevant probabilities from the medical literature and gaining a working understanding of Bayes' theorem allow a physician to better predict the outcome of different treatment options when diagnosis is uncertain.

Psychiatric Diagnoses Are Not Based on Self-Reported Symptoms Alone

One popular misconception used in attacks on criteria-based psychiatric diagnoses is the idea that modern diagnostic criteria, such as those of the DSM-IV, reduce the art of medical diagnosis to a mere checklist of symptoms endorsed by the patient. This is of course a caricature of modern psychiatric diagnosis. Several facts argue against this caricature.

First of all, psychiatric diagnosis occurs in the setting of a physician-patient relationship. Patients can hardly be expected to reveal valid information about their thoughts, hopes, mood, and intimate relationships to a cold stranger who reads questions from a list. Developing this trust is part of the physician's art and duty. Developing other skills needed for effective interviewing is also part of medical training.

Second, psychiatric diagnosis is based on reliable facts and not merely on a patient's reported symptoms. Although an individual's view of his life is meaningful and may even have diagnostic importance, it often does not accurately reflect objective history. The physician must keep straight whether she is dealing with verifiable history or with subjective history. Consider the following example:

> A woman comes to a physician and complains of lifelong depression. However, close friends and family members report that she sleeps and eats well, enjoys her usual activities, and usually appears happy. She does have brief minutes or hours every few days when she cries and feels hopeless in a difficult interpersonal situation.

In this case, the patient's distress is significant and may be an appropriate focus of clinical attention, but it does not reflect a major depressive episode. Discrepancies between symptom self-report and observation by others exist in all medical specialties. After all, different observers recall different facets of an experience and time blurs memory of past events. However, these discrepancies assume special importance in psychiatry, where patients often have disorders of perception, memory, thought, and insight. Additionally, information about past episodes of illness and health is often critical to an accurate psychiatric diagnosis. Thus when evaluating psychiatric complaints, symptoms must often be substantiated by objective observation.

Information to corroborate self-reported symptoms can come either from the physician's own observations or the observations of others. Medical records can be particularly valuable, since they contain written observations made by trained examiners. However, family members, close friends, co-workers, or even casual acquaintances can be better sources of information about a patient's functioning outside the hospital or office. Even when there is no inaccuracy in the patient's history, others often notice things about an individual that she does not notice about herself. Of course, a patient's permission must be obtained before the physician divulges confidential information *to* third parties. However, patients are often willing to allow the physician to obtain information *from* third parties once they understand how important this information can be to their diagnosis and treatment.

Whether or not third party observations are available, the physician is a trained observer. Good medical practice dictates examining for signs of illness in addition to eliciting symptoms. The mental status examination nearly always includes the assessment of certain signs; the physician observes the patient's appearance, behavior, speech, spontaneous movements, flow of speech, and emotional behavior. Memory and language are also examined. Certain presentations dictate further examination for other signs of illness, such as tachycardia, dilated pupils, goiter, apraxia, rigidity, catalepsy, or ataxia. When there is marked disparity between reported symptoms and visible signs, the physician should use caution in assigning a diagnosis. Therefore diagnosing schizophrenia is no more a rote checklist exercise than diagnosing rheumatic fever, since the examiner must know how to elicit and identify the signs of illness that form the criteria.

Third, psychiatric diagnoses are not based solely on self-report symptoms because diagnoses cannot be made as reliably on the basis of cross-sectional symptoms as they can through repeated observations. Sometimes the patient, her medical records, or third parties can supply adequate historical information for a confident longitudinal diagnosis. However, often patience and repeated follow-up examinations are required.

Fourth, medical history and signs of illness are elicited and interpreted by a physician. This is undoubtedly more important for certain diagnoses

PEARLS & PERILS

PSYCHIATRIC DIAGNOSIS

- Psychiatric diagnosis is based on clinical syndromes.
- Most psychiatric syndromes have a medical differential diagnosis.
- Psychiatric diagnosis is imperfect—just like diagnosis in any other medical specialty.
- Some psychiatric diagnoses are more valid (hence more useful) than others.
- Many psychiatric illnesses are both serious and treatable.
- The physician should do the following:
  (1) Consider psychiatric illnesses early in the differential diagnosis of both psychiatric and medical patients
  (2) Gather a longitudinal history from more than one source
  (3) Conduct a careful mental status examination, including appropriate items from the physical examination
  (4) Refer to the exact diagnostic criteria, especially where accurate diagnosis is crucial
  (5) Exercise diagnostic humility often in the form of undiagnosed, NOS, or provisional diagnoses
- The physician should not do the following:
  (1) Think of psychiatric illnesses only as diagnoses of exclusion
  (2) Lump all psychiatric patients together, denying them the benefits of careful diagnosis
  (3) Make a firm diagnosis based on symptoms alone
  (4) Make a firm diagnosis based on a cross-sectional presentation

(for instance, melancholia, delirium, somatization disorder, and schizophrenia), but these conditions are common and important and they are considered in the differential diagnosis of most psychiatric presentations.

Finally, psychological testing and the clinical laboratory can add valuable diagnostic information for certain presentations. Further discussion of how physicians elicit history, perform the mental status examination, and request psychological or laboratory testing is available in later chapters.

Case 2-1 is a fictitious but fairly typical case that illustrates many of the points discussed in this chapter.

Conclusion

Case 2-1 demonstrates many important points about psychiatric diagnosis (see the Pearls & Perils box on p. 24). Most importantly, the integration of psychiatric diagnosis into routine medical practice could have saved Ms. B. time, expense, invasive studies, and suffering. In other words, correctly diagnosing psychiatric illnesses is needed not only for education and research, but also for daily clinical work. Considering that good psychiatric diagnosis is really nothing more than a careful application of well-informed medical thinking to psychological symptoms, physicians owe their patients nothing less.

CASE 2-1

Ms. B. is a 35-year-old previously healthy woman who comes to the emergency room complaining of shortness of breath and inability to walk properly. She is agitated and appears frightened. Her physical examination is normal except for tachycardia and an abnormal gait. She falls consistently into the examiner, but after much reassurance she can walk normally. The symptoms resolve while diagnostic studies are underway. Arterial blood gases, a chest X-ray, and an electrocardiogram (ECG) are normal.

A similar episode occurs the following week. Ms. B. is admitted to the hospital and undergoes pulmonary function testing and studies to rule out recurrent pulmonary embolism. An intern elicits a history of several stressful events on the day of the first emergency room visit and wonders if the patient might have a psychiatric illness, but he is told that psychiatric illness is a diagnosis of exclusion only. However, after further testing and consultation with specialists, no "organic disease" is found and Ms. B. is referred to a psychiatrist for hysteria.

At this juncture, although Ms. B. has had thousands of dollars worth of medical care, she still has occasional episodes of dyspnea and anxiety and has taken a leave of absence from work. The psychiatrist, Dr. C., tries to substantiate the referring diagnosis. He knows that although the word *hysteria* tends to be a vague concept, criteria-based somatization disorder is a valuable diagnosis that can help avoid further costly or invasive laboratory testing. However, a systems review uncovers only a few medically unexplained symptoms. Other than the anxiety and difficulty walking, Ms. B.'s symptoms are largely limited to pulmonary and cardiovascular complaints. Her illness does not even approach DSM-IV criteria for somatization disorder. The psychiatrist realizes he could make a case for a diagnosis of conversion disorder, given her temporary inability to walk. However, Dr. C. knows that this less valid diagnosis is fairly meaningless, since up to 50% of patients with conversion disorder prove to have an underlying neurological or systemic illness. Thus hysteria does not explain the presenting symptoms, and there is still a concern that some serious or treatable illness may have been overlooked.

Since several of Ms. B.'s complaints were common symptoms of anxiety, Dr. C. probes further into possible anxiety diagnoses. These further questions reveal typical panic attacks in varied settings. The remainder of the mental status examination reveals no surprises, and Dr. C. makes a presumptive clinical diagnosis of panic disorder. He begins treatment and schedules a return visit in a few weeks.

After Ms. B. leaves the office, the psychiatrist looks up the DSM-IV criteria for panic disorder (since the exact defining symptoms are hard to remember) and finds that Ms. B. does in fact meet criteria for panic disorder with agoraphobia.

However, Dr. C. still feels uncomfortable with a definite diagnosis because of the patient's trouble walking, which is an unusual symptom in panic disorder. He knows that she still may have somatization disorder, since this diagnosis is often not detected on a single interview or by self-report alone. In his notes, he describes this concern and qualifies the DSM-IV diagnosis: "panic disorder with agoraphobia (provisional)."

With the patient's prior permission, he reviews her medical records and gathers diagnostic information from her family. These sources agree that she was quite healthy until recently; thus she does not meet criteria for somatization disorder. He considers insulinoma, pheochromocytoma, and other less common causes for recurrent anxiety attacks, but there is sufficient clinical information from the hospital chart that no further laboratory testing is indicated.

After several weeks of pharmacologic treatment and appropriate psychotherapy, Ms. B. has only rare, limited panic attacks; her fear of public places is greatly improved; and she is able to resume work. Over the ensuing years, she returns about twice a year and remains essentially symptom-free on modest doses of imipramine.

Annotated Bibliography

Goodwin DW, Guze SB: *Psychiatric diagnosis,* ed 5, New York, Oxford (in press).

This book provides a comprehensive review of the diagnostic validity of major psychiatric illnesses. The two brief prefaces discuss the importance of psychiatric diagnosis.

Robins E, Guze SB: Establishment of diagnostic validity in psychiatric illness: its application to schizophrenia, *Am J Psychiatry* 126:983-987, 1970.

This article discusses the rationale for the validation method summarized in Box 2-1.

Robins LN, Barrett JE, editors: *The validity of psychiatric diagnosis,* New York, 1989, Raven Press.

This is a multi-authored review of the evidence.

Sox HC Jr et al: *Medical decision making,* Boston, 1988, Butterworths.

This readable text brings clarity and relevance to mathematical decision making methods.

Widiger TA et al: *DSM-IV sourcebook,* vols 1-5, Washington, DC, 1994 (vol 1), American Psychiatric Association.

This multivolume work (some volumes are yet to be published) documents the rationale for the nosologic changes in DSM-IV. It serves as a convenient compilation of the literature on DSM-III, DSM-III-R, and DSM-IV diagnoses. Volumes 1 through 3 contain reviews of the literature on all major diagnostic categories, Volume 4 contains reanalyses of preexisting data sets to answer specific questions about certain diagnoses, and Volume 5 contains results of the DSM-IV field trials of new diagnostic criteria.

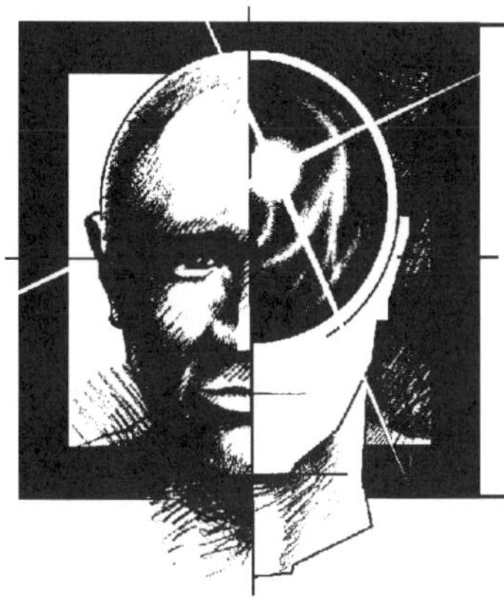

chapter 3

Examination of Patients

Richard W. Hudgens, MD and Daniel D. Pugh, MD

First, Make the Diagnosis

When a patient comes to a primary care physician complaining of symptoms, it is probable that this same physician will be the one who begins to treat him, even if he has a psychiatric illness. The first task in any case is diagnosis. Since a sizable minority of people who come to a physician are suffering from some psychiatric disorder, the physician must give the process of making a psychiatric diagnosis the same systematic attention as the process of diagnosing a medical or surgical disorder. This chapter serves as a guide to methods of interviewing that can make the processes of diagnosis and ongoing treatment of any disorder more effective and as a guide to the means of detecting psychiatric disorders specifically.

The Initial Interview

In the first contact with a patient (or with another informant when the patient is unable or unwilling to communicate) the physician's inquiry is driven by the chief complaint. Exploration of the chronology and details of that complaint, as well as of the immediate circumstances that brought the patient to the physician, is the beginning of the diagnostic process (see the Pearls & Perils box on p. 28).

An initial interview does not start as psychiatric, medical, or surgical, regardless of the specialty of the physician doing the questioning. An interview acquires a specialized character only as the types of symptoms are revealed, leading the physician to focus attention in particular areas. Ideally, an initial interview screens for all types of disorders and includes a review of systems wherein key questions are asked that extend beyond the boundaries of the chief complaint and present illness. In a nonemergency circumstance, such as the initial visit to a physician's office or a clinic, enough time should be scheduled for an extended interview with its screening questions. Even in situations where one clearly identified problem dominates the picture and requires urgent attention—for example, massive bleeding or a potentially lethal overdose—a

PEARLS & PERILS

EXAMINING THE PATIENT

- When a patient comes to a primary care physician with a complaint, it is probable that this same physician will be the one who begins to treat him, even if he has a psychiatric illness.
- Because so many of a primary care physician's new patients will have a psychiatric illness, the same systematic care must be given to psychiatric diagnosis as to the diagnosis of medical and surgical disorders.
- Failure to spend enough time with patients is a major cause of failure of both diagnosis and treatment of psychiatric illness.
- Physical symptoms are often the only spontaneous complaints offered by patients with major depression.
- Rapport is established by the physician's interested attention to the patient's complaints and not by talk of irrelevant pleasantries.
- If the patient is a concise and reliable historian, allowing him to give an uninterrupted history saves the physician time by eliminating the necessity for many routine questions.
- The specific reason a patient presents to a physician at a particular time may be just as important as the chief complaint itself.
- Depression occurring in patients with severe medical illness is not normal and requires specific treatment in its own right.
- The mental status examination is the sum of all observations made by the physician during the history-taking and not merely a list of questions tacked on at the end of the interview.

comprehensive history should be obtained as soon as possible. Important problems are often overlooked simply because the physician did not ask about them.

Exploration of the Chief Complaint

The interview should usually begin with an exploration of the symptoms that led the patient to seek help and the specific circumstances that brought the patient to the physician at this particular time. The latter subject may provide vital clues to the most important aspects of the problem. For example, the main symptom of abdominal pain may have been present for months, but a patient only seeks help after a week of being too weak to perform his job. It may turn out that the weakness is a result of occult bleeding that finally put the patient's red cell volume below a critical level. Another patient may have been hearing hallucinated voices for many years but was not motivated to seek help until the day they frightened her with commands to kill her family. The physician must not only ask what is wrong but also (if it is not obvious) how and why the patient chose that time to seek help.

When the patient or other informant is capable, the physician should encourage him to give a spontaneous account of the chief complaint and the circumstances surrounding it. To encourage spontaneity, from time to time the physician may need interject, "And then what?" or a similar phrase. When specific clarification is needed on some point, it is best for the physician to ask for information in a way that discourages brief answers. For example, "Tell me something about your marriage," elicits more information than, "Do you get along well with your wife?"

While the patient is giving his account, the physician should not interrupt him with a premature checklist of her own questions. If she does, important information may be missed and the diagnostic process may actually be prolonged. For instance, 5 or 10 minutes of a patient's spontaneous and relevant discourse may contain enough positive and negative information to make many review-of-system and mental-status questions unnecessary.

After the patient's spontaneous account of the chief complaint has been completed, the physician asks questions to complete a detailed chonological picture of the present illness. Further information is then elicited about the patient's medical and psychiatric history, review of systems, personal and social history, and family history of medical and psychiatric illnesses, especially in first degree relatives. Here the checklist method is essential; there are some things that should always be asked if the patient has not already mentioned them.

In almost all cases, collateral sources of history are helpful; in some cases they are indispensable. Whenever possible the physician should seek information from sources in addition to the patient. These sources may include relatives, other physicians, and hospitals, and the patient's permission should be obtained unless the absence of information poses a threat to the patient's life. It is usually best to talk with the patient first, but in some urgent situations that might not be practical.

Rapport

Much is written about the desirability for physicians and patients to have relationships of mutual trust and respect. In such circumstances patients are more comfortable, more likely to tell physicians what they need to know, and more likely to be compliant with treatment. Behavior by physicians that promotes good rapport is not only the kindest way to deal with patients; it is also the most medically effective way. This rapport is best established not by small talk about irrelevant pleasantries but by listening attentively to the patient talk about the things that trouble him most and by taking the patient's complaints seriously. The patient has come to the doctor because of a problem; nothing is more reassuring to him at the outset than the knowledge that it is this problem and nothing else in which the doctor is most interested. That is what it takes to get the physician and patient off to the right start.

Diagnosis of Psychiatric Disorders

The foregoing discussion is applicable to the assessment of patients with any type of illness. This section focuses on psychiatric disorders, including the clues that such disorders may be present, questions that should always be asked in such cases, and the mental status examination.

Clues to Psychiatric Disorders

1. Direct complaints of persistent emotional distress, such as depressed mood, fearfulness and excessive worrying, or behavior suggesting such distress, are indications that a psychiatric disorder may be present, even when there is an obvious medical disorder. Such symptoms do not automatically accompany even the most serious medical illnesses and demand further investigation. For example, it is a common mistake for physicians to think that depression is normal in people who are very sick with a medical illness. In fact it is not normal, and depression in such cases requires the same active treatment as major depressive illness occurring by itself.
2. Certain physical symptoms often accompany psychiatric disorders and may be the principal complaints. Prominent among these symptoms are chronic fatigue, chronic headache, chronic musculoskeletal pain without objective findings, panic attacks with feelings of breathlessness and chest discomfort, changes in eating behavior, changes in sleep pattern, any gastrointestinal complaint, and unexplained neurological complaints of weakness or altered sensation. Any of those symptoms can be part of the clinical picture of major depression, generalized anxiety disorder (GAD), and somatization disorder.
3. A change in the ability to think clearly, concentrate, or remember things occurs in a number of psychiatric disorders, most prominently major depression, schizophrenia, dementia, and delirium. Depression is the most common of these disorders, and the intellectual impairment in severe cases is unfortunately often mistaken for dementia.
4. Changes in behavior, even in the absence of complaints by the patient, often indicate that a psychiatric disorder is present. Irritability and temper outbursts occur in depression, delusional disorder, schizophrenia, dementia, and drug or alcohol dependence. This behavior may appear before any other symptoms. Lethargy, slovenliness, irresponsibility, or neglect of care for self may also be an early symptom of one of these disorders. In contrast, increased energy, excessive talkativeness, multiple projects hastily launched, impatience with restraint, and intense spiritual zeal in a person who was previously casual about religion may herald the onset of mania.
5. Whenever a prominent aspect of the history is peculiar or just does not make sense, the physician should be alert to the possibility that a psychiatric disorder is present, even if other symptoms are denied. In such cases further observation and information from reliable informants often reveal that the patient is suffering from delusions, is abusing drugs or alcohol, or is consciously making up stories for some gain of his own. The physician should always follow up histories that seem conspicuously weird. Something is going on that, for one reason or another, the patient does not want the physician to know about.

Questions That Should Always Be Asked

There are some items relevant to psychiatric illness that the physician should inquire about at the first contact with nearly every patient. There are additional items that should be asked about in any case where a psychiatric disorder is actually suspected. For each symptom the physician should not only ask about its presence or absence but also about its chronology—when it started and how it has developed—and the specific manner and extent of the symptom's interference with the patient's life.

In the first category, the physician should always ask about increases or decreases in energy, interest in things, sexual function, sleep, appetite, and weight; headaches, chest pain, dyspnea, and gastrointestinal dysfunction; a detailed history of drug and alcohol use and the effects of those substances; problems with motivation, attention, concentration, or memory; problems with co-workers or job performance; problems in marriage and family; and the presence of upsetting events and circumstances in the patient's life. At the end of the initial interview it is also well to ask if there is anything important that the patient has not mentioned. At this time patients often disclose material that they were reluctant to talk about.

If any psychiatric disorder is suspected, there are additional areas for the physician to explore. He should ask about *hopelessness leading to death wishes.* If such wishes are present, the doctor should inquire about their rationale. Reasons for wanting to die that are based on distortions of reality ("I'm guilty of the unpardonable sin") are most ominous. Patients who are considering killing themselves must be asked about specific suicide plans and the availability of the means of carrying them out. The physician should not be afraid of putting ideas in the patient's head; patients who are depressed have probably been thinking about this subject already. Exploring it in detail makes it possible to take measures to prevent suicide and gives the physician specific information that may govern the choice among types of treatment.

Obsessions and compulsions are often omitted from patients' spontaneous accounts of their histories; they are afraid of sounding foolish or "crazy." The incidence of obsessive-compulsive disorder (OCD) was greatly underestimated until epidemiological studies were done employing standarized comprehensive interviews wherein every question was asked of every subject. Similarly, the physician may miss this disorder, which is treated differently than the more common GAD or major depression, unless he asks the right questions. Is the patient bothered by repetitive thoughts that he tries to get out of his head but cannot? Does he feel compelled to spend time performing certain repetitive acts that he knows are illogical, such as excessive checking, washing, and counting, but if he tries to refrain from them, he becomes anxious?

Similar to OCD are some of the core psychological symptoms in *eating disorders* such as anorexia nervosa and bulimia nervosa. These symptoms are often concealed and sometimes denied even after specific questioning. The examining physician should particularly ask every anxious or depressed young woman, whether she is thin or not, about fears of fatness; compulsions to fast or to gorge on food; and compulsions to purge herself of feared weight by vomiting, taking laxatives or enemas, or taking diuretics.

The physician should ask about *delusions* in any patient who is severely depressed and anyone who is agitated, suspicious, hostile, or confused. This subject should be approached with tact but not avoided. The physician may begin by asking, "Is anything upsetting, scary, or strange going on in your life?" The physician may also ask about things that can happen to anyone and then move to questions about more bizarre experiences: are people bothering the patient, following him, trying to spread lies about him, or trying to harm him? Is he under electronic surveillance ("bugged")? Are comments on the radio or television aimed specifically at him? If the patient tells of events that could, in fact, be happening, the physician should inquire about the evidence for these occurrences. For example, a man who suspects his wife of infidelity on the basis of flashing lights from airplanes has something wrong besides a marital problem. Whenever a patient believes himself to be the object of harrassment or persecution, the physician should ask if he plans to do anything about it. In this way a need for immediate hospital care may be discovered, and harm to others may be averted. Physicians have a duty to report any credible threats to specific individuals so the targets of those threats can be warned.

Primary care physicians see many people who are preoccupied with fear of disease and who have repeated requests for reassurance, more tests, and so forth. Some of these people have hypochondriacal delusions, or the firmly held conviction that diseases are present despite all evidence to the contrary. These symptoms may occur in patients with severe depression and schizophrenia. They are ominous because they are relatively resistant to treatment and often accompanied by serious suicide risk. It is important for the primary care physician to be alert to the fact that persistent and unreasonable hypochondriacal beliefs may be the only spontaneous complaints from a person who is dangerously ill.

Hallucinations may occur in severe depression, mania, schizophrenia, drug intoxication, alcohol withdrawal, dementia, and delirium. Their presence should be inquired about in any of those conditions. The physician may ask the patient if he is seeing or hearing things, or more specifically, hearing voices or seeing visions. Even with detailed questioning it is often difficult and sometimes impossible to know whether or not a patient who answers those questions positively is experiencing a true hallucination (a perception in the absence of external stimuli) or only an illusion (a misinterpretation of actual external stimuli).

The great majority of hallucinations occurring in schizophrenia, mania, and major depression are auditory. Visual hallucinations usually indicate delirium or toxicity from medication or illicit drugs. Tactile hallucinations also occur in those circumstances. Olfactory hallucinations are rare and require a search for neurological disease, such as temporal lobe pathology. Taste is so often altered by food, the type of medication taken, and the amount of saliva that it is always difficult to be sure if true gustatory hallucinations are present.

The Mental Status Examination

The mental status examination is not merely a set of proverbs, current-event and orientation questions, or mathematical calculations tacked on at the end of a diagnostic interview. Rather it is the sum of all the observations made by the physician about the patient during the course of the evaluation. During this evaluation the physician should keep in mind the categories being assessed: appearance, behavior, mood, affect (expressed emotion), form of speech (and by inference, form of thought), content of thought, level of intelligence, sensorium (degree of alertness, memory, and orientation), quality of judgment, and degree of insight into the illness.

In the majority of cases in which a thorough history is obtained and the patient's speech, words, and behavior are carefully observed, the important requirements of the mental status examination are fulfilled. The physician will have a good enough idea about mood, memory, insight, the content of thought, rough intelligence level, judgment, and other attributes. There is no need to insert into the interview such awkwardnesses as the recitation of a reverse list of United States presidents or the serial subtraction of sevens from 100, and an artificial probe of judgment through questions about fire in a theater and the proper disposition of an unmailed letter are not necessary.

Patients in whom impairment of sensorium is suspected may require formal questioning to assess orientation, memory, and judgment. Orientation of the patient to his identity, the date, the place, and the specific significance of the current situation should be explored. Memory should be tested separately for recent and remote events. Impairment of a third function of memory, immediate recall, can be discovered by questions about items the patient was asked to remember a few minutes earlier in the same interview. Judgment and insight are best evaluated by asking the patient to tell about actual decisions he has made and about his understanding of the nature of his illness.

Follow-up Appointments

If a primary care physician is treating a patient for a psychiatric disorder, it is important to schedule enough time for each follow-up appointment. The physician must obtain an interval history that includes current symptoms, important life events, current mental status, and an evaluation of the therapeutic and toxic effects of medication. Even if the patient is in psychotherapy with someone else and the physician's role is simply to manage medication, she must devote enough time to acquire a comprehensive, if brief, understanding about what is going on in those areas. Time must also be allotted for the patient to ask questions. All this can rarely be well accomplished in fewer than 15 to 30 minutes, even if patients have completed a interval checklist questionnaire in the waiting room.

It is often the lack of time in a busy schedule, not lack of interest or knowledge, that leads the primary care physician to refer patients to a psychiatrist or other mental health professional. The process and rationale of such referrals, as well as community resources available to people with psychiatric disorders, are discussed in Chapter 7.

Annotated Bibliography

American Psychiatric Association: *The American psychiatric glossary,* ed 7, Washington, D.C., 1994, author.

This is an alphabetical listing of almost all the technical terms in current use in psychiatry along with their definitions.

Folstein MF et al: Mini-mental state: a practical method for grading of the cognitive state of patients for the clinician, *J Psychiatr Res* 12:189, 1975.

This is the most widely used clinical scale for assessing impairment of sensorium.

Hamilton M, editor: *Fish's clinical psychopathology: signs and symptoms in psychiatry,* ed 2, Bristol, U.K., 1985, John Wright & Sons Ltd.

This is a detailed synopsis of the German and Swiss contributions to descriptive psychopathology. The German language literature has always pioneered in this field.

Katzman R et al: Validation of a short orientation-memory-concentration test of cognitive impairment, *Am J Psychiatry* 140:734, 1983.

The *Short Blessed Test* contained herein is a clinical scale used to assess impairment of sensorium.

Pfeiffer E: A short portable mental status questionnaire for the assessment of organic brain deficit in elderly patients, *J Am Geriatr Soc* 23:433, 1975.

This clinical scale for assessment of impaired sensorium assesses orientation and memory almost exclusively, thus probing diffuse brain impairment uncontaminated by focal cortical signs.

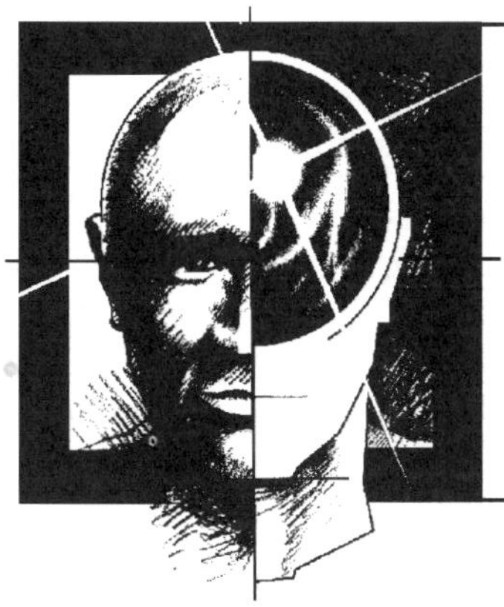

chapter 4

Psychological Testing

Richard D. Wetzel, PhD

What Is the Question? Testing Has to Make Sense Clinically

Testing Is a Part of Clinical History or Examination

Psychological testing in any branch of medicine is best understood by physicians when a psychological test is thought of as an expanded, detailed version of part of the patient's general examination. Depending on the type of test, the results can amplify the clinical history, the mental status examination, or the neurological examination (Table 4-1). The Logical Memory scale of the Wechsler Memory Scale-Revised may serve as a convenient example of the difference between the process a physician ordinarily uses in a mental status examination and the process a psychologist uses when testing. A physician typically tests memory by telling the patient three things and asking her to repeat them back. After an interval of approximately 5 minutes, the physician asks the patient to repeat the three items again. The physician thus has a quick measure of the patient's memory; it is quite informative if she cannot do the task. However, if the patient can recall three items after 5 minutes, the physician does not know a great deal more about her.

Testing Is a More Detailed History or Examination

What does a psychological test do? The Logical Memory Scale has two stories containing 25 pieces of information each. Thus there are 50 bits of information to remember. This allows the clinician to obtain a wide range, or distribution, of scores: 0 to 50 vs. the 0 to 3 range of the physician. The advantage is that the clinician can now describe a whole range of verbal memories from superb to terrible. One cannot judge whether the three-item approach or the 50-item approach is better until the clinical question to be answered has been determined. The physician must decide whether clinical interview or physical examination is adequate for the decision to be made. If one of these options is adequate, no testing is needed.

The data psychological tests obtain are merely gathered in greater detail, with more compulsive attention to procedure and comparison to explicit norms (standards) developed in some group of patients or people. Having developed a spread or range of scores, the psychological tester uses *normative data,* or statements about the distribution of scores (mean, standard deviation, skew, and kurtosis) in specific groups. Physicians tend to rely on implicit norms (for example, normal

TABLE 4-1

THE ROLE OF TESTS IN MEDICINE

Tests as clinical history	Inquire about
Beck Depression Inventory	Symptoms of depression
Minnesota Multiphasic Personality Inventory-2 (MMPI-2)*	Symptoms of anxiety, depression, psychosis, suicide ideation, etc.
Tests as mental status examination	**Measures**
Information scale-IQ test	Fund of information
Tests as physical examination	**Measure**
Finger tapping test	Motor speed
Hand dynamometer	Strength of grip

*The MMPI has been revised recently. The revised version is called the MMPI-2. The revision was substantial (about 30% of items). A new version for adolescents called the MMPI-A has also been published. Psychologists disagree among themselves over which version (MMPI vs. MMPI-2) is better.

BOX 4-1

HOW TO FIND OUT ABOUT A TEST

1. Consult the manual for the test. The makers of psychological tests are required by ethical standards for test construction to publish the relevant information about the reliability and validating studies done on the test.
2. Consult the Buros Institute's *Mental Measurements Yearbook*. This reference book is published every few years. It contains critical reviews (usually by more than one expert) of 300 to 400 tests. These are short, technical, and point out the flaws in a test in detail. This is a fast way to obtain information. The most recent edition, *The Eleventh Mental Measurements Yearbook,* was published in 1992. It contains 703 reviews on 477 different tests.
3. Call the author of the test, especially if it is an obscure test. Authors are usually glad when someone has heard of their tests and discuss them willingly. They usually provide selected reprints. The addresses and phone numbers of the authors can be obtained from the *Directory of the American Psychological Association*. The directory is available in many university libraries. Many psychologists also have one.
4. Almost all research on psychological tests can be found by consulting *PsychINFO* (computerized) or *Psychological Abstracts* (book), either online with a computer or in university libraries. This is the hard but thorough way.

people should be able to do this, and slow patients should be able to do that). Psychologists like explicit norms; that is, they want to be able to say what the average score is in some group and to be able to describe scores as near the tenth, twentieth, or eightieth percentile. The increased precision in measurement is sometimes valuable, depending on the clinical decision to be made.

Test Results as Laboratory Values with or without Consultation by a Psychologist

The second decision the physician needs to make is whether the goal is the additional information provided by a test alone or the opinion of a psychologist along with the data. More psychological testing is used directly by physicians (and their assistants) than by physicians consulting psychologists (Box 4-1).

If a physician knows what information is desired from a test and has enough experience with the test to know its clinical strengths and weaknesses, there is no need to involve a psychologist. Test makers and vendors recognize this and classify tests in terms of the training and experience required to purchase and use them. Many tests are directly available to physicians. More can be obtained if other requirements (such as courses and workshops) are met.

An interested physician, with a little effort, can develop enough skill and background to use some psychological tests (such as the MMPI-2, Millon Clinical Multiaxial Inventory-III [MCMI-III], and Temperament and Character Inventory [TCI]) as screening devices for a psychiatric or personality disorder. After a little experience, a physician can also use the simpler tests and rating scales (for example, the Beck Depression Inventory [BDI]; the Zung, Hamilton, and Yesavage depression inventories; and anxiety tests) to monitor response to treatment without direct consultation with a psychologist.

Reliability, Validity, and Norms

Psychologists are concerned about making errors. They often talk about reliability and validity when describing a test (Box 4-2). Both terms refer to the prob-

BOX 4-2

KEY TERMS IN TESTS AND MEASUREMENTS

Reliability: a measure (from 0.00 to 1.00) of how often the same answer is achieved under the same conditions of measurement. If a yardstick is used to measure a table, one would expect to get the same answer time and again. Giving the same test twice is the usual way to measure this. Some variables, such as depression, are expected to change over time. Statistical methods exist to estimate reliability in a variety of ways. Reliability is never a function of a test by itself; it is a function of a test being given under certain conditions to a certain population. A high reliability in the general population does not necessarily imply a high reliability in a special population; this is always an empirical question. The reliability of a test sets the upper limit of the validity of a test.

Validity: the degree to which a test measures what the tester wants it to measure with reasonable accuracy. A depression scale should measure depression and not anxiety or neuroticism. The validity of a test can be developed by using differing criterion groups and future outcomes or by the predictability from scientific theory of scores obtained on the test.

Distribution: If a useful test is given to a number of people, they will not all have the same score on the test. The tester can sort or order these scores and describe the way they spread out. The distribution of scores can be described in terms of their mean, standard deviation, skew, and kurtosis.

Mean: the mathematical mean of the scores, which is found by adding all the scores and dividing the total by the number of scores.

Standard deviation: a measure of how far the scores fall from the average. The differences between each score and the average are squared (the unsquared differences always add up to zero) and then added. The sum is divided by the number of scores and then changed back to the original units of measure by taking the square root.

Skew: a measure of whether one tail of the distribution is longer than the other. The difference between the scores and the mean is cubed (so one can see the difference between those above and below average).

Kurtosis: a measure of whether the distribution is too narrow or too wide. In other words, did the tester squeeze the distribution in or sit on it and flatten it out? The differences are raised to the fourth power, summed, and manipulated.

Normal curve, bell curve: a statistical or mathematical abstraction describing a theoretical distribution of scores. This is the result one would expect if scores have an infinite number of causes, all of which have a small effect. Scores on psychological tests never fit a normal curve perfectly. With a large enough number of scores, a statistically significant deviation from normality can always be found.

Standard score, T-score: standardized or transformed score. Remembering the mean and standard deviations of a number of different scales is difficult and bothersome. Test makers try to help by converting raw scale scores to a more easily remembered set of numbers. This is done by subtracting the mean score on the scale from the obtained score. The difference is then divided by the standard deviation. The original score has now been converted to a *Z-score,* with a mean of zero and a standard deviation of one. The Z-score is then multiplied by a constant. Then another constant is added. The Wechsler Intelligence Quotient [IQ] score is a standard score, or a T-score, with a mean of 100 and a standard deviation of 15.

Norms: the distribution (mean, standard deviation, skew, and kurtosis) of scores on a test in a specified population (for example, white males, college graduates, or patients with low back pain and no demonstrable pathology).

Standard error of measurement: Just as there is a distribution or range of scores within a large group of people taking a test, there is also a distribution or range of scores when a person (or a group) takes a test over and over again. The standard deviation in this situation is called the standard error of measurement. This is ordinarily much smaller than the standard deviation. The size of this statistic is a function of the number of times the test is taken or the number of people taking the test.

Difference scores: People like to compare a score on one test to that on another. For example, a person might like to say that he is better at math than spelling. This poses some problems, since the tester would like to be sure a difference between two scores is meaningful. In classic testing theory, a score on the first test is thought of as having two parts—a true measure of one trait and an error component. The score on the other test is a true measure of the second trait and its error component. When the two scores are compared, the result is the true difference between the first trait and the second trait plus two error terms. Difference scores are inherently less reliable (more influenced by error) than the scores from which they are derived.

State: a short-term condition, such as depression; a quickly changing trait.

Trait: a long-term condition or a slowly changing state. The distinction between state and trait is essentially arbitrary.

ability that errors influence a test score. A reliable test gives the same result again and again under the same conditions of measurement. The reliability of a test always sets an upper limit on the validity of a test. Validity in testing means that a test really measures what it claims to measure and nothing else. An unreliable test cannot be valid; a reliable test may be valid, or it may mismeasure something in a consistent fashion.

If the same test is given to the same person over and over again, he will have a personal average and a range of scores around that average. Psychologists often want to state that a score falls in a certain range rather than stating the score itself. This is because they are aware of the inability of psychological tests to measure precisely. However, physicians understand that error is not uniquely confined to psychological tests; other clinical tests have errors of measurement as well (although they are usually substantially smaller). Reticence about stating the exact score is a product of a psychologist's training not to appear overly precise; it is not ordinarily intended to frustrate physicians.

What psychological tests measure is almost always complex and affected by multiple influences. For example, the scores on a paper and pencil test can be affected by vision (reading), reading ability, hearing (directions), concentration, memory, motivation, testing situation, age, gender, race, socioeconomic status, birthplace, education, and more.

Because of this multifactorial issue, a test may not measure what its name suggests it measures, especially if it is used in a population different from that in which it was developed. Patients who are anxious have higher scores on depression scales than nonpatients even if they are not depressed; patients who are depressed have higher scores on anxiety scales. Psychological research does what any other science does. It develops increased confidence in the validity of a test by attempting to disprove that the test measures what it claims to measure. If a test purports to measure depression, researchers attempt to prove that it measures something else, such as anxiety or willingness to admit problems. Failure to prove that it measures some other attribute increases confidence in the test. Validation of a test often involves different procedures (interview vs. paper and pencil) and different constructs (anxiety vs. depression). A psychologist who uses a test should have a general knowledge of how it has been validated. He should also have some awareness of its problems and know when it makes mistakes and what the factors causing those mistakes might be.

Norms

Psychologists also deal with this multifactorial complexity by developing norms that show what the distribution of scores is in a given population. Generally, age, gender, race, and education affect test scores in important ways. The more extensive the norms are (that is, the greater the number of groups in which a test has been used and the distribution of scores described), the more psychologists tend to like or use a test. The goal is always to be able to describe with as much precision as possible where a person's score, ability, or dysphoric state fits in some distribution of scores.

The most common way to assess the validity of a test is through the use of criterion groups. Test scores are obtained from two groups of people. The most common design answers the question of whether nonpatients differ from patients on the test. Normals differ from patients in hundreds of ways; as a result, almost any test can pass this standard. The kind of validation a physician cares about in a clinical situation is whether a test can effectively discriminate among patients with disorders that are likely to be in a differential diagnosis (for example, depression vs. panic disorder vs. somatization disorder). Although this seems obvious to physicians, it is not necessarily part of the conceptual framework of psychologists, particularly those who do not interact with physicians often.

As a general rule, the clinical utility (validity) of psychological testing is greatly affected by the appropriateness of the norms used by the psychologist. A psychologist should always be able to state what norms were used and why they were chosen over other sets

PEARLS & PERILS

PITFALLS IN TESTING

- The most important decision a neuropsychologist makes is the estimate of how well the patient should be able to do on a test. The validity of all other conclusions depends on this conclusion.
- The diagnosis of mental retardation cannot be made solely from an IQ score. Social functioning is as important or more important than IQ scores.
- Screening for brain dysfunction with one test—usually a drawing test like the Bender-Gestalt Test—is not competent psychological or medical practice.
- The diagnosis of child sexual abuse offered to a physician solely or primarily on the basis of projective tests, art therapy products, or sand play should lead the physician to suspect that the person proffering the opinion is ignorant of the clinical and scientific literature, biased, or practicing out of their field of competence. An appeal to the person's experience in interpreting such material should confirm the suspicion.

of norms in the evaluation of a patient. A physician rarely has the background to know all the available tests of an ability or state and the norms developed for them, but if he asks, the physician will be able to understand whether the norms used by the psychologist are meaningful when they are applied to the patient.

Psychologists like to use cut-off scores (usually only one) to make diagnostic inferences. If the patient's score is above a certain score, she is likely to have something; if her score is below the cut-off point, she is less likely. At times, psychologists use the usual cut-off scores for a test in a mechanical way without thinking about the logic of the clinical situation. Statistical cut-off scores derived from a general population (such as the top 10%, 5%, or 1% of normals) are not necessarily good clinical cut-off scores. For example, the MMPI-2 graphically uses a T-score of 65 on its clinical scales, thus showing that 8% of the general population has scores above the upper line. The test makers required the same percentage of this population to be above this cut-off point on each scale: hypochondriasis, depression, hysteria, antisocial personality, paranoia, anxiety, schizophrenia, and mania. The rates of these disorders in the general population vary widely, yet the identical percentage is selected (see the Pearls & Perils box on p. 36). If 8% of the population is depressed, it is logical to use a cut-off score that selects 8% of the population. On the other hand, if only one person in 200 has antisocial personality or schizophrenia, selecting 8% of the general population makes little sense. Lyons and Keane have an excellent discussion on the difference between a statistically abnormal cut-off point (for the general population) and a different, clinically meaningful cut-off score on their MMPI-2 scale for posttraumatic stress disorder (PTSD).

Common Questions

Physicians tend to ask certain questions often. The following section addresses some of these questions.

How Intelligent Is My Patient?

Patients have to cope with the world, their diseases, and the medical regimen prescribed. Intelligence helps.

A Short Definition of Intelligence

Boring, a famous psychologist and historian of psychology, said, "Intelligence is what intelligence tests measure" (1923). Wechsler defined it as ". . . the aggregate or global capacity of the individual to act purposefully, think rationally, and to deal effectively with his environment" (Matarazzo, 1972). Kline stated that Spearman posed the question of why people who are good at one thing are generally good at another; his answer was *g*, a general factor of intelligence. Spearman invented factor analysis to explore the structure of abilities. In modern theories, *g* is broken into two parts: fluid intelligence and crystallized intelligence. Fluid intelligence is the basic reasoning ability of a person and is dependent on the neurological functioning of the person at the current moment. Fluid intelligence is basically what neuropsychological tests hope to measure in adults. Crystallized intelligence is reflected in the acquisition of skills valued in a culture.

The term intelligence quotient (IQ) was originally derived from a comparison of the cognitive level at which a child performed (mental age) with the child's chronological age. That concept has been abandoned. A deviation IQ (comparison with the population mean) is now used. Matarazzo (1972) notes, "The IQ merely states that a person's intelligence score at any given time is defined by his relative standing among his age peers." Standard IQ tests were developed, in part, to predict which children would require special help in middle-class grade schools. They are most accurate at the cut-off point between mental retardation and borderline intelligence (slow learners). They were not intended to discriminate well at the higher ranges of intelligence in older people (this is why students do not take IQ tests to get into medical school). Current IQ tests are culturally laden and measure both fluid and crystallized intelligence. It is well known that pupils from lower socioeconomic status (SES) groups have lower scores than those from higher SES groups. Kline (1991) states the case fairly:

> The bright and well-adjusted child who attends a good school and receives encouragement at home will invest most of her fluid ability in the crystallized skills of the culture. On the other hand, the equally bright child from a home where education is not valued and who attends a school of indifferent quality will not thus invest his fluid ability.

To say the apparent difference in IQ scores between groups differing in race, nationality, or SES is primarily the result of the biological determinants of intelligence is quite unsophisticated and naive. Less culturally laden IQ tests have been developed; they do not predict school success as well. Success in school is a function both of native intelligence (fluid) and the acquisition of culturally valued skills (crystallized). This explains, to a large degree, the continued use of scientifically problematic (factorially impure) tests.

What Can an IQ Test Tell Me?

When a patient is having problems at school, at work, or at home, a relative lack of intelligence should be considered as a potential cause or contributor to the problem. Intelligence test scores predict with some accuracy (10% to 25% of the variance, depending on the study) educational success, occupational success, and interpersonal effectiveness. Both physicians and psychologists tend to estimate IQ poorly because they adjust their estimates of average intelligence to their own patient population rather than the general population. Testing IQ is preferable to guessing if the answer is clinically important.

Is My Patient Mentally Retarded?

The diagnosis of mental retardation rests on several factors. IQ is important and should be measured. However, the diagnosis of mental retardation can not be made solely from an IQ score.* Social functioning is at least as important as the IQ score. Social functioning can be assessed formally with adaptive behavior scales. Two of the more widely used tests are the Vineland Adaptive Behavior Scale (VABS) and the adaptive behavior scale published by the American Association for Mental Retardation. A person who can care for herself in an age-appropriate way is not mentally retarded, whatever the IQ score. These adaptive behavior scales measure both positive and negative social skills and deficits. It is important to note that IQ scores should not be used in a mechanical or arbitrary way without good clinical judgment; of course, this is true of any other score, value, or finding a physician uses. When mental retardation is the question, both IQ and social adaptive behavior should be carefully evaluated.

Is My Patient Learning Disabled?

Learning disability is diagnosed when a patient's achievement does not match the level expected from the patient's IQ. A learning disability exists when a child or adult cannot learn as well as one would expect from his general IQ. The gap required between achievement expected for a person's IQ and his actual academic ability is usually fairly large. However, patients who are mildly mentally retarded can be learning disabled if their learning ability is significantly less than that expected for mildly retarded students. To make this diagnosis, a physician needs to assess IQ and academic achievement. Achievement tests measure the knowledge a person has acquired in limited areas (reading, writing, spelling, English, math, and so on). Since most schools do significant amounts of achievement testing, it is economical to obtain their test results. The norms on academic achievement tests widely used in public schools are such that as many as three fourths of children are above average on national norms. How a child or adult compares to the norms for the local school district is much more important clinically; these norms tend to be not nearly as inflated. They also define the level at which the patient is expected to perform. Elaborate diagnostic testing of academic abilities should be reserved for attempts at remediation or attempts to correlate academic difficulties with neuropsychological or neurological deficits.

Does My Patient Have Attention Deficits?

Many children and their parents are plagued with attention-deficit/hyperactivity disorder (ADHD). Many parents come to believe that they too have the disorder because the problems their children have are so similar to their memories of their own school experiences. The deficits of children with ADHD often persist into adulthood. To establish the presence of ADHD, the assessment of IQ is necessary. Attention deficit means at least that a patient's ability to attend is less than that expected for his IQ.

Multiple tests are available to measure attention and ADHD. This disorder has been approached psychometrically through tests assessing neglect in part of the visuospatial field, tests requiring continuous attention, and tests requiring selective attention. Other approaches have relied on parent questionnaires, teacher questionnaires, clinician checklists, self-report measures, and other similar evaluations. Research has shown relatively poor agreement among different approaches to problems with attention and concentration. It is generally accepted that the key to appropriate diagnosis of problems with attention and concentration is multimodal with multiple sources of information. Any single measure of attention is easily affected by transitory causes. The physician's goal is to establish that problems with attention exist relatively often in multiple settings under multiple conditions. If psychological assessment is to be used, it should be comprehensive and performed by an experienced practitioner with an interest in this area.

What Kind of Neurosis Does My Patient Have?

Objective tests to assess what used to be called *neurosis*—anxiety, depression, obsessive-compulsive disorder (OCD), phobias, panic disorder, and similar disorders—abound. Some widely used psychological tests still lump all these disorders together. Others split them into separate entities.

The most widely used clinical tests in psychology are the MMPI and the MMPI-2. They were developed from psychiatric interviews used in the United States before World War II. Items were constructed from the interview questions and tested on patient populations.

*A review of the diagnostic criteria established by the American Association on Mental Deficiency (AAMD) over the years is enlightening. At times, patients with IQs as high as 85 could be diagnosed as mentally retarded if their social functioning was sufficiently impaired. The current standard is an IQ of 75 or less. The criteria recommended by this association were accepted without revision in DSM-II, DSM-III, and DSM-III-R by the American Psychiatric Association. AAMD changed the criteria in 1992. DSM-IV accepts that change.

More than 10,000 different studies have been published with the MMPI and MMPI-2. Tested groups of larger than 10,000 participants from the general population exist to provide norms. As a result, a great deal is known about the test and its usefulness in many different populations when it is appropriately evaluated.

Initially the goal was to develop individual scales (for example, depression, schizophrenia, and mania) that could distinguish between patient groups and nonpatient groups. It quickly became clear that inspection of the scales one by one was not helpful. Psychiatric patients tended to score high on many scales. Specialists in the test moved to profile analysis, or looking at the pattern of scales (for example, determining the highest of the elevated scales).

This type of interpretation of the MMPI-2 is almost always based on *codetypes.* This term refers to the highest two or three scores on the standard 10 clinical scales of the MMPI-2 (1 equals hypochondriasis, 2 is depression, 3 is equal to hysteria, 4 relates to psychopathic deviance [antisocial personality], 5 corresponds to masculinity and femininity [interest patterns], 6 equals paranoia, 7 equals psychasthenia [anxiety disorders], 8 is schizophrenia, 9 corresponds to mania, and 0 is equal to social introversion or extroversion). If the highest two scores are psychopathic deviant (4) and mania (9), then the codetype is called *4-9.* Most computer interpretations of the MMPI-2 are based on these codetypes to a large degree. In no single codetype on the MMPI-2 do the majority of the patients who demonstrate it show a single diagnosis or group of diagnoses according to modern diagnostic criteria (DSM-III-R or DSM-IV).

The MMPI-2 can identify anxiety or depression quite well, although both are often present in the same patient. It can identify hypochondriasis and histrionic personality features (somatization disorder and hysteria) nicely.

If a physician wants to know how depressed or how anxious a patient is, the MMPI-2 is a poor choice. The depression or anxiety scales (such as those by Hamilton and Beck) are better. If a physician wants to know how many psychological problems a patient has, the MMPI-2 is excellent. It is important for physicians to recognize that at best the psychologist (or the computer) can only generate probabilistic statements based on a patient's answers to the MMPI-2. Again, we are dealing with hypotheses. If a patient has high scores on scales 2 (depression) and 7 (psychasthenia), there is a strong chance that he has a syndrome with anxiety or depression involved; it is never certain. It is often more interesting and more certain if the patient denies that a problem exists (no elevation on depression [2] or anxiety [7] equals euthymia).

Is My Patient Psychotic?

Psychological testing is not usually a reasonable way to answer this question. Test data takes time to analyze, and patients who are psychotic should not wait. However, if the patient can endure a session of testing, she is obviously less ill than many patients with psychosis. If testing is needed, a psychiatrist should order it after the situation has stabilized.

The MMPI was developed using a different system of nosology (current at the time of World War II) than that currently embodied in DSM-IV. The MMPI-2 standard scales reflect that older nosology. One example of this divergence can be shown by comparing the schizophrenia and depression scales. The MMPI-2 criterion group for schizophrenia was quite heterogenous. Therefore the content of the schizophrenia scale includes heterogenous content such as reported alienation from self and from others; perceived loss of control of thinking, emotions, and behavior; and reports of bizarre sensory experiences. This wide concept of schizophrenia is quite different than the much more narrow concept of schizophrenia reflected in the DSM-IV. On the other hand, the depression criteria group seemed to have rather severe endogenous depression with melancholic features. The DSM-IV concept of depression is broader. As a result, Ben-Porath, Butcher, and Graham showed that the MMPI-2 depression scale differentiates quite usefully between depressed and nondepressed psychiatric patients diagnosed by current criteria, but the MMPI-2 schizophrenia scale does not discriminate beyond the chance level between psychiatric patients who are schizophrenic and nonschizophrenic. Experienced users of the MMPI-2 allow for this. According to North et al., psychiatric patients with wide ranging problems (such as somatization disorder, borderline personality disorder, and dissociative identity disorder) tend to have their highest scores on the schizophrenia scale.

It is wise to assume that positive findings on the MMPI-2 represent possible clinical syndromes to be evaluated rather than anything stronger than that. If the test agrees with previous clinical findings, a physician's confidence in the findings increases. Using an objective personality test to screen for areas of concern other than the initial complaint is quite justifiable.

Some psychologists use projective techniques to diagnose schizophrenia or other psychoses. Projective techniques are tests that do not attempt to elicit structured answers (discussed on pp 41-43). The Exner criteria to identify schizophrenia on the Rorschach Inkblot Test are fairly reliable. The schizophrenia index depends to a considerable extent on verbalizations during the testing that are characteristic of thought disorder or disturbed thought content. The question is whether these kinds of tests are the best way to elicit this kind of material. The projective techniques are not sensitive or specific for diagnosing psychosis. Psychologists are usually better at identifying patients with schizophrenia than the tests are. Checklists (for the positive and negative symptoms of schizophrenia) are better than the more standard psychological assessment techniques.

Is My Patient Omitting, Exaggerating, or Embellishing? Validity Scales on Objective Tests

Objective personality tests usually have one almost indisputable advantage over clinical interviews and history taking. This is their quantified validity scales (for further discussion, consult Greene, 1988). These scales are designed to measure the patient's approach to taking the test. The standard validity scales on some tests look for carelessness, defensiveness, and exaggeration or malingering. Quantitative assessment of these variables has proved quite useful clinically. Carelessness has been measured by scales that look at the number of omitted or double marked (true and false) items, agreement on duplicate items scattered throughout a test, and logically paired items. Inconsistency associated with a bias to answer true or false has been assessed. Defensiveness indicates a patient's lack of willingness to disclose problems or faults. In some situations, this is intelligent (for example, during employment interviews), but when seeking treatment with a physician it may be harmful. Willingness to discuss problems tends to be a personality trait; that is, people tend to be somewhat consistent for a fairly long time across multiple situations. Again, exaggeration or malingering may reflect personality traits, special needs, or an attempt to manipulate the medical system to obtain nonmedical goals (such as drugs or money). Using a test with a good set of validity scales can confirm the suspicions of an astute physician, quantify reluctance, or bring a new problem to light.

Is My Patient with a Closed Head Injury Ready to Return to Work or School?

If a patient has a known neurological disorder, what can he do? What problems does he have? How is that likely to affect his social, educational, and occupational functioning? Research in these areas is currently somewhat limited, but the area is burgeoning. Testing also lends objectivity to recommendations about schooling, disability, and other social decisions.

Neuropsychological testing attempts to measure the patient's current level of fluid intelligence. The concern is with current ability to learn, remember, think abstractly, solve problems, draw, and complete other similar tasks. Neuropsychological tests are limited to those psychological tests that are recognized as sensitive to the integrity of the brain. Since the brain can do many different things, many different tests are generally needed. Screening for brain dysfunction with one test—usually a drawing test like the Bender-Gestalt—is not competent psychological practice. No conclusion can be reached other than what the test measures.

Neuropsychological tests differ in important ways from what a physician does in a neurological examination. The neurological examination uses simple tasks for the most part. Few options are available; the patient can do it, not do it, refuse to do it, or fake inability to do it. The interpretive possibilities are limited. Neuropsychological tests are generally quite complex. Multiple areas of the brain, clear sensory input channels, and clear motor output channels are required for successful performance on these tests. Performing sequential and complicated tasks using multiple brain areas is more like the demands of school or work than the neurological examination. If the patient is able to perform at the level expected for her IQ or education without undue fatigue, the answer is clear; the patient can function. Markedly impaired performance also leads to a clear recommendation. The neuropsychological examination in some cases, like any detailed examination by a specialist, picks up minor difficulties not previously noted. In that case, a partial return, a cognitive rehabilitation, or a delay may be indicated.

The most important decision a neuropsychologist makes is the estimation of how well the patient should be able to do on a test. The validity of all other conclusions depends on this conclusion. If a patient performs at an average level during neuropsychological testing, he is fine if he was average as a child. At the same level, he has overcome a handicap if a learning disability once caused him to perform poorly. At the same level, he has serious problems if he is a highly qualified medical specialist. To evaluate a neuropsychological opinion about a patient, a physician needs to understand how the estimate of premorbid ability was made and the effort that went into it. Some patients, of course, have preexisting problems that were undetected before an injury. The choice of tests is much less significant than the assumptions made about the expected level of performance.

Is My Elderly Patient Depressed or in the Early Stages of a Dementing Process?

A two-stage process can be recommended. The MMPI-2 can be a useful and inexpensive screening device when the differential diagnosis includes both depression and dementia. A patient who can complete

567* true and false items validly, presenting a typical profile for depression, has given a strong answer to the diagnostic question.

If the result of the MMPI-2 is not clear, then the physician can proceed with the evaluation. Neuropsychological testing has one advantage over the neurological examination in assessing how quickly a patient can do many different brain processes sequentially. This can be particularly useful when evaluating the early stages of progressive dementing illnesses. Tests that allow more precision in describing performance in the normal range are quite useful. Batteries for this purpose have been developed by Storandt et al., Benton et al., and many others. The logic is generally similar. A verbal comprehension test, a verbal fluency test, a construction task, a memory task, and an abstract-thinking task are used. Multiple brain areas are thus tested. The cut-off points are set so that poor performance in only one area is not sufficient to suggest dementia.

Psychological testing can be quite helpful in separating the cognitive impairment of depression (pseudodementia) from true dementia, because depressed patients are more depressed and less cognitively impaired than demented patients.

However, the ability of neuropsychological tests to identify most specific neurological problems independent of clinical history and other clinical tests is limited. An open-ended diagnostic question is not the best kind to pose to a psychologist. The diagnostic success of neuropsychologists depends in great part on the clinical information provided by physicians or information neuropsychologists obtain themselves. When the choices are sharply limited (depression vs. dementia), the probability of the correct diagnosis increases markedly. The diagnostic questions to neuropsychologists should be framed as carefully as the situation allows.

Special Problems to Avoid

A Lack of Definition of the Referral Question

Some physicians, uncomfortable with their lack of sophistication in testing, just order testing or a type of testing (such as projectives or psychometrics). With no clear direction or question, many psychologists perform their usual battery of tests. They then describe the patient in general terms and include some information not previously known to the physician. The relevance of the test results to the clinical decisions at hand will be marginal. The more precise the question, the more efficient, cheap, and helpful the testing will be.

Incomplete Assessment

The results of psychological tests should always become part of a comprehensive assessment. The clinical history and the examination of the patient should always control the interpretation of any psychological or other kind of test. All tests in medicine and psychology are subject to error and misinterpretation. A good physician always has to consider whether or not to believe the data. To be valid, data must fit the total picture, or the total picture must be reconsidered and reassessed. The user of a test must decide whether she knows enough about the test to use it knowledgeably and in the best interest of the patient. The physician needs to know how often a test makes mistakes, what kind of mistakes to expect, and what factors influence the error rate. It is equally important that the physician know enough about the patient to evaluate him knowledgeably in his best interest. Testing is not a substitute for the clinical interview and history; it is a supplement. One cannot separate the evaluation of the test from the evaluation of the patient.

The interpretation of a psychological test result is only a hypothesis to be considered in the context of all available information. This is particularly true of computerized test interpretations. Computer reports of standard personality tests usually contain 30 to 50 probability statements based on test answers and demographics. Assuming a 70% accuracy rate (a defensible assumption), 21 to 35 statements would be accurate and 9 to 15 would be inaccurate. The presence of a statement that really describes a patient based on one factor does not increase the likelihood that the next statement based on another factor is true. All test statements or hypotheses must be checked against the complete clinical picture.

Several professional associations (the American Counseling Association, the American Psychological Association, the American-Speech-Language-Hearing Association, and the National Association of School Psychologists) have generated standards for the responsible use of tests by their members. The first principle of competent use espoused by these psychologists, counselors, and speech pathologists is comprehensive assessment. Testing should always be integrated with all pertinent patient history and findings, according to these associations of testers. This must always be done by the physician and should usually be done by the psychologist as well.

Projective Personality Testing

Physicians who are not well versed in psychodynamic principles seldom, if ever, benefit from request-

*The MMPI-2 has one more item than the MMPI (with 566 items). One can tell which test it is in a second by looking at the answer sheet.

ing projective techniques. Psychologists usually enjoy interpreting projective test results. Projective techniques are those testing procedures that are relatively unstructured. The test is not attempting to elicit a specific answer or type of answer; there is no right or wrong answer. If someone asks what 2 plus 3 is, people agree that there is only one correct answer (in base 10). On the other hand, when a patient is shown a picture and asked to tell a story there is no clearly correct or incorrect answer. The patient brings his own history, abilities, traits, and penchants to the task. He projects himself into the material.

The best known projective technique is the Rorschach Inkblot Test developed by psychiatrist Hermann Rorschach in the hopes that it would help him study the disturbed perceptual processes of patients with schizophrenia. The Rorschach Inkblot Test has two phases. In the first phase, the patient is asked to identify what he sees on each of the cards. Initially, the patient is encouraged to make multiple responses to each card. After a few cards, the encouragement stops. After responses have been obtained for all of the cards, the examiner goes through the cards again with the patient to ascertain the location and basis for the patient's precept. The bases are called the determinants (that is, form, color, shading, texture, depth, and other aspects).

The responses and their determinants are coded. The current standard is the Exner system of coding. This system has supplanted the systems of Beck, Klopfer, Rappaport-Schafer, Hertz, and Piotrowski. It preempted the best and most reliable aspects of those older coding systems. The Exner system is now recognized, even by Ziskin and Faust, as the coding system of choice because it is both more comprehensive and much more reliable. Whereas the coding is not as reliable as that of objectively scored tests, it generally has quite good reliability.

The goal of the Exner Rorschach procedure, as it is generally used, is to describe the personality of the patient. The diagnosis of major psychiatric disorders (Axis I) or personality disorders (Axis II) is a less important goal. The results from the interpretation of a Rorschach Inkblot Test are of greatest interest to a psychodynamically oriented psychotherapist. In carefully selected patients, the Rorschach procedure can indicate the proper psychiatric diagnosis in a useful manner. However, if psychiatric diagnosis or patient management is the principal indication for psychological evaluation, the Rorschach Inkblot Test is both expensive and time consuming.

The other inkblot test is the Holtzmann Inkblot Test. This test allows only one response per card, but it uses more cards (40). As a result, it has significantly fewer psychometric problems than the Rorschach Inkblot Test. It has not attained significant popularity in the United States except in research; in 25 years of practice as a psychologist, I have never seen a report on a patient using the Holtzmann Inkblot Test.

The Thematic Apperception Test (TAT) is a widely used projective test. The patient is shown pictures on cardboard cards and asked to create a story using the scene in the picture as the middle of the story. The events leading to the scene and the outcome of the scene are left to the imagination of the patient. The test portrays interactions between parents and children, young and older adults, and men and women. A few pictures are bizarre in content. All could be described as somber. Unlike the Rorschach Inkblot Test, there is no generally accepted system for coding or scoring the responses. The test commonly provides interesting material for speculation about the ways in which the patient construes the world and interactions between people. Again, the information generated is of most use to a clinician contemplating extended psychotherapy.

A number of sentence-completion tests are available. These tests provide a sentence stem such as, "I like," which the patient completes with, "ice cream," "accomplishment," or "being left alone." Again, scoring or coding systems vary widely. The appeal of these tests is the amount of material they provide with little effort on the psychologist's part.

A number of procedures that involve drawing exist (such as the House-Tree-Person Test and the Draw A Person Test). These tests are not well standardized or well validated. They are easy to use. However, according to the studies of Cohen and Phelps, the scoring, coding, and interpretation are unreliable. Ratings by the same rater 3 months apart showed only a 70% agreement for criteria noted at either time. Interrater agreement averaged 42% in the most structured test. Furthermore, Cohen and Phelps (1985) reported, " these findings cannot be considered clinically significant. . . .The actual differences between the average number of markers for the two groups is too small to be detected without statistics." Sexually abused children averaged 1.28 of the 12 markers vs. 0.87 in the control group.

These techniques have been abused by untrained or poorly trained people working in the mental health field. Hagood (1992) comments appropriately, "At the present time, it has been consistently demonstrated that drawings alone cannot be used as evidence that sexual abuse has occurred." The diagnosis of childhood sexual abuse offered to a physician solely or primarily on the basis of projective tests, art therapy products, or sand play should lead the physician to suspect the person proffering the opinion is ignorant of the clinical and scientific literature, biased, or practicing out of his field of competence. An appeal to the person's experience in interpreting such material should confirm the suspicion. Rachel Klein, in particular, has questioned the usefulness of projective testing with children either for the purpose of describing personality or for clinical diagnosis. Klein (1987) states:

> In fact, there is very little evidence to document the belief that children's personality characteristics are well estimated by projective testing . . . . It is a grave error to make diagnostic or psychotherapeutic decisions on the basis of projective testing . . . . It is important to repeat that the very negative picture presented here pertains only to projective testing. There are other psychological testing procedures, such as tests of cognitive ability, that have great merit.

Cost of Testing

Some patient-answered scales and tests cost almost nothing because they can be scored in seconds by office personnel. Full-blown evaluations of personality or of neuropsychological functioning can cost a $1000.00 or more. The key to controlling cost is defining the testing request as sharply as possible and providing as much information as possible to the consulting psychologist.

Conclusion

A testing request always has a certain logic to it that should be as explicit as possible in the minds of both the referring physician and the psychologist receiving the referral. What is the clinical situation? What question will the testing answer? What are the relevant variables to be assessed (for example depression, memory, or something else)? Which test is the best measure of that variable? Was the patient able to cooperate as much as can be reasonably expected? Given the score on a test, how much confidence should the physician have in the result? What does the score suggest? How do these data fit into the whole clinical picture? Does it make sense? Should the physician believe it? Should he act on it? Going over a test result with a psychologist is just as appropriate as going over an x-ray with a radiologist.

Psychological testing can play a useful role in the practice of medicine. It can provide more careful assessment of significant features of the patient. Careful consideration of what information would be helpful in diagnosis, treatment, and monitoring of disease progress or disease response leads to the most efficient and profitable use of psychological testing or psychological consultation. Testing results should always be evaluated as part, and only part, of a comprehensive clinical evaluation.

CONSIDER CONSULTATION WHEN . . .

- The physician must decide whether clinical interview or physical examination is adequate for the decision to be made. If one of them is adequate, no testing is needed.
- The second decision the physician needs to make is whether the goal is the additional information provided by a test alone or the opinion of a psychologist along with the data. More testing is used directly by physicians (and their assistants) than by physicians consulting psychologists.

Annotated Bibliography

Greene, RL: *Assessment of malingering and defensiveness by objective personality inventories.* In Rogers R, editor: *Clinical assessment of malingering and deception,* New York, 1988, Guilford Press.

This is an excellent discussion of validity scales on a number of different objective personality tests.

Kline P: *Intelligence, the psychometric view,* New York, 1991, Routledge.

This book presents a careful argument about the nature of intelligence as revealed by factor analytic studies. It is not technical, and it can be readily understood by the nonexpert.

Kramer JJ, Conoley JC: *The eleventh mental measurements yearbook,* Lincoln, Neb., 1992, Buros Institute of Mental Measurements.

This is the latest in a series of books containing critical reviews of several hundred tests. It is the place to start looking up a test.

Spreen O, Straus E: *A compendium of neuropsychological tests; administration, norms and commentary,* New York, 1991, Oxford University Press.

This is an excellent source for reviewing neuropsychological tests. A new edition is scheduled in 1996.

Ziskin J, Faust D: *Coping with Psychiatric and psychological testimony,* ed 5, Los Angeles, 1995, Law and Psychology Press.

This is a biased, three-volume set of books that results from a careful search of the literature to cull out all negative evidence about psychological testing. If one wants to find out what is wrong with a test, this is an easy and good place to start. It offers little about the strengths of a test.

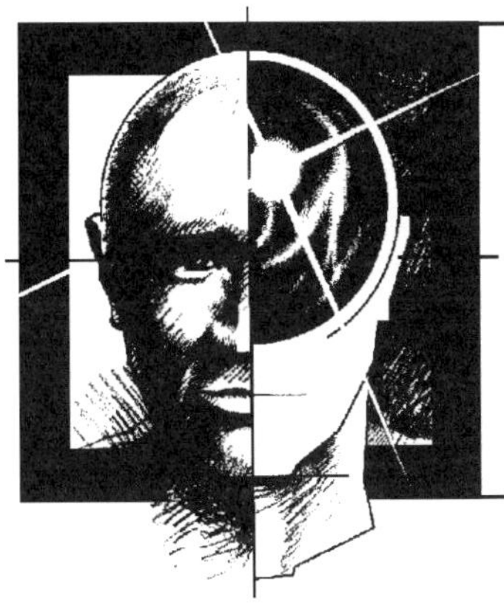

chapter 5

Clinical Rating Scales

Devna Rastogi-Cruz, MD and John G. Csernansky, MD

Rating Scales for Use in Particular Patient Groups
Rating Scales of General Psychopathology
Rating Scales for Drug Side Effects
Limitations of Using Clinical Rating Scales in Research
Clinical Rating Scales in Everyday Practice
Conclusion

In this chapter, the phrase *psychiatric rating scales* refers to standardized instruments used to quantify the symptoms and signs of psychopathology. Such scales facilitate the description of patients and their symptoms in terms that are replicable and easy to communicate (this definition does not include typical neuropsychological tests or instruments used to arrive at diagnoses; see Chapter 4 for further information in this area). Psychiatric rating scales can also provide quantitative data for sometimes difficult-to-grasp phenomena, and they are justly believed to be objective measures. There are three main types of rating scales: patient-rated, informant-rated, and professional-rated, which may also be called observer-rated. Although all of these scales are subject to certain biases, professional-rated scales are often felt to be the most objective.

All rating scales have certain advantages and disadvantages. Patient-rated scales render direct assessment of subjective internal states; however, the process of self-monitoring may have an effect on the target symptoms. These scales may also be more sensitive in identifying less severe pathological conditions. They require less professional time and are therefore less expensive. Disadvantages of patient-rated scales include difficulties completing the scales because of a patient's illiteracy, illness, unwillingness, or false answers. Completion of the patient-rated scales may also be problematic in cases where there are memory and attention problems.

Informant-rated scales, which can be completed by anyone who knows the patient well, have some of the same advantages and disadvantages as patient-rated scales. The main advantages include the ability to evaluate patients in their usual environments and distinguish between current symptoms and premorbid behavior. Such advantages may increase the sensitivity of these scales to recognize pathologic conditions. The shortcomings of informant-rated scales are similar to those of patient-rated scales and are related to biases of the rater.

Professional-rated scales can be done in different formats, including structured, semistructured, and unstructured interviews. Grebb, in his chapter titled *Psychiatric Rating Scales* in the 1989 edition of the *Comprehensive Textbook of Psychiatry,* has suggested that the more clinical judgment and inference are involved, the less reliable is the scale. Unstructured interviews may also allow different interviewing styles, experience, and theoretical beliefs to interfere with the reliability of assessment. Completely structured interviews that are standardized and involve specific ordering and wording of questions reduce variability and increase reliability. Grebb also noted that it is often the less experienced physicians who more reliably complete these scales, since they are more willing to follow instructions and defer their clinical judgment.

Psychiatric rating scales are used in clinical practice, in research, and for teaching. In clinical practice they can be used to document changes in symptoms during treatment. The practice of using such scales may become more prevalent as third-party payers require "hard" evidence of treatment benefits. The primary use of such scales is in research to characterize patient populations and to systematically evaluate the effects of experimental treatments. Therefore knowledge of commonly used psychiatric rating scales is needed to properly assess publications that report data derived from these scales. Another use of these scales is in teaching residents and students ways to evaluate particular groups of symptoms, anticipating that they may use these skills in clinical practice or research.

Psychiatric rating scales can evaluate symptoms selected *a priori* or the overall psychiatric picture. They can be used to assess internal states or observable behavior. Grebb, again, has stressed that for any rating scale, it is imperative that the time covered is specified and adhered to. It is also important that the answer scale is explicit. Clinical benchmarks to elucidate numerical scores are helpful in this regard. Rating scale scores may be either dichotomous (for example, absent or present and true or false) or continuous, where the rater has to describe frequency (never, rarely, occasionally, often, very often, always) or severity (absent, slight, mild, moderate, severe, extreme).

There are numerous psychiatric rating scales, and there are often many different types that can be used to evaluate the same symptoms or disorders. There is not a single best scale for each psychiatric disorder, so the first step in assessment is choosing the most appropriate scale. The choice of a rating scale should be based on its ability to accurately and reliably evaluate the specific symptoms and signs of the patient groups or disorder of interest and depends on whether the rater is the patient, an informant, or a professional. It is also important to consider why a rating scale is being used. Rating scales should be used to evaluate and monitor symptoms and signs; they should not be used for the purpose of establishing or supporting a diagnosis unless that is the intended purpose of the instrument.

It is beyond the scope of this chapter to discuss the merits and disadvantages of all psychiatric rating scales. Instead, the focus is to discuss the more widely used scales for use in particular patient groups and for assessing general psychopathologic states. In the interest of space, the scales themselves are not reproduced, but references are provided for all the scales discussed.

Rating Scales for Use in Particular Patient Groups

The Hamilton Rating Scale for Depression

The Hamilton Rating Scale for Depression (HAMD) is the most popular professional-rated scale that is used to evaluate the severity of depression and to demonstrate changes in such symptoms during treatment. The HAMD is not intended to be used as a diagnostic tool. The scale is completed based on an interview and considers observations of the patient and the patient's response to specific questions.

The classic HAMD consists of a 21-item list of symptoms that are evaluated on a severity rating of 0 to 4 or 0 to 2. Alternate 17- or 18-item versions (the last three or four items have been omitted) are also used. Guidelines are stated for each category to aid the rater in assigning a number to a symptom. For example, for agitation 0 corresponds to none; 1 equals fidgetiness; 2 is playing with hands, hair, etc.; 3 is moving about, can't sit still; and 4 equals hand wringing, nail biting, hair-pulling, and biting of lips. Hamilton advised that, if possible, two raters should administer the instrument. One rater should conduct the interview, and the second evaluator should ask supplementary questions. However, it is intended that they score the patient independently.

The HAMD has been commonly used for clinical and research purposes to quantify change in depressive symptoms and to evaluate the benefits of various treatments, including both antidepressant drugs, psychotherapy, and electroconvulsive therapy (ECT). Decreasing scores indicate improvement of symptoms. The HAMD has also been factor analyzed, with the result that two major factors were revealed—the vegetative factor (including sleep disturbance, loss of appetite, and similar symptoms) and the cognitive factor (with such symptoms as depressed mood and suicidal thoughts). These factors are compatible with current notions of the neurobiological dimensions of depression.

Beck Depression Inventory

The Beck Depression Inventory (BDI) is the most broadly used self-rating scale of depression, and like the HAMD it is the standard in its class. It was designed to measure the behavioral manifestations of depression based on the characteristic symptoms and attitudes of depressed patients in the literature. The original BDI, developed by Beck, Ward, Mendelson, Mock, and Erbaugh in 1961, contained 21 items that each consisted of graded responses ranging from 0 to 3 to indicate increasing symptom severity. Patients select the statement in each question that best describes their condition. In doing so, they have 84 statements to consider. The total score ranges from 0 to 63, and a particular score might indicate both the total number of symptoms present and the severity of symptoms. Six of the 21 items involve vegetative symptoms, and the rest refer to mood and cognitive symptoms.

Categories of symptoms covered by the BDI are mood, pessimism, sense of failure, lack of satisfaction, guilty feeling, sense of punishment, self-hate, self-accusations, self-punitive wishes, crying spells, irritability, social withdrawal, indecisiveness, body image, work inhibition, sleep disturbance, fatigability, loss of appetite, weight loss, somatic preoccupation, and loss of libido. This instrument is designed to measure varying degrees of depression along a continuum. It is not intended to distinguish among diagnostic categories, that is, the amotivation of schizophrenia or depression. However, if the BDI is used correctly to quantitate changes in the intensity of depression, it has been found to be internally consistent and stable and to have high degrees of reliability and validity.

Mania Rating Scales: The Beigel and Petterson Scales

The more widely used mania rating scales are all professional-rated scales, since using self-rating scales for a disorder characterized by uncooperativeness, poor judgment, distractibility, cognitive impairment, and denial of illness is not feasible. Self-rating scales may only be capable of differentiating hypomania from normality. Assessment of mixed states (both manic and depressive symptoms present simultaneously) necessitates using more than one scale. The different scales used to measure depression and mania have different emphases on cognitive, somatic, and behavioral aspects of the illness.

The Manic State Scale, developed by Beigel, was designed to be used by trained nursing staff and consists of 26 items that are rated from 0 to 5 to indicate intensity and frequency. The scale has been criticized for being too extensive to be serviceable, requiring too much time to finish, having some ambiguous items, and excluding some core features of mania, such as sleep changes.

The Petterson Scale is a shorter mania rating scale that consists of seven items and uses a five-point severity range. The behavior evaluated includes motor activity, pressure of speech, flight of ideas, noisiness, aggressiveness, orientation, and elevated mood. Because of the brevity of the scale, it can be readily used for even closely spaced serial ratings. The instrument also contains two global ratings that are also scored on a five-point scale and estimate the overall manic state and the overall change in the manic state since the previous rating. The Petterson Scale rates fewer symptoms than the Manic State Scale, but the items are more explicitly defined. It does not assess mixed states and does not address important aspects of mania, such as sleep and work disturbance.

Hamilton Anxiety Rating Scale

The Hamilton Anxiety Rating Scale (HAMA) is intended to assess the severity of anxiety symptoms and signs and to measure changes in anxiety in patients who have previously been diagnosed as having an anxiety disorder. It is a professional-rated scale that is recommended to be administered before treatment is started and periodically during treatment. The symptoms evaluated include anxious mood, tension, fear, insomnia, cognitive functioning, depressed mood, behavior at interview, somatic (sensory) symptoms, somatic (muscular) symptoms, cardiovascular symptoms, respiratory symptoms, gastrointestinal symptoms, genitourinary symptoms, and autonomic symptoms. The rating scale ranges from 0 to 4, with 0 equal to no symptoms and 4 corresponding to severe or grossly disabling symptoms.

The HAMA is used to evaluate a variety of anxiety symptoms. Besides the HAMA, there is no specific scale for generalized anxiety disorder (GAD). However, there are specific scales for phobias, panic disorder, posttraumatic stress disorder (PTSD), and obsessive-compulsive disorder (OCD). The only scale for a specific anxiety disorder discussed in this chapter is the Yale-Brown Obsessive Compulsive Scale (Y-BOCS).

Yale-Brown Obsessive Compulsive Scale

The Y-BOCS is a professional-rated scale that is designed to assess the severity of obsessive and compulsive symptoms, the cardinal manifestations of OCD. Again, it is not intended to be a diagnostic tool. The Y-BOCS has become the standard outcome measure in drug trials involving patients already diagnosed with OCD. Before administering the Y-BOCS for the first time, the rater should define the obsessions and compulsions to generate a Target Symptom List. The Y-BOCS contains a Symptom Checklist that has more than 70 examples of obsessions and compulsions to aid in the process of enumerating symptoms. Avoidance behaviors, which are often indicators of OCD symptoms, are also part of the Target Symptom List. Following completion of the Target Symptom List with the identification of avoidance behaviors, the interviewer uses the questions provided in the listed order to do the evaluation.

The main section of the Y-BOCS is a 10-item scale. Each item is rated from 0 (equal to no symptoms) to 4 (signifying extreme symptoms). The total range is from 0 to 40, but the subtotal of items 1 through 5 assesses the severity of obsessions and the subtotal of items 6 through 10 assesses compulsions. Symptoms are generally evaluated weekly, so the rating is based on the average occurrence of the symptom during the previous week. Both obsessions and compulsions are evaluated by how much they interfere with normal functioning, cause distress, take up the patient's time, are resisted by the patient, and can be controlled by the patient. The total Y-BOCS score is not directly affected by the type or number of obsessions or compulsions present. It is indicative of the total severity of the illness, which is based on the combination of the individual target symptoms and their effect on the patient. This characteristic enables the comparison of severity of illness in patients with different types of obsessions and compulsions. Another advantage of the scale is that it allows changes in obsessions and compulsions with treatment response to be evaluated separately.

The Y-BOCS is reliable, valid, and sensitive for use in assessing the severity of symptoms in patients diagnosed with OCD and is therefore useful for medication trials both in clinical and research settings. Decreases of 35% in the total Y-BOCS scores from the baseline are usually selected to signify clinically significant improvement. The indication for using Y-BOCS as an outcome measure in behavioral treatment studies has not been fully evaluated, but it is probably also suitable for these studies. The feasibility of using the Y-BOCS to evaluate OCD-related disorders, such as the repetitive pulling out of one's own hair (trichotillomania), is unclear. A computer-administered version of the Y-BOCS has been developed. A children's version, the CY-BOCS, is another modification of the Y-BOCS. The CY-BOCS resembles the Y-BOCS except for the use of easier language and the addition of those symptoms found more often in children to the CY-BOCS Symptom Checklist (for example, bedtime rituals). The CY-BOCS is also a reliable, valid, and sensitive instrument that is useful for drug-treatment studies.

SAPS and the SANS in Schizophrenia

The Scale for Assessment of Positive Symptoms (SAPS) and the Scale for Assessment of Negative Symptoms (SANS) provide standardized definitions and measurements of the positive and negative symptoms of schizophrenia, respectively. The positive symptoms of schizophrenia include hallucinations and delusions. The negative symptoms of schizophrenia include flat affect and the lack of volition. Recently, experts have suggested that illogicality of thinking, which is also characteristic of the disease, probably represents a third and separate dimension of the illness. Presently, different forms of this symptom are represented in both of the scales.

Neither the SAPS nor the SANS is intended as a diagnostic device. Their primary use has been in studies of the neurobiological correlates of symptom groupings. They are increasingly being used in drug treatment studies. The SAPS contains 34 items divided into four *a priori* subscales: hallucinations, delusions, bizarre behavior, and formal thought disorder (that is, loose associations among thoughts). The SANS comprises 25 items divided into five *a priori* subscales: affective flattening or blunting, alogia (paucity of apparent thinking and thought content), apathy, asociality, and inattention. Each item is scored from 0 (signifying no symptoms) to 5 (corresponding to severe impairment). Each category contains a global rating for that symptom group. The global ratings are also on the same five-point scale, and the addition of these scores from the global ratings of each category can comprise a total score for the SAPS and SANS. The possible range of total scores on the SAPS is 0 to 20, and on the SANS it is 0 to 25.

The Mini-Mental State Examination

The Mini-Mental State Examination (MMSE) is the most popular mental status screening examination in terms of how well it is known and how widely it is used. It is a quantitative assessment of the cognitive functioning and capacity of a patient. The MMSE assesses orientation, memory (registration and recall), attention, calculation, language (naming, repetition, ability to follow complicated commands, reading, and writing), and constructional ability. The instrument consists of 11 questions and takes only 5 to 10 minutes to administer. Therefore it can be used serially and routinely. It has been found to validly and reliably evaluate cognitive processes and distinguish patients with and without cognitive disturbances. It is reasonably sensitive to changes in the cognitive state.

As with the other scales discussed in this chapter, the MMSE should not be used diagnostically because it cannot determine the cause of the cognitive difficulties. Additionally, it may be insensitive to cognitive problems where the severity of the symptoms is slight (as in schizophrenia). There are different disorders in which cognitive impairments are present, and there are many other reasons for a low MMSE score besides delirium and dementia. These reasons include sensory deprivations such as blindness, deafness, mutism, aphasia or other language barriers, mental retardation or an educational level less than the eighth grade, or uncooperativeness. These reasons should always be taken into consideration when administering the MMSE, and patients should have their usual sensory aids such as glasses and hearing aids available during testing. The test is not timed, and the maximum total score is 30. Different scores indicate different levels of impairment. Mungas has proposed that a score of 25 to 30 indicates intact function or questionable impairment; 20 to 25 signifies mild impairment; 10 to 20 points to moderate impairment; and 0 to 10 implies severe cognitive impairment.

Rating Scales of General Psychopathology

The Brief Psychiatric Rating Scale

The Brief Psychiatric Rating Scale (BPRS), developed in the 1960s by John Overall, remains among the most widely used clinical rating scales in the world. It was originally intended for use in controlled clinical trials of new psychotropic drugs. However, it has also been widely employed in studies of the clinical (that is, symptom) correlates of cognitive and neurobiological phenomena. Eighteen individual items are rated by the physician on the basis of a semistructured interview, each describing a fundamentally different element of psychopathology. Each item is scored on a seven-point scale (from 0 to 6 or from 1 to 7 depending on the particular version being used).

The BPRS is somewhat unusual among rating scales in that it was first developed by polling experts in the testing of psychotropic drugs. They were asked what aspects of psychopathology, to be listed on a scale as items, were most characteristic of the major psychiatric syndromes (such as major depressive disorder [MDD], schizophrenia, and mania) and most likely to change in response to treatment with a psychotropic drug. After eliminating obvious redundancies, a prototype of the BPRS was used to rate large numbers of patients with diverse psychiatric disorders and then submitted to factor analysis to identify additional redundancies among the remaining items. In this way the final version of the BPRS was produced with a minimum number of items (18) that show little redundancy. The BPRS can be further factor-analyzed into five factors (hostility-suspiciousness, withdrawal-retardation, thinking disturbance, depression-anxiety, and activation). These factor scores, as well as the total score, are often used to evaluate changes in specific symptom groupings during treatment.

The Present State Examination

The Present State Examination (PSE), developed by John Wing, was developed in England for characterizing and classifying psychiatric disorders. Although it is popular in Europe, it is not widely used in the United States. Like the BPRS, it was not developed to rate the symptoms of any particular disorder. The items are rated by a physician who is conducting a semistructured interview and using clinical judgment to guide the use of specific questions. The instructions for the PSE indicate that the period to be assessed is 1 month. The PSE is most widely used to classify patients into likely syndromal groupings. It has also been used to characterize the response of patients to new psychotropic drugs.

The Clinical Global Impression Scale

The Clinical Global Impression Scale (CGI) is composed of three general items and is almost always used in the evaluation of new psychotropic drugs. The first item asks the rater to score the patient on a six-point scale according to the severity of illness in this patient compared with the physician's total prior experience with this type of client. Descriptors for the six items are as follows: 1 equals normal, not at all ill; 2 signifies that the patient is borderline mentally ill; 3 corresponds to the patient who is mildly ill; 4 signifies moderately ill; 5 equals markedly ill; 6 corresponds to severely ill; and 7 indicates that the patient is among the most extremely ill patients. The second item asks the rater to score the patient on a six-point scale to describe the degree of change since the last rating. For the second item, the descriptors vary from very much improved (a rate of 1) to very much worse (rated 7). The third item cross tabulates the degree of improvement with the global severity of side effects. In this way, the total utility of the drug treatment can be assessed.

During a clinical drug trial, patients may improve in ways difficult to detect using the scales of psychopathology chosen for the study. This may occur because the drug has unanticipated benefits for the patients and the scales required to assess them were not selected ahead of time, or because the changes in the patients' conditions cannot be recorded on any existing scales. At such times, the CGI can be invaluable and ultimately lead to the refinement and improvement of other clinical rating scales.

Nursing Observation of Inpatient Behavior

The Nursing Observation of Inpatient Behavior (NOSIE) was developed for nurses so their observations about the behavior of inpatients in clinical trials or other neurobiological studies of psychiatric illness could be recorded. Although it was originally intended for the assessment of patients with schizophrenia, it has been used for rating other types of patients as well. The NOSIE measures a variety of individual and social-interactive behaviors, as well as the severity of particular symptoms. It can be highly useful for recording the psychopathologic conditions of patients who cannot always articulate their own symptoms or whose behavior is rapidly changing.

Rating Scales for Drug Side Effects

Rating scales are available for a variety of specific drug side effects. In particular, there are scales for the neurological side effects of antipsychotic drugs, such as pseudoparkinsonism (the Neurological Rating Scale), akathisia (the Barnes Akathisia Scale), and tardive dyskinesia (the Abnormal Involuntary Movement Scale [AIMS]). These scales can divide the symptoms of a complex side-effects syndrome such as pseudoparkinsonism into components (for example, tremor and gait disturbance), or they can divide the assessment across the areas of the body, as does the AIMS. Global scores are usually also rated.

In addition to side-effect rating scales for known and defined syndromes, there are side-effect scales designed to rate common complaints (such as sedation and dizziness), regardless of the type of psychotropic drug being tested. The most common scales in this category are the Treatment Emergent Symptom Scale (TESS) and the Systematic Assessment for Treatment Emergent Events (SAFTEE). In both cases, the physician explicitly inquires about a long list of potential side effects. Another approach to eliciting side-effect complaints is for the physician to ask a nonspecific question, such as, "Have you noticed any unusual or troublesome sensations?" The latter approach is more likely to highlight serious (and unexpected) side effects, although many problems, such as complaints of sexual dysfunction, are notoriously underreported.

Limitations of Using Clinical Rating Scales in Research

Changes in the scores of particular rating scales, even those developed to rate the symptoms of a particular psychiatric disorder, do not always truly reflect a change in the severity of the target syndrome. This can occur because different clinical syndromes can overlap empirically. For example, many symptoms in patients with mood disorders and anxiety disorders are similar and nonspecific. Sleep disturbance in particular, although a specific symptom of depression, is also found in a variety of anxiety disorders and can be improved by any sedative drug. Therefore any sedative would appear to have anti-depressant effects if a change in this item were improperly interpreted.

PEARLS & PERILS

RATING SCALE GUIDELINES

- Nonspecific side effects of drugs (such as sedation) can affect the scoring of specific items on rating scales.
- Symptoms of specific psychiatric disorders can overlap.
- Statistically significant changes in rating scale scores may not be clinically significant.
- Rating scales can be used in everyday practice to record patterns of symptoms for review in the future.

As another example, aspects of depression and the negative symptoms of schizophrenia also overlap. In patients who have schizophrenia and no major mood disorder, assessments of decreased work, activities, and energy level can appear increased on scales used to assess either depression or negative symptoms. To avoid the interpretation of nonspecific drug effects as specific improvements for the intended disorder, overlaps among such clinical syndromes should be kept in mind when evaluating the results of clinical trials.

Another caveat that must be kept in mind when evaluating clinical rating scale data is that a statistically significant change in the scale score does not always indicate a clinically significant change (see the Pearls & Perils box above). In studies where the sample size is large, a statistically significant change may only represent a difference of 10% to 15% in the severity of the targeted group of symptoms. Whereas such changes may be important in the design of future drugs and future clinical trials, most physicians would be unimpressed. Additionally, physicians must keep in mind that in studies where the sample size is small, the measurement of change is unreliable, even when a reliable scale is used to assess it. This problem can often be encountered when reading small, uncontrolled, and unblinded trials or series of case reports.

Clinical Rating Scales in Everyday Practice

It is important for physicians to be familiar with clinical rating scales so they can properly interpret the clinical trial reports of new psychotropic drugs. However, physicians should also be familiar with these scales because they are useful in everyday practice. Often the physician may have difficulty grasping the most important symptoms of a patient and determining whether a drug treatment has worked. In this situation, the use of a clinical rating scale may clarify the most prominent symptoms of the patient and the degree to which they have changed during treatment. Additionally, patients themselves may find it difficult to articulate their symptoms without the benefit of being asked specific questions. When asking specific questions, it is difficult to find more appropriate ones than those recorded on a widely used scale. Reviewing such a list before and after treatment may offer the patient insight into the degree of her improvement.

Finally, anyone who has reviewed medical records searching for a record of a patient's prior response to treatment appreciates that in many records there are few specific or usable statements. A series of rating scales documenting the type and degree of the patient's response to a series of treatment interventions can become an invaluable record for review by the original physician or by others at a later date.

Conclusion

Clinical rating scales are widely used in epidemiological and neurobiological research to describe the characteristics of patients with psychiatric disorders and to record responses to treatment. Rating scales are available for specific psychiatric syndromes and treatments, and for global evaluations as well. Care should be exercised in the selection of rating scales so the goals of the study can be best achieved. Clinical rating scales can also be used in everyday practice to help the physician and patient articulate the most prominent symptoms of the patient and to make a record for the future.

Annotated Bibliography

Prien RF, Robinson, editors: *Clinical evaluation of psychotropic drugs,* New York, 1994, Raven Press.

This book contains an exhaustive review of information related to the design and implementation of clinical drug trials, including the selection and use of clinical rating scales.

Guy W: *NCDEU Assessment manual for psychopharmacology,* U.S. Department of Health, Education, and Welfare Publication (ADM)-76-338, Rockville, Md., 1976, Alcohol, Drug Abuse, and Mental Health Administration.

This manual contains example versions of a large number of the most commonly used clinical rating scales. The manual also contains reviews of reliability data for those scales available at the time.

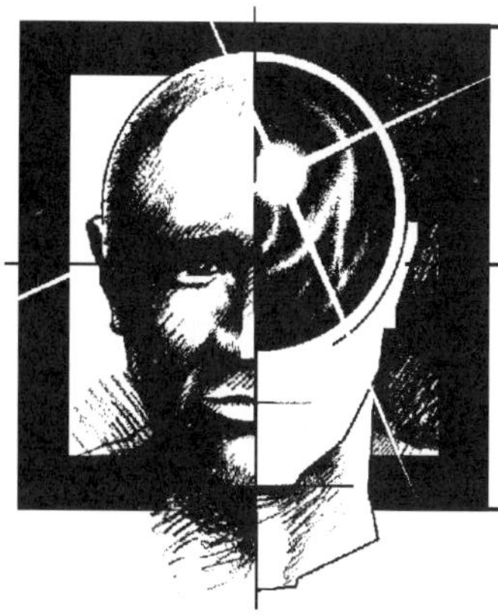

chapter 6

Neuroimaging in Psychiatry

Wayne C. Drevets, MD and Kelly Botteron, MD

Current Applications of Neuroimaging in Psychiatry

The application of modern neuroimaging technology in investigations of psychopathology holds the potential to transport psychiatry into an era in which pathophysiology, rather than signs and symptoms, guides the nosology of psychiatric disease. A variety of imaging techniques affords unprecedented opportunities to noninvasively examine brain structure and function, permitting elucidation of the neuroanatomical correlates of psychiatric disorders and of the emotional and cognitive processes disturbed in such disorders. Additionally, the trajectory of technology development in nuclear magnetic resonance spectroscopy (MRS) and ligand development for neuroreceptor imaging indicate that these neuroimaging techniques will provide increasingly powerful means of assessing the brain's chemistry, as well as its anatomy and physiology.

To date, the greatest utility of neuroimaging in psychiatry is found in its research applications, since its capabilities for determining diagnosis and guiding treatment decisions have not yet been established. Therefore this chapter emphasizes principles that are relevant to interpreting imaging research findings. Some of the consistently replicated findings in the literature are reviewed, and methodological issues germane to the resolution of apparent discrepancies across studies are discussed.

Neuroimaging Research

Neuroimaging encompasses techniques for mapping both the structure and the function of the brain. Structural imaging evaluates morphology and elements of tissue composition using magnetic resonance imaging (MRI) or computed tomography (CT). These techniques have revolutionized clinical diagnostic evaluation by affording the ability to noninvasively visualize gross neuropathological conditions in vivo, facilitating differential diagnosis in cases where psychiatric signs and syndromes may constitute manifestations of lesions or degenerative processes. Moreover, whereas in the primary psychiatric disorders qualitative inspection of MRI or CT images reveals gross pathological structures in only a minority of cases, research using quantitative neuromorphometric methods (that is, methods that quantify the size of cerebral structures) has provided compelling evidence that subtle differences in the size of cerebral structures exist between people who are psychiatrically ill and control subjects. Such studies have dispelled the notion that the major psychiatric disorders are purely functional in nature and are expected to guide postmortem histopathological analyses toward elucidation of the degenerative or neurodevelopmental processes underlying such disorders.

Functional imaging techniques permit noninvasive assessments of neurophysiology or neuroreceptor function. Compared with techniques involving lesion effects, electrical stimulation and recording, postmortem neuroreceptor assessment, cerebrospinal fluid (CSF) chemistry, or neuropsychological test performance, functional imaging affords superior spatial resolution and the ability to simultaneously measure the function of multiple brain structures in vivo. Functional imaging has generally involved either nontomographic multidetector systems or tomographic systems (which provide three-dimensional information) such as single photon emission computed tomography (SPECT) and positron emission tomography (PET). These cameras detect radiation emitted from the decay of radionuclides that are administered by inhalation or intravenous infusion. The most rapidly expanding area of imaging development involves functional MRI (fMRI), which detects nuclear magnetic resonance signals related to blood flow or metabolism that are not dependent on the administration of radiolabeled tracers.

Finally, one of the most promising areas for PET and SPECT imaging involves the quantification of neuroreceptor density and affinity. Ligands have been developed that permit imaging of dopamine, benzodiazepine, opiate, serotonin, and acetylcholine receptors. Complex receptor modeling problems are still being solved for most of these ligands.

Clinical Applications of Neuroimaging

The clinical utility of neuroimaging in psychiatry is currently confined to differential diagnosis, where it is used to rule out coarse brain diseases that present with psychiatric signs or symptoms (see Chapter 26). The most useful technology in this regard is neuromorphological MRI, which can sensitively detect areas of infarction or atrophy, tumors, or white matter lesions. Cases where anatomical MRI is generally indicated as part of the clinical evaluation include new onset of psychosis, new onset of mania after age 40, or new onset of psychiatric syndromes in patients with focal neurological deficits, seizures, cognitive impairment, or suspected metastatic disease.

In rare cases functional imaging has also been used in differential diagnosis. Examples have included cases in which PET was used to distinguish schizophrenia or mania from psychotic behavior associated with seizures because the electroencephalogram (EEG) was equivocal. However, functional brain imaging has generally not yet proven clinically useful in psychiatry. Although abnormalities in regional blood flow and metabolism have been consistently reported in carefully selected subgroups with psychiatric disorders, few studies have assessed the diagnostic sensitivity and specificity of such findings. This is partly because the magnitude of resting differences between psychiatric and control samples has been relatively low (between about 2% and 20%) and the variability of such measures has been high enough that the respective distributions of patient and control values overlap. Thus far, functional imaging abnormalities have not been shown to be detectable in most true positive cases and absent in most true negative cases (in other words, normative cases and cases with other psychiatric or neurological illnesses). Finally, repeated scanning of large numbers of subjects has not been performed to evaluate test-retest variability; duration of confounding medication effects; or the effects of nonspecific factors such as sleep deprivation, timing within the menstrual cycle, or caffeine and nicotine exposure.

In contrast to the relatively subtle resting blood flow and metabolic abnormalities identified in patients with psychiatric disorders, imaging techniques that quantify neuroreceptor binding or assess neurophysiological responses to pharmacological challenges may ultimately prove sufficiently robust to distinguish healthy and ill cases. For example, one study reported that in 9 of 10 subjects scanned in various phases of bipolar disorder, dopamine D_1-receptor affinity fell outside the distribution of control values. Another preliminary study found dramatic differences between five subjects with major depressive disorder (MDD) and six control subjects in the cerebral metabolic response to the serotonin releasing agent fenfluramine. Although such findings await replication in larger samples and assessments of specificity, they suggest that differences of the magnitude needed to differentiate target and normative populations may be achievable with functional imaging techniques.

Overview of Structural Imaging Technology

Computed Tomography

The development and application of x-ray CT afforded the first capabilities for in vivo examination of soft tissues such as the brain. In 1979 Cormack and Hounsfield described the analytical technique of projection reconstruction imaging, which enabled the development of CT and the other tomographic imaging techniques, MRI, PET, and SPECT. Although these technologies differ in the origin of the signals they detect, they share in common the reconstruction of two-dimensional views of a tissue slice from a set of one-dimensional projections taken at multiple angles. CT is based on delineation of the differential attenuation of x-rays by distinct tissue types.

The CT scanner consists of a rotating x-ray beam surrounded by a ring of x-ray detectors. Images are acquired slice by slice as the x-ray tube and detectors rotate 360° around the head. CT creates axial images of the brain parenchyma with a spatial resolution of 1 to 2 mm and is capable of identifying central nervous system (CNS) lesions such as tumors, infarction, and ventricular enlargement. Additionally, intravenously injected contrast agents may be administered during CT imaging to highlight areas of blood-brain barrier breakdown. CT is the preferred imaging modality when bony disease or lesions involving calcified tissue are suspected. However, CT is also susceptible to artifacts near bony surfaces that obscure visualization of the brain stem, the basotemporal cortex, and the posterior fossa (see the Pearls & Perils box below). Other disadvantages of CT relative to MRI include its low contrast resolution between gray and white matter, the risks associated with exposure to ionizing radiation, and the inability to acquire image slices in coronal or sagittal orientations.

PEARLS & PERILS

COMPUTED TOMOGRAPHY

- CT scans can identify gross neuropathological lesions such as structural malformations, ventricular enlargement, infarction, hemorrhage, and tumor.
- CT involves exposure to ionizing radiation.
- The intravenous contrast agents sometimes used in CT techniques may produce serious allergic reactions.
- CT is preferred over MRI for visualizing bony abnormalities.
- CT has poor gray-white matter contrast resolution, and some brain structures are poorly visualized with CT because of bony artifacts.

Magnetic Resonance Imaging

Of the in vivo brain imaging techniques, nuclear MRI provides the highest spatial and contrast resolution for neuroanatomical structures. MR images are generated using the inherent magnetic properties of atoms, which are amplified and enhanced for detection and visualization (Figures 6-1 and 6-2). The most common nucleus targeted for clinical MRI is hydrogen because of its abundant distribution in living tissue. Other nuclei such as phosphorus-31, carbon-13, sodium-23, and potassium-39 can also be imaged using nuclear MRS.

Tissues with different hydrogen concentrations and tissue relaxation parameters produce distinct resonance signals that underlie the characteristic appearances of CSF, gray matter, and white matter in MR images (Table 6-1). Moreover, alterations in the acquisition sequences can enhance the ability to examine particular types of tissue pathology. For example, T2-weighted images are more useful than T1-weighted images for examining white-matter pathological findings (see the legend for Figure 6-2).

MR images can be acquired in any plane of orientation. Standard clinical films generally consist of T1-weighted axial or coronal images and T2-weighted axial images. Whereas early techniques acquired MR images two-dimensionally, newer methods acquire data three-dimensionally, permitting visualization in any orientation desired. Examples of such acquisitions include fast low-angle shots (FLASH), gradient recalled

PEARLS & PERILS

MAGNETIC RESONANCE IMAGING

- MRI acquires images that can be visualized in any orientation.
- MRI is not susceptible to the bony artifacts associated with CT imaging, permitting visualization of the entire cerebrum, posterior fossa, and brain stem.
- MRI does not involve exposure to ionizing radiation.
- Compared with CT, MRI affords higher contrast between gray and white matter, superior delineation of white matter lesions, and greater spatial resolution (that is, small structures are better visualized).
- Image acquisition can be accomplished in fewer than 20 minutes.
- Subjects may develop claustrophobic anxiety in MR scanners that have a narrow cylindrical aperture.
- MR images are sensitive to motion artifacts, so patients who are unable to remain motionless may require sedation.

TABLE 6-1

TISSUE APPEARANCE OF MAGNETIC RESONANCE IMAGES

	T1-weighted	T2-weighted
Gray matter	Dark gray	Light gray
White matter	Light gray	Dark gray
CSF	Black	White
Inflammation/ demyelination	Darker	Brighter
Infarction	Darker	Brighter
Edema	Darker	Brighter
Solid tumor	Darker	Brighter
Hemorrhage (chronic)	Brighter rim	Brighter

acquisition in the steady state (GRASS), and magnetization prepared rapid gradient echo (MPRAGE).

MRI does not involve exposure to ionizing radiation and has no significant known biological risks at the magnetic field strengths currently employed for clinical use. Other advantages of MRI over CT include its higher spatial resolution (about 0.5 mm for newer scanners), superior gray-white matter contrast, ability to acquire images in any orientation, superior depiction of white matter pathologic findings, greater flexibility of image acquisition parameters to vary tissue contrast, and improved accuracy for volumetric measurements (see the Pearls & Perils box on p. 55). The disadvantages of anatomical MRI include its expense and sensitivity to motion artifacts. The known risks associated with MRI relate to the potential of the magnetic field to dislodge metallic objects (such as metal

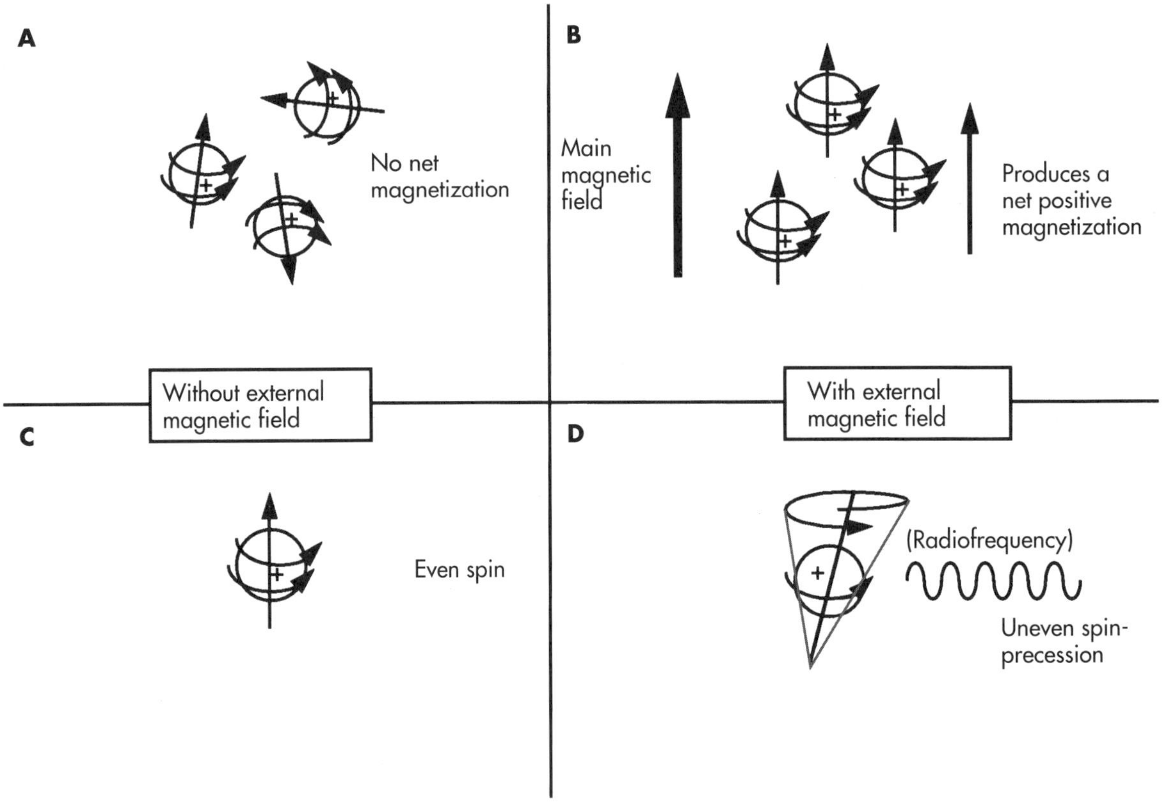

FIGURE 6-1 Physical principles of MRI. **A,** The atomic nuclei of elements that have an odd number of electrons or protons behave as spinning charged particles that create magnetic dipoles. In the natural state, these dipoles are randomly oriented so no net magnetization of tissue exists. **B,** When tissue is placed in the magnetic field of an MR scanner, these nuclei align parallel to the field and produce a net positive magnetization. In the natural state, such nuclei spin evenly **(C),** but within the magnetic field, the spinning nuclei wobble around the longitudinal axis of the field, precessing like a child's spinning top **(D).** The precession of molecules releases energy in the form of radio frequency pulses that are detected by the MR scanner. Each nuclear species has a characteristic precessional frequency known as its Larmor frequency. (Modified from Parmelee DX: *Child and adolescent psychiatry,* St. Louis, 1996, Mosby.)

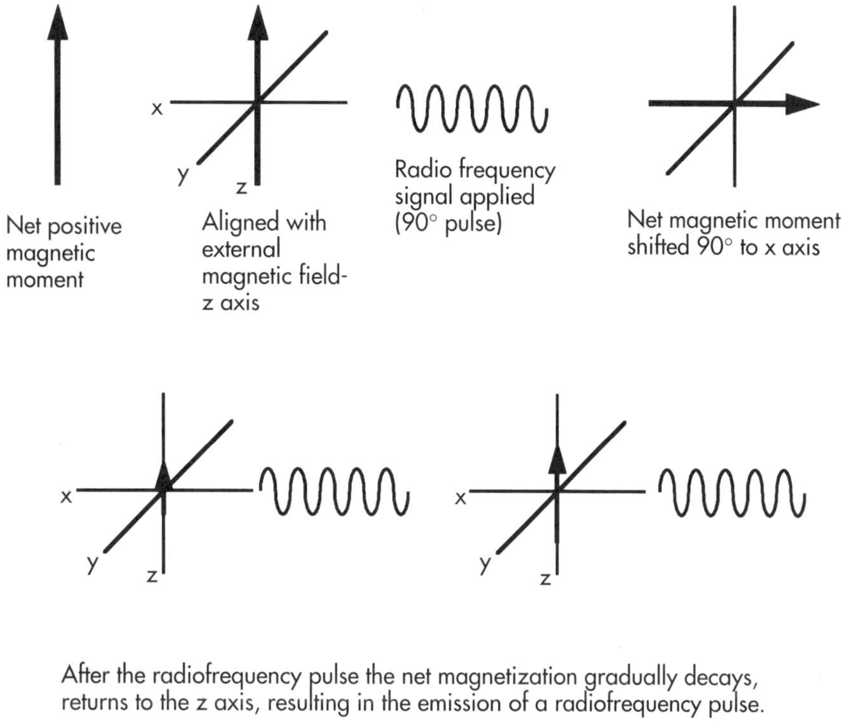

FIGURE 6-2 Continuing from Figure 6-1, to generate the MR image from nuclei precessing within the magnetic field, the nuclei are further excited by the application of a second magnetic field imposed by an external radio frequency pulse, which shifts the nuclei and net magnetization out of the plane parallel to the magnetic field (generally 90° perpendicular to the plane of magnetization). When the radio frequency pulse is removed, the nuclei return to their original planes within the magnetic field; this is known as the relaxation phase. Radio frequencies emitted during relaxation are detected by the receiver antenna and mathematically described by Fourier transformation to construct the MR image. Different relaxation parameters can be measured to alter the image appearance (see Table 6-1). In clinical medicine, T1 and T2 signal images are most commonly obtained; they refer to spin-lattice relaxation and spin-spin relaxation, respectively. T1-weighted images reflect the time taken by the nuclei to relax to their prior magnetized state, and they provide the best contrast between gray matter and white matter (CSF appears dark in such images). T2-weighted images reflect the dephasing of the nuclei during relaxation, and they generally provide the clearest delineation of lesions (CSF appears white in such images). (Modified from Parmelee DX: *Child and adolescent psychiatry,* St. Louis, 1996, Mosby.)

intracranial or aneurysmal surgical clips or intraocular metallic objects) and interfere with the operation of electrically or magnetically activated devices (for example, cardiac pacemakers and cochlear implants).

Overview of Functional Imaging Technology

Nontomographic Methods for Imaging Regional Blood Flow

Nontomographic methods used to measure regional blood flow in humans rely on the principles of inert gas exchange. After inhalation of air containing xenon-133, the gamma rays emitted during ^{133}Xe decay are counted by crystal multidetector systems placed over the scalp. Flow is quantitated by the rate at which the tracer clears from tissue rather than by the amount of tracer present. Since ^{133}Xe decays by emission of relatively low energy radiation (88 keV, compared with 511 keV for the annihilation photon emitted during ^{15}O decay; see the following section), detector sensitivity declines rapidly as tissue depth increases, and the recorded activity originates almost entirely from brain surfaces lying within 2 cm of the detector face. For this and other technical reasons, nontomographic methods employing ^{133}Xe measure blood flow exclusively from the cortical gray matter lying near the scalp. This is a major limitation in psychiatric studies, since measures cannot be obtained from the deep cortical (such as the ventral and medial portions of the frontal and temporal lobes), limbic, and basal ganglia structures that appear to participate in emotional processing, psychosis, and psychomotor activity.

Positron Emission Tomography

The PET camera images the annihilation radiation generated as positrons are absorbed in matter, recording highly accurate spatial representations of the distribution of a radionuclide that has been inhaled or infused (Figure 6-3). The PET image is effectively equivalent to a quantitative tissue radiogram in laboratory animals, but it affords the advantage of being noninvasive, permitting imaging in humans. The various positron-emitting radiopharmaceuticals available provide capabilities for imaging blood flow, blood volume, glucose or oxygen metabolism, neuroreceptor binding, or water extraction across the blood-brain barrier. Radioisotopes that decay by positron emission (and their respective half-lives) include ^{15}O (122 seconds), ^{13}N (10 minutes), ^{11}C (20 minutes), and ^{18}F (110 minutes).

The spatial resolution of PET is defined as the width of distribution of radioactivity at one half of the maximum counting rate for a point source, called *full-width at half-maximum* (FWHM). Although point sources smaller than one FWHM may be detected, two point sources of radioactivity cannot be discriminated from one another if they are separated by less than one FWHM. Newer PET systems have intrinsic resolutions of 5 mm FWHM. However, in most studies images are blurred with filters to reduce the statistical noise of the images, so data analysis is performed at resolutions of 10 to 20 mm FWHM. The ultimate resolution of PET has not been established, but it is limited by factors such as the 1 to 6 mm distance the positron travels in tissue before annihilation (see Figure 6-3).

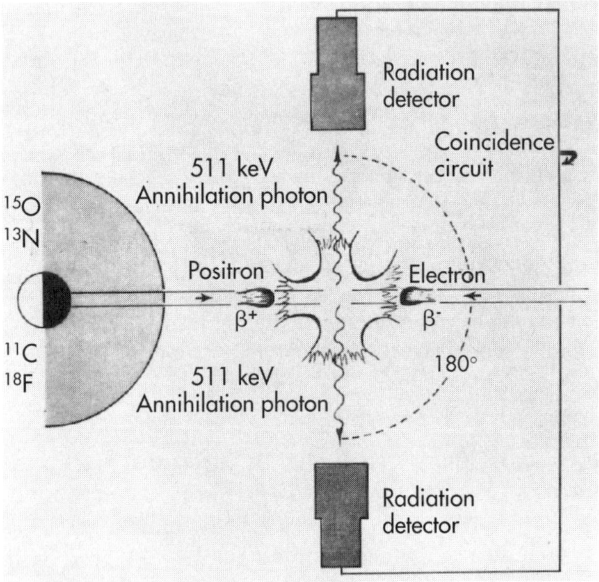

FIGURE 6-3 Detection scheme for PET. Radionuclides employed in PET decay by emission of positrons from a nucleus that is unstable because of a deficiency of neutrons. Positrons lose their kinetic energy in matter after traveling a finite distance (1 to 6 mm); when they are brought to rest they interact with electrons. The two particles are annihilated, and their mass is converted to two annihilation photons traveling at ~180° from each other with an energy of 511 keV. Annihilation photons are detected by the imaging device, using opposing radiation detectors connected by electronic coincidence circuits that record an event only when two photons arrive simultaneously. A major factor determining the ultimate resolution of PET is the distance traveled by a positron before its annihilation. (From Raichle ME: *Ann Rev Neurosci* 6:251, 1983.)

PET is superior to nontomographic measurements using ^{133}Xe, inhalation in that it provides three-dimensional data and the ability to image deep structures. Compared with SPECT, PET affords higher spatial resolution, greater sensitivity for deep structures, fewer artifacts from the scatter and attenuation of radiation, the ability to make both absolute and relative measures, and the potential for a greater variety of measurements. Finally, unlike fMRI, PET has the potential to measure characteristics of biological compounds (such as neurotransmitters and neuroreceptors), which exist in minute concentrations. The limitations of PET include its high expense and dependence on radiolabeled tracer administration.

Single Photon Emission Computed Tomography

SPECT systems measure the distribution of statically distributed radiopharmaceuticals (tracers trapped in the brain with a stable distribution over time) that reflect perfusion patterns. The radiopharmaceuticals for SPECT emit single gamma rays, in contrast to the two simultaneous gamma rays emitted by PET radiopharmaceuticals. This distinction leads to the instrumentation differences between SPECT and PET; SPECT cameras are designed to determine the point of origin of single photons (gamma rays) based solely on their trajectory. The spatial resolution of SPECT is nearly as high as that of PET, since recent innovations in SPECT instrumentation have led to systems capable of 8 mm resolution and imaging times as short as 2 to 3 minutes. Nevertheless, several technical problems reduce the sensitivity of SPECT for measuring changes (especially increases) in regional blood flow, particularly in deep structures.

SPECT radiopharmaceuticals fall into the following four categories: (1) diffusible indicators such as ^{133}Xe (quantitative analyses with SPECT are presently limited to dynamic ^{133}Xe blood flow imaging; the limitations of imaging with ^{133}Xe are described in the previous section); (2) iodine-123-labeled lipophilic agents, including ^{123}I-iodoamphetamine (IMP), which provide a relative distribution of blood flow but are not easily quantitated; (3) ^{99m}technetium-labeled lipophilic agents, including ^{99m}Tc-HMPAO, which distribute in a manner similar to IMP; and (4) ^{123}I-labeled neurotransmitter ligands that bind muscarinic choline, dopamine, serotonin, or benzodiazepine receptors. No pharmaceutical for SPECT is available for distribution in relation to glucose metabolism.

The major advantage of SPECT is that the instrumentation involved and the radiopharmaceuticals employed are routinely available in most nuclear medicine departments. The radiopharmaceuticals can be obtained from commercial manufacturers, obviating the need for an onsite cyclotron. Consequently SPECT imaging is lower in cost than PET.

Functional Magnetic Resonance Imaging

A variety of methods have been developed to image signals related to oxygen metabolism, blood volume, and blood flow with fMRI. The fMRI techniques for identifying the anatomical correlates of sensory or cognitive processing show regional changes that are similar in location to those identified in PET studies (Figure 6-4). The most commonly applied fMRI method for mapping brain function putatively detects shifts in local deoxyhemoglobin concentration. Unlike hemoglobin, deoxyhemoglobin is paramagnetic, a property that causes it to suppress the nuclear MR (NMR) signals from other substances in its immediate vicinity. When local neural activity increases sufficiently, local oxygen uptake, blood flow, and blood volume also increase. However, the increases in the latter two variables outpace the concomitant rise in oxygen utilization and cause the deoxyhemoglobin concentration to fall. The local water signal consequently becomes stronger than it was before the onset of the increased neuronal activity, providing a map of brain areas recruited by the experimental task.

There are several advantages of fMRI over PET and SPECT for blood flow imaging. For example, fMRI permits measurements with spatial resolution that is less than 1 mm, although the technical difficulties in distinguishing signal from noise are magnified at such high spatial resolutions. The temporal resolution of fMRI is also superior to that of PET, being at the approximate 0.5 second time required for the physiological signal to develop (MR scanners are capable of faster measurements, but the blood flow rise does not develop until about 0.5 seconds after the increase in cortical electrical activity) (Figure 6-5). Additionally, fMRI does not expose subjects to radiation and no deleterious effects have been associated with the magnetic and ra-

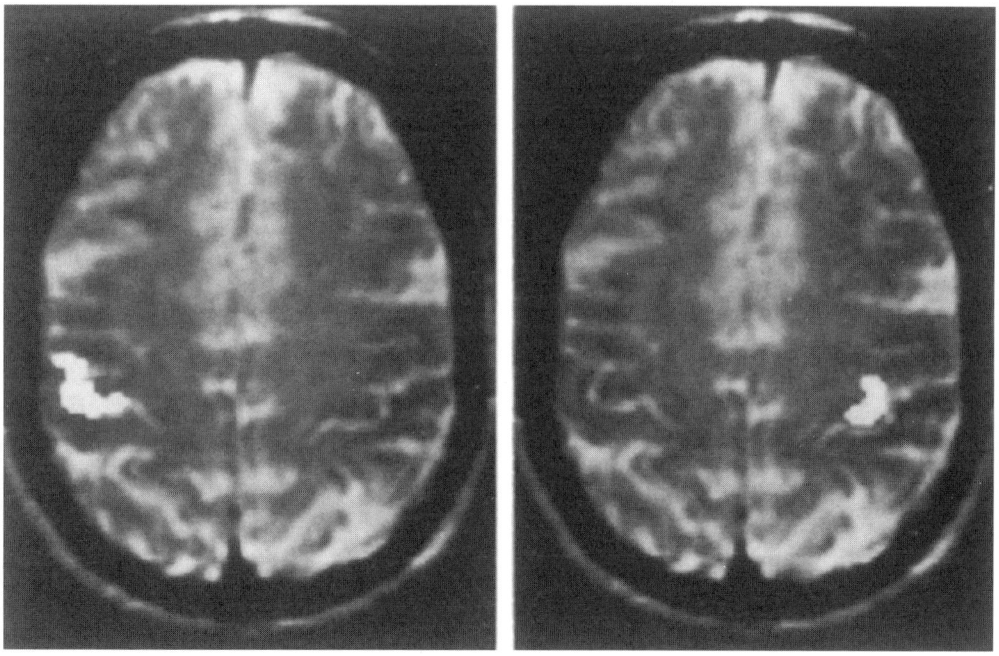

FIGURE 6-4 Activation of the contralateral motor cortex by repeatedly squeezing a sponge with each hand separately, detected by fMRI. Decreased deoxyhemoglobin concentration caused by increased local cerebral blood flow and blood volume was responsible for the bright regions in the motor cortices contralateral to the exercising left **(A)** and right **(B)** hands. The two images shown were produced by acquiring 16 single-excitation gradient echo images during left-hand squeezing, in alternation with 16 others made during right-hand squeezing. Images were obtained every 15 seconds, resulting in a total acquisition time of 8 minutes. The two groups of 16 images associated with left-hand or right-hand squeezing were summed separately and compared with each other by t-test mapping. Voxels different at a level of $p < 0.01$ comprise the bright regions, which are superimposed on a two-excitation spin echo anatomical image of the same brain made in the same session. (From Prichard JW: *The Neuroscientist,* 1:84-94, 1995.)

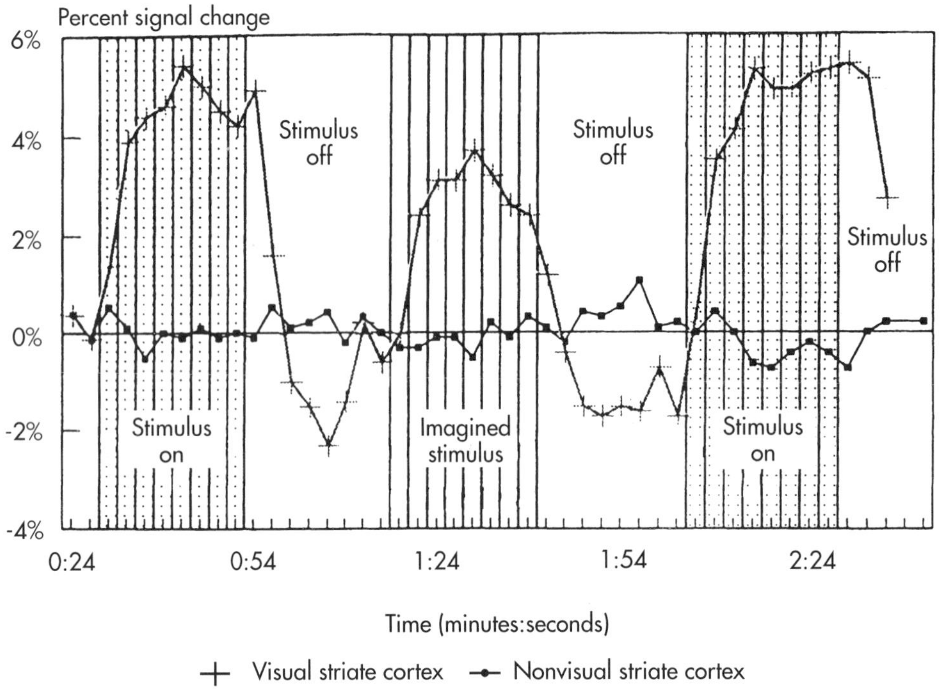

FIGURE 6-5 Activation of cerebrovascular changes by real and imagined visual stimulation, as detected using fMRI. The time course of signal intensity changes in visual and nonvisual cortex during two periods of actual photic stimulation by light flashing at 16 Hz and an intervening period during which the subject imagined the lights to be flashing. Images were obtained by pulse sequences sensitive to deoxyhemoglobin concentration in each voxel; the 5% intensity increases during actual photic stimulation and the 3% increase during imagined stimulation are all thought to reflect local increases in cerebral blood flow and volume related to neural activity in visual cortex. (From Le Bihan D et al: *Proc Natl Acad Sci USA,* 90:11802-11805, 1993.)

diofrequency fields applied, so subjects can undergo repeated study without risk. Finally, fMRI is more cost-effective than PET. The limitations of fMRI include its low sensitivity relative to PET, uncertainties regarding the nature of fMRI signals, and greater susceptibility to artifacts created by subject movement.

Magnetic Resonance Spectroscopy

In addition to the capabilities of nuclear MRI for examining anatomy and physiology, MR techniques also exist that provide in vivo information about the neurochemistry of brain tissue. MRS assays atoms that possess a net charge (for example, ^{31}P, ^{1}H, ^{19}F, ^{13}C, ^{7}Li, and ^{23}Na) and are present in sufficient concentration to produce an adequate signal. For example, ^{31}P-MRS can explore brain energy metabolism through assays of adenosine triphosphate (ATP) and related metabolites. MRS also permits investigations of the distribution of certain antidepressant and antipsychotic drugs via the use of ^{19}F-tagged medications.

MRS can be performed on standard MRI magnets with magnetic fields greater than 1.5 T. MRS is technically demanding, requiring rigorous standardization and prolonged scanning time. The latter constraint limits its utility for investigating rapid changes in metabolism related to neuronal activation. Nevertheless, MRS may be applied in comparisons across longer time frames (such as before and after treatment).

Methodological Issues in Structural Imaging Research

A wide range of qualitative and quantitative image analysis techniques have been applied in structural imaging studies. Qualitative evaluations rely on either standard clinical impressions or structured rating scales that are insensitive to subtle volumetric abnormalities. Quantitative techniques range from linear or area measures (for example, the ventricle-to-brain ratio, obtained by dividing the ventricular area in the axial slice where the ventricles appear largest by the area of the entire brain in that slice) to more sophisticated volumetric measures. Neuromorphometric techniques for measuring the volume of cerebral structures generally rely on either manual outlining of structures on sequential MR image slices or stereological sampling (point counting) methods. Semiautomated and automated techniques have also been developed; these either combine simple threshholding with manual editing or employ fully automated multispectral analytic methods to trace boundaries with uniform pixel intensity. However, the utility of these methods has been limited since the MR signal intensity is inhomogeneous across an MR image. Automated techniques that involve image warping (global deformation) models that reduce dependence on pixel intensity by utilizing shape information are being developed.

All of these methods struggle with problems of boundary definition for brain structures. The precise boundary of brain structures cannot be determined in MR images because unlike tissue sections, a CT or MRI pixel has a signal intensity that reflects an average of the signals from all of the tissues it contains, and structural borders are consequently blurred. Boundary definition becomes more difficult as image slice thickness increases, since more tissue types are included within and located adjacent to larger pixels. Early studies employed images with 5- to 10-mm slice thickness and an interslice gap between slices. More recent studies have employed new generation, high field (1.0 to 1.5 T) MRI scanners that produce 1-mm slices without interslice gaps. In addition to providing images of higher spatial resolution, the newer generation scanners also acquire images as three-dimensional sets that can be reformatted into standardized orientations. This allows uniform positioning of structures of interest within image slices across subjects, improving the accuracy and reducing the variability of area and volume measures.

Volumetric measures obtained by distinct techniques for a particular structure vary substantially, and individual laboratories have developed guidelines for defining regions that have adequate interrater and intrarater reliability within their own laboratory. However, since structures of interest such as the hippocampus, the amygdala, and the planum temporale have been defined differently across laboratories, it can be difficult to compare results across studies. Moreover, none of these techniques has been validated against tissue measures from monkeys or human cadavers, so true morphometric quantitation is not yet achievable.

Other experimental design issues critical to the interpretation of structural imaging results involve subject selection and sample size. Biological heterogeneity within a psychiatric disorder may result in dissimilar findings across studies. For example, in investigations of mood disorders, the polarity (unipolar vs. bipolar) and age of onset of the subject sample profoundly influence the results of both structural and functional imaging comparisons. Adequate matching of psychiatric and control subjects is also critical, since recent studies have shown that differences in age, sex, intelligence, socioeconomic status, or psychiatric comorbidity can lead to morphometric differences between groups. Finally, the high variability of human neuroanatomy reduces the sensitivity for replicating findings across studies, so studies involving relatively small samples may not have adequate power to test hypotheses based on previous results, contributing to apparent discrepancies across studies.

Principles of Functional Neuroimaging

In 1890 Roy and Sherrington published their pioneering observations that an "automatic mechanism" exists in the brain such that local variations in functional activity are accompanied by local variations in blood supply. This hypothesis has been corroborated by numerous experiments (both before and since the development of modern tracer methodology), which have additionally demonstrated that increases in neuronal activity are associated with rises in regional metabolism as well. By mapping regional blood flow or metabolism, functional imaging thus provides detailed pictures of local neuronal work.

The ability to noninvasively image regional blood flow and metabolism has afforded unprecedented opportunities to map the brain areas involved in cognitive processing. Using strategies that compare dynamic images obtained during experimental and control tasks, imaging studies have identified the anatomical correlates of motor, somatosensory, visual, auditory, linguistic, attentional, and memory tasks (for example, see Figures 6-4, 6-5, and 6-6). Such techniques are also beginning to elucidate the functional anatomy of human emotion, hallucinations, and psychomotor activity. Brain mapping studies involving induced emotional states have been particularly illuminating, since although animal research provides insights into the neural substrates of emotional behavior and autonomic expression, establishing the correlates of subjective emotional experience depends on human research.

Brain mapping studies using PET are generally limited to measurements of blood flow using ^{15}O-labeled water or butanol. This is because the short half-life of ^{15}O (2 minutes) permits image acquisition over a sufficiently short time (40 seconds) to capture physiological changes related to neuronal activity before the blood flow signal decays. In addition, the short half-life of ^{15}O permits repetition of measurements at 12-minute intervals, so scans can be acquired in multiple cognitive-behavioral states during the same session (see Figure 6-6).

In contrast, PET measures of glucose or oxygen metabolism are less suitable for activation paradigms. Changes in regional glucose metabolism and blood flow are tightly correlated during cortical activity, rising, for example, 51% and 50% respectively in the striate cortex during visual stimulation. However, measurements of glucose utilization employ radionuclides with long half-lives (about 2 hours for ^{18}F), mandating a longer image acquisition (45 minutes or more for ^{18}F-flurodeoxyglucose imaging) and limiting the ability to repeat measurements during the same session. This acquisition period is too long to sustain cognitive tasks because of subject fatigue, signal decay, and rehearsal effects over time. In contrast, the longer period for counting radioactive emissions during glucose metabolism imaging is an advantage in studies comparing resting neurophysiology between groups, since the larger number of radioactive counts per pixel in glucose metabolism as compared with blood flow images improves the statistical quality of metabolic images.

PET measures of oxygen utilization are less useful in mapping brain function, partly because they require sequential administration of three ^{15}O-labeled tracers: O_2, CO, and either H_2O or CO_2. Additionally, measures of oxygen metabolism are less sensitive in functional brain mapping because focal uncoupling of blood flow and oxidative metabolism occurs during at least the first 2 minutes of neuronal activation. For example, during somatosensory stimulation the mean blood flow elevation in the primary somatosensory cortex (29%) far exceeds the concomitant local increase in oxygen utilization (5%). Nevertheless, signal changes related to oxygen uptake are measurable with fMRI, which appear to have adequate sensitivity for mapping cortical activity during cognitive processing.

Brain Mapping During Cognitive Activation

The experimental strategies employed in brain mapping studies rely on paired comparisons between dynamic scans acquired in two different cognitive-behavioral states. Typically blood flow images in each task state are superimposed and then subtracted from one another to highlight regional blood flow changes that presumably reflect the mental events distinguishing the two states (Figure 6-6; see also Figures 6-4 and 6-5). Since each subject serves as his own control, nonspecific variations related to differences in anatomy and head positioning are minimized.

The number of possible interpretations for each area of observed blood flow change rises with the number of mental operations that differ between the experimental and control tasks. Thus complex cognitive processes are dissected into a series of simple, component steps. These elemental steps are imaged in successive control-activation subtraction pairs so that the distributed neural networks involved in each aspect of a more complex task can be isolated from one another.

This strategy for brain mapping studies is exemplified by the investigation of the cortical anatomy of single-word processing reviewed in Figure 6-6. In this experiment, knowledge in cognitive psychology, linguistics, and clinical neurology was used to parse single-word processing into three component steps, which were isolated from one another by scanning subjects in each of four behavioral conditions. The four behavioral tasks were used to form a three-level subtractive hierarchy such that each task state added a small number of mental operations to the previous task state.

The first level of comparison involved the subtraction between a blood-flow image acquired as the subject passively viewed nouns presented on a video screen and a blood-flow image acquired while the subject viewed a cross hair on the same screen. The blood-flow responses were interpreted as indicating two levels of computation: passive sensory processing (visual input), which was associated with blood flow increases in the primary visual (striate) cortex (other simple visual stimuli also produce blood-flow increases in this area), and modality-specific word-form processing, which was associated with blood flow increases in the extrastriate cortex. Subsequent experiments demonstrated that this latter area is also activated by words and pronounceable nonwords, but not by consonant letter strings or false fonts.

In a separate but parallel comparison, the nouns were presented aurally instead of visually. This resulted in blood flow increases in areas of the temporal cortex, where blood flow had not changed when the nouns were presented visually. However, in a subsequent experiment it was shown that blood-flow increases could be elicited in these temporal cortical regions using visual word presentation if a pair of words was shown and the subjects were required to judge in silence whether the two words rhymed.

In the second level of comparison, the subjects were again presented with a series of nouns, but this time they repeated the words aloud during the PET scan. The task in which the subjects passively viewed nouns served as the control task for comparison with the higher level "repeat-words" task. Flow increased in the brain areas related to motor output and articulatory coding: the mouth area of the primary sensorimotor cortex, the supplemental motor area, and a portion of the insular cortex (it was later demonstrated that blood flow increased in this insular area if subjects moved their mouths and tongues in the absence of visual word presentation or verbal output). These same brain areas were activated whether the nouns were presented aurally or visually.

In the third and final level of comparison, subjects were asked to view the nouns but to generate and state aloud a verb related to each noun. Whether the words were presented visually or aurally, blood flow increased in the inferior prefrontal cortex (PFC) and

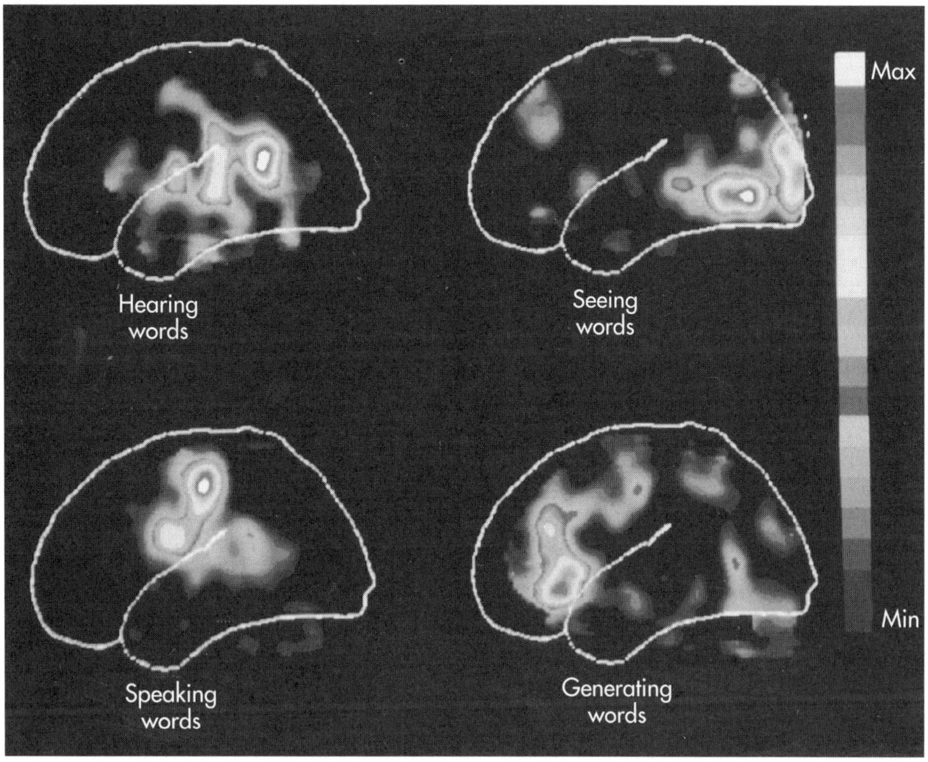

FIGURE 6-6 PET images of changes in regional blood flow show the cortical areas activated during single word processing. The image sections shown here are from composite images of mean blood flow changes in which images acquired with PET during the experimental task and the control task are superimposed and subtracted, and the resulting blood flow difference images from several subjects are then summed to enhance the signal-to-noise ratio. All of the sections shown are from sagittal slices through the lateral left hemisphere (the subjects were right-handed).

The *seeing words* image demonstrates areas in the occipital cortex where flow increases in a scan acquired as subjects passively view nouns presented on a video screen, as compared with one acquired as they view a cross-hair on the same screen. These blood flow responses indicate the functional anatomical correlates of passive sensory processing for visual input (striate cortex) and modality-specific word-form processing (extrastriate cortex). The *hearing words* image reveals areas in the temporal cortex where flow increases as nouns are presented aurally, rather than visually, during the experimental task. Thus at the level in which verbal input is passively received, distinct systems are activated for visual vs. auditory processing. In contrast, the *speaking words* comparison shows that as subjects repeat the nouns aloud, the same areas related to motor output and articulatory coding become activated whether the nouns have been presented visually or aurally. These areas include the mouth area of the primary sensorimotor cortex, the dorsal insular cortex (both shown) and the supplemental motor area (not shown); the task in which subjects passively viewed nouns served as the control task for comparison with this higher level "repeat-words" task. Finally, as subjects view or hear nouns and generate aloud a verb related to each noun *(generating words),* flow increases in the dorsolateral and inferior PFC (shown) and the dorsal portion of the anterior cingulate gyrus (not shown); the repeat-words task serves as the control task for this comparison. The anterior side is toward the left of each image, and the dorsal aspect is toward the top. (From Raichle ME. In Pechura CM, Martin JB, editors: *Mapping the brain and its functions,* Washington, D.C., 1991, National Academy Press.)

the dorsal portion of the anterior cingulate gyrus. This cingulate area was thought to participate in an anterior attention system engaged in selection for action, whereas the prefrontal area was thought to be involved in the process of semantic association.

It is noteworthy that the blood flow responses in the anterior cingulate and inferior PFCs during the verb generation task are most evident while the task is still novel and requires active attention. If subjects repeatedly practice generating verbs for the same noun list before the PET scan is acquired, significantly smaller blood-flow increases occur in these areas during verb generation, and a reciprocal blood-flow increase appears in the sylvian-insular cortex. The practice-related decrement in prefrontal and cingulate blood flow correlate with the practice-related decrease in reaction times associated with performing the task. This demonstration that the neurophysiology associated with a task changes as the performance of the task becomes more automatic with rehearsal introduces another level of complexity in the selection of behavioral tasks.

Functional Activation in Disease States

A potentially powerful strategy for investigating psychopathological conditions involves dynamic imaging during activated states. Differences in the regional blood-flow responses during cognitive or emotional tasks known to activate specific neural circuits may conceivably identify points within that circuit where dysfunction exists in psychiatric illness. Moreover, scans acquired during activated states may identify abnormalities in regions where blood flow or metabolism appears normal in the resting state. Finally, scans acquired during the performance of a neuropsychological task may demonstrate that psychiatrically ill subjects employ aberrant neural circuits in the processing related to that task.

However, the design of experimental tasks for dynamic imaging paradigms involving subjects with disease is complex, since experimental and control groups must be matched for stimulus and performance variables to conclude that any observed physiological differences relate to differences in cognitive processing. For example, elementary stimulus features such as repetition rate have profound effects on blood-flow responses. Somatosensory stimulation does not produce a measurable blood-flow response in the cat somatosensory cortex until the stimulus frequency reaches 3 Hz. This is apparently related to the limited spatial and temporal resolution of blood flow and metabolism measurements, since neuronally induced changes in blood flow or metabolism must occupy a sufficient portion of the measurement time and be present in a large enough area within the region of interest to produce measurable changes. Thereafter the measured blood flow declines until the frequency reaches 10 Hz, where it is again no longer measurable. A different relationship exists between blood flow and stimulus frequency in the human visual cortex, where photic stimulation produces a significant blood-flow rise in the striate cortex at less than 1 Hz, which peaks at 7.8 Hz and is still evident at 61 Hz.

An implication of these observations is that if behavioral performance differs between groups, one cannot be certain that stimulus rates involving the structure in question were identical. For example, one series compared blood-flow changes during performance of the Wisconsin Card Sort Test between control subjects and subjects with schizophrenia and found that the subjects with schizophrenic developed a blunted blood-flow response in the dorsolateral PFC while they were performing the task. However, they successfully completed an average of 1.5 categories during the scan, whereas the control subjects completed an average of 7.5 categories. Since the dorsolateral PFC is putatively involved in performing this task, the blood-flow response may have differed between groups because the rate at which the stimulus reached the dorsolateral PFC was unequal, the behavioral output was dissimilar, or the cognitive processing within the dorsolateral PFC is abnormal in schizophrenia. Thus unless stimulus and response variables such as performance rate and accuracy are similar between experimental and control groups, blood-flow response differences between groups cannot be interpreted as indicating regional dysfunction.

Abnormalities of Resting Physiology in Psychiatric Disorders

Resting differences in blood flow or metabolism between subjects who are psychiatrically ill and control subjects reflect a complex set of activations by the disease state. Regional metabolic differences may describe trait pathophysiological abnormalities associated with the genetic or environmental predisposition to a disorder, physiological state changes corresponding to symptoms (for example, hallucinations) or behaviors (such as obsessive thinking), or cytological changes that may cause or result from the illness or its manifestations (for example, the increased risk for alcohol abuse in bipolar disorder). Moreover, disparate states within a single diagnostic group may give varying functional patterns. For example, psychomotor agitation may have distinct functional anatomical correlates from psychomotor retardation, yet either may be present in MDD.

Another level of complexity relates to the nature of the metabolic signal. First, synaptic activity in the neuropil, rather than changes in the chemistry of cell bodies, accounts for nearly all of the metabolic changes observed during activation. Thus local changes in blood flow or metabolism in a specific region may occur either from increased interneuronal neurotransmission within that region or from increased afferent transmission from a projecting structure. Since local connections predominate in the cortex, blood flow and metabolic differences observed there are generally interpreted as reflecting local interneuronal activity. In contrast, physiological changes in the basal ganglia or the thalamus are more likely to reflect afferent transmission originating from neurons in a distal structure.

Second, both excitatory and inhibitory transmission result in increased metabolic activity in the neuropil because both result in activation of energy-consuming, ion-pumping activity at the postsynaptic membrane. The differentiation between excitatory and inhibitory transmission in terms of local metabolism would presumably be reflected one synapse away, where the postsynaptic neuron makes its efferent synapses. However, such efferent activity may be diffusely distributed and may not be evident in the functional brain image.

Abnormalities in functional images can also be accounted for by differences in cell number. Tomographic methods provide physiological measurements per volume unit of intracranial contents, such that image data are affected by the inclusion of metabolically inactive CSF spaces resulting from atrophy or hypoplasia (known as the partial volume effect). The presence of atrophy or hypoplasia in some psychiatric illnesses creates difficulties in the interpretation of functional imaging data, since it is unclear whether observed differences in blood flow or metabolism result from true changes in these parameters, atrophy, or a combination of the two. Studies are beginning to address this problem using MRI quantitation of anatomical differences to correct physiological images for partial volume effects, although such techniques await validation.

Other Issues in Image Analysis

Simple visual inspection of physiological images is generally not sensitive enough to detect the subtle abnormalities associated with psychiatric disorders, so comparisons of mean tracer uptake between psychiatric and control samples in specified regions are used to identify abnormalities. Deciding where to look in functional images is complicated, since an average PET slice is composed of about 7000 volume elements (voxels) and modern tomographic instruments obtain 15 to 47 slices during a single scan. Dealing with comparisons across so many data points poses serious statistical problems in distinguishing true differences from differences arising by chance alone. One approach for reducing the number of statistical tests is to limit comparisons to a few regions of interest in which the average value of all image voxels contained within each region of interest is compared between patients and controls.

To anatomically localize regional measurements within the relatively low-resolution functional brain images, the primary blood flow or metabolic images are commonly transformed into a standardized stereotaxic space using the coordinate system of a neurosurgical atlas. These methods allow stereotaxic placement of regions of interest across subjects. New methods rely on coregistration of PET and MRI images from the same subject, since anatomical detail is more easily seen in MRI images. Ultimately, methods under development that use anatomical information from the MRI scan to fluidly transform coregistered PET and MRI images into a standard three-dimensional space are expected to become the standard method for localization.

Although the region-of-interest method is currently superior to other approaches for assessing differences in small structures (such as the basal ganglia or limbic structures), it reduces sensitivity for identifying abnormalities in the cortex in studies of psychiatric disorders, since the uncertain knowledge regarding the pathophysiology of these disorders and the limited information regarding the cortical areas involved in the production of psychiatric symptoms reduce the likelihood of preselecting regions of interest where abnormalities exist. A more sensitive approach for assessing cortical areas involves the use of statistical maps in which image voxels are computed as either unpaired t-values for comparing the mean blood flow or metabolism of patient and control groups or as paired t-values for comparing mean differences across two distinct states in the same subject set (for example before and during a panic attack). Another type of statistical image that is used to explore relationships between clinical ratings and regional physiology involves the computation of correlational images (r-value maps). These methods rely on the aforementioned transformations of primary tomographs into standardized stereotaxic space, so images from different brains can be superimposed. Nevertheless, the generation of such statistical maps involves several thousand statistical comparisons (computations are performed for every image voxel), potentially leading to the statistical problem of obtaining significant differences by chance alone. Therefore conservative approaches confine the use of statistical maps to exploratory analyses in which areas of apparent significance in the statistical map generated from one subject set are used to generate candidate regions of interest, and the statistical probability that significant differences exist in such regions is tested in independent subject sets.

Neuroimaging Studies of the Major Psychiatric Disorders

Schizophrenia

Structural Imaging

Neuromorphometric studies have consistently shown that subjects with schizophrenia have enlarged lateral and third ventricles, widened cortical sulci, and reduced temporal lobe structure size relative to healthy control subjects, although the magnitude of these abnormalities is subtle relative to that of the corresponding changes in people with dementia (Figure 6-7). More than 50 studies have used CT or MRI to examine the lateral ventricles in schizophrenia, and 90% of the studies comparing subjects with schizophrenia against healthy controls found significant ventricular enlargement in the people with schizophrenia. The ventricle-to-brain ratio in schizophrenia correlates with negative symptoms (such as apathy, anhedonia, avolition, and paucity of speech), cognitive impair-

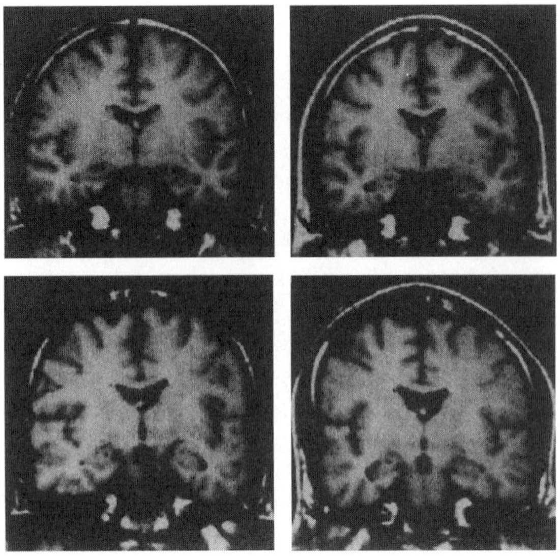

FIGURE 6-7 MRI coronal views from two sets of monozygotic twins discordant for schizophrenia showing subtle enlargement of the lateral ventricles in the affected twins (**B** and **D**) as compared with their unaffected co-twins (**A** and **C**). Differences are apparent even when the affected twin had small ventricles. (From Suddath RL et al: *New Engl J Med* 399:791, 1990.)

ment, poor premorbid adjustment, persistent unemployment, poor response to antipsychotic medications, EEG abnormalities, and incidence of extrapyramidal side effects with antipsychotic drug treatment. In contrast, the ventricle-to-brain ratio is inversely correlated with psychotic symptoms. Ventricular enlargement does not correlate with the extent or duration of neuroleptic treatment, the use of electroconvulsive therapy (ECT), or the length of previous hospitalization.

The portions of the lateral ventricles that appear enlarged to the greatest extent are the temporal horns, where enlargement is evident even in new-onset cases. This observation suggests that reduced tissue volume in the temporal lobe may account for enlargement of the ventricles, consistent with reports that temporal lobe volume is reduced in subjects with schizophrenia relative to healthy controls, particularly in the left hemisphere. Investigators that have segmented gray and white matter have also reported that the volume of temporal lobe gray matter is decreased in schizophrenia. Specific areas within the temporal lobe where volumetric reductions have been identified include the superior temporal gyrus, the hippocampus, and the parahippocampal gyrus (results in the amygdala have been conflicting). Postmortem neuropathological studies of schizophrenia have reported morphometric and cytoarchitectural abnormalities in some of these temporal lobe regions. The size reduction in the superior temporal gyrus, a putative auditory association area, correlates with the severity of auditory hallucinations, disordered thought flow, and reduced amplitude of the P300 component of the auditory event related potential.

The most compelling demonstration of these morphometric abnormalities involved a comparison between monozygotic twin pairs who were discordant for schizophrenia (see Figure 6-7). The unaffected twin served as a matched control for the affected co-twin regarding the anatomical variation that may be related to shared genetic factors and jointly experienced nongenetic factors (for example, socioeconomic status, early psychosocial stressors, and infections). Relative to their unaffected co-twins the twins with schizophrenia had significantly larger lateral and third ventricles, reduced left temporal lobe gray matter volume, and decreased hippocampal volume. The twins with schizophrenia could be differentiated from their unaffected co-twins inmost cases based on visual inspection of the images, suggesting that these subtle neuroanatomical differences are consistently present in schizophrenia, even though normal anatomical variability precludes sensitive separation of schizophrenic cases from less stringently matched control samples.

Third ventricle size is also consistently enlarged in subjects with schizophrenia relative to controls. This observation suggests that the tissue volume of structures lining the third ventricle, such as the thalamus and the midline forebrain limbic nuclei, may also be reduced in schizophrenia. Clinical correlates of the size of the third ventricle-to-brain ratio have been inconsistent, suggesting that third ventricle enlargement is present in a broader segment of patients with schizophrenia than is lateral ventricle enlargement.

The width of the cortical sulci appears increased in schizophrenia as determined by semistructured qualitative ratings or quantitative measurements of sulcal or gyral width. Sulcal widening has been shown in most studies comparing subjects with schizophrenia against healthy controls and in about one half of all studies comparing patients with schizophrenia against medical or neurological controls. Several studies report that sulcal widening is most pronounced in the PFC, compatible with postmortem evidence that neuronal organization is abnormal in parts of the PFC in schizophrenia. Nevertheless, in MRI studies the volume of the PFC has not differed between subjects who are schizophrenic and controls.

Changes in the volume of basal ganglia structures have been reported in MRI studies of schizophrenia. Two groups reported that the volume of the globus pallidus and the putamen are increased, but these findings were not replicated by others. A potentially relevant aspect of to these conflicting results is that one study found that although caudate volume was not abnormal in patients with new-onset schizophrenias who had never been medicated, when these subjects were rescanned after several months of antipsychotic drug treatment the caudate volume was enlarged.

In the cerebellum, 7 of 10 CT studies reported that on qualitative inspection, the cerebellar size is abnormally small in 5% to 17% of subjects with schizophrenia and in only 1% of controls. Consistent with the observation that reduced cerebellar size may exist in only a subset of patients with schizophrenia, MRI studies have not identified differences in the mean cerebellar volume when entire samples of subjects with schizophrenia and control subjects are compared.

In the corpus callosum (a white matter band containing the axonal fibers that connect the two cerebral hemispheres), studies have reported no differences, increases, or decreases in patients with schizophrenia relative to control groups. The monozygotic twin data suggest that changes may exist in the shape of the posterior corpus callosum, but that this difference reflects distortion from ventriculomegaly and not an actual change in callosal size.

Resting Blood Flow and Metabolism

Studies involving previously medicated patients who are chronically ill with schizophrenia have consistently demonstrated "hypofrontality," or lower frontal and whole brain blood flow and metabolism, relative to controls. In contrast, most studies using only patients who had never been medicated failed to confirm this finding. Pertinent to this discrepancy, several studies report that antipsychotic medications reduce frontal relative to nonfrontal blood flow or metabolism, suggesting that hypofrontality reflects a long-lasting effect of antipsychotic treatment rather than the pathophysiologic condition underlying schizophrenia. However, this issue remains controversial, since other studies find increases in absolute frontal blood flow and metabolism during treatment. An alternative interpretation of the reduced prefrontal blood flow and metabolism in schizophrenia was suggested by a study involving medicated subjects with chronic schizophrenia, which found that the abnormal reduction in dorsolateral prefrontal blood flow correlated with ratings of thought impoverishment (manifested clinically by a paucity of speech and an emptiness in the content of verbal communication). The authors hypothesized that subjects with chronic schizophrenia activate areas related to cognitive processing to a lesser extent than controls because they have are having fewer thoughts. They proposed that hypofrontality is less consistently seen in subjects who are acutely ill but have never been medicated, because thought impoverishment is less prominent early in the disease course and worsens during exposure to most antipsychotic drugs (see Chapter 13).

In the basal ganglia, one PET study demonstrated increased blood flow in the globus pallidus of subjects with schizophrenia who had never been medicated. A postmortem anatomical study reported that the volume of the pallidum is reduced in patients with schizophrenia, corroborating the potential importance of this structure in the pathophysiology of schizophrenia. Regional blood flow in a ventral striatal area located in the vicinity of the globus pallidus was shown to correlate with a "reality-distortion" factor that reflected psychosis ratings.

Finally, metabolism in limbic structures such as the hippocampus and the anterior cingulate gyrus is reportedly reduced in schizophrenia. Psychosis ratings have been shown to correlate positively with blood flow in the left medial temporal cortex (in the vicinity of the hippocampus) and negatively with blood flow in the posterior cingulate gyrus in medicated subjects with chronic schizophrenia. Metabolism increases in parts of the temporal lobe after treatment, although it is unclear whether this change extends to the hippocampus.

Limitations of Resting Blood Flow and Metabolism Studies

The interpretation of functional imaging data in schizophrenia are complicated by the neuromorphological abnormalities (that is, enlarged ventricles or reduced hippocampal and temporal lobe size) identified in structural imaging studies and the histopathological changes reported in postmortem studies of schizophrenia. The former may produce partial volume effects that potentially account for the blood-flow and metabolic decreases in the hippocampus and the temporal and frontal lobes. The cytoarchitectural abnormalities include changes in the organization of neuronal layers in the hippocampus and reductions in the quantity of axonal processes in cortical layer II of the anterior cingulate gyrus, which imply that early disturbances of neuronal migration play an etiological role in schizophrenia. Such cytoarchitectural abnormalities may alter the local synaptic activity and regional physiology, confounding the interpretation of functional imaging differences between schizophrenic and control subjects.

Activation Studies in Schizophrenia

One approach to dealing with such anatomical differences is to employ patients with schizophrenia as their own controls for dynamic imaging studies in which the functional responsivity of a region is probed by pharmacological agents or neuropsychological tasks. For example, a preliminary fMRI study reported that the signal change in the frontal lobe was decreased in subjects who were schizophrenic relative to controls during cognitive tasks thought to probe frontal lobe function. These data are similar to the results of studies performed with the nontomographic ^{133}Xe-inhalation method, which showed that subjects with schizophrenia demonstrate a blunted blood-flow rise in the dorsolateral PFC relative to controls while performing the Wisconsin Card Sorting Test. Unfortunately the interpretation of these studies has been obscured by performance differences across subject groups. For example, in one of these studies the subjects with schizophrenia successfully completed an average of 1.5 categories during the scan and the control subjects completed an average of 7.5 categories, so it could not be determined whether the difference in blood-flow response between groups was accounted for by a performance difference or by PFC dysfunction in schizophrenia. Potentially consistent with either interpretation, a recent study demonstrated reversal of this abnormal blood-flow response and improvement in task performance when amphetamine was administered before testing. Nevertheless, these pioneering endeavors may lead to simpler neuropsychological probes that can distinguish the functional responses of subjects with schizophrenic and control subjects without confounding performance differences.

Neuroreceptor Imaging in Schizophrenia

Several studies have assessed dopamine D_2-receptor density in the striatum in unmedicated subjects with schizophrenia. One group using PET and [^{11}C]N-methylspiperone found a two- to threefold elevation in receptor sites in the caudate nucleus bilaterally. Of other studies in which radiolabeled spiperone compounds were used to image dopamine D_2 receptor density, one using PET and [^{76}Br]-bromospiperone found no differences between untreated patients with schizophrenia and control subjects and another using SPECT and [^{77}Br]-bromospiperone found only a 10% increase in the striatal uptake in subjects with schizophrenia relative to controls. Another group using the more selective D_2-receptor antagonist ^{11}[C]-raclopride found no differences in receptor density or affinity in the striatum between subjects with schizophrenia and control subjects. The discrepancies across studies may be partly accounted for by dissimilarities in the specificity of these ligands, which have differential affinities for D_2, D_3, and D_4 receptors (all D_2 "family" receptors). Additionally, endogenous dopamine concentrations affect displacement of spiperone and raclopride differently, potentially contributing to the dissimilar results across studies.

D_1- and D_2-receptor ligands have also been employed to assess the receptor occupancy of antipsychotic drugs. Such studies have demonstrated that the majority of D_2 receptors are blocked by typical neuroleptic agents (such as haloperidol) and that the D_2 occupancy in the putamen correlates with the incidence and severity of extrapyramidal side effects (for example, dystonia and pseudoparkinsonism). Receptor imaging studies have also demonstrated that the atypical neuroleptic agent clozapine, which generally does not produce extrapyramidal effects, occupies only a minority of the D_2 sites in the striatum. Finally, receptor imaging has provided important information concerning the relationship between serum concentrations of antipsychotic drugs and D_2-receptor occupancy.

Magnetic Resonance Spectroscopy in Schizophrenia

One group has reported that the phosphomonoester signal is decreased and the phosphodiester signal increased in the dorsal PFC of patients with schizophrenia who have not been medicated relative to control subjects. Concentrations of these fatty acids are putatively related to the production and breakdown of cell membranes. In another study, alterations in the ratio of phosphocreatinine to inorganic phosphate that correlated inversely with symptom severity were identified in the temporal lobes of subjects with schizophrenia.

Significance of Neuroimaging Abnormalities in Schizophrenia

Both neurodevelopmental and neurodegenerative models have been proposed to explain the structural and functional alterations in schizophrenia. Observations that ventricular enlargement is not correlated with age or illness chronicity and is demonstrable in patients who are experiencing first episodes suggest that such changes are present early in the disease course and change little over time. Postmortem studies of schizophrenia have noted a conspicuous absence of gliosis (an overgrowth of neuroglia that accompanies neurodegenerative conditions), which is evidence against the presence of a neurodegenerative process. Instead, postmortem studies have found regionally decreased tissue volume along with abnormal cytoarchitecture, favoring neurodevelopmental hypotheses for the etiology of schizophrenia.

Mood Disorders

Mood disorders are particularly well suited for functional imaging studies, since they appear to be associated with neurochemical changes but not with clear histopathological changes (see Chapter 8). Their episodic nature and excellent response to treatment permit imaging in both symptomatic and asymptomatic states. Functional imaging studies may thus be capable of differentiating the physiological correlates of emotional symptoms from the pathophysiological changes that underlie the tendency to develop abnormal mood episodes. Additionally, since the symptoms of mood disorders represent exaggerations or extensions of cognitive and emotional states that can be expressed by subjects who are nondepressed, the nature of blood-flow or metabolic changes related to the depressed state can be explored by imaging control subjects during experimentally induced sadness, anxiety, or sleep deprivation.

Mood-disorder studies have largely been limited to subjects with depression because of the difficulties involved in scanning subjects in the manic state. The results of imaging studies of depression have appeared widely discrepant, with some studies reporting increases in PFC activity and others finding decreases or no differences in the PFC of patients with depression relative to control subjects. However, these discrepancies appear resolvable by attending to methodological issues such as the depressive subtype selected, the presence of medication effects, and the location of the region of interest within the PFC.

Methodological Issues in Neuroimaging Studies of Mood Disorders

Sample Selection: the Problem of Heterogeneity

A major challenge facing imaging studies of mood disorders stems from the likelihood that the major depressive syndrome encompasses a heterogenous group of disorders (see Chapter 8). Besides the obvious clinical heterogeneity extant within affective disease, biological heterogeneity also exists. For example, neuroendocrine and neurochemical abnormalities are typically present in subgroups but not entire samples of subjects with depression. If major depression is associated with multiple pathophysiological states, it is presumably associated with an assortment of different functional brain images and study results vary depending on the composition of the subject sample. The imaging literature confirms this hypothesis, since subtyping subjects with depression has proven critical for reducing the variability of image data. Broad categories that must be respected in the sample selection include the following distinctions: (1) unipolar vs. bipolar disorders; (2) primary depressive disorders vs. depressive syndromes occurring secondary to other psychiatric or medical disorders; and (3) late age of onset vs. early-onset depression (see Chapter 8).

Polarity of the Subject Sample

Bipolar disorder, in which both manic and depressive episodes occur, and unipolar depression (MDD), in which only depressive episodes occur, appear neurochemically, pharmacologically, and genetically distinct. Patients who have unipolar depression and those with bipolar depression also differ in their respective structural and functional imaging correlates. For example, enlargement of the lateral and third ventricles has been consistently found in both young and elderly adults with bipolar disorder, but the ventricles appear normal in relatively young patients with unipolar depression who are nondelusional. Additionally, unipolar and bipolar depression appear physiologically distinct in parts of the ventral PFC and the basal ganglia. In spite of such differences, most published studies have combined unipolar and bipolar depression without including separate comparisons based on polarity. The results from such studies are consequently difficult to interpret.

Primary vs. Secondary Depression

The results from studies of depressive syndromes that arise secondary to neurological disorders, drug withdrawal states, or other psychiatric disorders have in some cases differed from those reported for primary depressives syndromes that arise in the absence of other psychiatric or general medical conditions. One group reported that in subjects with either Parkinson's disease or Huntington's disease, ventral prefrontal metabolism was decreased in subjects who were depressed relative to subjects with no depression and the same neurological disorder. This finding differed from the results in young patients with primary depression (Table 6-2). Another group failed to confirm this finding in depressed patients with Parkinson's disease and instead found decreased blood flow in those patients relative to patients with Parkinson's who were not depressed. The differences were in the dorsal prefrontal and dorsal anterior cingulate regions, where they had also identified blood-flow decreases in subjects who were cognitively impaired and had primary depression. Finally, in another study, PFC activity did not differ between subjects who were depressed and subjects with no depression who had basal ganglia infarctions. These data suggest that functional imaging results in secondary depressive syndromes are more heterogeneous than those in primary depression (see Table 6-2) and that they may in some cases substantially differ between patients with primary and secondary depression. This parallels the functional imaging findings in primary and secondary obsessive-compulsive syndromes, in which ventral PFC metabolism is increased in the former but decreased or unchanged in the latter (see the related section in this chapter). Taken together, the neuroimaging results in primary and secondary depression support a neural model in which mood disorders are associated with dysfunctional interactions between multiple structures, rather than increased or decreased activity in a single structure (Figure 6-8; see also Figure 8-1).

TABLE 6-2

FUNCTIONAL IMAGING DATA IN PREFRONTAL CORTEX FOR UNMEDICATED PATIENTS WITH PRIMARY UNIPOLAR DEPRESSION[a]

Authors	Sample size: Depressed	Sample size: Control	Imaging technique	Result in depressed relative to control subjects: Ventral PFC	Result in depressed relative to control subjects: Dorsal PFC
Baxter et al., 1987	14	14	PET, ^{18}FDG	↑ Orbital gyrus (bilateral)[b]	N/A
Baxter et al., 1989	10	12	PET, ^{18}FDG	N/A	↓ Dorsal anterolateral (bilateral)
Bench et al., 1993	14[c]	23	PET, $H_2{}^{15}O$	N/A[d]	↓ Dorsolateral (left) and dorsal anterior cingulate
Biver et al., 1994	12	12	PET, ^{18}FDG	↑ Medial orbital and ↑ lateral orbital (bilateral)	↓ Dorsolateral (left)
Buchsbaum et al., 1986	4	24	PET, ^{18}FDG	↑ Frontal/occipital ratio (reportedly accounted for by ↑ ventral frontal metabolism)	N/A
Cohen et al., 1989	5	27	PET, ^{18}FDG	N/S	N/S
Drevets et al., 1992	13	33	PET, $H_2{}^{15}O$	↑ Ventrolateral, lateral orbital (left)	N/A
Drevets et al., 1995	22	10	PET, ^{18}FDG	↑ Ventrolateral, lateral, and medial orbital (bilateral)[e]	N/A
Ebert et al., 1991	10	8	SPECT, ^{99m}Tc-HMPAO	↑ Orbital (bilateral)[f]	↓ Dorsal anterolateral (in left superior frontal gyrus)
Mentis et al., 1995	11	12	PET, ^{18}FDG	↑ Orbital and lateral prefrontal	N/S
Trivedi et al., 1994	24	N/L	SPECT, ^{99m}Tc-HMPAO	↑ Inferior frontal gyrus (right)	↓ Superior and middle frontal gyrus (bilateral)
Uytdenhoef et al., 1983	16	20	Multidetector probes, ^{133}Xe	↑ Left frontal ratio (which included ventrolateral)	↑ Superior frontal gyrus (left)
Wu et al., 1992	15	15	PET, ^{18}FDG	↑ Ventral anterior cingulate[f,g]	N/A[g]

N/S, difference not significant; *N/A*, difference not assessed for region; *N/L*, not listed (study presented only in abstract form).

[a]Some studies also included subject samples with bipolar depression, the data for whom are not included here.

[b]Not reported as significant by analysis of variance, although the difference between patients with depression and controls in this region was similar in magnitude to that found in other studies using images with similar resolution and would be significant by t-test.

[c]An additional 19 subjects imaged in this study are not reported here because they were imaged while they were receiving medications.

[d]This study identified abnormalities using a statistical image that excluded pixels in the orbital cortex because image data had not been acquired for all subjects in this ventral structure (the PET camera gantry was ~10 cm).

[e]Abnormality specific to subgroup of subjects with depression (n = 11) meeting criteria for FPDD.

[f]Abnormality found only in subgroup that was responsive to sleep deprivation.

[g]No difference found in whole frontal lobe to occipital ratio.

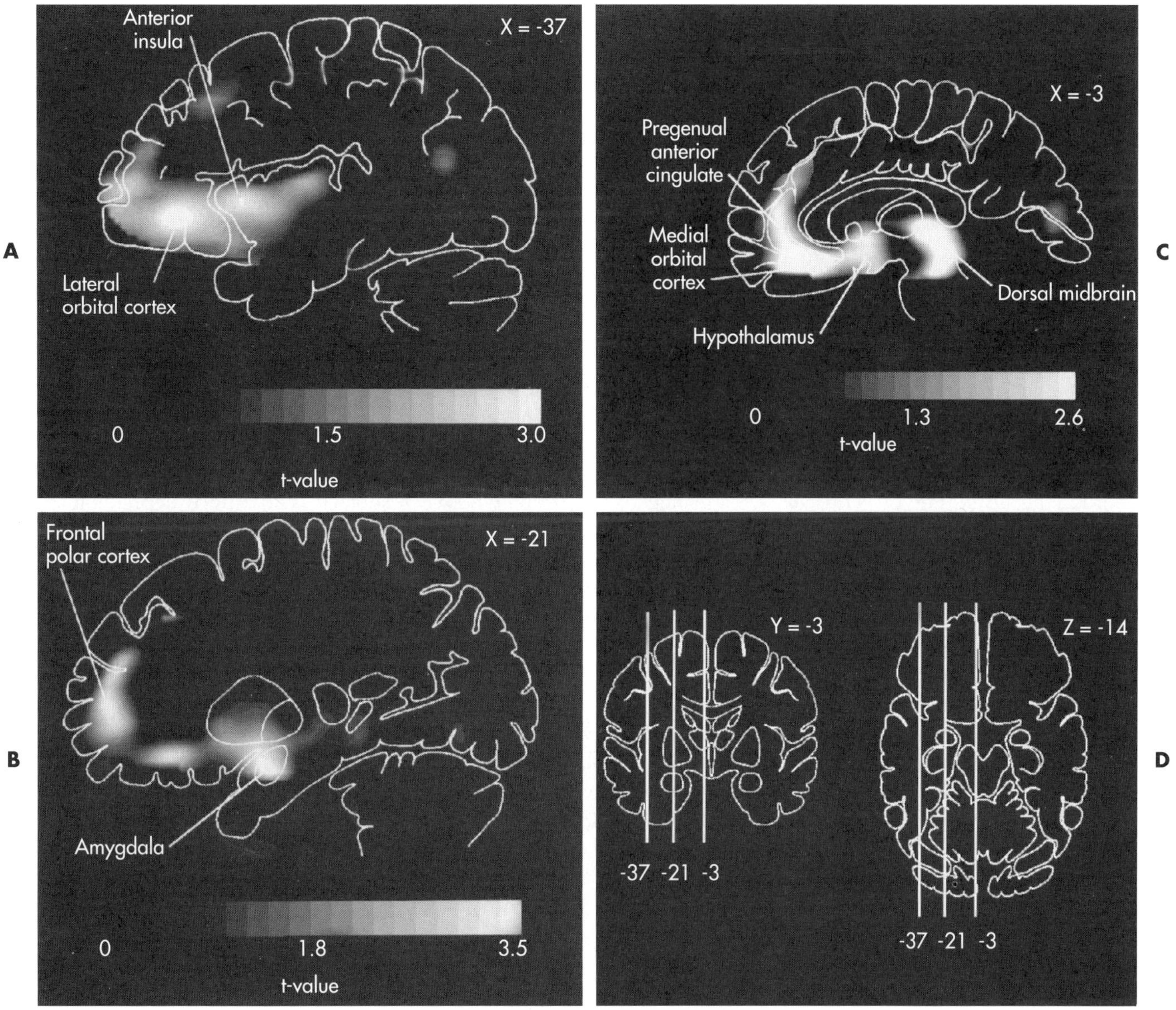

FIGURE 6-8 Regional blood flow increases in subjects with unipolar depression who have familial pure depressive disease (FPDD). The images shown are from an image of unpaired t-values, generated by subtracting composite images of mean blood flow from the subjects with depression and control groups and dividing the resulting difference image by the local variance. These statistical images were used to generate hypotheses regarding areas where regional activity may be abnormal in depression. The areas of significantly increased activity in patients with depression relative to controls in the lateral and medial orbital cortex, the anterior insula, the pregenual anterior cingulate gyrus, and the amygdala were subsequently confirmed twice using both regional blood flow and glucose metabolic image data from independent subject samples. Although no attempt was made to replicate the findings in the midbrain and hypothalamus because of the small size of these structures with respect to the spatial resolution of PET, both areas have been implicated in emotional expression and MDD by other types of information (see Chapter 8). The position of the three sagittal planes relative to the midline are indicated by the X coordinates, with negative X indicating the left hemisphere. Anterior is toward the left. (Corresponding atlas outlines from Talairach J, Tournoux P: *Co-planar stereotaxic atlas of the human brain,* Stuttgart, 1988, Thieme.)

Confounding Effects of Medications in Studies of Depression

Most functional imaging studies in depression have been confounded by medication effects. Administration of antidepressant, antipsychotic, or antianxiety drugs before scanning has been demonstrated to produce areas of decreased blood flow and metabolism in the PFC and limbic areas that are of interest in depression. It is thus unclear how the reports of blood-flow or metabolic decreases in medicated patients with depression can be interpreted if a baseline scan has not also been acquired before the patient began receiving medication.

Structural Imaging Studies

Neuromorphometric Abnormalities

Similar to the findings in schizophrenia, CT and MRI investigations report abnormal lateral and third ventricle size in adults with bipolar disorder (manic-depressive illness) and in some subgroups with unipolar depression (Figure 6-9). In subjects with bipolar disorder, the magnitude of ventricular enlargement is similar to that found in schizophrenia. The increased ventricle to brain ratio in these studies correlates with higher cortisol levels, hypothyroidism, CSF concentrations of the serotonin metabolite 5-HIAA, psychotic symptoms, poorer premorbid functioning, and cognitive impairment. Ventricular enlargement has not been identified in samples limited to relatively young patients with unipolar depression who are not delusional or to older patients with unipolar depression who experienced an early age of onset.

The specific regions where reduced tissue volume accounts for ventricular enlargement in some subgroups of patients with mood disorders remain under investigation. Frontal lobe volume was reported to be abnormally decreased in some but not all studies of adults with bipolar disorder or unipolar depression. MRI investigations in child and adolescent subjects have also suggested differences in the frontal lobe volume in bipolar disorder. The volume of the caudate and putamen is reported to be abnormally decreased in subjects with unipolar depression, but not in subjects with bipolar depression. Conversely, temporal lobe volume is reportedly reduced in subjects with bipolar depression but not those with unipolar depression. The area of the temporal lobe that is affected in bipolar disorder may not include the hippocampus, since one study found no differences in hippocampal volume between subjects with bipolar depression and controls and another found no differences between subjects with unipolar depression and controls.

In the cerebellum, the incidence of cerebellar atrophy was increased in CT investigations of affective disorders, similar to the findings in schizophrenia. Two MRI studies confirmed these observations by report-

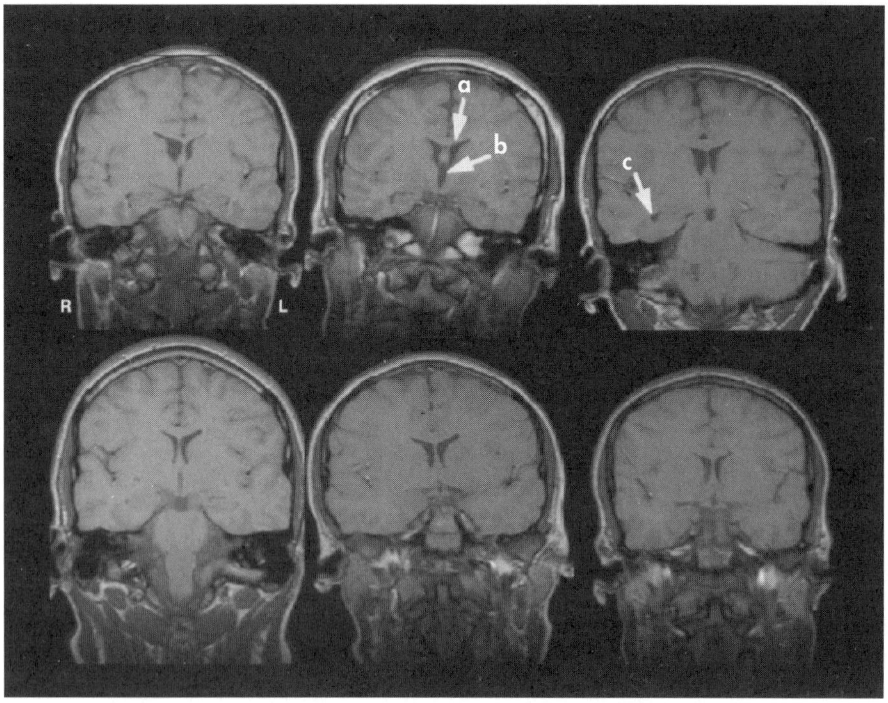

FIGURE 6-9 T1-weighted coronal MRI scans from adolescents with bipolar disorder *(top row)* compared with control subjects of similar ages *(bottom row)* demonstrating enlargement of the third ventricle *(b)*, and reversed asymmetry or prominence of the lateral ventricles *(a)*, and the temporal horn of the lateral ventricles *(c)*.

ing decreased cerebellar vermal area and decreased cerebellar volume in patients with unipolar depression relative to control subjects. Another MRI study failed to identify differences in cerebellar size between subjects with bipolar depression and controls.

Finally, the pituitary gland appears enlarged in the MR images of patients who are depressed. This may reflect a correlate of the hypothalamic-pituitary-adrenal axis hyperactivity that is demonstrable in patients with severe depression. Consistent with this hypothesis, the adrenal glands appear enlarged in abdominal MRI scans from subjects who are severely depressed.

Signal Hyperintensities

Another type of neuromorphological abnormality in patients with mood disorders is evident as signal hyperintensities in the deep white matter of T2-weighted MRI scans. These hyperintensities are found in 25% to 50% of MRI scans in healthy elderly subjects with no dementia and in approximately 5% of young healthy subjects. In contrast, they appear in one third of subjects with bipolar I disorder and in over two thirds of elderly subjects with unipolar depression who experienced the onset of depression at a late age (defined either as subjects who suffer the initial episode of depression after age 60 or who receive initial treatment for depression after age 60). The size of white matter hyperintensities is also increased in these patients with mood disorders compared with age-matched control groups (Figure 6-10). Other disorders in which deep white-matter hyperintensities appear larger and more prevalent include multiple sclerosis, multi-infarct dementia, CNS infections, and perinatal injuries. Thus the nature and origin of these hyperintensities may differ across disease states, reflecting pathophysiological changes in the white matter related to anoxia, ischemia, demyelination, or immune disorders.

In elderly patients with depression the presence of hyperintensities in the basal ganglia and the deep and periventricular white matter correlates with a late age of onset of depression and with atherosclerotic risk factors. In such cases the signal hyperintensities are predominantly located in the striatum, the thalamus, and the deep white matter of the frontal lobes in sites that correspond to the distribution of penetrating arterioles of the lenticulostriate, thalamoperforate, and medullary arteries (see Figure 6-10). Postmortem assessments of the tissue where MRI signal hyperintensities were apparent antemortem demonstrate ischemia-related changes such as edema, dilated perivascular spaces, and in the case of larger lesions, lacunar infarction. Moreover, their presence in elderly patients with late-onset depression is associated with enlargement of the cerebral ventricles, which may reflect ex vacuo changes that occur after ischemic damage. Such lesions are not clinically silent, since increased ventricular size correlates with cognitive impairment and psychomotor slowing, and the presence of caudate hyperintensities is associated with an elevated risk for the development of delirium during ECT or antidepressant drug therapy and for extrapyramidal side effects during antipsychotic drug treatment. As discussed in Chapter 8, the anatomical locations where cerebral infarction has been associated with poststroke depression are similar to the locations where signal hyperintensities are found in patients with late-onset depression (that is, in the frontal lobes and the caudate), and it is hypothesized that elderly patients with depression who had a late age of onset acquire a mood disorder from an arteriosclerotic source, homologous to the case of poststroke mood disorders.

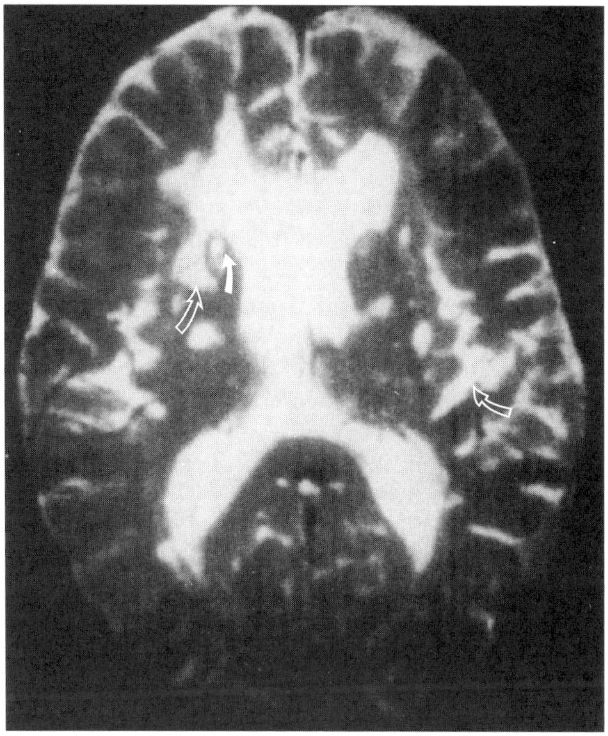

FIGURE 6-10 Brain MRI, axial view through base of lateral ventricles showing large, confluent, deep white matter hyperintensities *(open arrows)* and hyperintensity in the right caudate head *(closed arrow)* in an elderly patient with depression. (Courtesy of Figiel GS; from Drevets WC: *Brain imaging in psychiatry.* In Sierles FS, editor: *Behavioral science for medical students,* Baltimore, 1993, Williams and Wilkins.)

In contrast to these observations in elderly patients, white matter hyperintensities in young adults with bipolar disorder are not related to cardiovascular risk factors, age, past treatment, or illness duration. Moreover, increased rates of MRI signal hyperintensities have been reported in a study of children and adolescents with bipolar disorder. The cause of signal hyperintensities in young adults with bipolar disorder remains unclear, but it may differ from that associated with late-onset depression.

Implications of Structural Abnormalities for Functional Imaging Studies

The neuromorphometric abnormalities of ventricular enlargement in patients who are psychotic, elderly, or suffering from bipolar depression; reduced frontal lobe size in patients with bipolar depression or elderly patients with depression; and decreased amygdala size in subjects with bipolar depression may produce partial volume effects in or adjacent to these structures. Thus decreases in blood flow or metabolism in these areas in PET images from such subjects are difficult to interpret. Since studies evaluating young patients with unipolar depression who are not delusional or patients with unipolar depression characterized by a young age of onset have generally failed to identify these neuromorphometric abnormalities, the PET images from these groups must constitute the benchmark against which imaging findings in other depressive subtypes are compared. Nevertheless, preliminary evidence that even in young patients with unipolar depression the caudate and frontal lobe may be reduced in size indicates the importance of developing methods that correct PET measures for partial volume effects. This is particularly important for the caudate, where decreased blood flow and metabolism have been reported in young subjects with unipolar depression, which could reflect a partial volume effect of decreased caudate size.

The deep white matter and periventricular hyperintensities, caudate hyperintensities, and lacunar infarctions evident in the MRI images of elderly patients who are depressed present an even greater problem for functional imaging studies. Since these hyperintensities appear to reflect arteriosclerotic or ischemic areas based on postmortem and ^{31}P MRS evidence, they are presumably associated with reduced regional blood flow and metabolism on a cerebrovascular basis, irrespective of local synaptic activity. Consistent with the presence of ischemic and atherosclerotic changes, PET studies of elderly patients with depression demonstrate diffuse areas of decreased blood flow and metabolism in the frontal cortex and other cortical and subcortical areas (no attempt has been made in these studies to exclude subjects with MRI signal hyperintensities or lacunes). Since corrections for the effects of these lesions in PET images are not possible, functional imaging studies that include elderly subjects who are depressed and report areas of decreased blood flow or metabolism with respect to controls cannot be interpreted. In contrast, studies using such patients as their own controls by imaging them before and after treatment may provide interpretable information. For example, one group showed that in elderly patients with depression who were imaged before and after either ECT or antidepressant drug therapy, successful treatment resulted in a further decrement in blood flow in the left PFC. These findings converge with the findings in young patients who have unipolar depression, in whom left prefrontal activity is elevated in the depressed phase relative to the remitted phase and decreases during effective treatment (see Table 6-2).

Summary of Functional Imaging Findings in Mood Disorders

Abnormalities in the Prefrontal Cortex. The PFC comprises more than 40% of the human brain and contains numerous subdivisions based on anatomical connectivity and cytoarchitectonic distinctions. Additionally, lesion analyses, electrophysiological data, and PET studies indicate that the PFC has a myriad of functional components, with distinct areas activated during language, attention, memory, motor planning, and emotion. Therefore investigators must be as specific as possible when considering the location of PFC abnormalities.

Decreased blood flow and metabolism have been reported in the subgenual PFC (in the prelimbic portion of the anterior cingulate gyrus) of people with bipolar depression and people who have unipolar depression with FPDD. This abnormality could conceivably mediate the emotional, neurovegetative, autonomic, or neurochemical changes common to both unipolar and bipolar depression, since this region shares extensive connections with the lateral hypothalamus, the amygdala, the ventral striatum, and the midbrain nuclei that contain dopaminergic and serotoninergic neurons (see Chapter 8). Additionally, decreased blood flow and metabolism have been reported in both patients with unipolar depression and patients with bipolar depression in the dorsal anterolateral PFC, an abnormality that may be related to the neuropsychological impairment or cognitive slowing in depression.

In contrast, blood flow and metabolism are abnormally increased in the ventrolateral and orbital portions of the PFC and the pregenual portion of the anterior cingulate gyrus in unmedicated patients with primary unipolar depression (see Table 6-2 and Figure 6-8). These blood flow and metabolic increases in the ventral PFC are not found in all depressive subtypes, since patients who have bipolar depression, patients with unipolar depression who meet criteria for depressive spectrum disease (DSD), and patients with secondary depression have not demonstrated abnormal activity in the ventrolateral and lateral orbital portions of the PFC (see Chapter 8). Additionally, some elderly patients who are depressed and have late-onset depression have diffuse areas of decreased blood flow in the PFC (apparently accounted for by cerebrovascular changes). Nevertheless, in both young and elderly patients with unipolar depression, scans acquired in the asymptomatic state after successful treatment or spontaneous remission demonstrate that left ventral prefrontal activity is increased in the depressed phase relative to the remitted phase (that is, left prefrontal activity decreases during effective treatment).

The ventrolateral, orbital, and subgenual areas of the PFC are heavily connected with the amygdala, the ventral striatum, and the hypothalamus, areas that appear to participate in emotional processing or expression based on anatomical connectivity, electrophysiological data, and lesion analysis. Consistent with this evidence, PET images acquired during experimentally induced sadness and anxiety in subjects without depression or during induced anxiety and obsessional states in subjects with anxiety disorders demonstrate blood-flow increases in the ventrolateral, the ventromedial, and the orbital areas of the PFC and in the pregenual anterior cingulate gyrus. It is thus likely that the neuroimaging abnormalities found in these areas in depression are related to the core emotional and neurovegetative manifestations of mood disorders.

In contrast, the connectivity of the dorsolateral PFC and the types of cognitive tasks that activate this area make it difficult to relate to the core emotional features of depression. The dorsolateral PFC has sparse limbic connections with limbic structures (such as the amygdala), and areas of increased blood flow have generally not been reported in the dorsolateral PFC during emotional states. Instead, in the vicinity of the dorsal prefrontal areas where blood flow is decreased in depression, brain mapping studies in subjects without depression show blood-flow increases during tasks involving visuospatial memory, pictorial memory for visual objects, navigation of an unfamiliar maze, and manipulation of memorized verbal information (for example, word matching). It is thus unclear how decreased activity in the dorsolateral PFC in depression should be interpreted, though it could conceivably relate to some of the subtle neuropsychological impairments described in depression (for example, performance deficits on visuospatial tasks).

Decreased activity in the dorsal PFC in depression may reflect nonspecific slowing of cognitive processing. One group found that in both patients who were depressed and patients with schizophrenia, decreased blood flow in the dorsolateral PFC correlated with ratings of impoverished speech and thought content. This group proposed that the metabolic decreases in this region in a person with depression reflect depressive behaviors such as psychomotor retardation.

Alternatively, blood-flow decreases in the dorsolateral PFC in depression may reflect suppression of afferent transmission to nonlimbic regions while limbic structures engage in emotional processing. For example, during language processing, visuospatial attention, or maze navigation, blood flow decreases in the amygdala, the orbital cortex, and the pregenual anterior cingulate gyrus, areas where blood flow increases during emotional processing. Conversely, during severe anxiety and depressive states, blood flow decreases in the dorsal portion of the anterior cingulate gyrus, a region that is consistently activated during tasks requiring discriminative attention. These and other similar functional imaging observations support electrophysiological and behavioral data indicating that mechanisms exist in the brain for allocating cognitive processing resources by suppressing transmission to areas that are not immediately required for anticipated mental operations.

Abnormalities in Subcortical Structures. Functional anatomical abnormalities have also been reported in subcortical areas that share anatomical connections with the ventral and medial PFC. In the caudate, blood flow and glucose metabolism have been reported to be abnormally decreased in patients with unipolar, but not those with bipolar, depression. One morphometric MRI study demonstrated that the caudate volume is decreased in patients with unipolar depression relative to controls, suggesting that the abnormal reduction in caudate flow and metabolism in the PET images from such subjects could reflect a partial volume effect. In contrast to the findings in patients with unipolar depression, preliminary data in patients who have bipolar depression indicate that metabolism is increased in the ventral striatum regardless of the clinical phase in which subjects are scanned.

In patients who have unipolar depression with FPDD (see Chapter 8), blood flow and metabolism are abnormally increased in the left amygdala and the left medial thalamus, structures that share anatomical connections with the aforementioned ventral prefrontal and striatal regions (see Figure 8-1). In the left amygdala, regional blood flow appears abnormally elevated in both the depressed and the unmedicated or asymptomatic phases of FPDD, suggesting that the amygdala abnormality in FPDD could be related to the susceptibility to depressive episodes. Administration of antidepressant drugs to either subjects who are depressed or control subjects who are not depressed results in decreases in amygdala glucose metabolism, compatible with evidence in experimental animals that antidepressant drugs reduce both glucose uptake and neuronal firing rates in the amygdala. It is hypothesized that the depressant effect of these agents on amygdala function underlies their ability to both ameliorate and prevent depressive episodes.

Implications of Neuroimaging Findings: Anatomical Circuits Related to Mood Disorders. The neuroimaging data in primary and secondary mood disorders converge with evidence from lesion analyses to implicate circuits involving the ventral and medial PFC, as well as limbic structures such as the amygdala and related parts of the striatum and thalamus, in the pathophysiology of mood disorders (see Chapters 8 and 26). For example, the findings in patients with unipolar depression who have FPDD of abnormally increased blood flow and metabolism in the ventrolateral and orbital portions of the PFC, the amygdala, and the medial thalamus, coupled with indications of reduced flow in the medial caudate, suggest that two interconnected circuits are involved in the pathophysiology of FPDD: a limbic-thalamic-cortical circuit involving the amygdala, the mediodorsal nucleus of the thalamus (in the medial thalamus), and the ventral PFC; and a limbic-striatal-pallidal-thalamic circuit involving related parts of the striatum and the ventral pallidum as well as the components of the other circuit (see Figure 8-1). The amygdala and the PFC regions are interconnected by excitatory projections with each other and with the mediodorsal nucleus of the thalamus. Increased metabolic activity in the amygdala, the medial thalamus, and the PFC would presumably reflect increased synaptic activity in these areas, suggesting that synaptic transmission through the limbic-thalamic-cortical circuit is abnormally elevated in FPDD. Consistent with this hypothesis, neurosurgical procedures that ameliorate treatment-resistant depression interrupt projections within the limbic-thalamic-cortical or the limbic-striatal-pallidal-thalamic circuits. In ventral frontal lobe tissue removed from depressed patients undergoing these neurosurgical treatments, excitatory amino acid neurotransmitter concentrations are abnormally elevated, supporting the hypothesis of increased limbic-thalamic-cortical transmission. Antidepressant drugs may also compensate for the pathophysiology of FPDD by suppressing limbic-thalamic-cortical activity, since antidepressant drug administration is associated with decreased blood flow and metabolism in the amygdala, the ventral PFC, and the medial thalamus.

Clinical Correlations with Prefrontal and Amygdala Function. The functional imaging data gathered during depression in subjects with mood disorders and in control subjects during experimentally induced emotional states converge with the results of lesion analyses and single-unit recording studies to suggest specialized roles for the ventral PFC and the amygdala in depression. In the amygdala, regional blood flow and metabolism correlate positively with ratings of depression severity. The amygdala has been implicated by single-unit and lesion studies in assigning emotional significance to experiential stimuli. The associations formed in the amygdala between reinforcement and sensory stimuli are long lasting, and extinction of the behavioral responses to the associations formed in the amygdala may depend on modulatory projections from the ventral PFC.

In the left ventrolateral PFC and lateral orbital cortex, blood flow and metabolism are abnormally elevated during the depressed state of unipolar depression, but they are inversely correlated with ratings of depression severity and negative thought frequency. Similarly, PET studies performed in control subjects during induced sadness and in subjects with obsessive-compulsive disorder (OCD) or animal phobia during exposure to phobic stimuli have shown that blood flow increases in the orbital cortex during emotional induction. In each case, the magnitude of the blood-flow change correlates negatively with ratings of negative thought and emotion. These findings are consistent with electrophysiological data indicating that the orbital cortex plays a role in correcting behavioral responses that become inappropriate as reinforcement contingencies change. Impairment of this function associated with ventral prefrontal lesions results in perseveration of responses that are nonrewarded or nonreinforced. Ventral prefrontal damage may also result in perseveration within the emotional domain, since medial orbital damage interferes with the extinction of conditioned fear responses in experimental animals. Taken together, these observations suggest that parts of the ventral PFC are specifically activated in depressive and anxiety states to modulate or inhibit negative emotional responses or thought patterns.

The apparent functions of the amygdala and the ventral PFC suggest a model of depression in which the amygdala assigns negative emotional associations with thoughts, social interactions, or sensory stimuli and the ventral PFC mediates attempts to break these associations and convert nonrewarding thoughts or behaviors to rewarding ones. This model could account for biological heterogeneity, since the depressive syndrome could arise from dysfunction within either the amygdala or the PFC. For example, abnormally increased amygdala activity in FPDD may yield a state where negative affective labels are inappropriately assigned to all stimuli, or where neurons storing negative associations are excessively activated and as a consequence the left ventral PFC becomes activated to break these nonrewarding associations. In contrast to FPDD, other depressive subtypes may be associated with dysfunction within the ventral PFC so the ability to appropriately shift emotional or cognitive sets is impaired, resulting in perseveration of melancholic thoughts or emotions. This could account for the propensity of cerebrovascular lesions of the left PFC to induce a major depressive episode in poststroke or late-onset depressive syndromes. This hypothesis addresses the apparent paradox that orbital blood flow and metabolism are elevated in primary unipolar depression but reduced in some cases of secondary depression.

Imaging Neuroreceptors and Neurotransmitter Synthesis in Mood Disorders

One study of bipolar disorder showed that patients who are psychotic have an abnormally increased density of D_2-like dopamine receptor sites, as measured by $[^{11}C]$N-methylspiperone binding. This abnormality was present in patients with schizophrenia who were psychotic but absent in subjects with bipolar disorder who were not psychotic, suggesting it served as a correlate of psychosis rather than disordered mood. Consistent with this hypothesis, D_2 density correlated with psychosis ratings but not mood ratings in subjects with bipolar disorder who were psychotic. In another study, subjects with bipolar disorder had decreased affinity for dopamine D_1 receptors relative to controls, regardless of the clinical phase in which subjects were scanned.

In subjects with unipolar depression, one group imaged the uptake of a radiolabeled serotonin precursor, $[^{11}C]$5-hydroxytryptophan. Uptake was increased in the patients with depression relative to the controls in a ventromedial prefrontal area that included the pregenual anterior cingulate gyrus. Regional blood flow was increased in this area in patients with unipolar depression who had FPDD (see Figure 6-8).

Anxiety Disorders

The nature of anxiety disorders permits the acquisition of scans within a single session in both a resting condition and a state in which the anxiety syndrome is elicited or exacerbated. Moreover, by scanning during repeated anxiety inductions, in which patients typically develop the capacity to inhibit the fear response, functional imaging can be used to investigate the mechanisms of habituation. Finally, since psychiatrically healthy subjects can also experience anxiety, the anatomical correlates of experimentally induced anxiety can be compared in normal vs. pathological anxiety.

Obsessive Compulsive Disorder

Structural imaging studies have reported conflicting findings in caudate size in subjects with OCD. One study of adults with childhood-onset OCD reported that the caudate volume is abnormally reduced, whereas another study of adults with OCD found that the right caudate volume is abnormally increased. Other investigators found no significant differences between patients with OCD and control groups.

Most functional imaging studies of OCD found increased blood flow and glucose metabolism in the orbital gyri bilaterally, which in most studies decreases toward normal during effective treatment with antidepressant drugs. Some studies also reported that metabolic activity is abnormally increased in the caudate and the anterior cingulate gyrus. During symptom provocation by exposure to relevant phobic stimuli (for example, contact with soiled towels for patients with germ phobias), blood flow increases further in the orbital cortex, the caudate, and the anterior cingulate cortex. Thus the baseline metabolic changes may simply reflect the physiological concomitants of obsessive-compulsive symptoms or chronic anxiety. This observation is relevant to the interpretation of a study in which caudate metabolism decreased in subjects with OCD during either pharmacological or behavioral treatment. This reduction in caudate metabolism was only induced by effective treatment with either modality (that is, caudate metabolism was unchanged in people who did not respond to either treatment), suggesting that it reflects a physiological correlate of symptom resolution rather than a primary physical effect of treatment.

An intriguing study of secondary OCD described several cases of necrosis of the globus pallidus associated with induced obsessional symptoms. The PET images of these patients demonstrated decreased—rather than increased—metabolism in the ventral PFC. This case resembles the literature on depression, where primary unipolar depression is associated with increases in ventral prefrontal blood flow or metabolism (see Table 6-2), but secondary depression induced by some basal ganglia disorders has been associated with decreases in ventral prefrontal metabolism.

The similarities between the imaging findings in primary OCD and primary unipolar depression in the ventral PFC illustrate a case where two distinct disorders may involve an overlapping neural circuit, potentially accounting for the clinical features shared by both disorders. OCD and unipolar depression are distinct in their courses, prognoses, genetics, and neurochemical and neuroendocrine concomitants, and PET imaging data in some regions outside the ventral PFC differ between unipolar depression and OCD. Nevertheless, substantial co-morbidity exists between these disorders, since the major depressive syndrome arises in approximately 70% of patients with OCD and pathological obsessions can arise in unipolar depression. Moreover, the pharmacological and neurosurgical interventions that ameliorate OCD also effectively treat unipolar depression. Finally, the clinical phenomenology of unipolar depression and OCD is similar, since both conditions are characterized by persistent, intrusive, nonrewarding, or painful thoughts with an inability to switch to goal-oriented, rewarding, cognitive-behavioral sets.

The neuroimaging literature provides insight into these clinical similarities by implicating the cortical-striatal-pallidal-thalamic circuitry in the pathophysiology of both disorders (see above). This circuitry in general appears to be involved in the organization of internally guided behavior toward a reward, switching of response strategies, and habit formation. The cortical area of this circuit where activity is abnormally elevated in both OCD and unipolar depression is the medial orbital cortex, which appears to participate in correcting behavioral responses that have become inappropriate as reinforcement contingencies change. Dysfunction within the cortical-striatal-pallidal-thalamic circuit that interferes with the role of the orbital cortex could conceivably underlie the inability to inhibit unrewarded thoughts and behaviors in both disorders.

Panic Disorder

Patients with panic disorder have been scanned before and during panic attacks elicited by intravenous sodium lactate infusion. During the panic attack, regional blood-flow increases were identified in the anterior insula, the anteromedial cerebellum, and the midbrain. Blood flow also increases in these regions in subjects with animal phobias during exposure to the feared animal and in subjects without a specific phobia during the threat of a painful electrical shock, suggesting that the blood-flow increases in these regions reflect correlates of fear processing in general. Areas of increased blood flow are also evident in PET images in the facial muscles (for example, the temporalis and the masseter muscles) during panic attacks and other anxiety states, which in early PET studies were mistakenly described as being located in the pole of the temporal lobe (Figure 6-11).

The resting state in panic disorder is usually characterized by mild to moderate levels of chronic anxiety (termed *anticipatory anxiety*). In the resting state of panic disorder, blood flow is abnormally increased in an area of the midbrain (apparently the same area where blood flow further increases during lactate-induced panic) that contains multiple nuclei implicated in fear behavior (for example, the central gray nucleus), and blood flow and metabolism are elevated in the right lateral orbital cortex and the anterior insular cortex. In each of these areas, blood-flow increases have been reported in acute fear states, suggesting that the abnormalities observed in the anticipatory anxiety phase of panic disorder reflect activation of regions generally involved in anxiety processing. Regional blood flow and metabolism decrease in these areas, as well as in the anterior cingulate gyrus, during effective antipanic or antianxiety pharmacotherapy.

Simple Animal Phobia

Two recent studies have identified the functional anatomical correlates of phobic anxiety by acquiring blood-flow scans during exposures to the feared animal (for example, a snake). During the initial fearful scans, flow increases in the lateral orbital and anterior insular cortex bilaterally, the anteromedial cerebellum, and the pregenual portion of the anterior cingulate gyrus (see Figure 6-11). Blood flow increases in these areas in other anxiety states, suggesting that these changes reflect general correlates of anxiety processing.

In one of these studies, scans were acquired across enough exposures for habituation to develop during the scan session. Following the development of habituation, the magnitude of the blood-flow responses in the lateral orbital and anterior insular regions and the cerebellum diminished during exposures to the phobic stimulus, and blood flow increased in the left posterior orbital cortex in an area where blood flow had not changed during exposures that preceded habituation (Figure 6-12). Blood flow increases have also been identified in the posterior orbital cortex in subjects with no anxiety disorder during anxious anticipation of an electrical shock and in subjects with OCD during exposure to relevant phobic stimuli, suggesting that this region normally becomes activated during the anxiety syndrome. In all three studies (anxiety induction in subjects without anxiety disorders, subjects with animal phobias, and subjects with OCD), the increase in posterior orbital blood flow correlated negatively with anxiety or obsessional ratings, suggesting that the posterior orbital cortex plays a role in inhibiting anxiety responses. This hypothesis is compatible with single-unit recording and lesion studies in experimental animals, which show that orbital neurons subserve a mechanism for inhibiting behavioral responses to stimuli that are no longer reinforced, and that lesions of the posterior orbital cortex prevent extinction of the fear responses to conditioned stimuli. Taken together, these observations suggest the hypothesis that in simple animal phobia the posterior orbital cortex, an area that normally functions to extinguish fear responses to nonreinforced stimuli, fails to become acti-

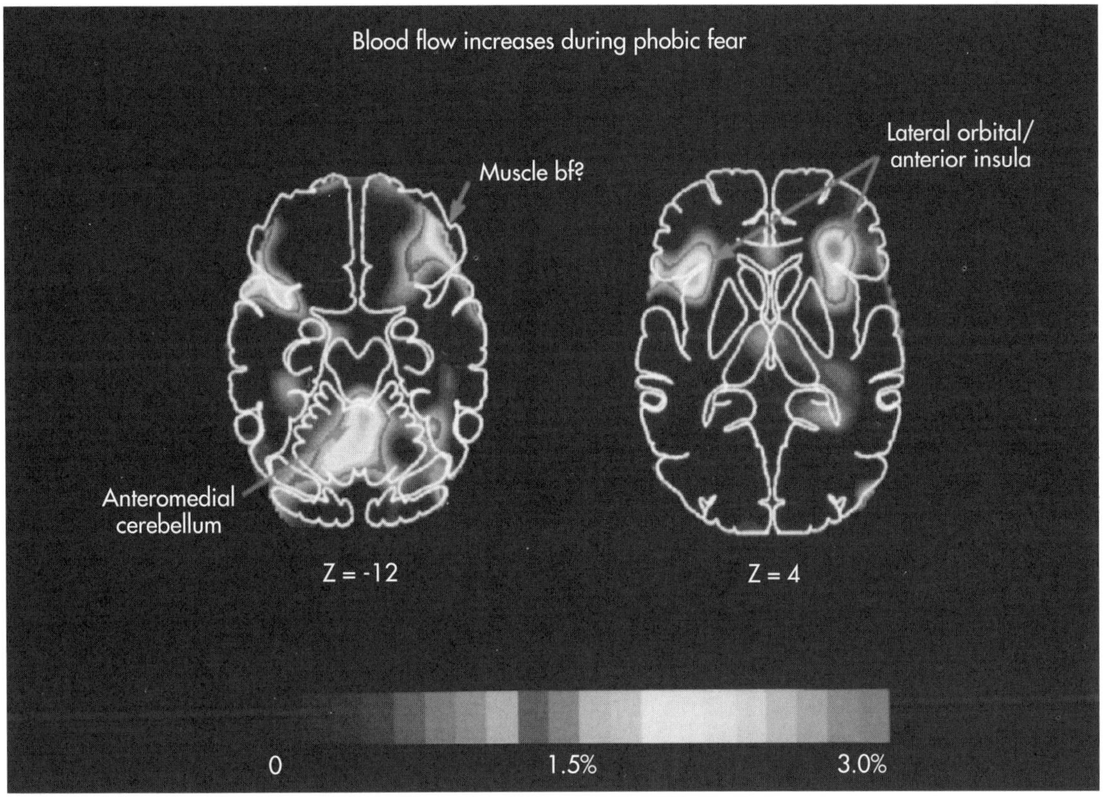

FIGURE 6-11 Regional blood flow increases in the lateral orbital and anterior insular cortex bilaterally and the anteromedial cerebellum during phobic anxiety. Blood flow also increases in these areas in subjects with panic disorder during a lactate-induced panic attack and in normal subjects during anxious anticipation of a painful electrical shock. The image shown is a composite image depicting the average changes in blood flow in the fearful condition relative to the nonfearful control condition from a group of subjects with simple animal phobias. Phobic anxiety was elicited by exposing subjects to a relevant phobic stimulus (such as a snake or a tarantula). The area of increased blood flow marked *Blood flow (bf)* has its center of mass located outside the brain over the temporalis and masseter muscles, where teeth clenching also produces increases in blood flow. This response presumably reflects increased flow in the facial muscles during anxiety, which is commonly seen in PET studies that involve anxiety induction. Only the medial edge of the blurred representation of this muscle blood-flow change is evident in this image section, which has been templated to exclude pixels outside the mean brain boundary. The patient's left is on the left side of the image, and the anterior aspect is toward the top. The color bar indicates the percentage of change in regional blood flow from the anxious condition to the control condition. The Z-coordinate provides the position (in mm) of each horizontal image plane relative to a plane containing the anterior and posterior commissures, with positive indicating the dorsal plane and negative indicating the ventral plane. (From Drevets WC et al: *J Cereb Blood Flow Metab* 15:S856, 1995b.)

vated during exposure to a specific animal type. However, repeated exposure to the phobic object facilitates the ability to activate the posterior orbital cortex, permitting inhibition of the fear response to the nonreinforced stimulus. This process could conceivably underlie the mechanism for the therapeutic effect of systematic desensitization.

Cocaine Dependence

Acute administration of cocaine produces a decrease in cerebral blood flow that particularly occurs in the frontal cortex. Other euphoriants (such as alcohol) produce similar effects acutely. In subjects who are cocaine-dependent, PET and SPECT studies reveal patchy perfusion defects in multiple areas of the cortex and the basal ganglia that persist for several weeks after cessation of cocaine use. These defects are more likely to be apparent in subjects who are dependent on both cocaine and alcohol than in subjects who are dependent on cocaine alone. In the areas where these perfusion defects are found, local blood flow decreases further during acute cocaine administration.

Neuroreceptor imaging has been used to assess the effects of chronic cocaine abuse on postsynaptic dopamine receptors and dopamine reuptake sites. PET studies demonstrate that chronic cocaine use results in downregulation of dopamine D_2-receptor density in the striatum for up to 1 month after cessation of

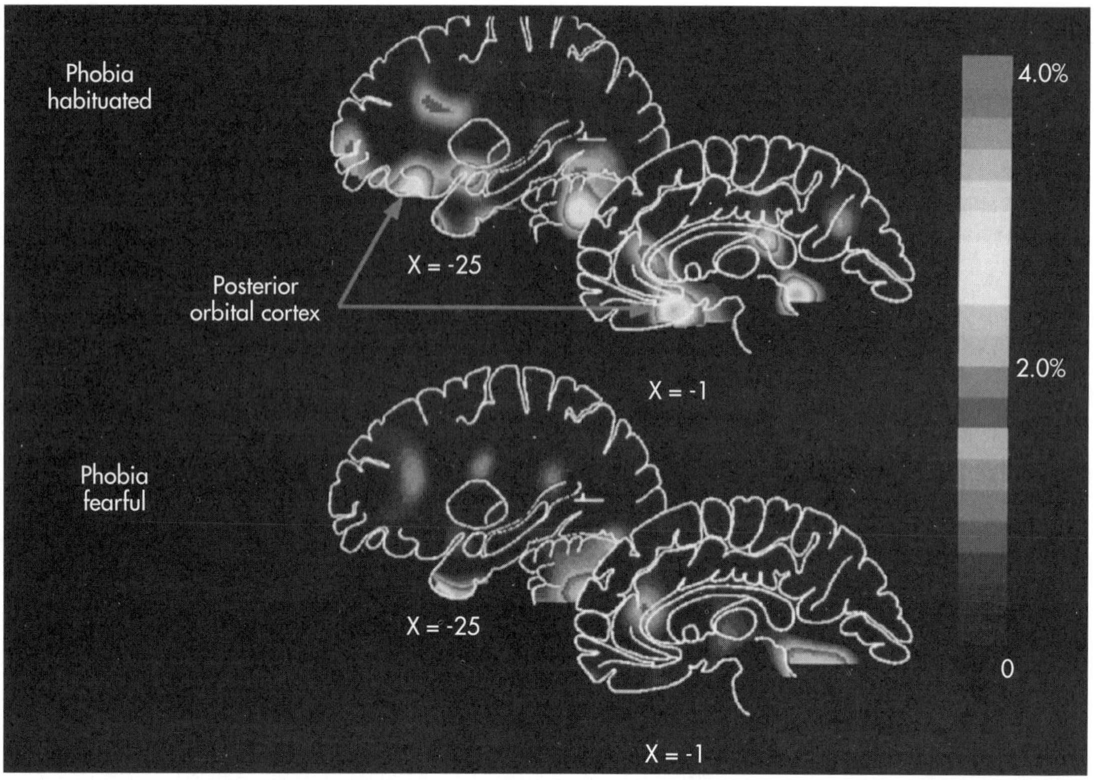

FIGURE 6-12 Habituation to a phobic stimulus was accompanied by the development of a blood-flow response in the posteromedial orbital cortex during repeated exposure to a phobic stimulus *(phobia habituated)*. The magnitude of the blood-flow change in this region correlated inversely with the accompanying changes in heart rate and anxiety ratings. In contrast, blood flow did not change in this area in the same subjects scanned during initial exposures to the same animal *(phobia fearful)*. The images shown are from the study described in Figure 6-11, with the habituated state referring to scans acquired during the fourth or fifth exposures to the animal when a markedly attenuated anxiety response was obtained relative to the initial exposures. Regional blood-flow changes during the initial exposures are reflected by the *phobia fearful* image slices here and by the image sections in Figure 6-11. In PET studies involving normal subjects and subjects with OCD who are exposed to anxiety-provoking stimuli, blood flow increases in the posteromedial cortex during the initial exposure to anxiogenic stimuli, with the magnitude of the blood-flow rise correlating inversely with symptom ratings. This inverse correlation is consistent with evidence from electrophysiological and lesion analysis studies suggesting that the posteromedial orbital cortex functions to inhibit or modulate nonreinforced anxiety responses. Subjects with phobias fail to activate this region until they have undergone repeated in vivo exposure to the phobic stimulus (as applied during the process of systematic desensitization, the treatment of choice for simple phobia). After the development of habituation, this region is successfully activated. Possibly in relation to this neurophysiological change, the anxiety response to the nonreinforced stimulus can be inhibited. The anterior side is toward the left of the illustration. The color bar indicates the percentage of change in regional blood flow from the anxious condition to the control condition. The X-coordinate provides the position (in mm) of each sagittal image plane relative to the midline, with negative X indicating left. (From Drevets WC et al: *J Cereb Blood Flow Metab* 15:S856, 1995b.)

cocaine use, consistent with evidence obtained in experimental animals. In cocaine users imaged after 1 month or more of abstinence, [^{18}F]-N-methylspiroperidol uptake in the striatum does not differ with respect to controls, suggesting that the density of postsynaptic dopamine receptors recovers from the effects of cocaine after a drug-free interval. SPECT imaging of the dopamine transporter using iodinated β-CIT, a cocaine analogue, shows abnormally increased density of these sites in subjects who are cocaine dependent, consistent with postmortem studies in cocaine abusers dying of overdose. Taken together, these findings suggest that chronic use of cocaine, which binds to dopamine transporter sites and blocks dopamine reuptake, results in downregulation of postsynaptic D_2 sites and upregulation of dopamine transporter sites. In the absence of repeated cocaine exposure, this state may produce a functional dopaminergic deficiency in the reward-related mesolimbic dopamine system, manifested by depressed mood, anhedonia, and cocaine craving.

Other Neuropsychiatric Disorders

Tourette's Disorder

MRI studies of adults and children with Tourette's disorder have reported decreased volume of the left basal ganglia and loss of the normal asymmetry between right and left basal ganglia structures with respect to controls. The basal ganglia have been implicated in the pathophysiology of this syndrome by other types of information. In addition to the motor and vocal tics that are the hallmark of Tourette's syndrome, a high proportion of patients with this disorder manifest obsessions and compulsions. In contrast to the functional imaging findings in primary OCD, the PET images of patients with Tourette's disorder show decreased metabolism in the ventral PFC and the caudate, providing another example in which the functional anatomy differs between a primary psychiatric disorder and a basal ganglia disorder that induces a clinically similar neuropsychiatric syndrome. The propensity of dysfunction in neural circuits formed by the basal ganglia, the thalamus, and the PFC for maintaining pathological cognitive and behavioral responses, manifested clinically by obsessive thoughts and compulsive behaviors, is discussed on pp. 76 and 77.

Attention-Deficit/Hyperactivity Disorder

Three MRI studies of children with attention-deficit/hyperactivity disorder (ADHD) have reported abnormal reductions in the size of the corpus callosum, which in one study correlated with classroom ratings of hyperactivity. Abnormal caudate asymmetry has also been reported in children with ADHD, and one group found that children with ADHD fail to demonstrate the normal developmental decrement in caudate volume over the preadolescent and adolescent years. A preliminary PET imaging study of [^{18}F]-fluorodopa uptake also implicated the striatum in ADHD, finding abnormally reduced uptake in the putamen. The potential importance of this finding is highlighted by the beneficial effects of agents that enhance dopamine function (such as methylphenidate) in treating ADHD.

Autistic Disorder

In a majority of subjects with autistic disorder the area of the cerebellar vermis has been found to be abnormally reduced in MRI images, a finding compatible with postmortem evidence that the numbers of Purkinje's and granule cells are abnormally reduced in the cerebellum of a person with autistic disorder. However, MRI studies have also suggested that a minority of subjects with autistic disorder have abnormal enlargement of the cerebellar vermis. Reduced parietal lobe size and increased incidence of developmental cortical malformations such as polymicrogyria, macrogyria, or schizencephaly have also been reported in autistic disorder.

Annotated Bibliography

Cohen MS, Bookheimer SY: Localization of brain function using magnetic resonance imaging, *Trends Neurosci* 17:268-77, 1994.
This article provides an overview of the technology development in and potential research applications of fMRI.

Keshavan MS et al: Magnetic resonance spectroscopy in psychiatry: potential, pitfalls and promise, *Am J Psychiatry* 148:976-984, 1991.
This article provides a review of MRS methodology. Included is a review of MRS applications in psychiatry to date and a discussion of future potential.

Pearlson GD, Marsh L: *Magnetic resonance imaging in psychiatry.* In Oldham JM, Riba MB, Tasman A, editors: *Review of psychiatry,* vol 12, Washington, D.C., 1993, American Psychiatric Press.
This is a review of current findings from structural MRI investigations of psychiatric disorders and discusses relevant technological and methodological issues.

Raichle ME: *Circulatory and metabolic correlates of brain function in normal humans.* In Brookhart JM, Mountcastle VB, editors: *Handbook of physiology: the nervous system,* vol V, Baltimore Md., 1977, American Physiology Society.
This is an overview of functional imaging that critically assesses the modalities available for blood flow and metabolism imaging and discusses constraints on the design and interpretation of brain-mapping experiments that relate to the nature of these physiological signals.

Zigun J, Weinberger D: *In vivo studies of brain morphology in schizophrenia.* In Lindenmayer JP, Kay SR, editors: *New biological vistas of brain morphology in schizophrenia,* New York, 1992, Brunner/Mazel.
This chapter reviews CT and MRI investigations of schizophrenia.

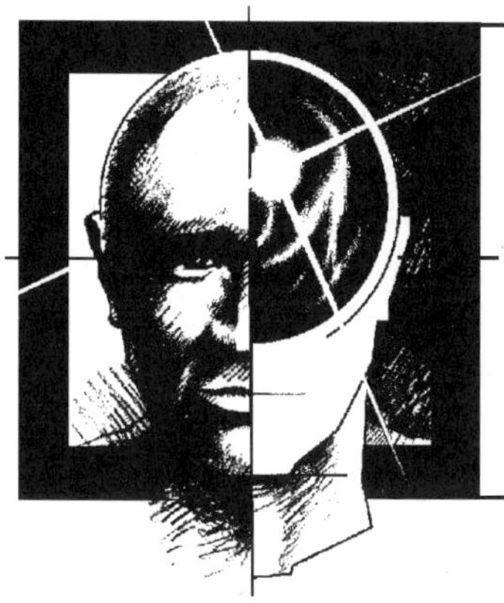

chapter 7

Referral of Patients: Mental Health Professionals; Family and Community Resources

Barry A. Hong, PhD, Barbara A. Koppe, MSW, and Richard W. Hudgens, MD

Recognition and Treatment of Psychiatric Disorders: Role of the Primary Care Physician

Most Americans who have psychiatric disorders are not treated for them, either because they do not seek help or because their illnesses are not diagnosed if they do seek help. When they do come to physicians with complaints, most of them go to their primary care physicians. If their illnesses are recognized and treated at all, it is usually by those same physicians and not by psychiatrists or other mental health professionals. Findings from the Epidemiologic Catchment Area Study, a comprehensive survey of psychiatric disorders, demonstrate that it is primary care physicians who are the front line of the mental health system in the United States.

Great numbers of people need psychiatric treatment. Physicians in the practice of general medicine are familiar with this fact because a large proportion of their patients have emotional complaints. Results of research confirm this; some recent studies of depression in general medical practices estimate depressive symptoms in 41% of medical patients studied over 6 months. In another epidemiological investigation, almost 10% of the population had significant depressive symptoms and 6% had general anxiety disorder (GAD) at some time in their lives.

The first task faced by the physician is diagnosis. This is made more difficult because patients rarely volunteer the complete story of their psychiatric problems. It is common for people to have complex histories, and they often have more than one psychiatric disorder, or a co-morbid condition. When they do, they may give an account of only one disorder. Thus patients who are depressed may tell of their depressive symptoms but not discuss their phobias, obsessions, or excessive drinking. Disruptions with work and family relationships may also go unmentioned by the patient and unnoticed by the doctor, even when a psychiatric illness has been identified. The physician must take a complete history to supplement the patient's spontaneous account. Only in that way will he diagnose the illness, understand its complexities, and make an informed decision about which patients to treat and which patients to refer to a psychiatrist or other mental health professional.

Which Psychiatric Patients Are Treated by Primary Care Physicians?

The answer to this question depends on the individual physician and the degree of his interest and comfort in treating psychiatric disorders, the amount of time available for dealing with problems that are time consuming, the availability of mental health professionals in the community, and the degree of the physician's confidence in those professionals. Primary care physicians who are the only resource in a large area find themselves treating more people with psychiatric illness than their colleagues in large cities.

In general, primary care physicians often treat patients who have symptoms of depression, anxiety, and obsessions, and complaints of physical symptoms in the absence of objective findings. They refer such patients to psychiatrists or other mental health professionals only when the symptoms do not improve or when the patients begin to take up a disproportionate amount of time. For these reasons primary care doctors need to be skilled in the use of several types of antidepressant, antiobsessional, and anxiolytic (tranquilizer) drugs. It is not unusual for a psychiatrist to receive the referral of a patient with depression who is considered a treatment failure after only one antidepressant has been tried and that at a dose so low that generally no response could be expected.

People with disruptive or bizarre behavior or people with delusions or hallucinations, whatever the psychiatric diagnosis, are rarely treated by their family physicians. The same is true for those who are *recognized* as suicidal or as having primarily drug or alcohol dependence (suicidal potential and drug or alcohol dependence often go unrecognized). Primary care physicians also seldom manage patients whose psychiatric disorders are of a type or severity requiring treatment with drugs that they are unaccustomed to prescribing, such as antipsychotic drugs or the mood stabilizer, lithium. At the other end of the severity spectrum, family physicians, irrespective of their degree of interest in psychiatry, almost always refer patients elsewhere for psychotherapy or for marriage and family counseling.

Preparing the Patient for a Mental Health Referral

Many patients are reluctant to ask for help with emotional problems or to begin treatment with a mental health professional. The primary care physician can do much to facilitate a successful mental health referral by assuming the appropriate attitude and behavior. First, the referring physician can reassure the patient that mental health and physical health are related and of equivalent importance. Second, she should be clear to the patient and to the mental health professional about the purposes of the referral. If the primary care physician is asking advice or guidance from a mental health professional, this perspective should be understood by the patient and the referral source. Should the patient be referred to a psychiatrist or to a nonmedical therapist? Will this patient benefit from marital therapy? Is this grief reaction abnormal?

In other situations, the primary care physician and the patient both request formal assessment and treatment. The referral mental health professional informs the primary care physician when the patient has been seen and that treatment will or will not begin. In some cases, assessment and treatment may be seen differently by the referring and primary physicians. Differences may occur because of different methods of assessment; for example, a person judged to be depressed by the primary physician may fall far short of fulfilling a psychiatrist's criteria for major depressive illness. In all instances, the confidentiality of the patient's information is respected. It is customary for psychiatrists and other mental health professionals to acknowledge that they have evaluated the patient referred to them and to give the information that the referring physician needs to know. However, if more detailed information about the assessment or treatment is to be sent to the referring physician, a formal release of information should be obtained. Even in those cases, personal information unconnected to medical aspects of the case is almost never disclosed. Patients should clearly understand these different types of referral so they can have full confidence in their treatment professionals.

Types of Mental Health Professionals

For the referral to be most beneficial to the patient, the primary care physician must be informed about the different types of mental health professionals available in the community and know what to expect from them. Referrals are often limited to a narrow range of professional acquaintances or by the patient's preference or bias (for example, the patient may say, "I'm not crazy," or "I won't take a drug that will affect my mind"). The problem is also vexing when considering a psychotherapy referral (as opposed to a referral to a psychiatrist for medication), since any type of mental health professional may be competent to provide psychotherapy.

The various types of professionals are described in brief, and their unique mental health training and skills are noted.

Psychiatrists are licensed physicians, doctors of medicine (MDs) or osteopathy (DOs), who admit patients to hospitals, order laboratory tests, and prescribe medications. Psychiatrists have completed medical school, a 1-year internship, and a 3-year residency program in psychiatry (usually 4 years for child psychiatry). Their expertise is the assessment and treatment of the whole range of psychiatric problems, particularly the most acute and severe psychiatric problems that might necessitate the resources of a hospital. Psychiatrists are also experts in differentiating psychiatric disorders that may in fact present as a medical illness. They may specialize in addition to their general clinical training. Specialties include forensic psychiatry, geriatric psychiatry, child psychiatry, psychopharmacology, alcohol and drug abuse, and other areas.

Psychologists are licensed providers of psychological services. They are generally trained at a doctoral level and have received a doctor of philosophy (PhD) degree from a university or a doctor of psychology (PsyD) degree from a professional school of psychology. Not all psychologists with doctoral training are eligible to provide psychological services. Psychologists who are clinically trained take additional clinical practicum courses in graduate school to prepare to become providers of psychological services, and they complete a year-long internship as part of their PhD training. Psychologists and psychiatrists are by law the only mental health professionals who can diagnose and treat mental disorders. Psychologists do not prescribe medications (although legislation has been introduced in some states that would permit them to do this), but they provide psychological services in hospitals and medical centers as hospital-based providers or as independent practitioners in the community. Training in psychology covers a wide range of psychological schools and theories, making psychologists skilled in more than one modality of psychotherapy. All states require psychologists to be licensed to practice.

In addition to their role in the treatment of patients, psychologists also perform cognitive and neurological assessments. Most clinical psychologists assess for cognitive function by means of tests and a clinical interview. *Neuropsychology* is a subspecialty of psychology for which psychologists have taken advanced training in brain-behavior relationships beyond the usual training of most clinical psychologists. Neuropsychologists work with other psychologists, psychiatrists, and neurologists to assess cognitive problems, including dementia and memory, attention, learning, and communication (that is, aphasia) disorders. In some communities, cognitive and neuropsychological assessment is available on a sliding scale basis through the clinical psychology departments of some universities.

Social workers, who have completed 2 years of postgraduate training for the master of social work (MSW) degree, are licensed in all states to provide social work services in agencies, hospitals, and independent practice. Because of their training in human service administration, community organization, and direct client services (that is, individual and group psychotherapy), social workers often direct or work in community organizations for the mentally ill or emotionally disturbed. Medical social workers work in hospitals coordinating human and financial resources. Additionally, they often provide brief individual counseling to medical or psychiatric patients. Psychiatric social workers have generally received specialized mental health training during social work school. It is also not uncommon for psychiatric social workers to have completed advanced training in psychotherapy beyond the MSW degree.

Nurses have an increasing role in the treatment of psychiatric patients beyond their traditional work on hospital staffs. Specialty training beyond the bachelor of science or registered nursing training qualifies them as, for example, advanced practice nurses or clinical nurse specialists. These nurses can work with psychiatrists in the initial medical and psychiatric assessments of patients, and in some jurisdictions they can even prescribe medication under supervision.

Marital and family therapists have become specialists among mental health providers. Generally, individuals, couples, or families who have communication or role problems are prime candidates for this type of therapy. The "patient" is usually the couple or the family unit. Assessment often includes the use of genograms, or family maps, that help trace the themes or generational markers of family psychotherapy. Psychologists and social workers, and less often psychiatrists, also conduct marital and family therapy, although psychiatric social workers and members of the clergy trained in pastoral counseling account for the majority of practitioners in this area. Formal training programs in marital and family therapy exist, and there are specific licensing requirements for such therapists in increasing numbers of states. Marital and family therapists may belong to the American Association of Marriage and Family Therapists (AAMFT). Therapists may often list AAMFT as their practice credential along with state licensure. Many clergy members who are therapists are members of the American Association of Pastoral Counselors (AAPC), a national organization that certifies religious counselors. Most mental health providers do not claim this as a specialty unless they have special interest and training.

Employee assistance programs (EAPs) work for businesses, companies, and industry. In these programs, mental health professionals, who are usually MSWs, work with individual employees in crisis or serve as the intermediary for a mental health referral. In many instances, an EAP counselor only sees an individual for a brief assessment and makes a referral if necessary. In other cases, the EAP counselor sees an employee for a brief number of psychotherapy interviews, usually six sessions or fewer. If a patient works for a company that provides EAP services, this may be a good starting point for a mental health referral. The EAP counselor is generally aware of community resources and knows about insurance coverage for mental health services. However, because of the relationship of an EAP counselor to an employee's company, some patients may be reluctant to use these services because they fear compromised confidentiality. In these cases, physicians should respect the patient's wishes and work toward other alternatives.

Some primary care physicians may not know specific mental health referral sources or may practice in an area with few mental health specialists. For these physicians, community resources still exist. The social work department of the county or of a local hospital is an important resource. The hospital social worker knows about other local resources and should be aware of "out-of-the-area" sources of help. In urban areas, a mental health association can provide information about providers, community agencies, and counseling programs with a sliding fee scale. For patients who at times need a "listening ear," mental health hotline and life-crisis phone services or suicide prevention hot lines can be valuable resources. Besides assisting with an acute problem, calls to the hot line can aid in referral to a mental health professional. The hot line can also send the police or paramedics to intervene in a suicide or serious threat of suicide. In some cases the primary care physician may need to call the police or paramedics.

Regional areas are often served by community mental health centers that are staffed by multidisciplinary mental health professionals and include the services of a psychiatrist. These centers provide acute and chronic care to the mentally ill and those in emotional crisis. They also provide community education and consultation. The centers especially encourage collaboration with primary care physicians.

There is a detailed discussion of various community resources in the second half of this chapter.

Some Special Referral Situations

Risk of Suicide or Homicide

Suicidal and homicidal behavior and communications should always be treated seriously by any physician. The referral of care to a psychiatrist is almost always indicated in those cases. A physician should never consider a suicide threat as a mere call for help or conclude that people who speak about suicide do not commit the act. A verbal agreement or contract with the patient not to commit suicide is not an effective way to deal with such threats.

In the case of suicidal or homicidal patients, the physician should be ready to ask if the patient has the means of suicide or homicide in their possession. It is not uncommon for individuals to surrender pills, knives, guns, and other items to a relative or even a physician. Furthermore, in the case of a threatened homicide, health care providers are obliged by law to warn the intended victims and to take action to protect them. Calling the police is a protective action. These laws derive from the case of *Tarasoff vs. University of California* (1976). When homicidal threats are made, confidential communications between the physician and the patient are no longer valid. Physicians must act to protect threatened lives and to prevent harm.

Referral of the patient to an emergency room of a hospital with a psychiatric division is usually necessary when there is a risk of a patient harming himself or others. Enlist the help and support of a family member or friend. This is especially important, since the family may be needed to transport the patient to a psychiatric treatment facility and to attest to his suicidal risk in case involuntary hospitalization is necessary. Patients whom the physician believes in good faith to be of danger to themselves or others can also be transferred to a hospital by ambulance in restraints.

Involuntary Hospitalization

Procedures for involuntary psychiatric evaluation and admission differ from state to state. Generally, individuals must be judged as imminently dangerous to themselves or others. The court allows individuals to be involuntarily evaluated for a specific time if the request has been made by a physician, mental health professional, or a state-appointed evaluator. The cooperation of relatives may be essential, since they may be the only ones who can give direct evidence of the threatening or troublesome behavior.

Health professionals must appear in court to formally request an involuntary admission for the purposes of evaluation. It should be noted that an individual can refuse treatment even if she is already in the hospital under court order, and an order for involuntary treatment must be separately specified by a court. Health care powers-of-attorney often do not apply to psychiatric treatment. In some states, alcohol and drug abuse may be excluded from involuntary procedures.

Abuse and Neglect

When neglect or abuse of a child or an elderly or disabled person is suspected, many professionals are mandated to report it to the authorities. Usually this is done by calling a state-run hot line that initiates an investigation. In cases of other abused adults, there is no legal mandate to report abuse. Some victims continue to remain in abusive relationships, covering up or minimizing what was done to them. Probably the largest group is battered women, who come to medical facilities for treatment of physical injuries, depression, or anxiety. However, after treatment they often return to their abusers. Such women are sometimes receptive to referrals to abuse organizations with specially trained counselors (usually women) who provide individual and group therapy related to breaking away from the abuser. These organizations may operate or be connected to emergency shelters for women and children. They can be found by contacting the local mental health center, United Way agency, or crisis line.

Disability Assessments for Mental Illness

Assessments for the degree of mental disability are performed by psychologists and psychiatrists. To be considered disabled, an individual needs to have a chronic psychiatric problem that impairs his ability to work and maintain a job. Additionally, a patient's psychiatric morbidity may incapacitate him for independent living in the community. Merely having a psychiatric disorder does not qualify an individual for a psychiatric disability. Even if an acute problem has a long duration and great severity, the psychiatric illness might not meet the definition of a chronic mental health condition and automatically qualify the patient as disabled. The impact of a psychiatric disability is often greater than the stigma of a psychiatric disorder. For many patients, *disability* means one is not a productive member of society and for that reason, some patients seek to end disability as the psychiatric illness improves. Unfortunately the threatened loss of disability benefits (supplementary income and in some cases Medicare) may undermine the patient's incentive to discontinue disability assistance and to rejoin the work force.

Alcohol and Drug Abuse Treatment Programs

Primary care physicians are often the first line of referral to self-help organizations such as Alcoholics Anonymous (AA) and Narcotics Anonymous (NA). These programs are not medical, but they are administered by people who are themselves recovering alcohol or drug abusers.

Formal, licensed treatment programs for chemical dependence have physicians on their staffs who may or may not be psychiatrists. The physician's level of involvement varies from program to program. Most of the active treatment—individual, group, and family therapy—is carried out by nonmedical therapists. Many of the counselors do not have advanced degrees. The old practice of inpatient hospital treatment programs lasting several weeks is giving way to short periods of detoxification that usually last fewer than 4 days and are followed by entry into a day hospital treatment program or intensive brief outpatient group therapy and follow-up sessions at longer intervals.

Some programs are not cooperative with physicians and are ignorant of or hostile to the medical model of psychiatric disorders. Such programs may advise against the use of any drugs for the treatment of psychiatric disorders and view any medication as antithetical to treatment. Fortunately this view is less common than in the past. A referral to a program with this philosophy could prove disastrous for patients who are severely mentally ill and whose health may depend on the maintenance of medication.

Because of the varying nature of different programs and their advantages and disadvantages for different individuals, the primary care physician might best serve patients by using intermediate referral sources. The physician should try to find a knowledgeable colleague—a physician, psychiatrist, psychologist, social worker, or alcohol and drug therapist—to give advice about the bewildering array of treatment programs.

Unfortunately, one treatment modality alone may not be adequate, so most programs strive to provide comprehensive help. For example, an alcoholic patient may need the help of AA, an outpatient day program, and an individual therapist. Treatments in this area need to be individually tailored, and often positive patient outcomes occur only after several attempts at treatment have failed. As with most treatments, psychological or medical, outcome is related to the level of motivation by the patient. Individuals with jobs and good family support maintain higher and longer levels of motivation with better treatment outcomes.

Pain Control and Management

Pain management programs are administered by multidisciplinary treatment teams. Neurologists and anesthesiologists often manage acute pain. Psychiatrists and psychologists often evaluate the personality variables and psychiatric symptoms associated with functional pain (for example, personality tests such as the Minnesota Multiphasic Personality Inventory-2 [MMPI-2] or the Temperament and Character Survey [TCI]). Often these mental health evaluations are used to determine how aggressively a medical cause of pain should be sought. Chronic pain programs are often directed by a psychiatrist or a psychologist. In these programs, patients are taught to live with their pain levels and are encouraged to resume as much of their normal activity as possible. Treatment programs measure progress in regaining strength, activities, and self-control and do not measure pain. Pain control programs are generally located at tertiary medical centers and often operate as day treatment programs or partial hospital programs.

Forensic Psychiatry and Psychology

These are emerging specialties within psychiatry and clinical psychology. Specialists in this area generally have advanced training beyond the educational requirements for general clinicians with an emphasis on integrating psychiatry, psychology, and mental health law. The area of concern for forensic specialists goes far beyond consideration of criminal cases to almost any area that might involve legal proceedings. For physicians or mental health providers who anticipate legal actions, consultation with a forensic psychiatrist or psychologist is especially encouraged, since these specialists are the most knowledgeable about the law and mental health. Forensic psychiatrists and psychologists generally work together as a team with legal professionals (see Chapter 28).

Child and Adolescent Mental Health Specialists

These psychiatrists, psychologists, social workers, and nurses concentrate on the problems of children and adolescents. Assessment and treatment approaches can be different and distinct from adult psychology and psychiatry. For children and adolescents, the family and school context make clinical work in this area time consuming and complex. Assessment can involve interviews with parents, teachers, other family members, and the family physician to understand the child's problem or psychopathologic condition. If a physician does not know of a specialist in child mental health, pediatricians generally know about local referral sources.

Behavioral Medicine Programs

Problems such as stress, smoking, sleep disturbance, weight control, shyness, and phobias are often treated by clinical or medical psychologists. These symptoms occur in psychiatric illness, in medical illness, or as isolated complaints. Patients with these behavioral problems are treated in individual or in group sessions. Most clinicians working in these areas use psychological approaches that emphasize behavioral, cognitive, and skill-training procedures. Anxiety-reducing medicines may or may not be used. When patients are treated in group sessions, treatment may resemble an educational class more than traditional group therapy. Hypnosis, biofeedback, and relaxation procedures may be part of the treatments employed. The goal of treatment is to enable patients to be more functional and to exercise greater control of their thinking, emotions, and behavior.

Behavioral clinicians and treatment programs are found in hospitals, in managed care settings, and in some colleges and universities. Clinical psychologists in private practice are trained to provide these treatments as well. In some communities, the clinical psychological services center or the clinic of the university psychology department provides for these services on a sliding scale basis. In these centers, advanced doctoral students provide assessment and treatment under the supervision of clinical psychology supervisors and professors.

Types of Community Resources

Most people who are treated for psychiatric disorders, especially those whose treatments are followed-up by primary care physicians, are not chronically disabled by their illnesses. Though major depression, the various anxiety disorders, and alcoholism are recurrent or even chronic, these common illnesses usually can be managed well enough to keep the periods of disability brief.

However, an unfortunate minority of psychiatric patients are disabled for long periods, even throughout their lives, and require a comprehensive system of support services. The rest of this chapter deals with these people's specific needs and the services available for them: help with stable housing, financial support, access to medical care, provision of medication, a support system, structured use of time, and special needs of the families of people with chronically disabling mental illness.

Every state has some services for the mentally ill, although the extent of these services varies. Information about what is available in a particular area can be obtained from a mental health association, the United Way referral service, a family and children's service, a suicide crisis line, or a community mental health center. Social workers in hospitals or clinics are good sources of information about these resources.

Housing

With the introduction of psychotropic medications in the 1950s, thousands of patients who were mentally ill were released from psychiatric hospitals into the community. Unfortunately, the community supports never adequately matched their needs and many patients were left to fend for themselves, either alone or with the help of their families. Two thirds of those released returned to their families, and those without families went to other resources or to the streets.

The process of deinstitutionalization continues, with state-run hospitals releasing more and more long-term patients into the community. For some of these individuals, this is the first time in decades that they have not lived within the confines of a structured and supervised world. It is now up to them to handle such basic skills as personal hygiene, meal preparation, money management, and—perhaps most important of all—taking their medications as prescribed.

The majority of people who are chronically disabled by mental illness still live with their families, who provide most of their care. However, many times it is in the best interests of the patient and the family for the person who is mentally ill to live elsewhere. This is especially important in promoting independence. It is hard for a patient to learn to take care of herself if the family will do it for her.

There has been a trend in recent years to divert money previously used for long-term hospitalization into the creation of more community supported services. The goals of these services are that everyone should have the right to live in their own homes, even if this requires comprehensive support services. This approach has led to the development of supervised apartment programs, case-management systems, and even live-in attendants whose job is to make sure the residents' needs are being met. Not surprisingly, these resources are limited and many who could benefit from them are not served.

A number of mentally ill people are able to live in their own apartments with little supervision or assistance. Others need more supervision, which may be provided by family members checking on them daily or weekly or from a case manager, who makes sure they get to medical and psychiatric appointments.

Even with support services, some people are unable to handle their business affairs, meals, and medications and need to live in a more supervised setting. Community programs such as group homes, halfway houses, boarding homes, residential care facilities, or sheltered care facilities are examples of such settings. The services offered vary, even among facilities with the same name. Most facilities provide meals and dispense medications to the residents. In some, the resident must do her own laundry; in others, this is a provided service. Some homes offer group therapy and behavioral management. Some offer regularly scheduled activities and field trips; others provide little stimulation other than television.

These homes are almost never locked facilities, so the patients are free to come and go within the limits of the house rules. For many patients who are mentally ill, even the least structured of these homes may still provide more structure than they would otherwise have on their own.

Many patients, despite the recommendations of psychiatrist, family, and case worker, refuse to live in a group setting. They offer many reasons, such as they do not want to share a room with another resident; they do not want to follow rules such as curfew; or they do not like institutional food. Perhaps the greatest reason is that they do not want to give up their monthly disability check, even when it has been explained to them that all of their needs will be taken care of.

Unless they have been judged in need of a guardian, people who are mentally ill can make their own decisions, even if these decisions are unwise in the opinion of family or mental health professionals. They can decide where they will live, how they will spend their time, and whether they will take their medication. Because their judgment is often impaired by the illness itself, this is one of the greatest frustrations for families.

Many patients prefer to live in subsidized apartments, where they are often mixed in with the elderly and with people who are physically and mentally disabled. But finding these apartments can be difficult because there may be a long waiting list for such housing (with variations from area to area). Housing is part of a complex system that may be difficult to navigate. If the client is already in a state's care system, he may have a case manager who can help.

Many people who are mentally ill and many people

with drug and alcohol dependence become homeless for a variety of reasons. Some cannot organize themselves enough to obtain and maintain an apartment. Many have refused referrals to group homes to increase the likelihood of medication compliance. Others spend their money on drugs or alcohol, or they give money away and are left with no resources.

Financial Support

People with a serious mental illness are usually eligible for disability payments and government-supported health insurance. If they have worked before becoming ill, they may have enough work credits to be eligible for Social Security Disability (SSD) payments, with the amount of the benefit determined by their earning history. After 2 years of receiving SSD benefits, they are eligible for Medicare, which is also the primary health insurance for the elderly.

Clients who are disabled and have no work history and low income may be eligible for Supplemental Security Income (SSI), which also provides a monthly check. The amount of the check is determined by government guidelines and varies from state to state. Financial eligibility also varies from state to state and often includes consideration of the total household income instead of just the income of the person who is mentally ill. Most clients who are eligible for SSI are also eligible for medical assistance, which is known as Medicaid (or by different names in different states). This is the medical insurance for the poor. It is possible to have both SSD and SSI (if the SSD payment is small), and it is possible to have both Medicare and Medicaid.

In some cases, individuals who become ill before the age of 23 can obtain SSD based on the work history of a parent. However, this is only possible when the parent is disabled, deceased, or retired. Some people who became mentally ill before age 19 and who continue to be dependent on parents can continue to be maintained on a parent's health insurance.

The Social Security Administration, which makes the rules for SSD and SSI, defines disabled as unable to perform any type of work for 12 months or longer. This means that individuals with episodes of depression are not likely to be eligible for disability unless their impairment continues for more than a year.

The impaired judgment of many people who are mentally ill prevents them from adequately handling their own finances. Social Security can appoint a payee (usually a family member) who must sign for the check and determine how it is to be spent.

Access to Medical Care

Finances and type of insurance strongly influence where a mentally ill individual receives psychiatric treatment. Many psychiatrists accept Medicare, but the patient is still responsible for the copayment for outpatient services.

In many states the number of private psychiatrists who accept Medicaid is much more limited, and many patients whose only insurance is Medicaid must use the state's mental health system.

There are countless types of private insurance, many of which are extremely limited in their coverage for psychiatric illness. Whereas a $1 million lifetime maximum in benefits for medical expenses is the norm for many large group policies, it is common for the same groups to limit psychiatric coverage to $25,000 to $50,000 for a lifetime. This maximum includes inpatient and outpatient treatment. At the rate of at least $500 a day for inpatient stays in private hospitals, $50,000 roughly pays for no more than 3 months of inpatient coverage. Although most hospitalizations are now extremely short, over the course of a lifetime a patient with schizophrenia can easily require many more than 90 days just for crisis stabilization of acute symptoms.

Additionally, coverage for outpatient psychiatric services is often set at a different rate than for medical services. For example, a patient's insurance may cover 80% of the cost of a medical doctor's visit; the same policy often pays only 50% for mental health treatment. Some patients with private insurance are also eligible for Medicaid, which can pick up the balance in such cases. However, many patients cannot receive Medicaid because their income is too large. A married person with no work history may not be eligible for SSI or Medicaid because the spouse's income is too high.

Many private insurances are Health Maintenance Organizations (HMOs) or Preferred Provider Organizations (PPOs), which dictate or strongly influence which provider a client may use. Individual insurance plans also determine which services are covered. Many exclude treatment for chemical dependency, alcoholism, or both. Other commonly excluded services are psychological testing and marriage and family therapy.

Community mental health centers must see any patient who lives in their catchment area. However, there may be a wait of weeks or even months for an initial appointment. Once in the system the client can expect regularly scheduled visits, primarily for medication supervision. Some centers may also provide psychotherapy, but many have increasingly limited their services to caring for patients with chronic mental illness.

Paying for medications is a major problem, not only for patients who are mentally ill but also for many who have physical illnesses. Medicare does not pay for prescription drugs of any kind. Those with Medicaid can usually obtain medications by making only a small copayment. However, states can determine which drugs they agree to pay for and which ones they wish to exclude from their approved list. Not every state provides every drug commonly used for psychiatric illness. Private insurances also vary tremendously in their coverage of medications.

Many psychiatric drugs, especially those developed more recently, can be extremely expensive. When clozapine (Clozaril) was first released, there were cost estimates of $9000 per year for the medication and the required weekly blood tests. This is much more than the entire annual income for most patients who are disabled. With approval for Medicaid coverage in at least some states, this drug has become available to those covered by Medicaid. However, it and other expensive drugs are still out of reach for many patients whose only insurance is Medicare.

Community mental health centers and the Veterans Administration (VA) facilities provide medications to their patients. But the prescriptions must be written by physicians at those facilities. If paying for medication is a problem, it may be in the best interest of the patient to go to a community mental health center or (when eligible) the VA facility, even if he has private insurance.

Compliance with Medication

Obtaining the medication is only one part of the overall issue of medication compliance. Patients must choose to take the medication. Reluctance to taking medication is not unusual for many people with physical disorders such as asthma, hypertension, or diabetes. Psychiatric patients feel this same reluctance, but their reluctance is also colored by the stigma about mental illness. Having to take psychiatric medications can be a confirmation that they "must be crazy." Such perceptions are enhanced by the illness itself, which often interferes with their thinking and robs them of insight into the need for medications.

Even if patients do not resist taking medications, their altered thinking may interfere with their ability to take them consistently. Simplifying the medication regime to once or twice a day has been found to greatly enhance the likelihood of medication compliance.

Once they begin to feel better, it is not uncommon for individuals to stop taking their medications because they feel they do not need it any more. Another factor in medication noncompliance is that the side effects are often unpleasant.

Haloperidol (Haldol) and fluphenazine (Prolixin), among the antipsychotic medications used in treating people with schizophrenia and the psychotic symptoms of bipolar affective disorder, are available in long-lasting injectable form. This eliminates some of the barriers to compliance.

Community Support Services

Many publicly funded programs for people disabled by chronic psychiatric disorders have developed a system of case managers, or individuals who are paid to take care of many of the day-to-day details necessary to keep a mentally ill person out of the hospital. This has been an invaluable service to patients who live independently in apartments. The kinds of services provided include medication supervision, with the case manager stopping on a daily basis in some cases to make sure the patients take their medications. The case manager may take a patient to appointments and grocery shopping or give reminders about the need to shower and wash clothes. He may help manage finances, pay bills, organize an apartment, and help develop a system to help the patient become more responsible for these things. In short, case managers act much like a surrogate family member.

Case managers are employed by state and private agencies. Access to their services is usually through the agency providing the service. Payment is often through Medicaid or the private funding of families. The case manager system has proven much less costly than the amount of hospitalization that would occur if the system did not exist.

Vocational Training

Some mentally ill people are able to hold full- or part-time jobs. The ability to go to work is a badge of normality and self-reliance, and many people see employment as the mark of success, even if it is only a minimum wage job washing dishes in a restaurant.

There are a number of vocational training possibilities. State-funded vocational rehabilitation programs can provide job training and even college for those who qualify and who can demonstrate the ability to benefit from them. Other private programs under the umbrellas of psychosocial rehabilitation provide job training.

Structured Use of Time

Many of the negative symptoms of schizophrenia and the apathy of chronic depression result in a lack of motivation. Structured use of time is an important part of treatment. It is too easy to spend days watching television or walking the streets for hours. Even if a patient is unable to work at a paying job, having a place to be at an expected time is also a sign of value and responsibility.

There are a number of day programs for the mentally ill. They vary in their activities, purpose, and eligibility requirements, but they all provide structured activities.

Partial hospitalization may be used on early signs of decompensation, to avoid inpatient hospitalization, or as a transition from inpatient treatment to the community. It offers individual and group therapy, medication adjustment, problem solving, and discharge planning. It is designed to be used as short-term crisis stabilization for patients requiring more intensive treatment than outpatient therapy. Funding is primarily through insurance.

Community partial hospitalization offers longer-term treatment for the chronic mentally ill who may be going through a difficult time or who need a medication adjustment. Through groups and individual therapy the focus is on problem-solving skills and stabilization. Patients may attend for longer periods than they can with the more acute partial hospitalization.

There are many day programs modeled after the Fountain House program in New York. This "clubhouse" approach is run by the patients themselves, who are called members. They are involved in specific work groups and tasks designed to teach responsibility and work skills. Many have additional programs, including job training and supported housing. The purpose is to maximize the functioning in the community of people who are chronically ill.

Adult day care is used primarily for elderly people who require supervision but who continue to live at home. Day care centers offer daytime activities designed to provide stimulation, nutrition, and socialization. Many also give baths and provide other basic types of care. Adult day care is paid for by Medicaid and private funding.

Volunteer work is available to some people who are mentally ill even if they cannot hold a paying job. The volunteer job helps promote a sense of self-worth and may teach certain skills that lead to actual employment. The local United Way chapter or Mental Health Association may be a source of information about finding volunteer work.

Support groups in the community run by volunteers supplement the professionally run programs discussed in the preceding paragraphs. They focus on coping skills needed for dealing with a specific problem or illness, and they have application to a much wider variety of people than the chronically ill or disabled population. There are a variety of "Anonymous" groups that use a 12-step approach to combat different forms of addiction (for example, AA, Cocaine Anonymous, Gamblers Anonymous, Overeaters Anonymous, and Emotions Anonymous).

Additionally, there are support groups that may help a person cope with such illnesses as cancer, strokes, Parkinson's disease, asthma, depression, or obsessive-compulsive disorder (OCD). These groups can be located by contacting agencies dealing with specific problems or by contacting the Mental Health Association.

Individuals who are grieving after the loss of a family member often benefit from bereavement groups, which are offered by hospitals, funeral homes, or private agencies. Repeatedly talking about an experience, especially with others who are similarly affected, seems to be a helpful part of the process.

The Role of Families

The majority of people who are chronically disabled by mentally illness live with their families, often at great financial and personal cost to themselves and their families. With the shorter hospitalizations of recent years, an ever-increasing burden of care falls on the family, and there are often few outside supports. Patients are being released to the care of their relatives in much sicker states; some patients are even still psychotic.

With some mental illnesses, such as depression, symptoms may eventually abate, giving the family a chance to regroup. Other illnesses last a lifetime. The effects of chronic illness on the family are profound and devastating. The literature describes it as nothing short of a catastrophe in that it disrupts normal family life through frequent crises. One of the most obvious effects lies in the upset of day-to-day functioning of the family. Families must reorganize their lives around the illness and deal with unusual and sometimes violent behaviors, as well as numerous emergencies involving hospitals, police, and the legal system. Families must try to provide 24-hour protection for their ill relative, sometimes in the face of legal obstacles that may shut them off from information about how to help. Lefley and Wasow comment that families are commonly made poorer and physically or mentally sicker themselves by the prolonged caregiving and case management responsibilities that befall them.

One of the most powerful ways that mental illness disrupts family life is by altering normal family roles. For example, schizophrenia often first appears in adolescence and disrupts ongoing human development, resulting in a perpetual adolescent who is forever dependent on her parents. Thus parental caregiving may continue on and on until the parents' death or incapacitation.

There is a great deal of sadness and grief that is often not expressed overtly about the lost potential of this child, who is locked forevermore into debilitating mental illness. Family members may also experience grief over the "normal" family that will never be or over the suffering of the person who is mentally ill. Many family members have described mental illness as worse than losing a child to death.

The burdens mentioned in the previous paragraph are magnified by the isolation that often results among families of the mentally ill. Although this may be the result of embarrassment or simply of limited energy from living in an unpredictable state of crisis, it means that families must shoulder their burden without the ongoing supports they might find with other difficulties.

Mental illness also disrupts marital relationships by upsetting the sense of partnership when one spouse is incapacitated (for example, by depression) and the other must pick up the slack. If the incapacity is severe or prolonged enough, the healthy spouse may also assume a parental role for the dependent spouse. He experiences many losses, such as those of intimacy and companionship and must also witness the suffering of the partner who is ill. Additionally, spouses must often bear alone the primary responsibility of raising children (who are in need of extra attention because of the mental illness in the family) and take on additional household duties. Shame and embarrassment, coupled with sheer fatigue, contribute to increasing isolation of the spouse who is not mentally ill. Being married to someone going through depression or another mental illness may demand superhuman patience, flexibility, and tolerance.

Children who grow up with a parent or sibling who is mentally ill may be (or feel) short-changed by the loss of a "normal" childhood. Whereas some children do well and even thrive under the chaos, studies have shown increased incidence of anxiety and depression in adult life. A child's reaction varies according to the severity and chronicity of the illness and the general level of stress and chaos at home. Lefley and Wasow (1994) liken mental illness to "a death in the family, which is complicated by stigma, the cyclical nature of the illness, and the continuing physical presence of the bereaved."

It is only recently that professionals have begun to understand and address the impact of mental illness on the family and to be aware of the important role families play. This is in contrast to previous approaches in which families were often viewed as the causes of mental illness and excluded from participation in treatment of patients. Much of earlier family involvement was considered family therapy and was designed to "cure" the family dysfunction that was suspected of causing the illness in the first place. With research more and more demonstrating a biological cause of mental illness, families are less and less blamed, although this tendency has not disappeared completely. Families are being included more often in their relative's treatment, and they have become more vocal about their needs.

What Do Families Need?

Families need information about the illness and its treatment. As the primary care givers, family members need to understand the diagnosis and treatment plan. They have often been excluded from receiving any information because of confidentiality issues. Although privacy and confidentiality need to be honored, it is necessary to balance one need against another and consider whether a delusional patient is really competent to make the decision to exclude his caregivers. Family members do not need to know all about the internal conflicts and personal issues experienced by their relative. But they do need to know the diagnosis, the prescribed medications and the reasons they are being given, and behavioral management techniques.

More and more professionals are including families in treatment planning, and there is a new approach of viewing families as partners in the treatment. Families may be seen as experts in their own right with valuable knowledge of their relative to share with the professionals. This new approach tends to assume that the family is healthy and functional apart from the impact of mental illness on its functioning.

Families need to know techniques for management of the illness. Families need information about how to handle difficult behaviors, such as the positive and negative symptoms of schizophrenia. Relatives can learn to tolerate bizarre or unusual behaviors that are not harmful or unacceptable, and they can learn how to gently confront or redirect the patient when the behavior cannot continue. Patients' families want to know how to deal with aggressive behavior, suicidal or self-destructive behavior, poor hygiene, social withdrawal, and refusal to cooperate with treatment. Families sometimes need a professional's permission to set limits, even to the point of refusing to allow the person to continue to live in their home.

A family can also learn to make changes in its environment that favorably impact the treatment of the illness. Research has shown that people with schizophrenia do better in a calm environment than in an environment where there are highly expressed emotions.

Families need to meet their own needs. Family members may need permission and encouragement to take care of their own needs. It is not unusual for them to neglect themselves out of guilt over the illness or pity for their loved one who is suffering from it. They may suffer from a variety of physical com-

PEARLS & PERILS

RESOURCES FOR PATIENTS AND FAMILIES

- Primary care physicians, not mental health professionals, are responsible for the treatment of most people with psychiatric disorders.
- If primary care physicians knew a little more about the use of antidepressant medications, psychiatrists would have a lot less to do.
- Suicidal and homicidal communications require referral to a psychiatrist and the resources of a hospital.
- Insurance coverage is usually much less adequate for psychiatric than for medical illnesses. This fact dictates and restricts the choice of the mental health professional and the type of treatment.
- Suspected abuse of a child or of an elderly or disabled person and threats of harm against another person must be reported to abuse hot lines. Considerations of confidentiality do not apply in these situations.
- Family members, not the mental health system, are responsible for the care of most people who are disabled by chronic psychiatric illnesses.
- It is essential to communicate with and often involve the family in the treatment of any patient who is seriously ill.
- One of the best sources of support for families is the National Alliance for the Mentally Ill (NAMI); 200 North Glebe Road, Suite 1015; Arlington, VA 22203-3754; (800) 950-6264.
- The nearest community mental health center and the social work department of the nearest hospital have the most up-to-date information on community support services for mentally ill patients.

plaints stemming from the stress of not meeting their own needs. Families benefit from maintaining a social life, regular exercise, good nutrition, and stress management.

Families need help with planning for the future. Parents of a person who is mentally ill worry a great deal about what will become of their child after their deaths. They are invariably relieved to learn about legal arrangements that can be made to provide ongoing care even after their deaths. The specifics of such arrangements vary tremendously depending on location, availability of other family members, and availability of financial resources.

One component of future planning addresses where the person who is mentally ill will live after the deaths of parents with whom he has always lived. There are differences of opinion about whether adult children should continue to live at home, given the impact on the family and the usual result of stifled independence. It is much more difficult to learn to live independently in later years, especially after being sheltered for an entire lifetime. It is generally felt that the move to independent living is smoother while the parents are still alive and in good enough health to be actively involved in the transition.

Families should play an active role in treatment. Perhaps more than anything, family members need to be listened to and taken seriously. In the more collaborative approaches to family involvement, families are viewed as having valuable information about the patient that is useful to professionals. If relatives are to continue treatment at home, they need to have input into what is feasible within their family.

Where Can Families Find What They Need?

Often a family's first introduction to ongoing assistance occurs when their relative is hospitalized and they talk to members of the treatment team. The psychiatric social worker at the hospital is a source of information about resources and support services in the community. Many hospitals also offer family education groups or seminars that address many of the issues mentioned in the previous section.

For many families, the greatest source of support has been the National Alliance for the Mentally Ill (NAMI), which was founded in 1979 (see the Pearls & Perils box above). Since then its mission has remained largely unchanged—support, education, advocacy, and research. NAMI has held to a number of guiding principles. The organization is a proponent of the disease model of mental illness rather than some of the environmental theories (such as family causation). The organization has also worked to improve funding for medical research and has served as an advocate for better services for the mentally ill.

NAMI's other guiding principle is that the best help is self-help. Its roughly 1000 chapters, with 140,000 members in 1993, are perhaps best known for the education and support components of its program. Family support groups, led by family members rather than professionals, are offered in many communities. They provide a place for families to exchange information and to support each other. Professionals are invited as consultants from time to time.

Annotated Bibliography

Depression Guideline Panel: *Clinical practice guideline no 5: depression in primary care,* vol 1: *Detection and diagnosis;* vol 2: *Treatment of major depression,* Agency for Health Care Policy and Research Publication 93-0550, Rockville, Md., 1993, U.S. Department of Health and Human Services, Public Health Service.

Volume 1 provides a general overview of mood disorders, including guidelines for detecting co-morbid psychiatric and medical disorders. Screening instruments and psychological tests are also discussed. Volume 2 provides a thoughtful and critical review of all the current treatments for depression.

Lefley HP, Wasow M, editors: *Helping families cope with mental illness,* Langhorne, Penn., 1994, Harwood Academic Publishers.

This book offers detailed information about the impact of mental illness on the family and about what families need from professionals. There is also useful information for professionals interested in implementing family education and support programs.

Mueser KT, Gingerich S: *Coping with schizophrenia,* Oakland, Calif., 1994, New Harbinger Publications.

This is an extremely useful book for families with members who are schizophrenic. It is written in everyday language and contains practical information about community resources and about ways of dealing with symptoms and behaviors stemming from the illness. It also offers suggestions about how to meet families' needs.

section two

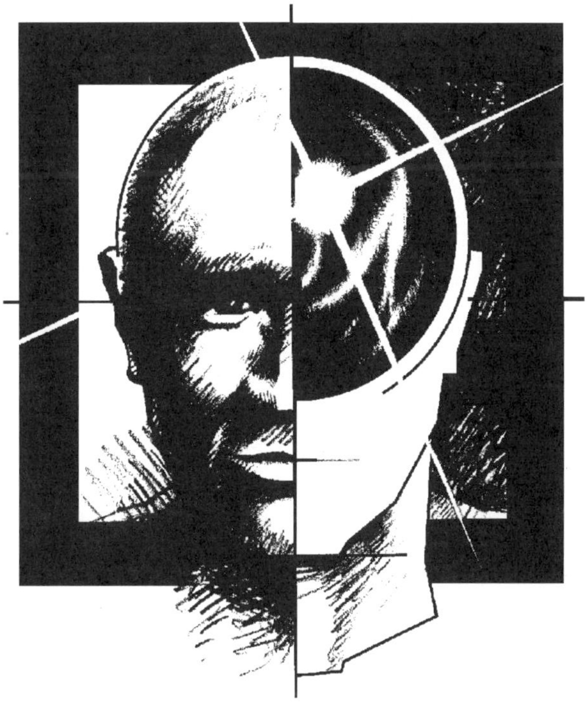

Psychopathology

Eugene H. Rubin, MD, PhD*

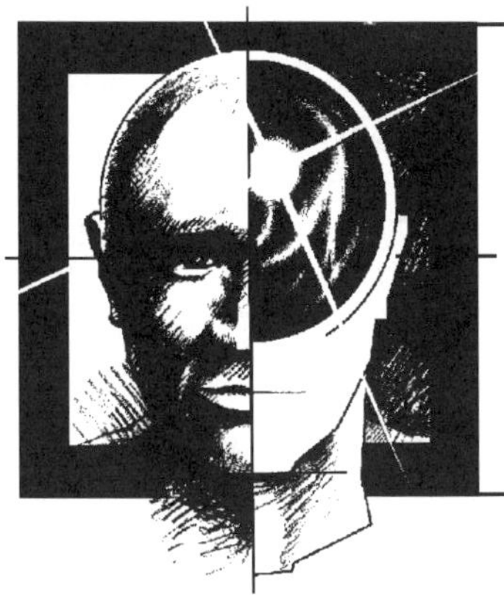

chapter 8

Depression, Mania, and Related Disorders

Wayne C. Drevets, MD and Richard D. Todd, PhD, MD

In this chapter the diagnosis and treatment of major depressive disorder (MDD), dysthymic disorder, bipolar disorder (manic-depressive illness), and cyclothymic disorder are discussed. Additionally, current knowledge regarding the etiology and natural history of these disorders is overviewed. Though these disorders occur in children and young adolescents, the comments in this chapter are limited to older adolescents and adults.

Phenomenology of Mood Disorders

MDD rivals hypertension as the most commonly encountered illness in primary health care. Nevertheless this and the other mood disorders remain among the most poorly understood human diseases. Factors that have hindered elucidation of the pathophysiology of these illnesses include the dearth of gross neuropathological changes in primary mood disorders, the lack of satisfactory animal models, the limitations in studying human brain function in vivo, and the complexity of studying interactions between psychosocial stressors and biological predisposition. Moreover, although scientific investigation has demonstrated that mood disorders are associated with genetic, neurochemical, neuroendocrine, and neurophysiological factors, biological markers have lacked the sensitivity and specificity needed to distinguish illness subtypes from one another or from normative states. Thus the nosology of mood disorders has been further prevented from advancing beyond the syndromatic level.

Because of this limitation, the syndromes identified as individual mood disorders do not reflect discrete disease entities but rather are presumed to encompass diverse groups of neuropsychiatric disorders. Heterogeneity is manifested by the ranges of behavioral signs (for example, from psychomotor retardation to agitation), symptoms (such as from insomnia to hypersomnolence), and biochemical abnormalities found within the same syndrome (for example, from abnormally low [in nonpsychotic depression] to high [in psychotic depression] cerebrospinal fluid [CSF] levels of homovanillic acid). Moreover, some patients experience phenomenologically distinct states over the illness course, suffering manic as well as depressive syndromes. Diverse biological antecedents appear capable of inducing mood disorders, since depressive or manic syndromes can be produced by dissimilar neurological disorders, endocrine disturbances, or pharmacological agents. Major depressive episodes can also occur in the absence of medical or psychosocial stressors as primary, familial, idiopathic disorders, or they may arise secondary to other psychiatric disorders in which neuropathological changes have been identified (such as schizophrenia). Finally, some cases of mood disorders do appear to have been initiated and maintained by psychosocial precipitants. Thus even though the pathophysiological correlates of mood disorder subtypes have not been established, mood disorders include a group of conditions stemming from a variety of genetic, neuropathological, or psychosocial factors working alone or in concert with one another.

The clinical heterogeneity within mood syndromes has enabled the coexistence of both psychological and biological theories regarding the origins and treatment of mood disorders. For example, Sigmund Freud studied mildly ill nonhospitalized patients and concluded that depression was rooted in a psychological reaction to the loss of a highly-valued "love object," thereby highlighting the similarities between depression and bereavement. More recently, competing hypotheses have arisen from behaviorist roots, which hold that depression results from thought patterns in which life events, social interactions, and self-perceptions are habitually viewed negatively, resulting in a lowered mood. The proponents of these cognitive-behavioral theories have also relied primarily on studies in less severely depressed outpatients (see the Environmental Factors section of this chapter). In contrast, the medical model approach adopted by most of the psychiatric research community emanates from the work of Emil Kraepelin, who described the symptoms of syndromes observed in severely ill hospitalized patients. Kraepelin coined the term *manic-depressive psychosis* to encompass both bipolar and unipolar mood disorders and insisted that the cause of such disorders was innate and independent of social and psychological forces.

Psychological theories follow logically from simple observations that mood is normally affected by social, medical, psychological, or spiritual and religious factors, leading to the assumption that mood disorders constitute reactions to psychosocial or medical stressors. However, in contrast to a normally reactive low mood, the major depressive syndrome does not simply arise in response to medical or psychosocial stressors. In most cases the role that adverse life events play in precipitating pathological mood episodes remains unclear. Furthermore, mood disorders persist for protracted periods of time, are not alleviated by positive life events, reach extremes in magnitude so function is impaired, and can be ameliorated and prevented by somatic treatments that do not affect mood states in people without mood disorders.

The extant scientific data support biological rather than psychosocial hypotheses regarding the pathogenesis of severe mood disorders. These data suggest that mood disorders constitute diseases that affect the brain circuits that modulate the set point and stability of emotion (see the section on pathophysiology in this chapter). The ultimate resolution of disagreements regarding the nature of mood disorders is expected to depend on elucidation of the pathophysiological correlates and the molecular genetics of the familial forms of mood disorders. Nevertheless in view of the clinical heterogeneity represented within the mood disorders, it should not be anticipated that every case falls into such categories, since some patients with mild or atypical forms of the major depressive syndrome may elude biologically based classifications.

Classification

In the progression of disease nosology from symptom to syndrome to pathophysiology to etiology (for example, symptoms: moodiness and forgetfulness → syndrome: general paresis → pathophysiology: pachymeningitis hemorrhagica, diffuse neuronal degeneration, and neuroglial proliferation → etiology: infectious involvement of the brain with *Treponema pallidum* [neurosyphilis]), psychiatric diagnosis largely remains at the syndromatic level. To differentiate mood disorders from feelings of sadness, despondency, or elation that occur normally in reaction to life circumstances, diagnostic criteria based on clusters of clinical symptoms and behavioral signs are used. Although such criteria are susceptible to the subjective interpretation of both the patient and the examiner, the diagnosis of MDD or bipolar disorder using this system has high interrater reliability and diagnostic stability across time. For example, about 84% of patients with unipolar depression retain the diagnosis of MDD after several years of follow-up study. Moreover, most patients for whom the diagnosis ultimately changes receive another mood disorder diagnosis, since about 10% of people initially diagnosed as having MDD convert to a diagnosis of bipolar disorder resulting from the subsequent development of mania. In either of these mood disorders, the diagnostic criteria for a major depressive episode are useful for demarcating a pathological mood state likely to respond to somatic antidepressant treatment.

Biological markers with adequate sensitivity and specificity to establish a mood disorder diagnosis are not available. Although laboratory analyses such as the dexamethasone suppression test and sleep electroencephalogram (EEG) studies can be confirmatory in ambiguous cases, a negative result on these assessments does not reliably exclude a mood disorder and a positive result does not delimit the diagnosis of a mood disorder (see the Pathophysiology section of this chapter). Laboratory analyses, EEG studies, neuroimaging results, and neuropsychological testing are instead used largely to exclude general medical or neurological illnesses that can present with depressive symptoms (see Chapter 26).

The absence of biological markers for disease can lead to diagnostic uncertainty when the severity of illness is mild, and the lower threshold for assigning a diagnosis and recommending treatment can be ambiguous. However, most patients who seek treatment from a physician are experiencing mood episodes of moderate to severe intensity and the diagnosis in these cases is relatively straightforward. When the diagnosis remains questionable, a family history of mood disorders weights the decision toward a positive diagnosis, since mood disorders follow a familial pattern of transmission.

The current diagnostic criteria for mood disorders are compiled in the DSM-IV. The symptom constellations fundamental to this classification are the *major depressive episode* as a pathological mood state characterized by dysphoric mood, the *manic episode* as a pathological mood state characterized by euphoric mood, and the *hypomanic episode* as a mild form of mania. The diagnostic framework built on these syndromes identifies *MDD* as single or recurrent depressive episodes (also called *unipolar depression*), *bipolar disorder* (manic-depressive illness) as a course in which manic episodes occur with or without depressive episodes, *dysthymic disorder* as a chronic subsyndromal depressive episode, and *cyclothymic disorder* as a milder expression of bipolar disorder.

The DSM-IV criteria for mood disorders are based on refinements of the criteria developed in natural history studies at Washington University by Eli Robins, Samuel Guze, and George Winokur. The older term *affective disorders* has been replaced in the DSM-IV by the term *mood disorders.* Affect is the mood state inferred by the physician from the patient's appearance, behavior, and verbally communicated emotional state, whereas *mood* indicates the subjective emotional state described by the patient. A feature of the Washington University criteria that was not adopted by DSM-IV but is applied and discussed in this chapter is the distinction of primary and secondary mood disorders. This concept is useful for both clinical and research approaches to mood disorders, just as this dichotomy has proven useful in other areas of medicine.

Major Depressive Disorder and Dysthymic Disorder

Diagnostic Criteria

The diagnosis of MDD is based on the presence of a major depressive episode and the absence of other medical or major psychiatric illnesses that might be associated with it, such as Parkinson's disease or schizophrenia (Box 8-1, Table 8-1). The major depressive episode consists of a pathological disturbance of mood and affect in which a persistent negative emotional state has been present for at least 2 weeks. Emotional changes alone do not warrant the diagnosis; they must be accompanied by changes in energy, sleep, appetite, activity, and cognition (Box 8-2, p. 104).

Dysthymic disorder is characterized by chronic, persistent, depressive symptoms of at least 2 years' duration (Box 8-3, p. 105). Too few depressive symptoms are present to warrant the diagnosis of MDD (that is, dysthymia is a "subsyndromal" depressive syndrome), and the depressed mood is less severe than that associated with MDD. Dysthymia is a heterogenous condition. Some people with dysthymia have a long history of being miserable and chronically unhappy; their condition has been classically termed *depressive neurosis.* Such patients generally respond poorly or incompletely to antidepressant treatment. Others appear to have a mild form of MDD and may later go on to develop full criteria for a major depressive episode. This latter group generally proves quite responsive to antidepressant pharmacotherapy.

Clinical Picture

The clinical presentation is variable, and the chief complaint may reflect an assortment of somatic, emotional, or neuropsychological symptoms. Since mood disorders follow an episodic course, a salient feature of mood syndromes is that the presenting symptoms constitute a clear deviation from the patient's usual mood, activity, and level of functioning. It can be helpful to have patients compare their current mood, desire to socialize, sleep pattern, libido, and concentration to their own baseline with questions such as, "Do you still enjoy ______ [The physician fills in the blank with items such as seeing grandchildren or engaging in hobbies, work, or sex.]?" However, episodes of depression may persist for several years, and some patients find it difficult to estimate their normal baseline.

DSM-IV DIAGNOSTIC CRITERIA

BOX 8-1 MAJOR DEPRESSIVE DISORDER, SINGLE EPISODE OR RECURRENT

A. Single episode: presence of a single Major Depressive Episode Recurrent: presence of two or more Major Depressive Episodes

Note: To be considered separate episodes, there must be an interval of at least 2 consecutive months in which criteria are not met for a Major Depressive Episode.

B. The Major Depressive Episodes are not better accounted for by Schizoaffective Disorder and are not superimposed on Schizophrenia, Schizophreniform Disorder, Delusional Disorder, or Psychotic Disorder Not Otherwise Specified.

C. There has never been a Manic Episode, a Mixed Episode, or a Hypomanic Episode. **Note:** This exclusion does not apply if all of the manic-like, mixed-like, or hypomanic-like episodes are substance or treatment induced or are due to the direct physiological effects of a general medical condition.

Specify (for current or most recent episode):
Severity/Psychotic/Remission Specifiers
Chronic
With Catatonic Features
With Melancholic Features
With Atypical Features
With Postpartum Onset

Specify (recurrent only):
Longitudinal Course Specifiers (With and Without Interepisode Recovery)
With Seasonal Pattern

Modified from American Psychiatric Association: *Diagnostic and statistical manual of mental disorders,* ed 4 (DSM-IV), Washington, D.C., 1994, American Psychiatric Press.

Emotional Manifestations

The emotional experience during a major depressive episode is marked by the intrusion of negative emotions and the absence of positive emotions. Since the pathophysiology of MDD remains obscure, the lay term *depression* has been applied to the group of neuropsychiatric disorders encompassed by this syndrome. Nevertheless, up to half of the patients who meet criteria for MDD do not endorse feeling sad or depressed (Table 8-2, p. 106). The more common emotional change is a pervasive loss of interest or pleasure in activities that previously produced positive emotion. For example, the enjoyment derived from interpersonal relationships, church activities, work, hobbies, food, or sex vanishes. This inability to experience pleasure is called *anhedonia* (see the Pearls & Perils box on p. 103).

Patients with MDD also experience anxiety, irritability, or despondence. Anxiety may be manifested as anxious mood, fear, worry, or motor tension, which may dominate the clinical picture. A minority of patients manifest panic attacks, obsessions, compulsions, or phobias (see Table 8-2). In primary MDD, such anxiety symptoms are usually delimited to the duration of the depressive episode and resolve during effective antidepressant pharmacotherapy. Irritability can be most troublesome for family members and may consequently serve as the presenting complaint of patients sent for treatment by their families. Women with MDD often experience increased irritability and dysphoria during the 1 to 2 weeks before menses, leading some to complain of having premenstrual syndrome. Patients may also describe feeling discouraged, worthless, or hopeless. Some report that simple emotional descriptors do not adequately characterize the mood phenomena and use terms such as *psychic pain* or *emotional deadness* instead (Boxes 8-4 and 8-5, p. 107).

Diurnal variation of the mood disturbance is relatively specific to mood disorders. This is usually manifested by severely depressed mood and anergia on awakening that persists throughout the morning but then progressively diminishes during the afternoon and evening. A reversal of this pattern can also occur, during which depressive symptoms are worse in the evening.

Neurovegetative Manifestations

The neurovegetative features of the major depressive episode are as critical to the diagnosis of mood

DIAGNOSIS

TABLE 8-1
MAJOR DEPRESSIVE DISORDER

Discriminating feature

1. Pervasive depressed mood or loss of interest or pleasure that constitutes a change from previous emotional state, lasting 2 weeks or longer

Consistent features

1. Episodic course
2. Fatigue or loss of energy
3. Change in sleep pattern, appetite, and libido
4. Excessive anxiety, worrying, and tension
5. Recurrent negative thoughts of guilt, self-reproach, death, or suicide
6. Improvement during somatic antidepressant treatment
7. Irritability
8. Impaired concentration
9. Diminished involvement in social and other motor activities
10. Apathy and amotivation

Variable features

1. Suicide risk
2. Psychotic or obsessional features
3. Panic attacks
4. Psychomotor retardation or agitation
5. Co-morbid substance abuse
6. Family history of mood disorder
7. Anorexia with weight loss
8. Hyperphagia with weight gain
9. Increased somatic complaints
10. Mood unreactive to positive events

PEARLS & PERILS

TIPS FOR DETECTING AND MANAGING DEPRESSION

- The most common emotional change associated with major depressive episodes is not depressed mood but rather the pervasive loss of interest or pleasure.
- The most common symptom associated with major depressive episodes is not an emotional symptom but rather a physical symptom: namely, fatigue or anergia.
- Major depressive episodes are associated with a significant risk of suicide, and patients suspected of suffering from a mood disorder should be asked if they are contemplating suicide.
- As a general rule, every patient who meets criteria for a major depressive episode deserves a trial of effective antidepressant treatment.

disorders as the emotional components. They facilitate distinctions between a major depressive episode and a "normal" low mood that is reactive to life situations. In many cases, changes in sleep, energy, or appetite precede the changes in emotion. The neurovegetative features can thus serve as harbingers of a recurrence in patients with a history of MDD.

The most common symptom associated with a major depressive episode is anergia (described as a loss of energy or easy fatiguability; see Table 8-2). This symptom is virtually always present and may constitute the chief complaint. Anergia is a common reason for patients who are depressed to consult physicians, highlighting the need for alertness to physical symptoms as presenting complaints for MDD.

Sleep disturbances are also almost always present. These include initial insomnia (difficulty falling asleep), middle insomnia (awakening during the night with difficulty returning to sleep), terminal insomnia (awakening early in the morning with inability to return to sleep), or hypersomnia (excessive sleeping). Sleep changes may also serve as the presenting complaint for MDD. Young adults or adolescents are more likely to experience initial insomnia, whereas terminal insomnia is more common in elderly patients.

Alterations in appetite and weight are also common components. Anorexia and weight loss can be observed in any patients who are depressed, but they are particularly prominent in elderly patients. Reduced oral intake during a major depressive episode may lead to dehydration and malnutrition in older adults who are depressed, contributing to the morbidity associated with geriatric depression. Additionally, hyperphagia with weight gain can be observed in younger patients. Dramatic weight fluctuations without other medical explanation should lead a physician to inquire about other depressive symptoms.

Finally, loss of libido and other types of sexual dysfunction are common. It is unclear whether this symptom reflects pathophysiological involvement of hypothalamic or neuroendocrine function or simply indicates another manifestation of anhedonia. The former explanation is suggested by observations that reduced libido may be the most persistent depressive symptom during treatment, continuing even after mood, hedonia, and self-esteem have returned to baseline. Moreover, some antidepressant drugs produce sexual dysfunction as side effects, necessitating monitoring for the development of new sexual problems during treat-

BOX 8-2 **MAJOR DEPRESSIVE EPISODE**

DSM-IV DIAGNOSTIC CRITERIA

A. Five (or more) of the following symptoms have been present during the same 2-week period and represent a change from previous functioning; at least one of the symptoms is either (1) depressed mood or (2) loss of interest or pleasure.

Note: Do not include symptoms that are clearly due to a general medical condition, or mood-incongruent delusions or hallucinations.

(1) depressed mood most of the day, nearly every day, as indicated by either subjective report (e.g., feels sad or empty) or observation made by others (e.g., appears tearful). **Note:** In children and adolescents, can be irritable mood.
(2) markedly diminished interest or pleasure in all, or almost all, activities most of the day, nearly every day (as indicated by either subjective account or observation made by others)
(3) significant weight loss when not dieting or weight gain (e.g., a change of more than 5% of body weight in a month), or decrease or increase in appetite nearly every day. **Note:** In children, consider failure to make expected weight gains.
(4) insomnia or hypersomnia nearly every day
(5) psychomotor agitation or retardation nearly every day (observable by others, not merely subjective feelings of restlessness or being slowed down)
(6) fatigue or loss of energy nearly every day
(7) feelings of worthlessness or excessive or inappropriate guilt (which may be delusional) nearly every day (not merely self-reproach or guilt about being sick)
(8) diminished ability to think or concentrate, or indecisiveness, nearly every day (either by subjective account or as observed by others)
(9) recurrent thoughts of death (not just fear of dying), recurrent suicidal ideation without a specific plan, or a suicide attempt or a specific plan for committing suicide

B. The symptoms do not meet criteria for a Mixed Episode.

C. The symptoms cause clinically significant distress or impairment in social, occupational, or other important areas of functioning.

D. The symptoms are not due to the direct physiological effects of a substance (e.g., a drug of abuse, a medication) or a general medical condition (e.g., hypothyroidism).

E. The symptoms are not better accounted for by Bereavement, i.e., after the loss of a loved one, the symptoms persist for longer than 2 months or are characterized by marked functional impairment, morbid preoccupation with worthlessness, suicidal ideation, psychotic symptoms, or psychomotor retardation.

From American Psychiatric Association: *Diagnostic and statistical manual of mental disorders,* ed 4 (DSM-IV), Washington, D.C., 1994, American Psychiatric Press.

ment. Disturbances of sexual function contribute to the strain that mood disorders place on marital relationships.

Psychological Manifestations

Disturbances of thought content, self-perception, and assessment of current and future circumstances also accompany depressive episodes. Negative thoughts intrude into the conscious thought processes and reverberate to the extent that the ability to inhibit such thoughts seems impaired. In patients who are severely depressed, psychotherapeutic attempts are unsuccessful at alleviating thoughts of guilt, death, suicide, or hopelessness, highlighting their obsessional or at times delusional nature. Ruminative ideation resolves relatively abruptly once a successful response to an antidepressant drug or electroconvulsive therapy (ECT) is achieved, which suggests that abnormal brain processes underlie and maintain such symptoms.

The most dramatic disturbance of the thought content is a preoccupation with death or suicide. Suicidal thoughts are present in about 60% of patients with MDD (see Table 8-2), and their appearance in patients with MDD should be taken seriously (see Chapter 27). Thoughts of death and suicide are often described as intrusive and difficult to interrupt. They are generally accompanied by a desire for death and the idea that only death will provide relief from the depressive epi-

DSM-IV DIAGNOSTIC CRITERIA

BOX 8-3 DYSTHYMIC DISORDER

A. Depressed mood for most of the day, for more days than not, as indicated either by subjective account or observation by others, for at least 2 years. **Note:** In children and adolescents, mood can be irritable and duration must be at least 1 year.

B. Presence, while depressed, of two (or more) of the following:

(1) poor appetite or overeating
(2) insomnia or hypersomnia
(3) low energy or fatigue
(4) low self-esteem
(5) poor concentration or difficulty making decisions
(6) feelings of hopelessness

C. During the 2-year period (1 year for children or adolescents) of the disturbance, the person has never been without the symptoms in Criteria A and B for more than 2 months at a time.

D. No Major Depressive Episode has been present during the first 2 years of the disturbance (1 year for children and adolescents); i.e., the disturbance is not better accounted for by chronic Major Depressive Disorder, or Major Depressive Disorder, In Partial Remission.

Note: There may have been a previous Major Depressive Episode provided there was a full remission (no significant signs or symptoms for 2 months) before development of the Dysthymic Disorder. In addition, after the initial 2 years (1 year in children or adolescents) of Dysthymic Disorder, there may be superimposed episodes of Major Depressive Disorder, in which case both diagnoses may be given when the criteria are met for a Major Depressive Episode.

E. There has never been a Manic Episode, a Mixed Episode, or a Hypomanic Episode, and criteria have never been met for Cyclothymic Disorder.

F. The disturbance does not occur exclusively during the course of a chronic Psychotic Disorder, such as Schizophrenia or Delusional Disorder.

G. The symptoms are not due to the direct physiological effects of a substance (e.g., a drug of abuse, a medication) or a general medical condition (e.g., hypothyroidism).

H. The symptoms cause clinically significant distress or impairment in social, occupational, or other important areas of functioning.

Specify if:
Early Onset: if onset is before age 21 years
Late Onset: if onset is age 21 years or older

Specify (for most recent 2 years of Dysthymic Disorder):
With Atypical Features

From American Psychiatric Association: *Diagnostic and statistical manual of mental disorders,* ed 4 (DSM-IV), Washington, D.C., 1994, American Psychiatric Press.

sode. The poor insight of depressed patients contemplating suicide is illustrated by their conviction that family members, including spouses and small children, would be better off without them. The determination of some depressed patients to commit suicide and the violent means they sometimes select bear testimony to the great suffering associated with MDD.

Other prominent distortions of thought content involve self-deprecatory ideation and hopelessness. Incessant ruminations of past failures or perceived shortcomings occupy a majority of the thought stream. Many patients describe waking up during the night to thoughts of self-reproach. In conjunction with such thoughts, self-confidence deteriorates and patients feel unable to handle conflicts or challenges at work or home that they have previously mastered. A sudden

TABLE 8-2

SYMPTOMS OF INDEX MAJOR DEPRESSIVE EPISODE

Symptoms*	Number and percentage of patients (n = 100)
Reduced energy level	97
Impaired concentration	84
Anorexia	80
Initial insomnia	77
Loss of interest	77
Difficulty starting activities	76
Worry more than usual	69
Subjective agitation	67
Slowed thinking	67
Difficulty with decision making	67
Terminal insomnia	65
Suicide ideation or plans	63
Weight loss	61
Tearfulness	61
Movements slowed (subjective perception)	60
Increased irritability	60
Feels will never get well	56
Diurnal variation	46
Difficulty finishing activities once started	46
Prominent self-pity	45
Inability to cry	44
Constipation	43
Impaired expression of emotions	42
Ruminations of worthlessness	38
Decreased libido	36
Anxiety attacks	36
Difficulty doing activities once started	35
Ruminations of guilt	32
Complains more than usual	28
Any type of delusion	27
Phobias during depression only	27
Multiple somatic symptoms during depression only	25
Communication of suicidal ideas, plans, or attempts	22
Place major blame for illness on others	19
At least one depressive delusion	16
Death wishes without suicidal ideation	16
Suicide attempts	15
Other delusions	14
Obsessions during depression only	14
Depersonalization and derealization	13
Ruminations of sinfulness	12

*The inclusion criteria for this study required that subjects had reported a mood change that they had described as either feeling depressed, blue, sad, low, discouraged, or that the future looked gloomy. The proportion of subjects endorsing each of these individual symptoms was not addressed, however.
From Winokur and Clayton, editors: *The medical basis of psychiatry,* Philadelphia, 1994, W.B. Saunders.

decrement in self-esteem is a usual concomitant of the depressive episode and can provide an important clue to its presence. Hopelessness regarding the future may develop in spite of evidence that the patient's social, economic, or medical status has not changed and appears positive to the examiner or the family. Hopelessness is reportedly associated with an elevated risk for suicide during a depressive episode.

Ruminations of guilt may achieve a delusional level. For example, patients may develop the belief that they have committed the "unpardonable sin" or have "lost their salvation," ideas that arrive with the onset of the depressive episode and depart with its remission. Patients may also describe persistent guilt regarding seemingly minor offenses they perceive having committed during interpersonal interactions. In many cases these involve statements made years earlier that have been forgotten by the recipient and are not con-

BOX 8-4

QUOTATION OF A DEPRESSED PHYSICIAN

Firstly, it is very unpleasant: depressive illness is probably more unpleasant than any disease except rabies. There is constant mental pain and often psychogenic physical pain too. If one tries to get such a patient to titrate other pains against the pain of his depression one tends to end up with a description that would raise eyebrows even in a medieval torture chamber.

Naturally, many of these patients commit suicide. They may not hope to get to heaven but they know they are leaving hell. Secondly, the patient is isolated from family and friends, because the depression itself reduces his affection for others and he may well have ideas that he is unworthy of their love or even that his friendship may harm them. Thirdly, he is rejected by others because they cannot stand the sight of his suffering.

There is a limit to sympathy. Even psychiatrists have protective mechanisms for dealing with such cases: the consultant may refer the patient to an outpatient clinic; he may allow too brief a consultation to elicit the extent of the patient's suffering; he may, on the grounds that the depression has not responded to treatment, alter his diagnosis to one of personality disorder—comforting, because of the strange but widespread belief that patients with personality disorders do not suffer.

Fourthly, and finally, the patient tends to do a great cover-up. Because of his outward depression he is socially unacceptable, and because of his inward depression he feels even more socially unacceptable than he really is. He does not, therefore, tell others how bad he feels.

Most depressives, even severe ones, can cope with routine work—initiative and leadership are what they lack. Nevertheless, many of them can continue working, functioning at a fairly low level, and their deficiencies are often covered up by colleagues. Provided some minimal degree of social and vocational functioning is present, the world leaves the depressive alone and he battles on for the sake of his god or his children, or for some reason which makes his personal torment preferable to death.

From Price, JS: Chronic depressive illness, *Br Med J* 1:1200-1201, 1978.

templated by the patient outside the context of a depressive episode. Finally, pathological guilt may target behaviors or events that the patient has not normally associated with guilt.

Psychotic features such as delusions or auditory hallucinations are present in about 20% of patients with a depressive episode and occurring most commonly in elderly patients or patients who are bipolar depressive. Depressive delusions are usually mood congruent in that they involve typical depressive themes of personal inadequacy, guilt, disease, death, nihilism, or deserved punishment. Delusions in the setting of a major depressive episode have important treatment implications, with the most effective treatments being either ECT or a combination of an antidepressant drug plus an antipsychotic drug. Additionally, a diagnosis of MDD is associated with a decreased risk of violence relative to the base rate for the population; however, when patients with MDD commit violent acts against other people, it commonly occurs in response to persecutory or nihilistic delusions. Auditory hallucinations are less common in MDD and usually convey persecutory content. Visual, tactile, or olfactory hallucinations are exceedingly rare in mood disorders, and their presence should prompt a search for metabolic, toxic, or neurological disturbances.

Psychosomatic Symptoms

Patients who are depressed often complain of headache, pains, gastrointestinal disturbances, or cardiovascular symptoms. Headache is present in the majority of cases; when it is associated with a depressive episode, it resolves along with the other depressive symptoms. Headaches may be related to increased contraction of the head and neck musculature. For example, psychophysiology studies demonstrate that the frontalis muscles have greater electromyographic activity in resting patients who are depressive than can be elicited in subjects who are not depressed and intentionally contracting their facial muscles. Gastrointestinal complaints are also common and include functional (irritable) bowel syndrome, constipation, and abdominal pain (possibly reflecting a heightened sensitivity to visceral sensation). When medical workup for somatic complaints has proven negative, the alert physician should attempt to elicit other criteria for major depression.

BOX 8-5

SUFFERING IN DEPRESSION

Now that I've had both depression and cancer, I'd have to say the cancer has been easier to deal with. Cancer is something tangible that you can understand and describe to other people. With major depression you suffer horribly, but you can neither comprehend why you feel the way you do nor communicate your suffering to others. When you talk about the pain of major depression with others it makes no sense to them.
(stated by a patient after successful treatment of her depression with doxepin, before her death from breast cancer)

Psychomotor Manifestations

Psychomotor agitation and retardation are striking clinical features of severe depressive episodes. Agitation occurs more commonly in elderly patients with depression, and retardation is found more often in younger patients who have unipolar or bipolar depression. In half of cases, the psychomotor activity is not disturbed, so a relatively normal appearance does not rule out MDD. Agitation is evident in about 30% of patients with depression who are hospitalized. When present, it may dominate the clinical presentation as patients pace, wring their hands, or incessantly complain of worries and nervousness. Such patients may repeatedly bemoan their fate, ask for reassurance, or beg for help, yet they cannot be consoled. Psychomotor retardation is observed in about 20% of hospitalized patients as a decrease in the rate and the amount of movement and speech or as a latency in the onset of speech. The slowing can sometimes be elicited by having patients perform simple motor tasks. In outpatients, psychomotor retardation is less commonly evident on the mental status examination but may nevertheless be described by the patient as a sense that the rate of their thought flow has slowed.

Neuropsychological Manifestations

Patients who are depressed often complain vociferously of impairments in concentration, memory, or ability to make decisions. However, in many cases employers, family members, and friends are unaware of any deficits in thinking or performance. In other cases school or work performance deteriorates, reflecting the combined impact of diminished motivation; preoccupation with obsessive ruminations, severe anxiety, or insomnia; and impaired concentration. Occasionally, the lack of effort and motivation on the part of the patient during the mental status examination may give the appearance that memory is impaired. This presentation has been referred to as *pseudodementia* or *dementia of depression,* in which manifestations of the memory impairment resolve with effective antidepressant treatment (see Chapter 25). Core dementing signs such as aphasia, anomia, acalculia, agraphia, or apraxia are not associated with mood disorders, and their presence suggests that if the depressive syndrome is present, it has occurred in the setting of a neurological disorder (see Chapter 26). In contrast, neuropsychological testing in patients who have MDD alone reveals only subtle impairments that in most cases cannot be differentiated from the effects of diminished effort during testing.

Impairment of Insight and Judgment

Insight may be impaired to the point that patients deny that they are ill or that their illness is treatable. Even patients who have experienced excellent antidepressant treatment responses during previous episodes may maintain that only death will relieve their suffering. Patients may also cry profusely or discuss suicide plans with the physician but deny feeling depressed or being ill. Such cases require intervention by the family and the physician to initiate and complete treatment.

Impaired insight can result in poor judgment, and depressed patients may attempt to change jobs, discontinue school, or seek divorce because they think that such a change will relieve their symptoms. It is generally prudent for the physician to advise against making such changes until the depressive episode has been effectively treated. Other examples of failures in judgment include the propensity of some patients to act on depressive delusions or to self-medicate with illicit drugs or alcohol.

Alcohol and Illicit Drug Use

Some patients increase alcohol use during depressive episodes, describing a desire to self-medicate their anxiety, insomnia, or dysphoria. Others decrease alcohol use after experiencing a worsening of such symptoms or an increase in suicidal behavior related to alcohol consumption. The former group generally admits that any relief obtained from alcohol is short-lived and usually succeeded by an exacerbation of the depressive symptoms. New onset of alcohol abuse, particularly after age 40, should prompt a careful evaluation for signs and symptoms of a mood disorder.

Illicit drugs are also employed to alleviate depressive symptoms. Marijuana and cocaine are the most common agents abused by patients with mood disorders. Cocaine can produce a depressed mood as a withdrawal symptom, making the differential diagnosis between cocaine dependence with secondary depression versus primary depression with secondary cocaine abuse difficult.

Diagnostic Subtypes

In an attempt to address the clinical heterogeneity of MDD, the depressive syndrome has been subdivided in numerous classification schemes. The DSM-IV recognizes melancholic and seasonal subtypes of MDD. The other subtypes described in the following paragraphs have proven useful in selecting relatively homogenous subject samples for mood disorders research and have noteworthy clinical implications as well.

Melancholic Type

The DSM-IV criteria for melancholic subtype are thought to identify a more severe form of MDD (Box 8-6). These criteria emphasize nonreactive mood, pervasive anhedonia, prominent neurovegetative symptoms, psychomotor signs, and freedom from characterological disturbances. A substantial body of evidence

BOX 8-6 **MELANCHOLIC FEATURES SPECIFIER**

DSM-IV DIAGNOSTIC CRITERIA

Specify if:

With Melancholic Features (can be applied to the current or most recent Major Depressive Episode in Major Depressive Disorder and to a Major Depressive Episode in Bipolar I or Bipolar II Disorder only if it is the most recent type of mood episode)

A. Either of the following, occurring during the most severe period of the current episode:

(1) loss of pleasure in all, or almost all, activities
(2) lack of reactivity to usually pleasurable stimuli (does not feel much better, even temporarily, when something good happens)

B. Three (or more) of the following:

(1) distinct quality of depressed mood (i.e., the depressed mood is experienced as distinctly different from the kind of feeling experienced after the death of a loved one)
(2) depression regularly worse in the morning
(3) early morning awakening (at least 2 hours before usual time of awakening)
(4) marked psychomotor retardation or agitation
(5) significant anorexia or weight loss
(6) excessive or inappropriate guilt

From American Psychiatric Association: *Diagnostic and statistical manual of mental disorders,* ed 4 (DSM-IV), Washington, D.C., 1994, American Psychiatric Press.

suggests that this cluster of signs and symptoms predicts a good outcome during ECT or treatment with antidepressant drugs.

Seasonal Depression

The course of depressive episodes exhibits a seasonal pattern in some cases, with depression onset occurring in fall and winter and symptom remission ensuing in the spring. Most studies of seasonal depression have been conducted in northern locations (such as Scandinavia, Canada, New England, or the Pacific Northwestern states), suggesting that it is more prevalent at latitudes where sunlight exposure substantially shortens during winter. Up to half of such patients have bipolar disorder. Winter seasonal depression may respond to phototherapy.

Primary vs. Secondary Mood Disorders

A mood disorder is considered *primary* when the pathological mood episode arises in the absence of other psychiatric disorders or chronic debilitating medical disorders that might be associated with it. In contrast, a major depressive episode is considered *secondary* to another psychiatric disorder if the first depressive episode historically ensued after the onset of the other disorder. Similarly, if the first major depressive episode ensues after the onset of a major medical illness, it can be considered secondary. This does not necessarily signify that the depression is etiologically related to the other disorder. The concept of comorbidity also attempts to characterize multiple, concomitant psychiatric syndromes, but such knowledge is less useful without the hierarchical information provided by the primary vs. secondary distinction.

The knowledge of whether a depressive episode is primary or secondary to another illness holds prognostic and therapeutic implications. As discussed below, treatment selection is generally directed toward the primary rather than the secondary disorder. Additionally, whereas primary mood disorders are often associated with a return to the premorbid baseline (that is, relative normalcy) between episodes, many secondary depressions are not, since the preexisting primary disorder is often a chronic illness (such as schizophrenia or obsessive-compulsive disorder [OCD]). Furthermore, the risk of suicide is significantly higher in primary MDD than in secondary depression (with the exception of depression secondary to alcoholism, which also carries a high risk for suicide). Finally, the sleep EEG, neuroendocrine, and neuroimaging abnormalities found in people who have primary depression with MDD or bipolar disorder are usually not found in people who have secondary depression.

Classification of Primary Unipolar Depression Using Family History

A classification that has proven useful in selecting relatively homogenous samples of subjects with unipolar depression for neuroimaging studies identifies three subtypes based on family history. Familial pure depressive disease (FPDD) is defined as primary unipolar depression in an individual who has a parent, sibling, or offspring with primary unipolar depression but no family history of alcoholism, antisocial personality disorder, or mania. Depression spectrum disease (DSD) is unipolar depression in a patient who has a first-degree relative with alcoholism or antisocial personality disorder. Sporadic depressive disease (SDD) is unipolar depression in a subject who has no first-degree relatives with a history of depression, alcoholism, or antisocial personality disorder. Patients with FPDD have been associated with abnormal dexamethasone-suppression test results in 70% to 85% of cases, regional cerebral blood flow (rCBF) abnormalities in limbic-thalamic-cortical circuits in 75% to 90% of cases, and preferential responsiveness to antidepressant drug therapy (see the related section in this chapter). In contrast, subjects with DSD are less likely to demonstrate abnormal neuroendocrine, sleep EEG, or neuroimaging results. Patients with DSD are more likely to have life events that provoke a depressive episode or a history of multiple personality difficulties and a stormy social history (such as multiple marital and social problems) that culminate in a depressive episode. Moreover, as a consequence of having family members with alcoholism or sociopathy, they are more likely to have been exposed to psychosocial traumas such as childhood abuse and may need referral for psychotherapy to address the sequelae of such events. The specificity of this taxonomy is limited by the high prevalence of alcoholism, since some severely depressed, melancholic patients who otherwise resemble subjects with FPDD are assigned to the DSD category because they have an alcoholic relative.

Late-Onset Depression

As the age of depression onset increases, the degree of familial aggregation of depression decreases, implying that genetic risk factors become less important and acquired factors grow more important in late-onset depression. Insight into the nature of these acquired factors has been provided by magnetic resonance imaging (MRI) evidence that signal hyperintensities appear in the frontal lobe, the caudate, and the white matter adjacent to these structures in 70% to 80% of subjects with depression onset after age 60. Postmortem and magnetic resonance spectroscopy (MRS) data have demonstrated that these signal hyperintensities probably reflect arteriosclerotic or ischemic lesions, and the occurrence of such abnormalities in patients who have depression correlates with both atherosclerotic risk factors and age. As expected in the presence of such lesions, positron emission tomography (PET) images from elderly patients with depression show decreased blood flow in diffuse areas of the frontal lobe that decreases further with treatment (see Chapter 6). The cerebral ventricles are also enlarged in elderly patients with depression onset after age 60 (an abnormality that persists after successful treatment), which may reflect *ex vacuo* changes after ischemic damage. It is noteworthy that the anatomical locations where signal hyperintensities are found in subjects with late-onset depression are similar to those where cerebrovascular infarction has been associated with an elevated risk for the development of poststroke depression, namely the frontal lobes and the caudate. Therefore it is thought that patients with late-onset depression who show such MRI abnormalities constitute a subgroup acquiring a mood disorder secondary to arteriosclerotic damage in the emotional circuitry that is homologous to the case of poststroke mood disorders.

A late onset of depression carries several clinical implications. Such patients commonly have neuropsychological impairments that persist after depressive symptoms have remitted. They tend to have a single chronic episode and are less likely to have recurrent episodes after symptom remission. Finally, they are less likely to respond completely to antidepressant drug treatment and prove more susceptible to the development of delirium during treatment with ECT or tricyclic antidepressant agents (TCAs).

Prevalence and Natural History

Age of Onset

The onset of MDD can occur throughout the life span, although the first depressive episode usually occurs after puberty. The median age of onset is about 34. About 20% of patients experience illness onset during the teenage years. As described in the previous section, depression onset after age 60 is associated with a distinct set of risk factors, clinical course, neuroimaging abnormalities, and treatment responsiveness as compared with early-onset illness.

The median age of onset has been decreasing, and the lifetime risk of MDD is increasing in individuals who were born more recently. The reasons for these secular trends are unclear, but they do not appear to be accounted for by changes in diagnostic methods. Similar changes in the age of onset and lifetime prevalence of MDD have been observed worldwide.

Epidemiology

The limitations in establishing diagnosis have contributed to substantial variability across epidemiological studies. In a large population-based study, the lifetime prevalence (proportion of individuals in a population who had experienced a disorder up to the time of assessment) for a major depressive episode varied between 3.7% and 6.7% over 3 catchment areas in the United States. The lifetime prevalence for dysthymia varied between 2.1% and 3.8%. Other studies have reported higher lifetime prevalence rates of MDD, ranging from 8.1% in an Iowa study to 18% in a Connecticut study. The prevalence rates reported from other countries have generally fallen within this same range.

Reported annual incidence figures for MDD vary widely, ranging from 247 to 7800 cases per 100,000 per year. In one series, 82 to 201 males and 320 to 500 females per 100,000 per year began receiving antidepressant treatment. This gender difference is not limited to the population seeking treatment, since all studies of unipolar depression show that females are about twice as likely to be affected as males, including those studies that identify both treated and untreated cases.

In the otherwise healthy elderly population, it remains controversial whether the point prevalence of MDD differs from that found in the general population. However, the point prevalence of MDD is clearly higher in special elderly populations, rising to 13% in elderly patients with concomitant medical illnesses admitted to acute care facilities and to 20% in elderly persons free of cognitive impairment who are confined to long-term care facilities. Psychosocial and physiological stressors are increased in these subgroups, and their higher prevalence of mood disorders is likely to have a multifactorial explanation (see sections in this chapter on bereavement, mood disorders induced by medical disorders, and late-onset depression). The management of geriatric depression is often complicated by treatment resistance, intercurrent medical disorders, psychotic features, and increased disability, which can necessitate relatively protracted periods of intensive treatment. Related in part to such issues, this age group requires a disproportionately high percentage of the inpatient beds devoted to depression treatment.

Family Clustering

A number of studies have examined the risk to relatives of patients with depression for developing mood disorders or other psychiatric problems. As mentioned, MDD is often co-morbid with alcoholism or anxiety disorders. The lifetime risk of a first-degree relative developing depression is about 30% (2 to 10 times the risk in the general population). The risk for a first-degree relative developing bipolar disorder is about 1% (about the same as in the general population). Earlier age of onset of MDD is associated with higher rates of both unipolar and bipolar illness in relatives. This familial clustering is thought to represent the contribution of genetic elements to liability to develop illness.

The risk of alcoholism and anxiety disorders in the relatives of patients with depression is 10% to 20%. Relatives of people who have early-onset depression are at an even higher risk for developing alcoholism. Controversy exists regarding the explanation for the increased prevalences of substance abuse and anxiety disorders in the relatives of adults with depression. Current data support the independent transmission of alcoholism and depression in families but indicate a complex interaction between depression and anxiety disorders.

Course

The usual course of MDD consists of recurrent depressive episodes that are separated by a return toward the premorbid baseline (that is, feeling back to normal). Single-episode cases are seen, but with follow-up periods of 15 or more years, most individuals have at least one recurrence. After an initial episode, the average number of episodes over the next 20 years is 5 or 6. After either spontaneous remission or discontinuation of antidepressant drug treatment, about 35% of patients experience recurrence of the depressive syndrome within 1 year. When only those patients who have had 3 or more prior episodes are considered, relapse occurs more rapidly, with 40% of patients having relapsed by 15 weeks. Thus the physician must always warn the recovered patient and her family that additional episodes are likely and educate them about early warning signs of recurrence. Periodic follow-up examinations are generally indicated.

Treatment clearly affects some aspects of the natural history of MDD. In studies performed before the use of antidepressant drug treatment, the average length of episodes ranged from 6 to 13 months and only 50% of patients had recovered at a 1-year follow-up examination. At a 3- to 5-year follow-up examination, 70% of untreated patients with depression had recovered, and at a 15-year follow-up study, 85% of patients had recovered. Thus chronicity of depressive episodes generally does not continue indefinitely. With antidepressant treatment the duration of depressive episodes is shortened and chronicity is less of a problem. One study showed that with treatment, 63% of patients had recovered at 4 months. Of patients who were chronically depressed for 2 years, 80% recovered with treatment in the ensuing 3 years. Between episodes patients may report a complete return to normalcy or simply a lessening in the severity of residual depressive symptoms. In either case, the level of functioning usually improves between episodes in patients with unipolar depression. Nevertheless, up to 20% of patients who have unipolar depression develop a chronic illness that is difficult to treat.

Ten to fifteen percent of patients who initially experience a depressive episode eventually have a manic episode. The risk factors for converting to a bipolar course include family history of bipolar disorder, psychotic features accompanying the depressive episode, and early age of onset. Patients with such risk factors should be warned about the risk for developing mania during treatment with antidepressant drugs.

Complications

Primary MDD carries a substantial risk of suicide. About 15% of patients hospitalized for a major depressive episode commit suicide (see Chapter 27). A major depressive episode is the most significant precursor of suicide and is recognized in about one half of completed suicides. Mortality from other causes is also elevated in patients with mood disorders. For example, MDD is associated with excessive mortality caused by accidental death, which may in part reflect suicides that cannot clearly be established as such. Moreover, the risk of cardiovascular mortality is doubled in patients who are depressed vs. patients with no depression who have been approximately matched for atherosclerotic risk factors or heart disease. This observation could relate to decreased medical compliance in patients who are depressed, to the autonomic changes associated with MDD, or to indications that late-onset depression, which appears to be associated with cerebrovascular disease, serves as a marker for more extensive atherosclerosis. Depression may also result in reduced oral intake, which results in dehydration or malnutrition and diminished physical activity. Such problems may predispose patients to medical complications such as falls, hip fractures, or pulmonary embolism.

Depressive episodes are accompanied by substantial suffering, disability, and social impairment. Most aspects of life are adversely affected by the reduced interest, energy, and motivation; the incessant preoccupation with negative ideation; and the impaired concentration associated with a depressive episode. As a result, major depressive episodes can lead to job loss, scholastic failure, divorce, and social isolation.

Differential Diagnosis

Bereavement

The normal emotional state that most closely resembles a major depressive episode is acute bereavement. Since up to one third of all people bereaving a spouse meet criteria for a major depressive episode within 3 months of their spouse's death, the recent death of a loved one is considered an exclusion criterion for the diagnosis of MDD (see Box 8-2). Bereavement is less persistent than major depression and is generally associated with fewer depressive symptoms. MDD differs from bereavement in that its depressive episodes may appear in the absence of precipitants and it may respond to antidepressant drug treatment, follow an episodic course, appear co-morbidly with other psychopathological signs (such as mania, psychosis, obsessions, compulsions, suicide, or pathological guilt), and be associated with neurochemical and neuroendocrine abnormalities (for example, nonsuppression of cortisol release after dexamethasone administration is common in depression but not in bereavement).

Although DSM-IV permits the presence of acute bereavement to exclude a diagnosis of MDD for only 2 months, grieving patients are generally not treated with antidepressant therapy unless they have maintained criteria for a major depressive episode beyond 6 to 12 months of losing their loved one because somatic antidepressant treatments do not significantly alter the emotional state associated with uncomplicated grief. However, suicide ideation or delusional guilt are rare in bereavement, and their presence in a bereaved person indicates a need for more aggressive treatment. People who are bereaved and meet criteria for a major depressive episode beyond 1 year (complicated bereavement) are likely to have had a psychiatric disorder before their loved one's death.

Secondary Depression

The psychiatric disorders commonly associated with secondary depression are schizophrenia, OCD, panic disorder, somatization disorder, substance abuse and dependence, and personality disorders (for example, antisocial personality disorder). The application of *secondary* also encompasses major depression associated with debilitating medical illnesses (such as chronic pain syndromes or paraplegia from long neuronal track damage). The psychiatric disorders commonly associated with secondary depression along with their implications for treatment are discussed in the following sections.

Obsessive-Compulsive Disorder

About one half of all patients with OCD develop major depressive episodes (see Chapter 10). The antidepressant drugs that potently inhibit serotonin reuptake (clomipramine, fluoxetine, fluvoxamine, sertraline, and paroxetine) are significantly more effective for OCD than those that do not, making them the agents of choice for secondary depression in patients with OCD. These antidepressant agents may also be relatively more effective for patients with primary MDD who have secondary obsessions.

Panic Disorder

About 50% of patients with panic disorder develop major depressive episodes after the onset of panic disorder (see Chapter 9). Since about one third of patients with primary MDD develop panic attacks after the onset of the mood disorder, the determination of whether a patient has primary depression with secondary panic or primary panic with secondary depression can be difficult. The family history is instructive, since relatives who have mood disorders predominate in the former case and relatives with anxiety disorders occur more often in the latter. Additionally, primary panic disorder usually has an onset before age 40. Panic attacks arising after this age in a patient with depression usually indicate that the mood disorder is primary.

The diagnostic dilemma between primary panic vs. primary MDD need not translate into a treatment selection problem as long as effective antidepressant dosages of an antidepressant drug are prescribed. In addition to their antidepressant effects, antidepressant drugs exert prophylactic effects against panic attacks. A benzodiazepine such as alprazolam can be added to the antidepressant on a "take-as-needed" basis for acute management of panic attacks. This is especially useful early in treatment, since the antipanic effect of antidepressant drugs does not appear until the third week of treatment. Although benzodiazepines can be effective monotherapy for primary panic disorder with secondary depression, they are generally not sufficiently effective for managing primary MDD with secondary panic.

Schizophrenia

At least one half of all patients with schizophrenia develop major depressive episodes (see Chapter 13). Since delusions and hallucinations can also occur in primary mood disorders, a diagnostic dilemma can exist between primary MDD with psychotic features and schizophrenia with secondary depression. The diagnosis usually becomes clear with longitudinal follow-up studies. The diagnosis is more likely to be MDD with psychotic features if remission of delusions or hallucinations is maintained after discontinuation of the antipsychotic drug or if the illness course is episodic rather than chronic. In contrast, schizophrenia is typically accompanied by progressive social deterioration and negative symptoms (for example, impoverished speech and thought content, blunting of the affect and personality, loss of initiative, and apathy). Finally, the family history provides diagnostic clues, since MDD with psychotic features typically occurs in patients who have relatives with mood disorders. Initial management of either MDD with psychotic features or schizophrenia with secondary depression usually involves combined treatment with an antipsychotic drug and an antidepressant drug, although the addition of the antidepressant drug is usually minimally effective for depressive symptoms associated with schizophrenia.

Somatization Disorder

Patients with somatization disorder (see Chapter 16) complain as dramatically of depressive and anxiety symptoms as they do of somatic symptoms. They tend to score highly on depression rating scales because they endorse most symptoms. However, their affect is usually not appropriate to the severity level indicated by their complaints. Even though they describe suicidal thoughts and intense dysphoria they may smile, jest, or demonstrate *la belle indifférence.* They often report resolution of their depressive complaints after only a few days of evaluation—before treatments are expected to be effective.

Patients with primary MDD can also develop somatic complaints that are not explained by the medical evaluation. These complaints seldom spread throughout the entire review-of-systems as they do for patients with somatization disorder. Additionally, conversion symptoms (unexplained neurological symptoms) are uncommon in primary mood disorders. Finally, the unexplained somatic complaints have generally not been present outside of the historical context of a depressive episode and resolve completely with effective antidepressant treatment. In contrast, patients with somatization disorder have long histories of unexplained somatic complaints dating to adolescence or early adulthood that have been present even in the absence of secondary depression.

Alcohol Dependence

Patients with primary alcoholism may develop secondary depression. The differential diagnosis in this case includes primary MDD with secondary alcohol dependence, since some patients who are depressive increase their drinking behavior during episodes of illness. In either case a major goal of treatment involves the discontinuation of the alcohol use. Antidepressant drugs may benefit either condition, and the new generation agents that are nonlethal in overdose and not potently sedating are preferable (see the section in this chapter on treatment).

Alcohol may produce depressive symptoms by direct and withdrawal effects. During intoxication the mood can become labile or dysphoric, judgment is impaired, and patients become disinhibited and impulsive. In this condition patients may come to the emergency room after a suicide attempt or complaining of suicidal intention. While they are intoxicated they may endorse criteria for the major depressive syndrome. When reinterviewed during sobriety, many of these patients deny any further suicidal ideation or death wish and neither demonstrate nor endorse the emotional and neurovegetative manifestations of the depressive syndrome. Depressive symptoms associated with alcohol withdrawal commonly last 2 weeks or more.

Cocaine and Amphetamine Dependence

Depressed mood and anhedonia are observed in the first few weeks or months after withdrawal from cocaine or amphetamine dependence. These agents respectively block reuptake or facilitate release of dopamine in the mesocorticolimbic dopaminergic projections that are thought to subserve a reward-related system in the brain. During repeated exposure to cocaine the postsynaptic dopamine receptors in the mesolimbic system become desensitized. It is thought that this subsensitive receptor state may be associated with anhedonia once dopamine transmission is no longer being facilitated by cocaine. These emotional symptoms generally resolve within 1 week to several months, which is the postulated time needed to reflect the restoration of dopamine receptor sensitivity toward the precocaine baseline. Depressed mood and anhedonia may increase risk for relapse during cocaine withdrawal and may be reduced by antidepressant drug treatment (although antidepressant treatment does not appear to substantially alter the relapse rate of cocaine dependence).

Depressive Disorders Induced by Pharmacologic Agents or Medical Disorders

The DSM-IV includes a category of mood disorders related to medical disorders, which are referred to when a mood syndrome, based upon "the history, physical examination, or laboratory findings, is the direct *physiological* consequence of a general medical condition" and is not better accounted for by an "adjustment disorder with depressed mood in response to the stress of having a general medical condition" (DSM-IV, 1994). The term *adjustment disorder* is applied to depressive symptoms that do not meet criteria for MDD but are felt to constitute maladaptive psychological responses to the disability, pain, or terminal nature of a medical disorder. Ideally, the determination that a secondary major depressive syndrome arises as a pathophysiological consequence of the primary condition is based on literature establishing an increased risk for the development of the major depressive syndrome when that primary condition is compared with control conditions that are matched for disability, suffering, and prognosis (see Chapter 26). Such studies are difficult to accomplish.

Conceptually, the category of mood disorders related to medical disorders is applied to specific conditions that are thought to induce depressive or manic episodes through their neuropathological or neurochemical effects in the neural systems that subserve emotional processing and modulation. For example, Parkinson's disease is associated with a twofold to fourfold increase in the risk for the depressive syndrome compared with quadriplegia resulting from long track damage and a fourfold to eightfold increase in the risk when compared with severe degenerative arthritis. In Parkinson's disease the degeneration of mesolimbic (in addition to nigrostriatal) dopaminergic projections is thought to affect central reward-related systems. In contrast, it is less clear that the chronically debilitating medical conditions mentioned in the discussion of secondary depression exert a direct effect on the limbic circuitry or produce elevated rates of the major depressive syndromes relative to similarly debilitating medical conditions. The physiological and psychological effects of chronic stress may play a role in such secondary depressive syndromes. For example, elevated activity within the hypothalamic-pituitary-adrenal axis during stress may result in sustained release of corticosteroids or corticotropin releasing factor, which have both been implicated in producing depressive symptoms. Alternatively, some chronic diseases that are commonly associated with secondary depression, such as diabetes mellitus, may produce diffuse changes in small vessels or neurons in the limbic system that have not yet been identified. Such secondary mood disorders may eventually be thought of as being directly induced by the underlying medical condition. Similarly, some psychiatric disorders that are associated with secondary depression have also been associated with neuropathological changes (for example, schizophrenia) or functional anatomical changes (such as in OCD) in the same neural systems implicated in the pathophysiology of the primary mood disorders (see Chapter 6). They thus may also be inducing depressive episodes on a similar pathophysiological basis.

In summary, the distinction between induced mood syndromes and secondary depressive syndromes remains nebulous since the pathophysiology of these conditions is not understood. The uncertain knowledge regarding the neural substrates of human emotion and of primary mood disorders permits only hypotheses and unclear pathophysiological links between medical disorders and induced mood syndromes. Since current knowledge does not permit reliable distinctions between mood disturbances that are physiological responses from those that are psychological responses to a medical stressor, some advocate grouping depressive syndromes arising in the setting of any medical condition under the general category of secondary mood disorders.

The medical diseases that can putatively induce depressive syndromes based on their increased risk of being associated with depressive episodes relative to similarly debilitating conditions include endocrine disturbances (such as hypothyroidism or Cushing's syndrome); degenerative basal ganglia disorders (for example, Parkinson's, Huntington's and Wilson's diseases); epileptic foci involving the temporal lobe; and structural lesions (such as tumors, infarcts or, injury) involving the striatum, the frontal lobe, or the mesiotemporal cortex (see Chapter 26). The association between these diseases and pathological mood syndromes holds implications for the pathophysiology of the primary mood disorders, as discussed in the pathophysiology section of this chapter. For example, in Huntington's disease the major depressive syndrome may arise before motor manifestations and before the patient has knowledge of his risk for the disease. The striatal neuronal degeneration occurring in this early period of Huntington's disease may thus provide an important insight into the pathophysiology of the primary mood disorders, which are also associated with striatal abnormalities in neuroimaging studies (see Chapter 6).

The DSM-IV category for mood effects related to pharmacologic agents is *Substance-Induced Mood Disorder,* with specification added as to whether the major depressive syndrome appears associated with the direct effects of the drug or with its withdrawal effects. This category largely consists of agents that putatively induce similar neuroendocrine or biochemical abnormalities found in the primary idiopathic mood disorders. Examples include corticosteroids (such as prednisone) and catecholamine depleting agents (such as reserpine). Mild to moderate depressive symptoms are also reported by some women who are taking oral contraceptive agents. No clear mechanism is evident for other medications, such as cimetidine, that are associated with an increased risk for developing depressive episodes. The drug withdrawal states associated with depressive symptoms include withdrawal from sedative-hypnotic agents (for example, barbiturates and alcohol) or psychostimulants (cocaine or amphetamine).

The Bipolar Disorders and Cyclothymic Disorder

Bipolar affective disorder (or manic-depressive illness) is often a severe, chronic illness characterized by periods of depression and elation. If untreated, patients suffer prolonged distress and impairment. Manic and depressed phases are both associated with significant morbidity and mortality. Cyclothymia represents a clinically milder but distinct disorder. For the majority of patients with bipolar affective disorder effective treatments exist. However, even with optimal treatment most patients need some level of long-term medical care. Because of the variable presentation, course, and severity of these relatively common disorders, suspected cases of bipolar disorder should have comprehensive psychiatric evaluations for diagnosis and initial treatment planning.

Diagnostic Criteria

Bipolar disorder is defined by the presence of a manic episode alone or by a hypomanic episode with a history of one or more depressive episodes (see Box 8-2; Boxes 8-7, 8-8, and 8-9, pp. 116-119). As defined in DSM-IV, a manic episode represents a distinct period of abnormally and persistently elevated, expansive, or irritable mood lasting at least 1 week. During mania, patients experience psychomotor restlessness, an inflated sense of self-esteem or grandiosity, a decreased need for sleep, a sense that their thoughts are racing, and pressured speech (Table 8-3, p. 120). Distractibility is common, and the flow of speech demonstrates rapid changes in the content of thought (flight of ideas). Individuals often show an increased interest in or an excessive involvement in pleasurable activities (for example, sexual indiscretions) or activities of questionable judgment (such as spending sprees). Psychotic features such as paranoia or delusions may be present. The disturbance in mood must be severe enough to cause impairment in occupational or social functioning and cannot be directly related to the effects of a pharmacological substance or a medical condition (such as stroke or hyperthyroidism).

The criteria for a hypomanic episode are similar to those for a manic episode except that the disturbance of mood is not severe enough to cause marked impairment in occupational or social functioning. Additionally, no psychotic features are present. Hypomania is characterized by a distinct period of persistently elevated or irritable mood lasting at least 4 days and different from the individual's usual mental state. During the mood disturbance there is persistent inflated self-esteem or grandiosity, decreased need for sleep, increased talkativeness, flight of ideas, or racing thoughts. Distractibility, increased goal-oriented activity, and excessive involvement in pleasurable activities are common. As with mania, symptoms cannot be attributed to the effects of medications, substances of abuse, or general medical conditions.

Bipolar disorder is usually divided into two forms—I and II. The diagnosis of bipolar I disorder requires a manic episode. The individual may also have experienced depressive episodes or mixed episodes of manic and depressive symptoms. The diagnosis of bipolar II disorder requires at least two major depressive episodes and a hypomanic episode. Once an individual qualifies for the diagnosis of bipolar I or bipolar II disorder, the diagnosis during subsequent mood episodes continues to be bipolar disorder, with the most recent episode being described as depressed or manic.

In contrast to the bipolar disorders, cyclothymic

DSM-IV DIAGNOSTIC CRITERIA

BOX 8-7 MANIC EPISODE

A. A distinct period of abnormally and persistently elevated, expansive, or irritable mood, lasting at least 1 week (or any duration if hospitalization is necessary).

B. During the period of mood disturbance, three (or more) of the following symptoms have persisted (four if the mood is only irritable) and have been present to a significant degree:

(1) inflated self-esteem or grandiosity
(2) decreased need for sleep (e.g., feels rested after only 3 hours of sleep)
(3) more talkative than usual or pressure to keep talking
(4) flight of ideas or subjective experience that thoughts are racing
(5) distractibility (i.e., attention too easily drawn to unimportant or irrelevant external stimuli)
(6) increase in goal-directed activity (either socially, at work or school, or sexually) or psychomotor agitation
(7) excessive involvement in pleasurable activities that have a high potential for painful consequences (e.g., engaging in unrestrained buying sprees, sexual indiscretions, or foolish business investments)

C. The symptoms do not meet criteria for a Mixed Episode.

D. The mood disturbance is sufficiently severe to cause marked impairment in occupational functioning or in usual social activities or relationships with others, or to necessitate hospitalization to prevent harm to self or others, or there are psychotic features.

E. The symptoms are not due to the direct physiological effects of a substance (e.g., a drug of abuse, a medication, or other treatment) or a general medical condition (e.g., hyperthyroidism).

Note: Manic-like episodes that are clearly caused by somatic antidepressant treatment (e.g., medication, electroconvulsive therapy, light therapy) should not count toward a diagnosis of Bipolar I Disorder.

From American Psychiatric Association: *Diagnostic and statistical manual of mental disorders,* ed 4 (DSM-IV), Washington, D.C., 1994, American Psychiatric Press.

disorder (Box 8-10, p. 121) is characterized by numerous fluctuating periods of hypomanic and depressive symptoms that occur for at least 2 years (1 year for adolescents). None of the episodes of either hypomanic or depressive symptoms meet the full criteria for a manic, hypomanic, or major depressive episode. By definition, cyclothymia is a chronic disorder that often progresses to the development of bipolar I or bipolar II disorder.

Clinical Picture

The emotional, neurovegetative, psychological, psychosomatic, psychomotor, and neuropsychological manifestations of the depressed phase of the bipolar affective disorders are the same as those for MDD. However, the manic or hypomanic stages of bipolar affective disorder possess a unique constellation of features.

Emotional Manifestations

As described in the diagnostic criteria of DSM-IV, a principal feature of the manic or hypomanic state is a distinct change in mood state characterized by a persistently elevated, expansive, or irritable mood. The patient does not describe herself as having a problem but as feeling better than ever or being full of energy and drive. Patients often describe feeling powerful or indestructible. Family members or acquaintances describe them as being more active, upbeat, euphoric, or irritable than usual and as not recognizing normal social boundaries. In contrast to the depression disorders where the primary feeling is one of either sadness or anhedonia, individuals in manic or hypomanic states feel elated and are overly optimistic. The primary distinction between the emotional disturbances of individuals who are manic, hypomanic, or cyclothymic is one of degree. In a manic state the mood disturbances result in marked impairment of occupational social functioning, whereas in hypomanic or cyclothymic states euphoria does not cause significant impairment. As in the major depressive syndrome, irritability is often present. However, in contrast to the irritability noted in depression, irritability in manic syndromes is associated with increased energy and drive, as well as feelings that others are inhibiting the individual's progress or recognition.

Neurovegetative Manifestations

In MDD the most common neurovegetative symptoms are easy fatiguability and loss of energy. The reverse is true for mania. Patients generally describe

BOX 8-8 HYPOMANIC EPISODE

DSM-IV DIAGNOSTIC CRITERIA

A. A distinct period of persistently elevated, expansive, or irritable mood, lasting throughout at least 4 days, that is clearly different from the usual nondepressed mood.

B. During the period of mood disturbance, three (or more) of the following symptoms have persisted (four if the mood is only irritable) and have been present to a significant degree:

(1) inflated self-esteem or grandiosity
(2) decreased need for sleep (e.g., feels rested after only 3 hours of sleep)
(3) more talkative than usual or pressure to keep talking
(4) flight of ideas or subjective experience that thoughts are racing
(5) distractibility (i.e., attention too easily drawn to unimportant or irrelevant external stimuli)
(6) increase in goal-directed activity (either socially, at work or school, or sexually) or psychomotor agitation
(7) excessive involvement in pleasurable activities that have a high potential for painful consequences (e.g., the person engages in unrestrained buying sprees, sexual indiscretions, or foolish business investments)

C. The episode is associated with an unequivocal change in functioning that is uncharacteristic of the person when not symptomatic.

D. The disturbance in mood and the change in functioning are observable by others.

E. The episode is not severe enough to cause marked impairment in social or occupational functioning, or to necessitate hospitalization, and there are no psychotic features.

F. The symptoms are not due to the direct physiological effects of a substance (e.g., a drug of abuse, a medication, or other treatment) or a general medical condition (e.g., hyperthyroidism).

Note: Hypomanic-like episodes that are clearly caused by somatic antidepressant treatment (e.g., medication, electroconvulsive therapy, light therapy) should not count toward a diagnosis of Bipolar II Disorder.

From American Psychiatric Association: *Diagnostic and statistical manual of mental disorders,* ed 4 (DSM-IV), Washington, D.C., 1994, American Psychiatric Press.

needing only a few hours of sleep a night, or they do not sleep at all for several days. They have more energy and drive than usual. Alterations in appetite and weight are less predictable than in MDD, although weight loss is common in manic states secondary to increased activity levels. Such overactivity and weight loss in the elderly can contribute to a marked worsening of other medical conditions or lead to malnutrition. Also in contrast to the depressive syndromes, people who are manic or hypomanic often describe increased libido and increased enjoyment of pleasurable activities. This commonly involves increased interest if not outright promiscuity in sexual activities. These behaviors can put the individual at increased risk for sexually transmitted diseases and for legal difficulties.

Psychosomatic Symptoms

Whereas psychosomatic symptoms are common in people who are depressed, most manic or hypomanic individuals describe themselves as having no physical complaints or problems.

Psychomotor Manifestations

Psychomotor agitation is common in manic and hypomanic states. Patients have increased motoric activity, pacing, or tapping behaviors. Psychomotor retardation is uncommon, although it can be associated with manic catatonic states in which there is immobility. Such catatonic states can be life threatening because of the decreased intake of food and fluids and must be aggressively treated with hospitalization.

Neuropsychological Manifestations

Most patients who are manic or hypomanic feel that their concentration, memory, and ability to make decisions are markedly improved. These self-observations are commonly belied by their inappropriate and self-destructive behaviors. Although work and school performance may improve and productivity may increase in the initial stages of a manic episode, work and school performance deteriorate as the manic state worsens. In contrast to the mechanism of lack of motivation in depression, deteriorated work and school performance in manic states are secondary

DSM-IV DIAGNOSTIC CRITERIA

BOX 8-9 BIPOLAR I DISORDER

Single manic episode

A. Presence of only one Manic Episode and no past Major Depressive Episodes.

Note: Recurrence is defined as either a change in polarity from depression or an interval of at least 2 months without manic symptoms.

B. The Manic Episode is not better accounted for by Schizoaffective Disorder and is not superimposed on Schizophrenia, Schizophreniform Disorder, Delusional Disorder, or Psychotic Disorder Not Otherwise Specified.

Specify if:
Mixed: if symptoms meet criteria for a Mixed Episode

Specify (for current or most recent episode):
Severity/Psychotic/Remission Specifiers
With Catatonic Features
With Postpartum Onset

Most recent episode hypomanic

A. Currently (or most recently) in a Hypomanic Episode.

B. There has previously been at least one Manic Episode or Mixed Episode.

C. The mood symptoms cause clinically significant distress or impairment in social, occupational, or other important areas of functioning.

D. The mood episodes in Criteria A and B are not better accounted for by Schizoaffective Disorder and are not superimposed on Schizophrenia, Schizophreniform Disorder, Delusional Disorder, or Psychotic Disorder Not Otherwise Specified.

Specify:
Longitudinal Course Specifiers (With and Without Interepisode Recovery)
With Seasonal Pattern (applies only to the pattern of Major Depressive Episodes)
With Rapid Cycling

Most recent episode manic

A. Currently (or most recently) in a Manic Episode.

B. There has previously been at least one Major Depressive Episode Manic Episode, or Mixed Episode.

C. The mood episodes in Criteria A and B are not better accounted for by Schizoaffective Disorder and are not superimposed on Schizophrenia, Schizophreniform Disorder, Delusional Disorder, or Psychotic Disorder Not Otherwise Specified.

Specify (for current or most recent episode):
Severity/Psychotic/Remission Specifiers
With Catatonic Features
With Postpartum Onset

Specify:
Longitudinal Course Specifiers (With and Without Interepisode Recovery)
With Seasonal Pattern (applies only to the pattern of Major Depressive Episodes)
With Rapid Cycling

From American Psychiatric Association: *Diagnostic and statistical manual for mental disorders,* ed 4 (DSM-IV), Washington, D.C., 1994, American Psychiatric Press.

DSM-IV DIAGNOSTIC CRITERIA

BOX 8-9 **BIPOLAR I DISORDER—CONT'D**

Most recent episode mixed

A. Currently (or most recently) in a Mixed Episode.

B. There has previously been at least one Major Depressive Episode, Manic Episode, or Mixed Episode.

C. The mood episodes in Criteria A and B are not better accounted for by Schizoaffective Disorder and are not superimposed on Schizophrenia, Schizophreniform Disorder, Delusional Disorder, or Psychotic Disorder Not Otherwise Specified.

Specify (for current or most recent episode):
Severity/Psychotic/Remission Specifiers
With Catatonic Features
With Postpartum Onset

Specify:
Longitudinal Course Specifiers (With and Without Interepisode Recovery)
With Seasonal Pattern (applies only to the pattern of Major Depressive Episodes)
With Rapid Cycling

Most recent episode depressed

A. Currently (or most recently) in a Major Depressive Episode.

B. There has previously been at least one Manic Episode or Mixed Episode.

C. The mood episodes in Criteria A and B are not better accounted for by Schizoaffective Disorder and are not superimposed on Schizophrenia, Schizophreniform Disorder, Delusional Disorder, or Psychotic Disorder Not Otherwise Specified.

Specify (for current or most recent episode):
Severity/Psychotic/Remission Specifiers
Chronic
With Catatonic Features
With Melancholic Features
With Atypical Features
With Postpartum Onset

Specify:
Longitudinal Course Specifiers (With and Without Interepisode Recovery)
With Seasonal Pattern (applies only to the pattern of Major Depressive Episodes)
With Rapid Cycling

Note: The Bipolar II Disorders are comparable, with these inclusion criteria requiring the presence of a hypomanic episode rather than a manic episode in a subject who has never experienced a manic episode.

to the loss of normal social boundaries and judgment. Patients in severe manic states may appear as if they have schizophrenia because of their disorganization of the thought stream and the presence of delusions and auditory hallucinations. Patients who are manic also describe a sensation of racing thoughts that interferes with their ability to organize activities. This is clinically apparent as pressured or rapid speech or as numerous tangential shifts in the topic of conversation (flight of ideas).

Impairment of Insight and Judgment

A classic manifestation of manic states is the loss of economic and social judgment. Many patients engage in spending sprees or convince other individuals that they have large resources even though they are buying far beyond their means. In untreated states, people who are manic may ruin their family's financial position. Additionally, there is a clear lack of social judgment and inhibition that may result in spousal or child physical abuse or other violent behavior. Violent be-

DIAGNOSIS

TABLE 8-3

BIPOLAR DISORDER, MANIC OR HYPOMANIC PHASE

Discriminating feature

1. Distinct period of abnormally and persistently elevated, expansive, or irritable mood, lasting 1 week or longer

Consistent features

1. Episodic course
2. Labile mood and affect
3. Elevated self-esteem, inflated assessment of personal capabilities
4. Elevated psychomotor activity: agitation, restlessness, increased energy, racing thoughts
5. Speech faster, louder, or more voluminous
6. Insomnia with decreased subjective need for sleep
7. Family history of mood disorder
8. Distractibility
9. Increased involvement in goal-directed or pleasurable activities
10. Impaired insight and judgment

Variable features

1. Threatening speech or behavior
2. Auditory hallucinations, persecutory or grandiose delusions (consistent in mania)
3. Co-morbid substance abuse
4. Religiosity exceeds usual baseline, religious ideas bizarre relative to group norms
5. Catatonic features

havior is more common in the presence of psychotic symptoms. As mentioned, poor judgment with respect to sexual contacts may place the individual at great risk for sexually transmitted diseases or pregnancy.

Alcohol and Illicit Drug Use

Patients in manic or hypomanic states commonly abuse alcohol or other substances. This may represent attempts to self-medicate with alcohol or sedating drugs of abuse, or it may reflect increased engagement in pleasurable activities along with diminished judgment. In today's culture, manic or hypomanic patients most commonly abuse alcohol, cocaine, amphetamines (or related stimulants), marijuana, and sedative-hypnotics. At times, it becomes difficult to distinguish a manic episode from drug-induced or drug-withdrawal related behaviors.

Prevalence and Natural History

Age of Onset

Controversy exists regarding the age-of-onset distribution of the bipolar disorders. Historically, the average age of onset has been reported as being in the early twenties, with approximately 20% of cases arising in adolescence. However, the age of onset is often obscure, since patients with bipolar disorder may suffer symptoms for several years before formal diagnosis. Moreover, patients with bipolar disorder typically suffer one or more depressive episodes before the first manic or hypomanic episode. Hence these individuals receive a formal diagnosis at a later age than their true onset of illness. Consistent with this concern, new studies of children and young adolescents have suggested that the incidence of bipolar disorder with early onset has been underestimated. Moreover, as with MDD there is evidence that the age of onset of bipolar disorder is decreasing among individuals born more recently. In contrast to MDD, the onset of bipolar disorder after age 40 is rare and should prompt a full medical evaluation. Much less is known about the age of onset distribution for cyclothymia. Many well-documented cases of cyclothymia developed several years before the onset of the more clear-cut bipolar disorder.

Epidemiology

Bipolar disorders occur in between 1.5% and 3% of the general population. Based on community samples the lifetime prevalence is approximately 0.8% for bipolar I disorder, 0.5% for bipolar II disorder, and 0.5% for cyclothymic disorder. Unlike MDD, the prevalence of these disorders is the same for men and women. Also in contrast to MDD, there is little evidence that the prevalence of the bipolar disorders is changing. There is no association with race, ethnic group, or socioeconomic class of the parents, although affected individuals commonly drop in social class. Although the bipolar disorders are much less common than MDD per se, the marked degree of personal and familial morbidity and mortality associated with these disorders makes them important public health problems.

Familial Clustering

As with MDD the bipolar disorders cluster in families. The risk among first-degree relatives is 6% to 7% for bipolar I disorder, 2% to 5% for bipolar II disorder, and 25% to 35% for MDD. In contrast, first-degree relatives of bipolar II patients are at significantly increased risk for developing bipolar II disorder and MDD but not for developing bipolar I disorder. For early-onset cases of bipolar I or bipolar II disorder, the number of

DSM-IV DIAGNOSTIC CRITERIA

BOX 8-10 CYCLOTHYMIC DISORDER

A. For at least 2 years, the presence of numerous periods with hypomanic symptoms and numerous periods with depressive symptoms that do not meet criteria for a Major Depressive Episode. **Note:** In children and adolescents, the duration must be at least 1 year.

B. During the above 2-year period (1 year in children and adolescents), the person has not been without the symptoms in Criterion A for more than 2 months at a time.

C. No Major Depressive Episode, Manic Episode, or Mixed Episode has been present during the first 2 years of the disturbance.

Note: After the initial 2 years (1 year in children and adolescents) of Cyclothymic Disorder, there may be superimposed Manic or Mixed Episodes (in which case both Bipolar I Disorder and Cyclothymic Disorder may be diagnosed) or Major Depressive Episodes (in which case both Bipolar II Disorder and Cyclothymic Disorder may be diagnosed).

D. The symptoms in Criterion A are not better accounted for by Schizoaffective Disorder and are not superimposed on Schizophrenia, Schizophreniform Disorder, Delusional Disorder, or Psychotic Disorder Not Otherwise Specified.

E. The symptoms are not due to the direct physiological effects of a substance (e.g., a drug of abuse, a medication) or a general medical condition (e.g., hyperthyroidism).

F. The symptoms cause clinically significant distress or impairment in social, occupational, or other important areas of functioning.

From American Psychiatric Association: *Diagnostic and statistical manual of mental disorders,* ed 4 (DSM-IV), Washington, D.C., 1994, American Psychiatric Press.

relatives with mood disorders is especially high. Cyclothymic disorder has not been as well studied, but the prevalence of bipolar disorders and MDD among first-degree relatives of patients with cyclothymia also appears increased.

For all of these mood disorders, the familial risks for substance-abuse disorders (especially alcoholism) are elevated. Hence, the identification of a patient as having a bipolar disorder identifies a family with a markedly increased risk for both affective disorders and substance-abuse disorders. It is prudent to screen family members for these conditions.

Course

Bipolar patients commonly experience multiple major depressive episodes before their first manic or hypomanic episode. Early in the illness course, episodes of depression or mania are often separated by relatively long periods of normal behavior; without treatment, subsequent episodes occur more often. Untreated manic or depressive episodes typically last several months. However, with treatment both manic and depressive episodes decrease in length and severity.

The course of the bipolar disorders shows marked variability both within and between individuals. For 10% to 15% of patients with bipolar I or bipolar II disorder the number of episodes increases to four or more per year. This "rapid cycling" form carries a relatively poor prognosis, because such patients are less responsive to treatment and suffer greater social and occupational morbidity, as well as higher suicide rates. Some patients develop episodes that have prominent features of both mania and depression. These mixed episodes may confuse physicians regarding response to treatment. Psychotic symptoms may develop during any manic episode, but once they are present, subsequent manic episodes are more likely to be accompanied by psychotic features. Approximately 20% to 30% of patients with bipolar I disorder and 15% to 20% of patients with bipolar II disorder do not experience total recovery between episodes. These patients manifest continued mood liability, irritability, and occupational and social impairment.

The course of cyclothymic disorder is chronic by definition (see Box 8-10). Of patients with cyclothymic disorder, 20% to 50% develop bipolar disorder over the next few years.

Complications

Bipolar disorder, like primary MDD, carries an increased risk of suicide and accidental death. Suicides are more common during depressed or mixed manic/

depressive episodes and while patients are intoxicated. Accidental injury and death are more common when patients are in manic and hypomanic states because of their poor judgment and increased risk-taking behavior. Mania in the elderly is associated with increased medical morbidity caused by malnutrition and exhaustion states that result from increased activity and decreased sleep. Manic episodes in patients with atherosclerotic vascular disease or other serious medical problems are particularly likely to increase mortality and morbidity.

Mania, hypomania, and cyclothymia are all associated with marked occupational, scholastic, and social impairment. The risks of substance abuse, divorce, spousal abuse, child physical abuse, truancy, school failure, job loss, and financial distress are markedly increased in untreated mania. Whereas individuals in hypomanic episodes are often described as being more creative and productive, irritability and difficulties getting along with family or peers may result in numerous job changes or divorce. The morbidity associated with depressive episodes is similar to that as described for MDD. Individuals with mixed manic/depressive episodes appear to have the highest psychosocial morbidity.

Differential Diagnosis

The differential diagnosis of the bipolar disorders is dependent on the phase of illness. The depressed phase of bipolar I or bipolar II disorder must be distinguished from MDD. This differential is critical, since the treatment implications for depressive episodes with or without a history of mania differ. The depressed phase of bipolar disorder must also be distinguished from depressive syndromes induced by general medical conditions or pharmacological substances. The substance-induced depressive disorders can be particularly difficult to distinguish from depressive episodes with a history of mania when only cross-sectional information is available. In this case, the identity of the medication class ingested or detection in the drug screen may suggest a substance-induced mood disturbance. Agents that can produce such syndromes include alcohol, cocaine, barbiturates, and corticosteroids.

When the manic phase of bipolar I disorder is accompanied by psychotic features, it must be distinguished from other psychotic disorders such as schizoaffective disorder and schizophrenia. These disorders can all present with irritability, grandiosity, hallucinations, delusions, or paranoia. Marked changes in mood and a history of prior manic and depressive episodes are more typical of bipolar disorder. In contrast, the other psychotic disorders are characterized by primary disturbances in perception that exist, at least for a significant time, in the absence of changes in mood. Additionally, the family histories usually differ between the bipolar and psychotic disorders. The distinction of mania from schizophrenia or schizoaffective disorder can prove especially difficult in adolescents or in cases where the past psychiatric and family history are unavailable.

Manic-like or hypomanic-like episodes may also be associated with general medical conditions or with substance abuse. For example, hyperthyroidism may result in an agitated state that is clinically indistinguishable from mania. Mania has also been reported after stroke or traumatic injury, and it may rarely arise in patients with Huntington's disease or cerebral tumors (see Chapter 26). Manic-like or hypomanic-like symptoms are commonly associated with intoxication or withdrawal from a variety of illicit drugs (such as cocaine, phencyclidine [PCP], or amphetamine). Manic-like episodes may also be precipitated by antidepressants.

Etiology

Environmental Factors

Environmental factors are presumed to play a role in the genesis of mood disorders, although the identity of these factors and the nature of their effects in the brain remain poorly understood. Family studies of bipolar disorder and MDD indicate that among monozygotic twin pairs in which one twin is affected, the concordance rates for bipolar disorder and MDD in the co-twins are only about 75% and 50%, respectively, suggesting that nonheritable as well as heritable factors are involved in disease expression. Environmental factors are also suggested by the decreasing age at onset for both MDD and bipolar disorder in successive birth cohorts.

Since some aspects of a major depressive episode resemble a severe stress response (for example, bereavement), it has been presumed that stressful events constitute one type of environmental factor that may play a role in the development of mood disorders. However, such a link has been difficult to establish. Depressed patients may or may not mention life events or situations that they consider important in precipitating their depressive symptoms. Many patients state that they have no reasons to feel depressed since their social, economic, medical, or spiritual status has not significantly changed, an observation that may be corroborated by family members. In particular, patients with recurrent depressive episodes learn that their pattern of depressive or euphoric symptoms is inappropriate to and not explained by life situations. Other patients report stressors that seem trivial and difficult for the physician to take seriously, suggesting that patients attempt to account for depressive symptoms on the basis of a psychological response to a stressor. Furthermore, when a more substantial precipitating event is reported by a patient, a critical evaluation of the chronology of the patient's symptoms often reveals that the depressive symptoms preceded the event. This is partly because stressful events such as job loss and marital conflict may occur as consequences of a depressive episode. In other cases the importance of life events to depressive episodes is difficult to evaluate because the onset of the mood episode cannot be determined. Until the onset of depressive episodes can be better defined, it will remain difficult to assess the strength of the contribution of life events to the development of mood disorders.

Chronology is less of a problem in studies that have examined the relationship between adult-onset depression and traumatic events occurring in childhood. For example, parental loss in childhood has been associated with an increased risk for the development of MDD in adulthood in some studies. However, most of these studies failed to control for the possibility that early parental loss occurred because of parental affective illness that led to suicide, accidental death, or disturbed family relationships. Having parents with mood disorders increases the risk for developing MDD on a genetic basis, confounding attempts to assign etiological significance to childhood bereavement experiences.

Nevertheless, some patients who meet criteria for MDD do appear to consistently develop depressive symptoms on the basis of adverse psychosocial events. Depressive episodes in this subgroup have been termed *neurotic-reactive* or *exogenous* by some classifications to distinguish them from *endogenous* episodes that appear to have a pathophysiological basis. This distinction may have theoretical utility, but its clinical utility remains elusive since behavioral signs and symptoms that sort pathophysiologically-based depressions from psychologically-based depressions or reliably predict response to pharmacological vs. psychotherapeutic treatments have not been identified.

Life events that are associated with the development of pathological mood syndromes in patients with endogenous MDD or bipolar disorder include pregnancy and delivery. The postpartum period in particular constitutes the epoch of greatest risk for the onset of mood disorders and for the recurrence of mood episodes. In one series 37% of women with bipolar disorder and 17% of women with unipolar depression experienced their first major depressive episode during pregnancy or the post-postpartum period. The increased susceptibility to mood disorders during these times suggests an effect of the hormonal changes accompanying these events. Such an interaction may also account for the twofold increase in the incidence of depression in women relative to men and for the exacerbations of depressive symptoms that commonly occur in depressed women in the 1 to 2 weeks preceding menses.

Although the data do not establish a simple relationship between psychosocial stressors and the development of mood disorders, a complex interaction between stress and individual biological predisposition may exist. For example, one of the heritable factors for mood disorders may be an increased susceptibility to the effects of stress. This hypothesis is supported by recent twin and recurrence studies. Post et al. have specifically hypothesized that the genetic risk for mood disorders is conferred by an anomalous susceptibility of limbic neurons (such as those in the amygdala) to the development of long-term sensitization in response to stress. In this model, episodes of stress induce permanent changes in the strengths of the synaptic connections of limbic neurons in such a way that they may subsequently develop the entire stress response spontaneously in the absence of a new stressor. This type of behavioral sensitization finds an analogy in the kindling-related phenomena that are demonstrable in limbic neurons. Stress-sensitization hypotheses appear particularly intriguing in view of positron emission tomography (PET) imaging findings that amygdala blood flow may be abnormally elevated in both the unmedicated-depressed and the unmedicated-remitted (asymptomatic) phases of MDD. According to such models, antidepressant drugs may exert their prophylactic effects against depressive episodes by preventing abnormal amygdala activity from inducing spontaneous recurrences of the major depressive syndrome. Antidepressant drugs have been shown to decrease metabolic activity in the amygdala in depressed patients with MDD, in nondepressed control subjects, and in experimental animals, and to decrease amygdala neuron firing rates after chronic administration in nonhuman animals, suggesting that they may exert direct effects in the amygdala.

Genetics and Family History

Heritability of Bipolar Disorder and Major Depressive Disorder

Twin, adoption, and family studies indicate that genetic factors substantially contribute to the liability for developing bipolar disorder and MDD. Moreover, earlier age of onset appears to increase the transmissibility of both bipolar disorder and MDD. Family studies attempting to subdivide bipolar and unipolar illness have established that the first-degree relatives of adults affected with bipolar disorder are at increased risk for both bipolar and unipolar disorders when compared with relatives of people who have unipolar disorder or with general population rates. These studies have also shown that the bipolar genotype can be manifested as both bipolar and unipolar illness. Nevertheless, even though it is clear that there is some shared genetic liability between bipolar and unipolar disorder, the data also suggest that bipolar and unipolar disorders are transmitted to some extent independently.

Taken at face value, adult twin and adoption studies indicate that the familial transmission of bipolar disorder is largely related to genetic factors and that genetic factors are more important in the development of bipolar disorders than of MDD. Recent twin studies of adults with MDD report a heritability of approximately 40%, which corresponds to a monozygotic twin correlation of 0.4 and a dizygotic twin correlation of 0.2. These estimates of the heritability of MDD should be considered low, since recent examinations of the stability of the reporting of depressive symptoms indicate that approximately 50% of the variability in reporting diagnoses of MDD may represent fluctuation of symptom reports in mild cases. If heritability estimates for MDD are corrected for the assessment error associated with this type of reporting attenuation, the heritability of MDD may equal that of bipolar disorder.

Putative Genetic Loci in Mood Disorders

There is little evidence that familial forms of affective disorders are the result of simple genetic defects such as autosomal dominate or recessive mutations. However, just as for other complex medical conditions with prominent genetic components (such as hypertension, diabetes mellitus, or Alzheimer's diseases), there is great interest in identifying genetic factors. Searches for the genes involved in the origins of affective disorders have taken one of two general strategies. The first is linkage (which is usually agnostic about what gene is involved). The second is testing of specific candidate genes by association studies.

Over the last decade there have been several claims of linkage of particular genetic loci to the affective disorders. Most notable among these have been a number of genetic linkage studies of bipolar disorder reporting conflicting findings on the involvement of chromosome 11 and the X chromosome. More recently, there have been claims of linkage to loci on chromosome 18, chromosome 21, and a new X chromosome locus. Other investigators have used case-control association approaches for testing the involvement of specific genes in the development of bipolar disorders. At present none of the putative linkage locations or associations are widely accepted, and they have not been replicated in general positive studies. Currently there are no genetic tests that help with the diagnosis of the depressive or manic disorders.

Pathophysiology

Neurochemical, neuroendocrine, neurophysiological, and neuropsychological abnormalities have all been demonstrated in mood disorders, suggesting that several systems within the brain are affected in these illnesses. Moreover, biological differences appear to exist across subgroups of subjects meeting criteria for the MDD, suggesting that this syndrome is associated with multiple pathophysiological states. This section highlights some of the brain systems implicated in mood disorders that likely relate to their core features.

Anatomical Correlates of Mood Disorders

Neuroimaging Findings

Brain imaging technologies have demonstrated that mood disorders are associated with a variety of abnormalities in brain regions that have already been implicated in emotional processing or modulation by other types of evidence (see Chapter 6). For example, in most depressive subtypes, abnormalities have been reported in portions of the ventral prefrontal cortex (PFC) where cerebral blood flow (CBF) increases during emotional states induced in psychiatrically healthy subjects. In unmedicated patients with primary, unipolar depression and who are under age 60, CBF and metabolism are increased in the ventrolateral and orbital portions of the PFC (Figures 8-1 and 8-2; see also Figure 6-8, p. 71). Scans acquired in the asymptomatic state after successful antidepressant treatment or spontaneous remission demonstrate normalization of the CBF and metabolic abnormalities in these areas. However, these abnormalities have not been found in patients with bipolar or late-onset depression (see Chapter 6). An abnormality that appears common to the depressed phase of both bipolar and unipolar illness has been identified in the subgenual PFC (the portion of the anterior cingulate gyrus ventral to the genu of the corpus callosum), where CBF and metabolism are decreased in subjects with depression relative to nondepressed or manic control subjects. The ventrolateral, orbital, and subgenual prefrontal areas are all heavily interconnected with limbic structures (such as the amygdala) that have been implicated in emotional processing. The subgenual PFC also has extensive connections with the lateral hypothalamus and the midbrain nuclei that contain dopaminergic and serotoninergic neurons, which appear to function abnormally in depression.

Abnormalities are also found in subcortical areas

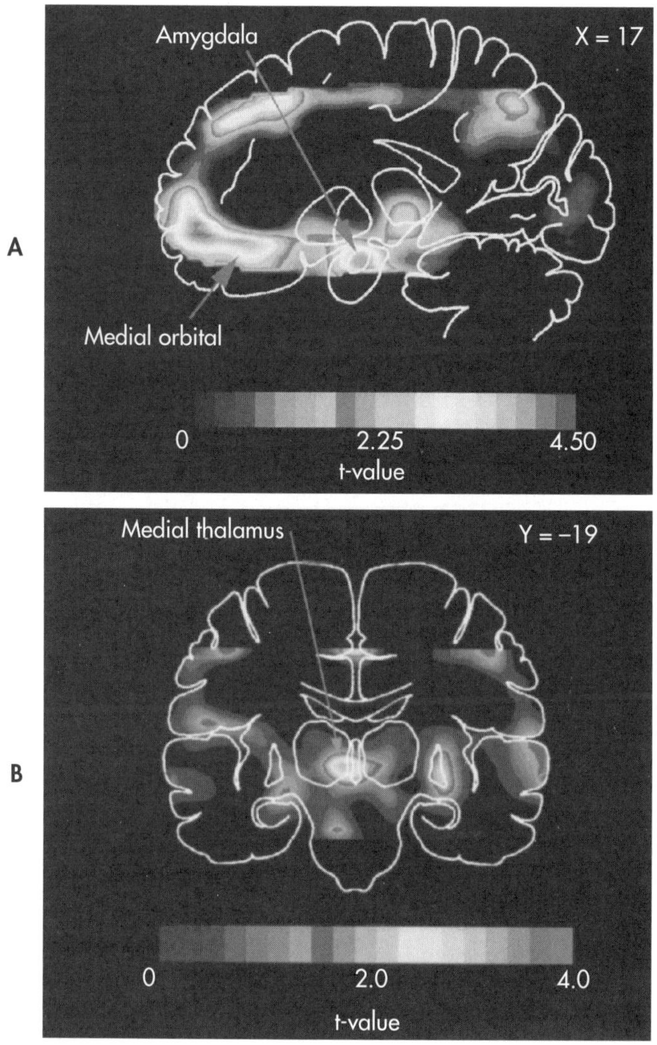

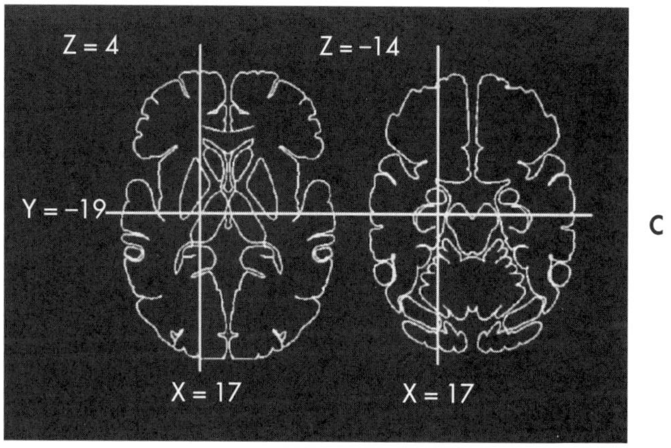

FIGURE 8-1 Areas of increased blood flow in the left amygdala and the medial orbital cortex of subjects with unipolar depression who have FPDD. The sagittal and coronal image slices shown are from an image of t-values, produced by a voxel-by-voxel computation of the t-statistic, and they indicate areas where flow is increased in the subjects with depression relative to the control group. This t-image was used to generate hypotheses regarding the regions that might contain differences between depressed and control subjects. The presence of abnormal activity in these regions has subsequently been confirmed using both rCBF and glucose metabolic image data from independent subject samples. The area of increased flow in the left PFC extends from the medial orbital cortex to the lateral orbital cortex, (the tissue immediately caudal to the frontal pole) and the pregenual portion of the anterior cingulate gyrus. These limbic prefrontal areas interconnect with the amygdala and the medial dorsal nucleus of the thalamus to form the limbic-thalamic-cortical circuit (Figure 8-2). The number above each image locates the section in mm from the anterior commissure, with negative Y = posterior, positive X = left hemisphere, and negative Z = ventral to a plane containing both the anterior and the posterior commissures. The orientations of the sagittal and the coronal image slices are indicated on horizontal atlas tracings at the level of the amygdala ($Z = -14$) and the medial thalamus ($Z = 4$). Left is on the left for the coronal section, and anterior is toward the left for the sagittal section or the page top for the horizontal tracings. (Modified from Price JL, Carmichael ST, Drevets WC: *Prog Brain Res* 107:523-536, 1996 and Talairach J, Tournoux P: *Co-planar stereotaxic atlas of the human brain,* Stuttgart, 1988, Thieme.)

that share anatomical connections with these ventral prefrontal areas. In people who have unipolar depression, CBF and glucose metabolism are abnormally increased in the left amygdala and the left medial thalamus, structures that have been shown in electrophysiological studies to participate in emotional processing. In the left amygdala, rCBF appears abnormally elevated in both the depressed and the unmedicated-asymptomatic phases of FPDD, leading to the hypothesis that FPDD may be associated with an abnormality related to the trait of being susceptible to depressive episodes in the amygdala. During successful treatment with antidepressant drugs, amygdala activity decreases toward normal.

The amygdala and the ventral PFC also project to the medial caudate and the ventral striatum, areas implicated in emotional modulation. In the caudate, CBF and metabolism are abnormally decreased in patients with unipolar depression, and morphometric MRI studies have demonstrated that the caudate head is abnormally small in subjects who are depressed. In patients with bipolar depression, caudate flow and metabolism are not abnormally reduced, and preliminary data indicating that metabolism is increased in the ventral striatum in both the depressed and the manic phases of bipolar disorder were recently reported.

In cortical regions that are not clearly related to emotional processing, such as the dorsolateral PFC and the temporoparietal cortex, metabolic activity is also decreased in depression. These abnormalities may be related to the subtle performance deficits exhibited by

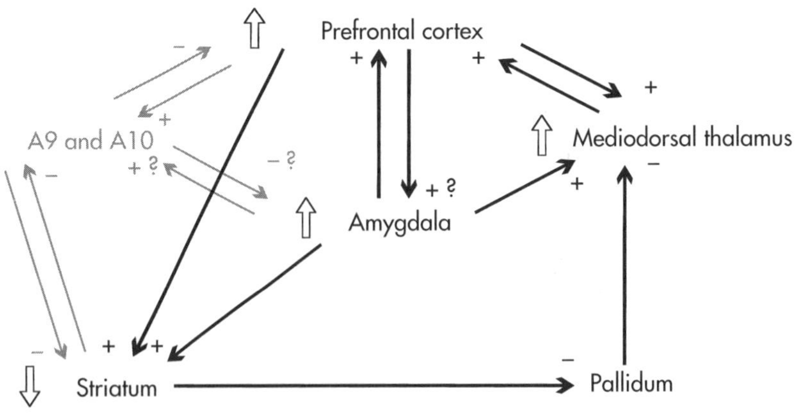

FIGURE 8-2 Neuroanatomical circuits hypothesized to participate in the functional anatomy of MDD based on functional neuroimaging and lesion analysis studies. The open arrows adjacent to each region indicate the direction of significant differences in blood flow and glucose metabolism in patients with unipolar depression who have FPDD relative to healthy controls. The regions' monosynaptic connections with each other are illustrated *(closed arrows)*, with + indicating excitatory, − showing inhibitory projections, and *?* indicating limited experimental evidence. These portions of the PFC involve primarily the lateral and medial orbital cortex. The parts of the striatum under consideration are the ventral medial caudate and the nucleus accumbens, which particularly project to the ventral pallidum. In this primary mood disorder the findings of increased flow and metabolism in the amygdala, the medial thalamus, and the limbic PFC are compatible with other evidence suggesting that synaptic transmission through the limbic-thalamic-cortical circuit is abnormally elevated. In contrast, in major depressive syndromes arising secondary to some neurological disorders, blood flow and metabolic abnormalities have been reported in some of these regions that are opposite in direction with respect to the normative baseline as those shown here. This observation is consistent with evidence from lesion analysis studies that mood disorders may arise by a variety of functional or structural lesions occurring at multiple points within these circuits that affect the synaptic transmission through them in diverse ways.

The major dopaminergic projections from the black substance *(A9)* and the ventral tegmental area *(A10)* to these structures are illustrated with the shaded tone. Serotoninergic, noradrenergic, and cholinergic projections into this system also exist as well and likely contribute to its overall modulation. Whereas somatic antidepressant therapies influence each of these systems, their therapeutic mechanisms may be associated with enhancing dopaminergic and serotoninergic (especially serotonin$_{1A}$ relative to serotonin$_2$ receptor) function. Both effects would putatively inhibit transmission through the limbic-thalamic-cortical circuit. Other structures and neurotransmitter systems likely play important roles in mood disorders as well, and the circuit shown here is simplified both for clarity and for lack of knowledge. (From Drevets WC et al: *J Neurosci* 12:3628-3641, 1992.)

patients with depression on some neuropsychological tests, rather than to the emotional features of mood disorders. For example, the dorsolateral prefrontal areas where flow and metabolism are decreased in patients with either unipolar or bipolar depression have sparse limbic connections and are activated during tasks involving visuospatial processing, visual object memory, eye movements, or maze navigation. The reduction of metabolic activity in this region in depression has been hypothesized to reflect either the nonspecific effects of psychomotor slowing or the gating of brain processing resources away from such cognitive functions and toward the perseverative negative mood and self-evaluative states of depression (see Chapter 6).

People with late-onset depression have frontal lobe abnormalities of a different nature. MRI signal hyperintensities appear in the frontal lobe, the caudate, and the white matter adjacent to these structures in over 70% of subjects with depression onset after age 60 (see Chapter 6). Postmortem and MRS data have demonstrated that these signal hyperintensities probably reflect arteriosclerotic or ischemic lesions. As expected in the presence of such lesions, PET images from such elderly patients with depression show diffuse areas of decreased CBF in the PFC that are presumably accounted for by reduced vascular supply and damaged tissue, rather than by the shifts in local synaptic activity that are thought to dictate the regional metabolic changes in younger patients with depression. When elderly patients are used as their own controls by acquiring scans before and after ECT or antidepressant drug treatment, remission of the depressive syndrome is associated with further CBF decreases in the left PFC. Thus in patients with young-onset or late-onset depression, left prefrontal activity appears to be elevated in the depressed phase relative to the remitted phase of MDD, and conversely, left prefrontal activity decreases during effective antidepressant treatment.

Anatomical Circuits Related to Mood Disorders

The neuroimaging data in both normal emotional states and in primary and induced mood disorders converge with evidence from lesion analyses to implicate circuits involving the ventral and medial PFC along with limbic structures such as the amygdala and related parts of the striatum and thalamus. For example, the findings of abnormally increased CBF and metabolism in the ventral PFC in patients with unipolar depression who have FPDD, the amygdala and the medial thalamus coupled with indications of reduced flow in the medial caudate suggest that the following two interconnected circuits are involved in the pathophysiology of FPDD: a limbic-thalamic-cortical circuit involving the amygdala, the mediodorsal nucleus of the thalamus (in the medial thalamus) (MD), and the ventrolateral and medial PFC; and a limbic-striatal-pallidal-thalamic circuit involving related parts of the striatum and the ventral pallidum, as well as the components of the other circuit. The first of these circuits can be conceptualized as an excitatory triangular circuit whereby the amygdala and the PFC regions are interconnected by excitatory projections with each other and with the MD. Increased metabolic activity in the amygdala, the medial thalamus, and the PFC presumably reflect increased synaptic activity in these areas, suggesting that synaptic transmission through the limbic-thalamic-cortical circuit is abnormally elevated in FPDD. In ventral frontal lobe tissue removed from patients with depression undergoing these neurosurgical treatments, the concentration of the neurotransmitter (aspartic acid) is increased, supporting the hypothesis of increased limbic-thalamic-cortical transmission. Also consistent with this hypothesis are neurosurgical procedures that ameliorate treatment-resistant depression to interrupt projections within the limbic-thalamic-cortical and the limbic-striatal-pallidal-thalamic circuits. Other somatic antidepressant treatments may also compensate for the pathophysiology of FPDD by suppressing limbic-thalamic-cortical activity, as antidepressant drug administration is associated with decreased CBF and metabolism in the amygdala, the ventral PFC, and the medial thalamus in patients with depression and with decreased amygdala neuronal firing rates in experimental animals.

This circuitry model provides a useful conceptual framework for approaching the depressive syndromes induced by neurological lesions. Induced mood syndromes may also stem from dysfunction within limbic-cortical-striatal-pallidal-thalamic circuits, since lesions involving the PFC (that is, tumors or infarctions) and diseases of the basal ganglia (such as Parkinson's disease or Huntington's disease) are associated with higher rates of depression than other similarly debilitating conditions (see Chapter 26). Although these disorders all affect limbic-cortical-striatal-pallidal-thalamic circuits, the point of dysfunction is different in each condition, implying that abnormal interaction between elements of this circuit, rather than increased or decreased activity in any single structure, can produce major depressive episodes. The hypothesis that lesions affecting various points within neural circuits that subserve and modulate emotion can give rise to mood disorders is analogous to the case in the motor circuitry (involving the primary and supplemental motor cortices, the dorsal striatum, the dorsal pallidum, and related parts of the thalamus) in which dysfunction at multiple sites results in movement disorders.

Distinct abnormalities within limbic-cortical-striatal-pallidal-thalamic circuits could account for clinical differences between depressive subtypes. For example, the sites where lesions can induce bipolar or manic syndromes differ from those where lesions are associated with unipolar depressive syndromes. Cerebrovascular lesions associated with induced manic or bipolar syndromes involve the right ventral PFC, the right striatum, the right thalamus, or the right basotemporal cortex (which may include the amygdala), whereas lesions involving the left PFC and the left caudate are associated with induced unipolar depressive syndromes. Furthermore, degenerative disorders of the basal ganglia associated with unipolar versus bipolar mood syndromes affect synaptic transmission through the limbic-cortical-striatal-pallidal-thalamic circuitry differently. For example, in Parkinson's disease increased striatal-pallidal transmission results from the loss of the inhibitory effects of nigrostriatal dopaminergic neurons, and the course of the induced depression is unipolar and nondelusional (similar to FPDD, where increased striatal-pallidal transmission is hypothesized). In contrast, in Huntington's disease decreased striatal-pallidal transmission results from the degeneration of striatal neurons, and the course of the secondary mood disorder can be bipolar with or without psychotic features. Finally, the dissimilar rCBF patterns in bipolar as compared with unipolar depression provide an example of primary depressive subtypes that are associated with distinct abnormalities within the limbic-cortical-striatal-pallidal-thalamic circuitry.

Neuroendocrine Abnormalities in Major Depression

Mood disorders have been associated with neuroendocrine disturbances in the hypothalamic-pituitary-adrenocortical axis, the thyroid axis, and the growth hormone axis. These abnormalities may be related to the neurochemical changes described in the following paragraphs and to the involvement of the ventral prefrontal and limbic structures already described. Both the amygdala, where increased metabolism was found in unipolar depression, and the subgenual PFC, where decreased metabolism existed in both unipolar and bipolar depression, have extensive connections with the lateral hypothalamus. Disruption of the functional interactions between these structures and the hypothalamus could partly underlie some of the neuroendocrine and autonomic manifestations of mood disorders, as well as the neurovegetative symptoms of the major depressive syndrome (such as disturbed sleep, appetite, libido, and energy).

For example, severe depression is associated with hyperactivity of the hypothalamic-pituitary-adrenocortical system as indicated by increased CSF levels of corticotropin-releasing factor (CRF), hypersecretion of adrenocorticotropic hormone (ACTH) and cortisol, and pituitary and adrenal gland enlargement (in MRI scans). These abnormalities suggest that CRF is hypersecreted in a major depressive episode. In actions compatible with this hypothesis, the ACTH response to intravenously administered CRF is blunted in depression and CRF receptor density is decreased in the frontal cortex of suicide victims (presumably reflecting compensatory desensitization or downregulation of CRF receptors caused by CRF hypersecretion). Additionally, premature escape from the cortisol suppressant effects of dexamethasone is found in 70% to 85% of patients with bipolar depression and unipolar depression who have FPDD, suggesting that CRF release is disengaged from control by glucocorticoid feedback inhibition. Abnormal dexamethasone suppression is not observed in bereaved subjects with depressive symptoms, so this phenomenon does not simply appear to reflect a correlate of stress.

Elevated CRF release could result either from subsensitivity of the glucocorticoid feedback inhibition mechanisms in the hippocampus and the hypothalamus or from excessive stimulation of CRF-containing neurons (such as those in the amygdala). The latter possibility is compatible with the PET imaging evidence of elevated amygdala activity in FPDD (see Figure 8-2). During successful (but not unsuccessful) treatment with antidepressant drugs or ECT, serum cortisol levels normalize, cortisol secretion becomes suppressible by dexamethasone, and CSF levels of CRF normalize. Similarly, successful (but not unsuccessful) antidepressant drug treatment reduces amygdala metabolism, potentially inhibiting a pathological stimulatory influence on CRF release. Antidepressant drugs also increase corticosteroid immunoreactivity and binding capacity and raise glucocorticoid receptor messenger ribonucleic acid (mRNA) levels in the brain, presumably augmenting feedback inhibition of CRF release.

Some depressive symptoms could directly reflect neuropsychiatric manifestations of elevated CRF or cortisol levels. For example, the clinical features of Cushing's syndrome include fatigue (100%), anergia (97%), irritability (86%), depressed mood (77%), decreased libido (69%), middle (69%) or terminal (55%) insomnia, anxiety (66%), impaired concentration (66%), crying (63%), appetite disturbance (54%), hopelessness (43%), and guilt (37%). These symptom rates are similar to those found in MDD (see Table 8-2). Less commonly, elevated glucocorticoid administration (such as prednisone treatment) or release (in Cushing's syndrome) induces manic symptoms. It remains unclear whether increased corticosteroid levels directly induce emotional and neurovegetative symptoms or instead trigger mood syndromes via a separate mechanism.

Neurochemical Systems Implicated in Depression

Neurochemical abnormalities have been consistently identified in the central norepinephrine, serotonin, dopamine, acetylcholine, γ-aminobutyric acid (GABA), and neuropeptide (that is, CRF and opiate) systems in the primary mood disorders. Dysfunction within these integrated systems likely contributes to the functional anatomical and neuroendocrine abnormalities described in this chapter, as well as to the neuropsychiatric manifestations of mood disorders. However, it remains unclear whether these neurochemical alterations are fundamentally involved in the origins of mood disorders or instead reflect compensatory changes caused by pathologic conditions in other systems.

Norepinephrine

The central noradrenergic system has been implicated in major depression by several lines of evidence. Urinary concentrations of the norepinephrine metabolite 3-methoxy-4-hydroxyphenylglycol (MHPG) are consistently decreased in patients with bipolar depression and in some patients with unipolar depression. Additionally, responses of the neuroendocrine (such as growth hormone release) and autonomic (for example, heart rate changes) systems to α-adrenoreceptor agonists (such as clonidine) are blunted during both the depressed and remitted phases of MDD. Adenylate cyclase responses to β-adrenoreceptor agonists are also diminished in patients who are depressed, but this abnormality returns to normal with treatment. Finally, β-adrenoreceptor density is abnormally increased in the frontal and temporal cortical tissue of suicide victims. Treatment may also reverse this abnormality, since most antidepressant drugs downregulate β-adrenoreceptor density in experimental animals.

Serotonin

Serotoninergic function also appears to be altered in depression, as indicated by evidence of deficient serotonin presynaptic activity and alterations in postsynaptic serotonin$_{1A}$ and serotonin$_2$ receptor density and sensitivity. Some of these changes may not be specific to MDD, since decreased concentrations of the serotonin metabolite 5-hydroxyindoleacetic acid (5-HIAA) in the CSF antemortem and in the brainstem postmortem are found in both victims of suicide and people who have attempted suicide and who were depressed and nondepressed. These data have lead to the hypothesis that lower serotoninergic function is associated with suicidal behavior that involves planning and results in greater medical damage but is not specifically associated with MDD.

Postmortem studies in suicide victims have demonstrated decreased serotonin transporter sites in the orbital and lateral PFC areas but not in other prefrontal areas, resembling the regional specificity of the CBF and metabolic abnormalities found in PET imaging studies of MDD (see Figures 8-1 and 8-2). Moreover, increased serotonin$_2$ receptor density has been demonstrated in the PFC in patients with depression who died either from suicide or from natural causes. In contrast to the serotonin$_2$ receptor changes, the functional responsiveness of the serotonin$_{1A}$ system is attenuated in depression, and the density of serotonin$_{1A}$ receptors is decreased in the hippocampus and the lateral orbital cortex in patients with depression who died from suicide or from natural causes. Notably, cortisol upregulates expression of serotonin$_2$ receptors but downregulates expression of serotonin$_{1A}$ receptors, so the postmortem patterns of serotonin receptor changes in subjects with depression could reflect the effects of hypercortisolism (see pp. 127, 128). Notably, many antidepressant drugs reverse these serotonin receptor abnormalities by increasing the sensitivity of postsynaptic serotonin$_{1A}$ receptors (apparently through an effect on G-protein synthesis) and by downregulating or antagonizing serotonin$_2$ receptors. Antidepressant drugs also increase serotonin transmission, potentially reversing the deficient presynaptic serotonin activity evident in MDD.

Dopamine

The dopamine projections from the ventral tegmental area and the substantia nigra into the limbic striatum (the medial caudate and the nucleus accumbens) and the medial PFC appear to subserve a reward-related system that mediates motivation, hedonia, behavioral reinforcement, and psychomotor activity. Since the emotional experiences and behaviors that appear to be mediated by this mesolimbic dopamine system are disturbed in mood disorders, it has been implicated as a system where hypofunction could yield the anhedonia, psychomotor retardation, and amotivation characterizing a depressive episode and where hyperfunction could account for the euphoria, psychomotor restlessness, and hypermotivation observed in mania. The available data support this hypothesis, since reduced dopamine function in depression is suggested by the consistent findings that antidepressant drugs enhance dopamine receptor sensitivity in limbic structures and that CSF concentrations of the dopamine metabolite, homovanillic acid, are reduced in patients who are nondelusional and depressed. Moreover, mania has been associated with increased dopamine function by findings that manic symptoms are reduced by dopamine receptor antagonists or dopamine synthesis inhibitors and can be precipitated in euthymic or depressed bipolar patients by dopamine receptor agonists. Finally, one study showed that in subjects with bipolar disorder who were psychotic the density of D_2-like dopamine receptor sites is abnormally increased. However, this abnormality may be related to psychosis rather than mood, since it was also found in patients with schizophrenia who were psychotic but not in subjects with bipolar disorder who were not psychotic and its magnitude correlated with psychosis ratings but not mood ratings.

Altered Sleep Stages in Mood Disorders

Among the most consistent physiological changes found in MDD or bipolar disorder are abnormalities in the sleep EEG. During a depressive episode, most adults with primary mood disorders demonstrate reduced slow wave sleep (stages 3 and 4, or deep sleep), reduced rapid eye movement (REM) latency (time between sleep onset and REM onset), and increased REM density (time spent in REM sleep). These changes are consistent with the subjective impression of patients with depression that their sleep is restless and that they fail to sleep deeply.

The implications that these sleep abnormalities hold for the pathophysiology of mood disorders are unclear. Insomnia and sleep EEG abnormalities have been hypothesized to correlate with decreased serotoninergic function or with alterations in the ratio of cholinergic-to-aminergic neurotransmission. Sleep EEG changes have also been postulated to corroborate neuroimaging evidence of PFC dysfunction in mood disorders, since the PFC has been implicated in the regulation of sleep architecture.

However, sleep EEG changes are absent in children and early adolescents with depression (who otherwise resemble depressed adults), indicating that such changes are not fundamental to the development of mood disorders. They may reflect secondary phenomena associated with effects of affective illness, or they may be associated with an increased risk for the development of depression relatively late in life, given their strong correlation with age. Some sleep EEG changes encountered in depression may reflect epiphenomena of depressive symptoms, since reduced REM latency has been reported in subjects who were not depressed but who were sleep-deprived. Moreover, a contribution of stress or sadness to altered REM density is suggested by studies of elderly patients who were not depressed bereaving their spouses, and like patients with depression who had MDD, showed elevated phasic measures of REM sleep even though they did not differ from controls on other sleep EEG measures or on subjective evaluation of sleep quality. In contrast, elderly people who are bereaved and who also meet criteria for a major depressive episode show reduced slow-wave sleep, reduced REM latency, and diminished sleep efficiency, similar to patients with MDD who are depressed. Since people who are either depressed or bereaved may experience insomnia, the extent to which nonspecific effects of sleep deprivation account for such sleep EEG changes is unclear.

An intriguing observation regarding sleep disturbances in mood disorders is that a night of total sleep deprivation can transiently alleviate depressive symptoms. Moreover, some subjects with bipolar disorder report that sleep deprivation can precipitate hypomanic or manic episodes. A link between sleep deprivation and antidepressant drug effects (which can both ameliorate depression and precipitate mania) has been afforded by observations in experimental animals indicating that both treatments increase the sensitivity of dopamine$_2$-family receptors. Moreover, a successful response to either sleep deprivation or antidepressant drugs has been associated in PET imaging studies with reductions in baseline glucose metabolism in limbic structures such as the amygdala and the anterior cingulate (see Chapter 6). These observations have led to speculation that insomnia may reflect a physiological mechanism to combat depression and that administration of hypnotic drugs to patients with MDD before the onset of antidepressant drug efficacy is not indicated. Additional data are required to test these hypotheses.

Treatment

Management of Major Depressive Disorder

General Considerations

The conservative approach to managing mood disorders mandates that patients who meet criteria for a major depressive episode receive antidepressant treatment. The risk of not treating mood disorders is high, and the risk associated with antidepressant treatment is in most cases quite low.

Depression management requires office visits that are long enough to educate, support, and reassure patients. Frequent follow-up visits are usually needed to ensure that the treatment is tolerated and effective, since patients are often too ill to make decisions or to act on their own behalf. Family members and ancillary healthcare staff may need to be involved in the management of a depressed patient because of the impaired insight and judgment that often accompany mood disorders. Follow-up visits should occur at semiweekly to monthly intervals, depending on severity, until the patient's symptoms have at least partially remitted. Once a complete or nearly complete remission has been established, this interval can be increased to 2 to 6 months. Follow-up visits must include monitoring for the development of suicide ideation, psychotic features, or mania (antidepressant drugs can precipitate mania or hypomania in 0.3% to 1.0% of cases).

Need for Hospitalization and Psychiatric Referral

A primary reason for hospitalization is suicide prevention. Patients who are at a significant suicide risk ought to be hospitalized until they can be safely managed on an outpatient basis. The assessment of suicidal risk and the management of suicidal behavior are discussed in Chapter 27. Other reasons to hospitalize patients with mood disorders include mania, psychosis, refusal to eat or drink, and inability to manage other medical problems because of depressive symptoms.

As a general rule, patients with depression who require hospitalization also warrant referral to a psychiatrist. Outpatients with depression who develop suicidality, psychosis, or mania, or those who fail to care for their medical needs also require psychiatric referral. Failure to respond to two 6- to 8-week treatment trials, at least one of which involves antidepressant pharmacotherapy, should also prompt referral or consultation with a psychiatrist.

Length of Treatment

Once symptom remission has been achieved, maintenance treatment with antidepressant drugs is continued for a variable time. The data from long-term studies lasting as long as 5-years suggest that antidepressant drugs not only ameliorate the current depressive episode but that they can also prevent relapse and recurrence in a majority of cases (Figure 8-3). Nevertheless, guidelines for the duration of maintenance therapy have not been established. The decision regarding the length of treatment involves consideration of the severity and frequency of previous episodes.

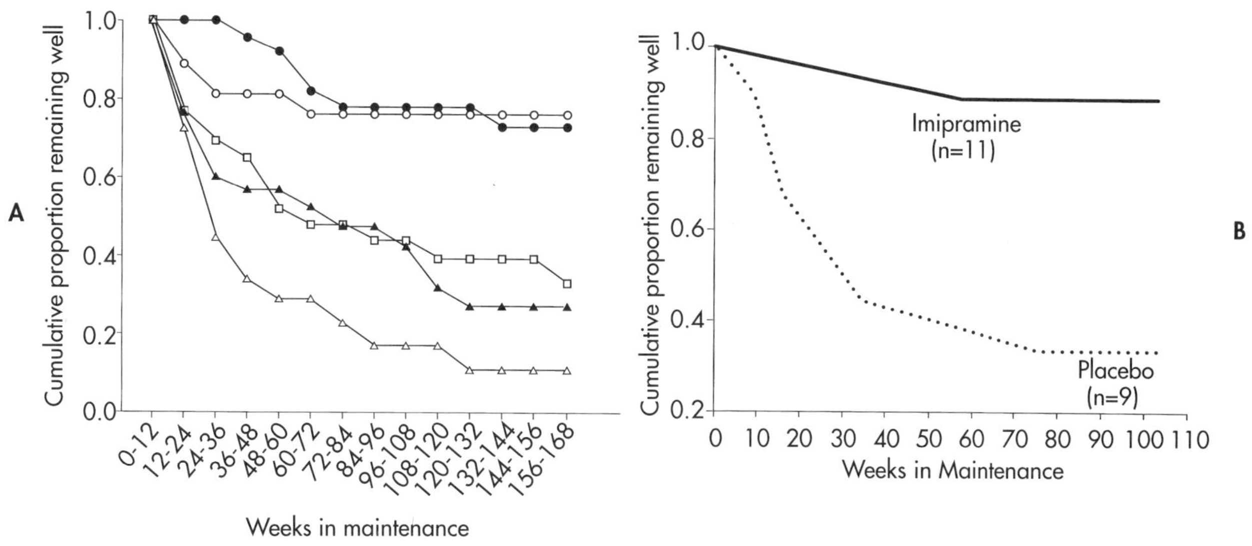

FIGURE 8-3 **A,** Outcome of maintenance therapies in recurrent depression shown as the cumulative proportion of subjects remaining in remission during the 3-year treatment period. Open circles represent a group that underwent medication clinic and active imipramine (a TCA); solid circles depict the results of a group treated with both interpersonal psychotherapy and active imipramine; squares represent a group treated with interpersonal psychotherapy alone; solid triangles show the results of a group treated with interpersonal psychotherapy and placebo; and open triangles correspond to a group that underwent medication clinic and placebo. **B,** Outcome of maintenance therapies in recurrent depression shown as the cumulative proportion of subjects remaining in remission during the years 4 and 5. At the conclusion of the 3-year study summarized in **A,** 20 subjects from the two groups that had received active imipramine were recruited for an additional 2-year study in which they were randomized to either continued imipramine treatment or placebo. Although subjects had been in remission for 3 years before being converted to placebo, most relapsed within 1 year of imipramine discontinuation. In contrast, 10 of the 11 subjects maintained on imipramine treatment remained free of a recurrence of a depressive episode through year 5. (**A** from Frank et al: *Arch Gen Psychiatry* 47:1093-1099, 1990; **B** from Kupfer et al: *Arch Gen Psychiatry* 49:769-773, 1992.)

Redevelopment of the depressive syndrome within 6 months of treatment discontinuation is usually called *relapse;* beyond 6 months it is called *recurrence.* The relapse rate increases as the duration of maintenance treatment decreases. Previously, 6 months was considered an acceptable length of maintenance therapy for most patients. However, the relapse rate for such a short treatment duration is unacceptably high. Twelve to 18 months of maintenance treatment may prove more beneficial for the first one or two episodes of depression.

For the third and later episodes, longer treatment periods are indicated unless each episode has been separated from the others by several years of remission. Frequent episodes are increasingly being considered a reason for chronic treatment, given the recurrent nature of MDD and its risk of excess mortality and indescribable suffering. The importance of chronic treatment for such cases is highlighted by preliminary indications that up to 30% of patients fail to respond to the antidepressant drug that proved effective in the previous episode if it has been discontinued before the current episode. This is an ominous event for physicians, since identifying another effective agent for such a patient can require trials of several antidepressant drugs.

Selection of Treatments

Several safe, effective, and well-tolerated therapeutic options exist for the treatment of major depression. Biological markers or clinical criteria capable of predicting treatment outcome for a specific treatment do not exist. Consequently the approach to identifying an effective regimen is empirical (trial-and-error), and in many cases a myriad of pharmacological and nonpharmacological interventions are tried before a successful treatment response is obtained. It is thus imperative that ineffective trials of pharmacotherapy or psychotherapy be amended (for example, by increasing the dosage) or discontinued to permit initiation of new treatments.

Psychological Treatments (Psychotherapy)

Management of depression always involves supportive and rehabilitative psychotherapy (see Chapter 20). More specific psychotherapeutic techniques that may prove beneficial in treating MDD include cognitive behavior therapy (CBT) and interpersonal psychotherapy

(IPT). These techniques have shown greater efficacy for treating MDD than other forms of psychotherapy in controlled studies. In contrast to CBT and IPT, insight-directed psychotherapies that involve examination of subconscious motives, repressed memories, and deep feelings have not clearly been shown to be effective in depression and may exacerbate a patient's guilt and self-depreciation.

The theoretical bases for CBT and IPT are distinct. CBT is based on the hypothesis that depressive emotions arise because patients develop cognitive distortions, in which they view themselves and their circumstances in a consistently negative light. The therapist attempts to help the patient logically challenge such perspectives to train her to recognize such negative thoughts as unrealistic (for example, changing the thought from "I can't do anything right," to "I do several things well, and no one does everything perfectly"). The patient is thereby guided to develop more positive, realistic, and constructive means of assessing her own capabilities and circumstances.

The goal of IPT is to enhance the patient's social functioning by improving his ability to effectively deal with stressors and to manage the personal and social consequences of his depressive episode. Within IPT, special techniques have been developed for managing patients who are dealing with grief or loss, interpersonal deficits, or marital problems. The most beneficial psychotherapeutic approach in most cases is likely to be an eclectic one in which elements of all of these techniques are brought to bear on the patient's behalf.

Psychotherapy vs. Pharmacotherapy as a Single Treatment

The efficacy of CBT and IPT has been compared with that of pharmacotherapy for the treatment of MDD. Most studies showing similar efficacy for psychotherapy and pharmacotherapy appear to have suffered from an ascertainment bias, in that most patients referred to such studies have been considered good candidates for psychotherapy by the referral source. The general expectation among physicians is that patients who are relatively mild in severity, are "psychologically-minded," and have retained mood reactivity are more likely to respond to psychotherapy. *Mood reactivity* means that a patient is able to feel better when positive life events occur and that a depressive episode may have been precipitated by life events. Patients who are more severely depressed and who demonstrate prominent psychomotor disturbances, neurovegetative signs, anhedonia, nonreactive mood, and biological markers for depression are generally not referred for psychotherapy alone.

This distinction has been demonstrated in studies that included a wide variety of patient types to assess the psychobiological correlates of psychotherapy response. For example, an older study divided patients into exogenous and endogenous groups and found that exogenous patients were at least as likely to respond to CBT as to medications but that endogenous patients were far more likely to respond to antidepressant drug therapy than to CBT. Similarly, a recent study included inpatients ($n = 32$) as well as outpatients ($n = 110$) and found that a poor outcome with CBT was associated with greater pretreatment symptom severity, unemployment, and sleep EEG abnormalities. Among the inpatients in particular, poor outcome to CBT was associated with elevated urinary free-cortisol levels, male gender, and diagnostic co-morbidity. In contrast, people with relatively mild, nonchronic depression who did not demonstrate biological markers for depression were more likely to respond to CBT.

Finally, in a large multicenter trial that compared CBT, IPT, and imipramine, imipramine proved superior to either psychotherapeutic technique for patients who were more severely depressed and functionally-impaired. In contrast, significant differences between treatments could not be demonstrated for the subgroup that was less severely depressed and less impaired.

It is likely that the heterogeneity within MDD is responsible for the controversy over whether mood disorders can be treated with psychotherapy alone. A simplistic hypothesis in this regard is that patients with biologically-based depressive episodes need somatic antidepressant treatments with or without psychotherapy, whereas patients with psychologically-based (neurotic-reactive) depressive episodes can be treated with either medication or psychotherapy alone. For example, in preliminary PET studies, the patient types in whom metabolic and blood flow abnormalities were identified (patients who were moderately or severely depressed and had FPDD or bipolar depression) typically did well with antidepressant drugs but failed trials of psychotherapy. Nevertheless, such data are preliminary, and at present no reliable means exist for distinguishing patients with biologically-based mood disorders or for predicting response to psychotherapy as opposed to pharmacotherapy.

Reasonable clinical guidelines based on the extant data are that more severely ill patients or patients with the melancholic subtype should receive antidepressant pharmacotherapy with or without psychotherapy. For patients with mild nonmelancholic cases and who are not suicidal and not functionally impaired, a trial of psychotherapy may be a viable option. However, if such patients do not respond to psychotherapy within 8 weeks, they should be offered a trial of antidepressant drug treatment.

Psychotherapy as an Adjunctive Treatment to Pharmacotherapy

In addition to the supportive and educational psychotherapy that all patients should receive, adjunctive psychotherapy using more specific approaches such as CBT or IPT can prove invaluable in many cases where patients are receiving antidepressant drugs. Established guidelines for identifying patients likely to benefit from combined therapy are not available. Studies assessing the differential efficacy of using combined antidepressant drug and psychotherapy for randomly selected samples have yielded mixed results, with some showing a significantly greater response for combined treatment than for drug therapy or psychotherapy alone and others showing no benefit for combined therapy over antidepressant drug therapy alone. Thus it cannot be concluded that all patients require combined therapy. Patients for whom referral for adjunctive CBT or IPT may be indicated are included on the following list: (1) patients with depression who have inadequately responded to somatic treatments; (2) patients who have improved as a result of taking antidepressant drugs but need more intensive rehabilitation for persistent effects of the depressive episode on self-esteem or interpersonal relationships; (3) patients exhibiting chronic patterns of cognitive distortions (for example, focusing exclusively on the negative aspects of situations) that have been present irrespective of major depressive episodes; and (4) patients with a history of traumatic life events that have chronically affected self-esteem, emotional stability, or social relationships (for example, experiences of physical or sexual abuse).

Pharmacological Treatments for Depression

General Considerations

Efficacy. Management of MDD usually includes treatment with antidepressant drugs because of their relatively high efficacy and relatively mild adverse-effect profile. When all patients with MDD are considered together, the efficacy across antidepressant drug classes is similar. Of patients who complete a 6- to 8-week drug treatment trial, about 60% to 70% experience substantial improvement. However, the literature suggests that efficacy may be lower for some subgroups. For example, patients older than age 75 commonly experience only modest therapeutic responses to antidepressant drugs, and patients with depression who are hospitalized or elderly and have the melancholic subtype may be less responsive to selective serotonin reuptake inhibitors (SSRIs) than they are to tricyclic antidepressants (TCAs).

Minimizing Adverse Effects. Since in most cases the efficacy of antidepressant agents appears similar across classes, selection of antidepressant drugs is largely based on their risk in overdose, side-effect profile, and potential for drug interactions. The importance of considering the latter two categories is magnified for elderly and medically ill patients. For example, cardiovascular effects are of greater concern in the elderly because of the increased prevalence of concomitant cardiovascular disease and the more limited capacity of the elderly to adjust to perturbations in cardiovascular function. The TCA agents have Type IC antiarrhythmic effects, which in patients with bundle branch disease can result in potentially lethal atrioventricular conduction block and ventricular arrhythmias. Additionally, the most common cardiovascular effect of antidepressant drugs (occurring with the TCAs, the monoamine oxidase inhibitors [MAOIs], and trazodone) is orthostatic hypotension. Whereas in younger patients this side effect is usually inconsequential, orthostatic hypotension in the elderly increases the risk of falls and hip fractures. Consequently, agents without cardiovascular effects are generally used as first choices in elderly patients.

The anticholinergic effects of the TCAs provide other examples of problems that become exaggerated with old age. Urinary retention or paralytic ileus resulting from TCA use is almost exclusively seen in the elderly. Additionally, whereas younger patients are annoyed by dry mouth and constipation, these side effects can become serious management problems in the elderly, since constipation can lead to impaction and dry mouth can preclude the wearing of dentures. Anticholinergic effects can also contribute to acute confusional states or memory impairment in the elderly patients who are depressed, although these are rarely seen in younger patients. People with late-onset depression, in particular are at increased risk for developing delirium during treatment with either TCAs or ECT that is possibly related to the neuropathological changes reflected in their MRI scans. The newer generation antidepressant drugs that are less likely to produce anticholinergic effects or CNS toxicity are consequently better choices for initial therapy.

Pharmacokinetic Considerations in Elderly and Medically Ill Patients. Several factors associated with normal aging affect the pharmacokinetics of psychotropic drugs. First, the volume-of-distribution (VOD) for most psychoactive drugs, which are highly lipophilic, increases with the patient's age, since the ratio of fat to muscle increases with age. Second, the clearance of most psychotropic drugs by the liver and the kidney decreases with age (the polar metabolites of some psychotropic drugs that are generated by hepatic metabolism are excreted by the kidney). Since the elimination half-life of a drug varies in proportion to its VOD and in inverse proportion to its clearance, both the increasing VOD and the decreasing clearance associated with advancing age work to prolong a drug's half-life in an elderly patient. The steady-state concentration of a drug is also inversely proportional to clearance. Thus as the clearance of most antidepressant drugs decreases in old age, either the magnitude of the dose or the frequency of administration must be reduced in elderly patients to prevent excessive elevations in plasma concentration (see Chapter 25).

An additional factor that may alter pharmacokinetics in the elderly is the increasing prevalence of disease in multiple organ systems with advancing age. This increases the likelihood that hepatic or renal dysfunction may contribute to changes in pharmacokinetics. It also raises the potential for pharmacokinetic and pharmacodynamic drug interactions, since elderly patients are more likely to be receiving multiple medications.

Classes of Antidepressant Agents

Six major classes of antidepressant drugs are now available: the TCAs (for example, nortriptyline, desipramine, amitriptyline, imipramine, and doxepin), the SSRIs (such as fluoxetine, sertraline, paroxetine, and fluvoxamine), the phenylpiperizines (such as trazodone and nefazodone), the MAOIs (such as phenelzine, selegiline, and moclobemide), the aminoketones (that is, bupropion), and the phenethylamines (such as venlafaxine). Although each class contains effective antidepressant agents, substantial differences exist both across and within classes in side-effect profiles, propensity for drug interactions, and the extent to which the pharmacokinetics are affected by aging.

Tricyclic Antidepressants. The TCAs are thought to exert their antidepressant effects by inhibiting the reuptake of serotonin, norepinephrine, and to a lesser extent dopamine across the presynaptic membrane. Their efficacy is well established in patients of all ages. However, the multiple pharmacodynamic actions of the TCAs can result in adverse effects that are particularly problematic in elderly and medically ill patients. However, their main liability is their lethality in overdose.

The TCAs inhibit Na^+,K^+-dependent adenosinetriphosphatase (ATPase), which accounts for their ability to stabilize excitable membranes. This membrane-stabilizing effect slows cardiac conduction and can precipitate arrhythmias or heart block in patients with bundle-branch disease. The risk of cardiac toxicity is highly correlated with plasma levels, accounting in part for the lethality of a TCA overdose. Moreover, unintentional TCA overdose may occur at standard oral doses in patients who metabolize TCAs at anomalous slow rates. Thus the narrow therapeutic index of the TCAs necessitates plasma drug level monitoring in all patients. Plasma level monitoring is particularly important in pediatric and elderly patients, in whom the hepatic metabolism of the TCAs is even more variable.

High TCA levels have also been associated with the development of delirium and seizures. Advanced age increases the risk for CNS toxicity because the plasma level required for the development of TCA-induced delirium decreases as age increases. The incidence of delirium appears particularly increased in the presence of cerebrovascular disease (that is, in poststroke or late-onset depression).

The TCAs also block muscarinic cholinergic, histaminergic, and α-adrenergic receptors, accounting for a variety of problematic side effects in elderly patients. The anticholinergic effects of the TCAs can result in delirium, memory impairment, confusion, sinus tachycardia, urinary hesitancy, constipation, dry mouth, blurred vision, and increased intraocular pressure in the presence of narrow angle glaucoma. The anti-α_1-adrenergic effect presumably accounts for the orthostatic hypotension and the consequent two- to threefold increase in the risk of falls and hip fractures associated with TCA use in the elderly. The antihistaminic effects of the TCAs are thought to confer their potential for producing sedation, which often limits the ability to achieve therapeutic doses in elderly patients. Finally, treatment with the TCAs is commonly associated with weight gain.

Besides the cognitive impairment associated with the anticholinergic and sedative properties of the TCAs, impaired mentation or arousal can also result from pharmacodynamic interactions between the TCAs and other drugs that exert sedative (such as alcohol and benzodiazepines), anticholinergic, or antihistaminic effects. Pharmacokinetic interactions can occur with agents that inhibit the activity of the hepatic isoenzymes P-450 2D6 and 3A4 (for example, the SSRIs), which slow the metabolism of TCAs and may increase plasma concentrations to toxic levels. Conversely, agents that induce the activity of the P-450 enzymes (such as phenobarbital and carbamazepine) can lower TCA concentrations to subtherapeutic levels.

The sedative and anticholinergic effects associated with the tertiary amine TCAs (for example, amitriptyline, doxepin, and imipramine) are generally greater than those of the secondary amine TCAs (such as nortriptyline and desipramine), making the latter agents better choices for most patients. In the elderly, dropout rates commonly exceed 50% in clinical trials in which tertiary amine TCAs are used. In contrast, dropout rates are often less than 10% in trials using the secondary amine nortriptyline. Nortriptyline may also be less likely to produce orthostatic hypotension than other TCAs.

Selective Serotonin Reuptake Inhibitors. The SSRIs exert relatively selective inhibition of the reuptake of serotonin into presynaptic terminals. After chronic administration this effect results in persistent enhancement of serotonin neurotransmission through desensitization of the presynaptic serotonin$_{1A}$ autoreceptor. With the exception of paroxetine, which has weak affinity for muscarinic cholinergic receptors, the SSRIs exhibit no significant binding to peripheral or central neurotransmitter receptors. They are consequently free of the troublesome anticholinergic, antihistaminic, and antiadrenergic effects of the TCAs. Additionally, the SSRIs lack the membrane stabilizing effects of the TCAs and thus do not affect cardiac conduction. Finally, the SSRIs are not associated with CNS toxicity (that is, the potential for causing seizures) and are unlikely to produce delirium. Therefore the SSRIs have a wide therapeutic index and are free of many of the adverse effects associated with other classes of antidepressants.

The side effects of the SSRIs are generally limited to the relatively mild adverse effects accompanying excessive blockade of peripheral and central serotonin reuptake. These most commonly include sexual dysfunction and gastrointestinal effects such as nausea, vomiting, and loose stools. Treatment with the SSRIs can also result in insomnia, anxiety, and restlessness, which are most commonly associated with fluoxetine. Sedation is less common during SSRI treatment and occurs more commonly with paroxetine than with other SSRIs. Fluoxetine-induced nausea and anorexia has been associated with significant weight loss in people over age 75 with depression who are medically ill.

The incidence of side effects during SSRI treatment rises proportionally with drug dose or plasma levels, whereas the curve relating antidepressant response to dose or plasma levels remains relatively flat. Consequently, bothersome side effects can sometimes be eliminated without sacrificing clinical efficacy by decreasing oral dose. Such adjustments can be accomplished within a few days for sertraline and paroxetine, which have elimination half-lives of about 1 day and require less than 1 week for new steady-state plasma drug levels to be reached after each dose change. In contrast, achieving a new steady-state for norfluoxetine, the active metabolite of fluoxetine, requires 8 to 10 weeks.

The SSRIs also differ in their potential for causing pharmacokinetic interactions between drugs. All of the available SSRIs inhibit cytochrome P-450 2D6 and thereby slow the metabolism of other drugs cleared by this enzyme system. These drugs include the TCAs, the phenothiazines (such as thioridazine), the Type IC antiarrhythmics (such as propafenone, flecainide, and ecainide), bupropion, valproate, and carbamazepine. Paroxetine, fluoxetine, and norfluoxetine are more potent inhibitors of cytochrome P-450 2D6 than sertraline and fluvoxamine. Consequently, coadministration of paroxetine or fluoxetine with the TCAs, bupropion, or the Type IC antiarrhythmics (which have narrow therapeutic indexes) requires extreme caution. Fluoxetine and fluvoxamine also appear to inhibit the cytochrome P-450 enzyme 3A4, and fluvoxamine additionally inhibits the P-450 enzyme 1A2 (see Chapter 26). When prescribing SSRIs, physicians should review with patients the drugs that may potentially interact with SSRIs. Of the SSRIs, sertraline appears least likely to produce clinically important drug interactions.

Whereas several studies have now documented the antidepressant efficacy of SSRIs in outpatients who are depressed, concerns have been raised that the SSRIs may be less effective than the TCAs in inpatients with depression and in elderly patients who are melancholic. The first studies to report a differential efficacy found significantly higher response rates in hospitalized patients with depression who were treated with the TCA clomipramine than in those treated with the SSRIs citalopram and paroxetine. A more recent study reported that the proportion of elderly patients with depression whose symptoms remitted during treatment with nortriptyline (82%) was significantly higher than that for matched patients treated with fluoxetine (28%). This difference was magnified in the subset of subjects meeting criteria for the melancholic subtype, where 20 of 24 (83%) patients experienced remission during nortriptyline treatment compared with only 1 of 10 (10%) who had remission during fluoxetine treatment. These studies have been criticized for their inherent inability to maintain the investigators' blind to the drug administered because of the differences in side-effect profiles between the TCAs and the SSRIs. However, a recent study comparing fluoxetine with venlafaxine, which has a similar side-effect profile to that of the SSRIs, also found superior efficacy for venlafaxine relative to fluoxetine in inpatients who were melancholic. Until additional research establishes a differential efficacy for subgroups of patients with depression, a reasonable recommendation may be that patients who are severely depressed or melancholic and who fail to respond to an SSRI or relapse when they are taking an SSRI ought to receive a therapeutic trial of an agent from another antidepressant drug class.

In summary, the SSRIs generally produce fewer and more benign adverse effects than the TCAs. Of the SSRIs, sertraline possesses pharmacokinetic advantages over fluoxetine or paroxetine for the treatment of elderly and medically ill patients, since its pharmacokinetics are the same in both elderly and younger patients and its inhibitory effects on the activity of the hepatic isoenzyme P-450 2D6 are substantially weaker than those of paroxetine, fluoxetine, or norfluoxetine. Additional research is needed to assess the significance of the aforementioned concerns that the SSRIs are less efficacious in subgroups with more severe depression than agents that block both serotonin and norepinephrine reuptake.

Monoamine Oxidase Inhibitors. MAOIs inhibit the oxidative enzymes located within synaptic terminals that degrade monoamine neurotransmitters, resulting in increased concentrations of norepinephrine, serotonin, and dopamine within the synaptic cleft. The clinical use of these agents has generally been limited to patients who are refractory to other antidepressant drugs because of their potentially life-threatening pharmacodynamic interactions with sympathomimetic drugs or foods and beverages containing tyramine. The former include the sympathomimetic amines, phenylpropanolamine, and pseudoephedrine, which are contained in some over-the-counter decongestant preparations. The use of MAOIs in the elderly is also limited by the more common cardiovascular effect of MAOIs, orthostatic hypotension.

The enzyme responsible for the metabolism of tyramine is MAO-A, and blockade of MAO-A is thus responsible for the production of acute hypertensive crisis after tyramine ingestion. The MAOIs previously available in the United States were irreversible inhibitors of both MAO-A and MAO-B (that is, phenelzine, isocarboxazid, and tranylcypromine). Although it was initially hoped that selegiline, a selective inhibitor of MAO-B, may not have this liability, selegiline loses its specificity for MAO-B in the doses required to achieve antidepressant effects (that is, in high doses, selegiline can also inhibit MAO-A).

More recently, reversible inhibitors of MAO (RIMAs) (such as moclobemide and brofaromine) have been developed. They may have a lower potential for dangerous interactions with tyramine. Moclobemide also appears to have better tolerability than either the irreversible inhibitors of MAO or the tertiary amine TCAs amitriptyline and clomipramine. Thus the enhanced safety and tolerability of the RIMAs may expand usage of MAOIs as they become more widely available.

Bupropion. Bupropion is an aminoketone that weakly inhibits dopamine reuptake, has multiple and complicated effects on noradrenergic function, and has no pharmacologically relevant effects on serotonin. Because of its novel mechanism, bupropion commonly proves useful in patients who have failed other treatments. Bupropion produces no significant effects on the cardiovascular system and does not cause sedation or cognitive impairment.

Bupropion is associated with the development of seizures in approximately 0.4% of patients treated at doses up to 450 mg/day (patients with seizure disorders or bulimia may be at increased risk for seizures). However, the incidence of seizures increases sevenfold between 450 and 600 mg/day. Although these doses exceed the recommended upper limit of 450 mg/day, this disproportionate increase in seizure risk causes concern in elderly patients, in whom the pharmacokinetics are not well studied (large interindividual variations in metabolism exist even among young subjects). This is an important concern, since the metabolism of bupropion is complex and higher levels of its three metabolites may contribute to the risk of seizures. Therapeutic drug monitoring has not been adequately established for bupropion as a means to guide dose adjustments to avoid the increased risk of metabolite accumulation. Because of its narrow therapeutic index in regards to the development of seizures, bupropion's use has commonly been limited to patients who are refractory to the SSRIs or other new generation antidepressant drugs.

Phenylpiperazines. Trazodone is a triazolopyridine, which is a potent $serotonin_2$ receptor antagonist (its ability to block serotonin reuptake at clinical doses is negligible). Trazodone and its metabolite m-chlorophenylpiperazine also block α-adrenoreceptors. Trazodone lacks anticholinergic effects and exerts minimal effects on cardiac conduction, although it has been associated with arrhythmias in patients with preexisting cardiac disease. Trazodone is unlikely to cause clinically significant pharmacokinetic interactions between drugs and has a pharmacokinetic profile that is not substantially altered by age or intercurrent disease. Trazodone's use has been limited by its most common side effect, sedation, and by its propensity to cause orthostatic hypotension (presumably the result of antagonism of α-adrenoreceptors). These effects can also result in clinically significant pharmacodynamic interactions with other drugs that decrease arousal or impair cognitive performance, or with adrenergic agents that affect blood pressure.

Nefazodone, a chemical analog of trazodone, is less likely to produce sedation or orthostatic hypotension than trazodone. Like trazodone, nefazodone blocks $serotonin_2$ receptors, but unlike trazodone, nefazodone (along with its active metabolites) also appears to exert significant reuptake inhibition of both serotonin and norepinephrine at clinical doses. Similar to trazodone, nefazodone possesses minimal affinity for muscarinic cholinergic or histaminergic receptors. However, nefazodone has substantially weaker affinity for α-adrenoreceptors than trazodone, presumably accounting for its decreased risk for producing orthostatic hypotension. Relative to other new generation antidepressant drugs, such as the SSRIs and venlafaxine, nefazodone appears less likely to produce sexual dysfunction or sleep disturbances. Nefazodone does not inhibit cytochrome P-450 2D6, but it can lead to clinically important drug interactions through its inhibition of cytochrome P-450 3A4.

Venlafaxine. Venlafaxine is a phenethylamine that inhibits uptake of serotonin, norepinephrine, and to a lesser extent dopamine. Venlafaxine is devoid of affinity for brain muscarinic cholinergic, histaminergic, or adrenergic receptors, and it appears to lack any propensity to produce arrhythmias or seizures. Its side-effect profile resembles that of the SSRIs, with nausea, dizziness, insomnia, dry mouth, and sexual dysfunction being the most common adverse effects. Less commonly, patients treated with venlafaxine may develop sustained diastolic blood pressure elevation, necessitating regular blood pressure monitoring during treatment. The incidence of this adverse effect is dependent on dosage.

In one study venlafaxine demonstrated greater efficacy than fluoxetine in hospitalized patients with major depression of the melancholic subtype. These data taken together with the aforementioned evidence that the SSRIs may be less effective than the TCAs in inpatients who are depressed and in elderly patients with melancholic depression suggest that these subgroups may preferentially respond to agents that inhibit reuptake of both serotonin and norepinephrine (that is, TCAs, venlafaxine, and nefazodone). Finally, several studies report that the antidepressant efficacy relative to placebo is significant after only 2 weeks of venlafaxine treatment (using relatively high doses), suggesting that this agent may produce clinical improvement earlier than other antidepressant agents.

Other Somatic Therapies for Depression

Electroconvulsive Therapy

ECT remains the most effective treatment for major depressive episodes. The indications for ECT, along with its safety, efficacy, and side effects are discussed in Chapter 22. This treatment is often life saving for patients with depression who fail to respond to antidepressant drugs or who because of suicidal intent or refusal to take in food or liquids cannot safely await the 3 weeks required for the onset of antidepressant drug efficacy. After ECT most patients require maintenance antidepressant pharmacotherapy to prevent relapse.

Phototherapy

Phototherapy is used in cases of MDD where a winter-related seasonal pattern of depressive episodes is evident. This involves daily exposure to ultraviolet light at wavelengths similar to sunlight with phototherapy devices marketed for this purpose. Data assessing dosage and long-term adverse effects are still accumulating. The mechanism of action is thought to involve suppression of nighttime melatonin production from the pineal gland.

Management of Bipolar Disorder

General Considerations

The recurrent nature of the bipolar disorders and the high morbidity and mortality associated with them make it imperative that patients with bipolar I or bipolar II disorder receive aggressive treatment. The treatment imperative for cyclothymic disorder is less clear. Although the depressive phases of these disorders can often be managed on an outpatient basis, full manic episodes or the presence of psychotic symptoms in manic or depressive phases are indications for hospitalization. With aggressive management, approximately 85% of patients with bipolar disorder show marked improvement. The main impediments to successful treatment are recognition of the diagnosis by physicians and compliance with medications by patients.

The mood stabilizing agents, such as lithium, valproate, or carbamazepine, constitute the mainstay of medical management for the bipolar disorders, particularly for maintenance treatment. During acute phases of either manic or depressive episodes, antipsychotic medications, minor tranquilizers, antidepressant medications, or ECT may also be indicated. Initial treatment approaches for acute manic and depressive episodes and for maintenance therapy are outlined in the following sections. These have recently been described in detail by the American Psychiatric Association in the form of Practice Guidelines.

As with all serious psychiatric or behavioral disorders, medications should be part of a comprehensive treatment plan involving education, family therapy, and behavioral management. Management of severe manic episodes can pose difficult challenges. As described in the next paragraphs, there is ample evidence for the rational choice of pharmacological agents to manage each of the phases of bipolar disorder. In contrast, few formal studies have addressed the application of specific social or psychotherapeutic interventions. Brief family therapy that includes the goal of acceptance of the illness by the patient and his family is usually helpful. Though there is no evidence that psychosocial factors cause bipolar disorder, stressful life events may influence the timing and severity of episodes. The identification of potential precipitating stress factors and the exploration of possible future stressors is a major goal of family-based intervention. This involves the family in plans to minimize future stresses and enhances their acceptance of the need for continued treatment after resolution of the acute episode. In the absence of appropriate pharmacological management, there is no evidence for the efficacy of individual or family psychotherapeutic interventions.

Classes of Pharmacological Agents for Bipolar Disorder

The main pharmacological intervention for acute manic and acute depressive episodes in bipolar I disorder and for depressive episodes in bipolar II disorder involves the use of the mood stabilizing agents lithium, valproate, and carbamazepine.

Lithium

Lithium has been shown to be effective in the acute treatment of manic and depressive episodes and in the prevention of recurrence. Lithium may also decrease mood instability in general and can be useful in the treatment of cyclothymia and hypomania. Lithium is available as the carbonate or the citrate salt and comes in tablet, capsule, or liquid form.

The correlation between oral dosage and serum lithium levels is variable across patients, but it is relatively stable within individuals. Peak serum levels occur 1½ to 2 hours after ingestion, except for the slow-release form, which reaches peak levels in 4 to 4½ hours. Since both the therapeutic and the toxic effects of lithium correlate with serum levels, serum level monitoring is required. Steady-state levels are reached 5 to 7 days after initiation of therapy or change of dosage. Serum levels should be measured approximately 12 hours after the most recent dose.

Lithium is secreted principally by the kidneys and has a half-life between 14 and 30 hours. The clearance of lithium decreases with age in association with diminished glomerular function. Lithium levels can change with hydration, and episodes of dehydration may lead to toxic serum levels. Additionally, renal failure or sodium deficiency increases lithium serum levels. Thiazide diuretics increase lithium levels by 30% to 50%, and nonsteroidal antiinflammatory agents or angiotensin-converting enzyme-inhibiting antihypertensive agents may also increase serum levels.

The majority of patients taking lithium experience side effects. Most are of little clinical significance or can be reduced by lowering the dosage. Dose-related side effects include polyuria, polydipsia, weight gain, poor concentration, tremor, sedation, and gastrointestinal disturbance. Patients may also experience hair loss, acne, and edema. Nausea, vomiting, and diarrhea can be managed by giving lithium with meals or using lithium citrate rather than carbonate. Polyuria and polydipsia can be moderated by the use of amiloride. A small proportion of patients may develop hypothyroidism after several months of lithium treatment. Lithium-induced hypothyroidism can usually be reversed by the administration of levothyroxine or the discontinuation of lithium. Notably, patients who develop lithium-induced hypothyroidism are at increased risk of experiencing a depressive episode and possibly the onset of rapid cycling between manic and depressive episodes. A commonly debated topic is whether long-term lithium use results in irreversible kidney damage. Up to one fifth of patients treated for more than 10 years display morphological changes in the kidney on histological examination. However, these changes have not been related to the development of renal insufficiency or to changes in glomerular filtration rates. It is prudent to measure thyroid hormone and creatinine levels once or twice per year during lithium treatment.

The usual 12-hour postdose therapeutic serum level of lithium is 0.8 to 1.2 mEq/L. Serum levels of 0.6 to 0.8 mEq/L may be adequate in some elderly patients and reduce the risk of CNS side effects in this age group. The daily dose necessary to achieve this trough level is variable across individuals but usually ranges between 900 and 1800 mg/day of lithium carbonate. This can be divided in two to three doses to decrease gastrointestinal side effects. However, many individuals are able to tolerate one dose per day, which is usually administered at bedtime.

Toxic side effects are usually encountered at trough blood levels above 1.5 mEq/L. Early indicators of intoxication include nausea, vomiting, diarrhea, blurred vision, vertigo, confusion, and marked tremor of the extremities. If serum levels rise above 2.0 mEq/L, life-threatening adverse effects, which may include seizures, cardiac arrhythmias, or coma, are more likely. For severe toxicity or overdosage, the only reliable method of rapidly removing excess lithium is dialysis. However, at lower levels of toxicity the patient may be treated with fluids, electrolyte management, and prevention of further gastrointestinal absorption.

Anticonvulsant Therapy

More recently, anticonvulsants have become established as mood-stabilizing agents. They have proven particularly useful for patients who experience significant adverse effects with lithium or who are poorly responsive to lithium. The two most widely studied agents are valproate and carbamazepine.

Valproate is available in capsule and liquid form, with the most commonly prescribed formulation for bipolar disorder being divalproex. Although it has not been as extensively studied as lithium, the therapeutic range for the treatment of either acute mania or maintenance therapy for mania is the same as or higher than that considered effective for epilepsy (50 to 125 μg/ml, with some patients requiring levels up to 150 μg/ml). Divalproex is usually initiated at 750 to 1000 mg/day in two or three divided doses, and the total daily dosage is then increased as tolerated to between 1000 and 2500 mg/day. Valproate is rapidly absorbed, and peak serum levels are usually reached within 2 hours. The plasma half-life is 6 to 16 hours. Valproate is extensively metabolized by the liver and is highly protein bound in serum. Drug interactions may occur with other medications that are metabolized by the liver or are extensively protein bound. The common side effects of valproate include sedation and gastrointestinal distress, which usually resolve with dose adjustment or continued treatment. Valproate has rarely been associated with hepatotoxicity (which has been fatal in some children under age 10) and blood dyscrasias (such as thrombocytopenia), so baseline liver function and hematologic screening is indicated before initiating treatment, once during the first few weeks of treatment, and every 6 to 12 months during maintenance treatment.

Carbamazepine is available in a variety of forms. Treatment is generally aimed at achieving serum levels between 4 and 15 μg/ml. Maintenance doses range from 200 to 1600 mg/day and average about 1000 mg/day. Carbamazepine is principally metabolized by the liver and induces hepatic microsomal enzymes such that, with continued treatment, its half-life decreases from between 20 and 60 hours to between 5 and 25 hours. The total daily dosage and frequency of administration may thus require adjustments over time to maintain efficacy. Carbamazepine also has important interactions with drugs that inhibit microsomal enzyme induction or with drugs that are also metabolized by hepatic cytochrome P-450 enzymes (such as 3A4). Additionally, carbamazepine is highly protein bound and may interact with drugs that are extensively protein bound. Carbamazepine may produce neurological side effects such as ataxia and blurred vision. These are usually dose-limited and transient in nature, except in elderly patients, who are typically more sensitive to these effects. Most patients develop a mild asymptomatic leukopenia. Rarely, serious agranulocytosis, aplastic anemia, or hepatic failure may develop. During the first few months of treatment, frequent monitoring of complete blood counts, platelet counts, and liver function tests is recommended. During maintenance treatment the frequency of these laboratory analyses may be reduced to every 3 to 4 months.

Antipsychotic Agents and Benzodiazepines

Antipsychotic agents (for example, haloperidol, thiothixene, trifluoperazine, clozapine, and risperidone) and benzodiazepine agonists (such as clonazepam and lorazepam) have been shown to be useful adjunctive treatments for acute mania. Antipsychotic agents are especially helpful when the manic or depressive phases are associated with psychotic features. In the absence of psychotic symptoms, the benzodiazepines may be effective for reducing motor hyperactivity and agitation. The benzodiazepines offer sedation without the extrapyramidal side effects associated with the antipsychotic drugs (such as dystonia, dyskinesia, akathisia, or parkinsonian-like syndromes). However, chronic use of benzodiazepines may result in the development of tolerance, and the withdrawal syndromes associated with benzodiazepine dependence may cloud the clinical picture by resembling an exacerbation of manic symptoms.

Antidepressants

Although antidepressant medications have been well studied in the treatment of MDD, their use in the depressed phase of bipolar disorder is controversial. Antidepressants are more effective than placebo in treating bipolar depression, but there is little evidence that they are more effective than lithium or other mood-stabilizing agents. Additionally, virtually all antidepressant agents have been reported to precipitate mania in some patients with bipolar disorder, and some studies have suggested that the use of antidepressants in patients with bipolar disorder who are depressed may increase the risk of developing rapid cycling or mixed bipolar states. Nevertheless, some patients with bipolar disorder require the combination of an antidepressant agent and a mood-stabilizing agent to alleviate or prevent depressive episodes. The dosing of antidepressant drugs in patients with bipolar depression is more complicated than in patients with unipolar depression, since some people with bipolar depression improve on relatively low dosages but become manic at modestly higher dosages. Generally, the treatment of bipolar depression with antidepressant drugs requires consultation with a specialist.

Electroconvulsive Therapy

ECT is effective for both the depressed and the manic phases of bipolar disorder. ECT may be the treatment of choice for managing acute manic episodes when mood-stabilizing agents or antidepressant drugs are contraindicated (such as in pregnancy or in the presence of serious medical disorders). The usefulness of ECT for maintenance treatment of bipolar disorder has not been established.

ECT may have interactions with other antimanic treatments. The use of ECT in the presence of lithium therapy may result in confusional states. Consequently, lithium is usually discontinued before ECT. The use of the anticonvulsant mood stabilizers, valproate and carbamazepine, may decrease the efficacy of ECT by raising seizure threshold. These issues are discussed in Chapter 22.

Treatment of Acute Mania

The initial treatment of an acute manic episode involves the use of either a mood-stabilizing agent (for example, lithium) or ECT. Antidepressant medications should be discontinued, since they may worsen the manic state. It is imperative that an adequate serum level of a mood-stabilizing agent be achieved rapidly. Underlying medical conditions such as hypothyroidism should be identified and treated. Benzodiazepines may be used for severe agitation. If psychotic features are present, antipsychotic agents are usually indicated.

Acute Treatment of Depressive Episodes

If a patient is not taking a mood-stabilizing agent such as lithium, one should be aggressively instituted (see the Pearls & Perils box above). For patients who are receiving adequate dosages of mood-stabilizing agents, additional treatment with ECT or antidepressant drugs may be required (with or without or specific psychotherapy). If the depressed phase includes psychotic features, adjunctive treatment with antipsychotic drugs is usually necessary.

Treatment of Rapid Cycling or Mixed Episodes

Most studies suggest that patients experiencing mixed episodes of manic and depressive symptoms should be treated as if they were manic. Antidepressant drugs should be avoided. Similarly, patients undergoing rapid changes between depressed and manic states should be treated primarily with mood-stabilizing agents such as lithium or ECT, but not with antidepressant drugs. Care should be taken to ensure that thyroid function is adequate and that other general medical disorders are identified and treated.

Prophylaxis or Maintenance Treatment

Overwhelming data suggest that prophylactic treatment of patients with bipolar disorder decreases the frequency and severity of subsequent manic and depressive episodes. The best studied mood-stabilizing agent for long-term maintenance therapy is lithium. However, studies from patients being treated for both epilepsy and bipolar disorder suggest that valproate and carbamazepine are effective maintenance treatments. A critical aspect of maintenance therapy is continued patient education and supportive psychotherapy. Education and supervision are necessary to improve medication compliance. One of the most common reasons for recurrent mood episodes is self-discontinuation of medication after periods of improved health. Compliance appears particularly important in light of anecdotal evidence suggesting that patients who experience episodes after discontinuing lithium may be less responsive to the reinstitution of lithium therapy. If maintenance therapy is terminated, discontinuation should be gradual to minimize the risk of relapse.

PEARLS & PERILS

IMPORTANT CLINICAL CONSIDERATIONS

- Common errors committed during management of mood disorders include failure to detect and diagnose major depressive disorder, prescription of subtherapeutic doses of antidepressant drugs, and prescription of sedative-hypnotic rather than antidepressant drugs.

CONSIDER CONSULTATION WHEN . . .

- A patient develops:
  - Serious suicidal ideation, intent or plans
  - Delusions or hallucinations
  - Mania
  - Violent or threatening speech or behavior
  - Malnutrition or dehydration due to reduced food or fluid intake
  - Disability
  - Noncompliance with treatments for other life-threatening medical disorders
  - Catatonia
  - Agitation inadequately controlled by current intervention
- A patient with depression has failed to respond to two trials of antidepressant treatment, involving pharmacological agents from two distinct antidepressant drug classes, taken at adequate therapeutic doses for a sufficient time (usually 6 weeks)
- The physician is uncomfortable with managing the symptoms, signs, or risks associated with the major depressive or the manic syndrome or with assessing the response to treatment or the adverse effects associated with treatment
- A manic episode occurred while the patient was receiving a therapeutic dose of lithium (as documented by serum levels)
- A patient with mania is under age 16 or the current manic episode is the patient's first

Annotated Bibliography

American Psychiatric Association: Practice guideline for major depressive disorder in adults, *Am J Psychiatry* 150(4 Suppl):1-26, 1993.

This article provides an overview of current viewpoints regarding the treatment in major depressive disorder.

American Psychiatric Association: Practice guideline for the treatment of patients with bipolar disorder, *Am J Psychiatry* 151(Suppl):1-36, 1994.

This article is a succinct overview of the state-of-the-art in bipolar disorder treatment.

Bloom FE, Kupfer: *Psychopharmacology: the fourth generation of progress,* New York, 1995, Raven Press.

This text contains a current and comprehensive compendium of reviews of various aspects of the pharmacological management of mood disorders and the extant data regarding neuroendocrine, neurophysiological, and neurochemical studies in depression and mania.

Goodwin FK, Jamison KR: *Manic-depressive illness,* New York, 1990, Oxford University Press.

This is a comprehensive overview of the clinical presentation, natural history, epidemiology, and treatment of bipolar disorder.

Preskorn SH: *Outpatient management of depression,* Durant, Okla., 1994, Professional Communications, Inc.

This is a pocket-sized text that offers practical guidelines for primary care physicians in the diagnosis and pharmacological management of major depressive disorder. Dr. Preskorn includes clinically relevant pharmacokinetic and pharmacodynamic information regarding the newer generation antidepressant agents.

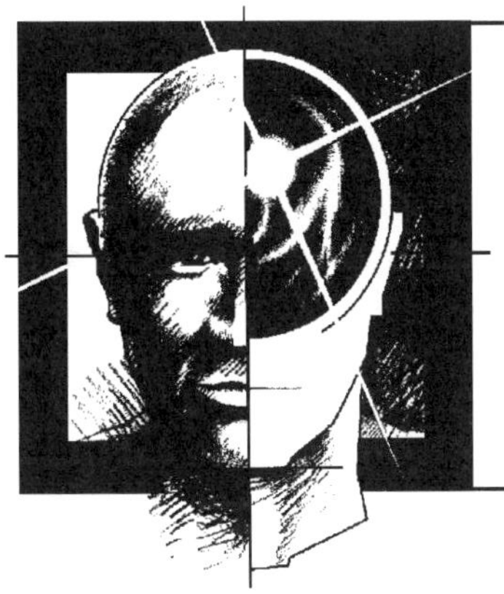

chapter 9

Anxiety Disorders

Laura Jean Bierut, MD

Anxiety, a feeling of fear and apprehension, may be a component of any psychiatric illness or may represent an independent anxiety disorder. Anxiety disorders are chronic illnesses that cause significant social and occupational impairment. Two factors significantly associated with these illnesses are female gender and low socioeconomic status.

Anxiety disorders are among the most common psychiatric disturbances and affect up to one sixth of the general population in a year. Unlike mood disorders and substance dependence, this rate has remained stable over the years. Given the incidence of anxiety disorders in the general population, primary care physicians often care for patients who have these disorders. This chapter describes the diagnosis and management of three anxiety disorders: panic disorder, phobias, and generalized anxiety disorder (GAD).

Panic Disorder

Clinical Features

The hallmark of panic disorder is panic attacks. These episodes of severe acute anxiety develop abruptly and reach their zenith within minutes. Related to this fear are numerous physical symptoms associated with autonomic nervous system arousal. These symptoms include a pounding heart, chest pain, shortness of breath, sweating, lightheadedness, and more (Box 9-1, Table 9-1). These physical symptoms subside and completely resolve within a short time, although some residual anxiousness can last for hours or days.

Many individuals are able to distinctly recall their first episode of panic. Initially, this can be triggered by

DSM-IV DIAGNOSTIC CRITERIA

BOX 9-1 PANIC ATTACK

Note: A Panic Attack is not a codable disorder. Code the specific diagnosis in which the Panic Attack occurs (e.g., Panic Disorder With Agoraphobia.

A discrete period of intense fear or discomfort, in which four (or more) of the following symptoms developed abruptly and reached a peak within 10 minutes:

(1) palpitations, pounding heart, or accelerated heart rate
(2) sweating
(3) trembling or shaking
(4) sensations of shortness of breath or smothering
(5) feeling of choking
(6) chest pain or discomfort
(7) nausea or abdominal distress
(8) feeling dizzy, unsteady, lightheaded, or faint
(9) derealization (feelings of unreality) or depersonalization (being detached from oneself)
(10) fear of losing control or going crazy
(11) fear of dying
(12) paresthesias (numbness or tingling sensations)
(13) chills or hot flushes

From American Psychiatric Association: *Diagnostic and statistical manual of mental disorders,* ed 4 (DSM-IV), Washington, D.C., 1994, American Psychiatric Press.

DIAGNOSIS

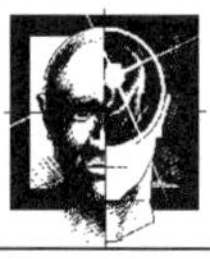

TABLE 9-1 PANIC ATTACKS

Discriminating feature

1. A discrete period of intense fear

Consistent features

1. Pounding heart
2. Sweating
3. Chills or hot flashes
4. Trembling
5. Sensation of smothering
6. Feeling of choking
7. Chest pain
8. Numbness
9. Feeling faint
10. Feelings of unreality or being detached
11. Fear of losing control
12. Fear of dying
13. Nausea

Variable features

1. May occur at any age
2. Initial attacks can be triggered by an event, but subsequent attacks have no precipitant

an event, such as an intimidating social situation, a physically dangerous situation, or the loss of a loved one; subsequent panic attacks can then occur without any precipitant. For instance, many patients report being awakened from their sleep by panic attacks.

Panic attacks alone do not automatically lead to the diagnosis of panic disorder. A clustering of recurrent, unexpected panic attacks along with concern of future panic attacks, worry of the results of panic attacks, or a significant change in behavior must occur for the diagnosis of panic disorder (Box 9-2, Table 9-2). Case 9-1 highlights the onset of panic disorder years after a first panic attack.

Panic disorder can unfortunately lead to further impairment. Recurrent panic attacks can cause anticipatory anxiety about future attacks, and as a result, an individual limits activities in an attempt to avoid potential attacks. This can lead to the development of agoraphobia, or a fear of situations from which escape might be difficult or in which help may not be available. Panic disorder is associated with agoraphobia in 25% to 50% of cases.

Another complication of panic disorder is depression. Panic disorder and major depression co-occur more often than expected by chance alone. Major depression occurs in 50% to 65% of individuals with a history of panic disorder. It is often difficult to determine whether the clinical presentation of panic disorder and depression represents two individual disorders or one disorder causing the other. Nevertheless, when

DSM-IV DIAGNOSTIC CRITERIA

BOX 9-2 PANIC DISORDER WITH/WITHOUT AGORAPHOBIA

A. Both (1) and (2)

(1) recurrent unexpected Panic Attacks
(2) at least one of the attacks has been followed by 1 month (or more) of one (or more) of the following:

(a) persistent concern about having additional attacks
(b) worry about the implications of the attack or its consequences (e.g., losing control, having a heart attack, "going crazy")
(c) a significant change in behavior related to the attacks

B. The presence/absence of Agoraphobia

C. The Panic Attacks are not due to the direct physiological effects of a substance (e.g., a drug of abuse, a medication) or a general medical condition (e.g., hyperthyroidism).

D. The Panic Attacks are not better accounted for by another mental disorder, such as Social Phobia (e.g., occurring on exposure to feared social situations), Specific Phobia (e.g., on exposure to a specific phobic situation), Obsessive-Compulsive Disorder (e.g., on exposure to dirt in someone with an obsession about contamination), Posttraumatic Stress Disorder (e.g., in response to a stimuli associated with a severe stressor), or Separation Anxiety Disorder (e.g., in response to being away from home or close relatives).

Modified from American Psychiatric Association: *Diagnostic and statistical manual of mental disorders,* ed 4, (DSM-IV), Washington, D.C., 1994, American Psychiatric Press.

CASE 9-1

Ms. A. first had a panic attack in high school. Subsequently she had an attack about once a year, but she had no associated worries and she continued all her usual activities. When she was in her mid-20s, Ms. A. had another panic attack at a workplace meeting where she had to participate in a group discussion. After this attack, she had several panic attacks per week with no precipitant. She grew anxious about having further attacks and began avoiding meetings at work. Fearful that she had heart problems, she visited her physician; at that time she was diagnosed with panic disorder.

DIAGNOSIS

TABLE 9-2 PANIC DISORDER

Discriminating feature

1. Recurrent unexpected panic attacks

Consistent features

1. Persistent concern about additional attacks
2. Worry about the consequences of attacks
3. A significant change in behavior

Variable features

1. Onset usually in late adolescence through mid-30s
2. Waxing and waning lifelong course
3. Often associated with major depression, substance misuse, and agoraphobia
4. May run in families

symptoms of major depression and panic occur, both illnesses should be diagnosed and treated appropriately.

Panic disorder and substance dependence also co-occur more often than expected. About one third of individuals with panic disorders suffer from substance abuse or substance dependence in their lifetime. Both disorders must be recognized and treated for successful results.

Suicide attempts have been identified as a complication of panic disorder independent from co-morbid major depression and alcohol dependence. In a general community survey, 20% of subjects with panic disorder had made a suicide attempt. Thus panic disorder may have a lethal potential.

Panic disorder has a variable long-term course. In follow-up studies of individuals who had been treated for panic disorder, 30% were recovered, 40% to 50% were improved, and 20% to 30% were the same or had worsening of symptoms. Overall, panic disorder remains a lifelong illness with a waxing and waning course.

CASE 9-2

Mr. J. is a 56-year-old man with a history of hypertension, diabetes, and coronary artery disease who comes to the physician with chest pain and tachycardia. Over the last 4 months, Mr. J. has had four emergency room visits for similar complaints. Other than a mildly elevated blood pressure, his physical examination is unremarkable. His blood glucose level is normal and his electrocardiogram (ECG) shows no significant changes. Since these episodes have recurred within a short time, further history of these episodes is obtained.

Mr. J. reports that these episodes come out of the blue. On further probing, it becomes clear that Mr. J. had similar episodes beginning in his 20s and occurring a few times per year, but he sought no medical treatment at that time. Since he now has medical problems, he assumes he is having a heart attack when he has these symptoms. Given this history, panic disorder is strongly suspected.

Since it is impossible to accurately apportion the cause of these symptoms to each illness, a multipronged approach is taken to optimize the management of each illness. Mr. J.'s blood pressure is closely monitored for several weeks, and pharmacological control is optimized. Similarly, his blood glucose level is monitored to avoid hypoglycemic episodes. At the same time, treatment for panic disorder is initiated. Over the next several months, Mr. J.'s condition stabilizes and he has only rare episodes of tachycardia and chest pain.

Differential Diagnosis

Panic attacks are a common feature of many psychiatric disturbances, such as major depression, substance dependence, substance withdrawal, psychosis, and other anxiety disorders. In the initial evaluation of panic attacks the presence of other potential psychiatric illnesses must be determined as potential causative or co-morbid disorders.

Medical causes for panic attacks, such as hyperthyroidism and pregnancy, must be eliminated. In medically ill patients an evaluation of panic attacks and panic disorders is difficult, since many disorders may be contributing to anxiety symptoms. In these patients, a review of their anxiety symptoms that focuses on the first time symptoms occurred is helpful. Since panic disorder is a lifelong illness with an onset generally before age 40, a history of previous panic attacks at a young age is crucial in making a diagnosis of panic disorder. Case 9-2 highlights the evaluation of panic disorder in a medically ill man.

The key feature in the diagnosis of panic disorder is the unexpected, untriggered panic attacks with the subsequent development of anxiety. Panic attacks are differentiated from phobias by the absence of a triggering factor for panic attacks. Panic disorder differs from GAD by the discrete episodes of panic.

Family History

There is a striking clustering of panic disorder within families. Family members of an individual with panic disorder are at a 4 to 7 times greater risk of developing panic disorder compared with the general population. Twin studies also support a genetic component to panic disorder, with monozygotic twins more often afflicted than dizygotic twins who have co-twins with panic disorder.

Epidemiology

Panic disorder is a relatively common disorder with a 2.3% 1-year prevalence and 3.5% lifetime prevalence in the general population. Women are 2 to 3 times more likely to be affected than men. The onset of panic disorder is typically in the age range of adolescence through the mid-30s.

PEARLS & PERILS

PANIC DISORDER

- The onset of panic disorder is usually from late adolescence through the mid-30s.
- Panic disorder is a lifelong illness that waxes and wanes.
- The lifetime prevalence is 3.5% (2 to 3 times more women than men are affected).
- The risk of panic disorder in first-degree relatives is 4 to 7 times greater than in the general population.
- Panic disorder is often associated with major depression, substance misuse, and agoraphobia.
- The treatment of panic disorder includes TCAs, MAOIs, SSRIs, and benzodiazepines.

Treatment

After the diagnosis of panic disorder, there are three major treatment approaches: pharmacological management, cognitive behavior therapy (CBT), and a combination of both. The responses to pharmacotherapy and CBT are similar, and combination therapy has a somewhat superior response. Patient choice and availability of therapy direct treatment.

Effective pharmacological management includes tricyclic antidepressants (TCAs), monoamine oxidase inhibitors (MAOIs), selective serotonin reuptake inhibitors (SSRIs), and benzodiazepines (see the Pearls & Perils box above). The TCAs are the most studied medication class, and imipramine is the most studied member of the group. MAOIs are also a standard treatment for panic disorder. SSRIs, a new group of antidepressant medications, have recently been shown to be ef-

CASE 9-3

Ms. S. is a 35-year-old woman who went to her family physician complaining of headaches and stress. She reported that she had been stressed over the last 4 months and was unable to give any specific precipitants to this stress. She developed an abrupt fear that she was going to die. She also had sweating, hot flashes, palpitations, and lightheadedness. These episodes lasted approximately 20 minutes and then completely resolved. She worried that something terrible was wrong with her, so she limited her activities.

Ms. S. denied any alcohol or substance use; however, she endorsed low mood over the last several years. She described crying spells, decreased energy, poor concentration, and feelings of guilt. She had trouble falling asleep. There were no weight changes, no psychotic symptoms, and no thoughts of hurting herself.

Ms. S. had both panic disorder and major depression. In an attempt to treat both groups of symptoms, she was treated with an antidepressant medication, 20 mg of fluoxetine per day. She had worsening of her anxiety with the first dose, so the medication was restarted at 2 mg per day with daily 2-mg increases until she reached a dose of 20 mg per day. Over several weeks, there was a gradual reduction in both depressive symptoms and panic attacks. She has remained free of symptoms for several months, and she and her physician have decided to continue long-term pharmacological treatment.

fective in the treatment of panic disorder. Although fluoxetine has been the primary SSRI studied, others in this group are likely to have similar effectiveness. High-potency benzodiazepines, along with other benzodiazepines, are also effective.

Referral to a therapist trained in CBT may be used. Brief CBT is effective in the treatment of panic disorder. The cognitive aspect includes the reframing of thoughts, so the patient no longer immediately assumes that he will die when autonomic nervous system symptoms begin. Behavioral treatment includes relaxation techniques.

Case 9-3 describes the co-occurrence of panic disorder and major depression.

Phobias

Clinical Features

A phobia is an excessive fear surrounding a specific event or object. This event or object almost invariably provokes an immediate anxiety response even though the individual recognizes that the fear is unreasonable. As a result of this excessive fear, situations are avoided and activity may be limited. Phobic disorders have been divided into the following three major categories: specific phobia, social phobias, and agoraphobia.

Specific phobias are fears targeted at specific objects or situations; for instance, a fear of heights or a fear of animals (Box 9-3). Specific phobias that occur in childhood are often transitory and not clinically significant. However, phobias that persist into adulthood do not often remit. An isolated fear may not significantly affect an individual's lifestyle; however, a specific phobia can cause significant impairment in occupation or relationships, depending on the phobic stimulus and the person's daily responsibilities.

Social phobias are fears caused by specific social situations (Box 9-4). For example, a social phobia can be the fear of eating in public, speaking in public, or embarrassing oneself in some way. Social phobia is the most common type of phobia and can be extremely impairing, since it impinges on relationships and social interactions.

Agoraphobia is the fear of being in a situation from which escape might be difficult or in which help may not be available (Box 9-5, Table 9-3). Historically, agoraphobia is linked with panic disorder and has generally been considered a complication of panic disorder. However, recent epidemiological surveys demonstrate the existence of agoraphobia without panic disorder. Agoraphobia causes impairment since an individual does not attempt an activity or requires a companion for an activity.

Case 9-4 describes an isolated fear that is life long but does not meet criteria for phobic disorder because of the lack of impairment in social and occupational functioning.

Case 9-5 illustrates a case of social phobia with a significant restriction of social activities.

Phobias are commonly associated with co-morbid psychiatric illness, primarily major depression, substance dependence, and other anxiety disorders. The lifetime prevalence of major depression is about 20% in individuals with phobias. Substance abuse or dependence complicates about one fourth of phobic disorder cases. Phobias are also commonly associated with panic attacks and GAD.

Differential Diagnosis

Patients are often able to clearly describe phobias when asked. The symptoms of the phobia can be consistent with a panic attack, but the episodes are always triggered by the phobic stimulus as opposed to untriggered panic attacks in panic disorder. Since there are often co-morbid illnesses with phobias, disorders such as major depression and substance abuse must be evaluated.

DSM-IV DIAGNOSTIC CRITERIA

BOX 9-3 SPECIFIC PHOBIA

A. Marked and persistent fear that is excessive or unreasonable, cued by the presence or anticipation of a specific object or situation (e.g., flying, heights, animals, receiving an injection, seeing blood).

B. Exposure to the phobic stimulus almost invariably provokes an immediate anxiety response, which may take the form of a situationally bound or situationally predisposed Panic Attack. **Note:** In children, the anxiety may be expressed by crying, tantrums, freezing, or clinging.

C. The person recognizes that the fear is excessive or unreasonable. **Note:** In children, this feature may be absent.

D. The phobic situation(s) is avoided or else is endured with intense anxiety or distress.

E. The avoidance, anxious anticipation, or distress in the feared situation(s) interferes significantly with the person's normal routine, occupational (or academic) functioning, or social activities or relationships, or there is marked distress about having the phobia.

F. In individuals under age 18 years, the duration is at least 6 months.

G. The anxiety, Panic Attacks, or phobic avoidance associated with the specific object or situation are not better accounted for by another mental disorder, such as Obsessive-Compulsive Disorder (e.g., fear of dirt in someone with an obsession about contamination), Posttraumatic Stress Disorder (e.g., avoidance of stimuli associated with a severe stressor), Separation Anxiety Disorder (e.g., avoidance of school), Social Phobia (e.g., avoidance of social situations because of fear of embarrassment), Panic Disorder With Agoraphobia, or Agoraphobia Without History of Panic Disorder.

Specify type:

Animal Type
Natural Environment Type (e.g., heights, storms, water)
Blood-Injection-Injury Type
Situational Type (e.g., airplanes, elevators, enclosed places)
Other Type (e.g., phobic avoidance of situations that may lead to choking, vomiting, or contracting an illness; in children, avoidance of loud sounds or costumed characters)

From American Psychiatric Association: *Diagnostic and statistical manual of mental disorders,* ed 4 (DSM-IV), Washington, D.C., 1994, American Psychiatric Press.

CASE 9-4

Dr. J. had the onset of a fear of heights in childhood. As a result, she never climbed trees with her friends. In adulthood, she is able to function well in her occupation as a physician and she has an active social life. She still feels slightly queasy when crossing a high bridge, but this fear has had no significant impact on her functioning.

CASE 9-5

Mr. M. had the onset of social phobia in high school. He became anxious whenever he had to speak with someone new. Although he had excellent grades, he chose not to attend college but instead began working at a loading dock. He was able to function adequately in this job, since he had little contact with new people. At the age of 40, he still lived at home and had few friends. The friends he did have all dated back to childhood.

CASE 9-6

Ms. D. is a 40-year-old executive with a severe phobia about flying who avoids flying whenever possible. When a family reunion was planned several thousand miles from her home, she was confronted with either flying or not attending. She discussed this with her physician and was prescribed 1 mg of alprazolam to be taken before each flight. Although she did experience some anxiety, she was able to tolerate the flight and enjoy her family reunion.

BOX 9-4 SOCIAL PHOBIA

DSM-IV DIAGNOSTIC CRITERIA

A. A marked and persistent fear of one or more social or performance situations in which the person is exposed to unfamiliar people or to possible scrutiny by others. The individual fears that he or she will act in a way (or show anxiety symptoms) that will be humiliating or embarrassing. **Note:** In children, there must be evidence of the capacity for age-appropriate social relationships with familiar people and the anxiety must occur in peer settings, not just in interactions with adults.

B. Exposure to the feared social situation almost invariable provokes anxiety, which may take the form of a situationally bound or situationally predisposed Panic Attack. **Note:** In children, the anxiety may be expressed by crying, tantrums, freezing, or shrinking from social situations with unfamiliar people.

C. The person recognizes that the fear is excessive or unreasonable. **Note:** In children, this feature may be absent.

D. The feared social or performance situations are avoided or else are endured with intense anxiety or distress.

E. The avoidance, anxious anticipation, or distress in the feared social or performance situation(s) interferes significantly with the person's normal routine, occupational (academic) functioning, or social activities or relationships, or there is marked distress about having the phobia.

F. In individuals under age 18 years, the duration is at least 6 months.

G. The fear or avoidance is not due to the direct physiological effects of a substance (e.g., a drug of abuse, a medication) or a general medical condition and is not better accounted for by another mental disorder (e.g., Panic Disorder With or Without Agoraphobia, Separation Anxiety Disorder, Body Dysmorphic Disorder, a Pervasive Developmental Disorder, or Schizoid Personality Disorder).

H. If a general medical condition or another mental disorder is present, the fear in Criterion A is unrelated to it, e.g., the fear is not of stuttering, trembling in Parkinson's disease, or exhibiting abnormal eating behavior in Anorexia Nervosa or Bulimia Nervosa.

Specify if:
Generalized: if the fears include most social situations (also consider the additional diagnosis of Avoidant Personality Disorder)

From American Psychiatric Association: *Diagnostic and statistical manual of mental disorders,* ed 4 (DSM-IV), Washington, D.C., 1994, American Psychiatric Press.

Family History

The rates of phobic disorders in families are less well studied than for many other psychiatric disorders. Family studies demonstrate a familial aggregation with up to a three-fold risk to relatives. Twin studies have shown evidence of a genetic predisposition to phobias.

Epidemiology

Phobic disorders are common in the general population. A recent epidemiological survey estimated the following 1-year and lifetime prevalences: agoraphobia without panic disorder—2.8% and 5.3%; specific phobia—8.8% and 11.3%; and social phobia—7.9% and 13.3%. Women are affected 1½ to 2 times more often than men. The onset of phobias are in childhood to early adulthood. The natural history for phobias that persist into adulthood is a chronic and lifelong course.

Treatment

Treatment for phobias include both pharmacological and psychotherapeutic interventions, singly or in combination. A treatment approach is often based on the chronicity and intensity of the phobia. For instance, an isolated phobia that does not impinge on an individual's everyday life may require only episodic treatment with no long-term management necessary. On the other hand, if the phobic disorder is causing distress often, a long-term treatment approach should be considered. Case 9-6 describes treatment of a fear of flying with mild impairment.

Effective long-term treatment for phobias includes treatment with MAOIs, benzodiazepines, and beta blockers (see the Pearls & Perils box on p. 150). A promising treatment option that has not been extensively studied is treatment with SSRIs. Psychotherapeutic approaches rely primarily on behavior therapy as a

DSM-IV DIAGNOSTIC CRITERIA

BOX 9-5 AGORAPHOBIA

Note: Agoraphobia is not a codable disorder. Code the specific disorder in which the Agoraphobia occurs (e.g., Panic Disorder With Agoraphobia or Agoraphobia Without History of Panic Disorder).

A. Anxiety about being in places or situations from which escape might be difficult (or embarrassing) or in which help may not be available in the event of having an unexpected or situationally predisposed Panic Attack or panic-like symptoms. Agoraphobic fears typically involve characteristic clusters of situations that include being outside the home alone being in a crowd or standing in a line; being on a bridge; and traveling in a bus, train, or automobile.

Note: Consider the diagnosis of Specific Phobia if the avoidance is limited in one or only a few specific situations, or Social Phobia if the avoidance is limited to social situations.

B. The situations are avoided (e.g., travel is restricted) or else are endured with marked distress or with anxiety about having a Panic Attack or panic-like symptoms, or require the presence of a companion.

C. The anxiety or phobic avoidance is not better accounted for by another mental disorder, such as Social Phobia (e.g., avoidance limited to social situations because of fear of embarrassment), Specific Phobia (e.g., avoidance limited to a single situation like elevators), Obsessive-Compulsive Disorder (e.g., avoidance of dirt in someone with an obsession about contamination), Posttraumatic Stress Disorder (e.g., avoidance of stimuli associated with a severe stressor), or Separation Anxiety Disorder (e.g., avoidance of leaving home or relatives).

From American Psychiatric Association: *Diagnostic and statistical manual for mental disorders,* ed 4 (DSM-IV), Washington, D.C., 1994, American Psychiatric Press.

DIAGNOSIS

TABLE 9-3 PHOBIA

Discriminating feature

1. Marked, unreasonable fear cued by a specific object or situation

Consistent features

1. Exposure to the stimulus almost invariably provokes anxiety
2. The phobic situation or object is either avoided or endured with intense anxiety
3. There is impairment in occupational or social functioning

Variable features

1. Onset usually in childhood through early adulthood
2. Childhood fears often transient
3. Adolescent and adulthood fears often last lifelong
4. Commonly associated with major depression and substance misuse
5. May run in families

PEARLS & PERILS

PHOBIA

- The onset of phobias is from childhood through early adulthood.
- The course of a phobia is chronic.
- The lifetime prevalence of specific phobia is 11.3%; it is 13.3% for social phobia and 5.3% for agoraphobia without panic disorder.
- There is some familial clustering of phobias.
- Phobias are often associated with major depression and substance misuse.
- The treatment for phobias includes MAOIs, benzodiazepines, and beta blockers.

long-term treatment approach. A patient is exposed to the feared stimulus, either through imagery or actual exposure, until the associated anxiety diminishes.

Generalized Anxiety Disorder

Clinical Features

GAD is a diagnostic category that has recently been added to the family of anxiety disorders. As opposed to panic disorder and phobias, which are characterized by discrete episodes of anxiety, GAD is a chronic, continuous, low-grade anxiety syndrome. Symptoms of GAD are out of proportion to the situation and cause

DSM-IV DIAGNOSTIC CRITERIA

BOX 9-6 GENERALIZED ANXIETY DISORDER

A. Excessive anxiety and worry (apprehensive expectation), occurring more days than not for at least 6 months, about a number of events or activities (such as work or school performance).

B. The person finds it difficult to control the worry.

C. The anxiety and worry are associated with three (or more) of the following six symptoms (with at least some symptoms present for more days than not for the past 6 months). **Note:** Only one item is required in children.

(1) restlessness or feeling keyed up or on edge
(2) being easily fatigued
(3) difficulty concentrating or mind going blank
(4) irritability
(5) muscle tension
(6) sleep disturbance (difficulty falling or staying asleep, or restless unsatisfying sleep)

D. The focus of the anxiety and worry is not confined to features of an Axis I disorder, e.g., the anxiety or worry is not about having a Panic Attack (as in Panic Disorder), being embarrassed in public (as in Social Phobia), being contaminated (as in Obsessive-Compulsive Disorder), being away from home or close relatives (as in Separation Anxiety Disorder), gaining weight (as in Anorexia Nervosa), having multiple physical complaints (as in Somatization Disorder), or having a serious illness (as in Hypochondriasis), and the anxiety and worry do not occur exclusively during Posttraumatic Stress Disorder.

E. The anxiety, worry, or physical symptoms cause clinically significant distress or impairment in social, occupational, or other important areas of functioning.

F. The disturbance is not due to the direct physiological effects of a substance (e.g., a drug of abuse, a medication) or a general medical condition (e.g., hyperthyroidism) and does not occur exclusively during a Mood Disorder, a Psychotic Disorder, or a Pervasive Developmental Disorder.

From American Psychiatric Association: *Diagnostic and statistical manual of mental disorders,* ed 4 (DSM-IV), Washington, D.C., 1994, American Psychiatric Press.

DIAGNOSIS

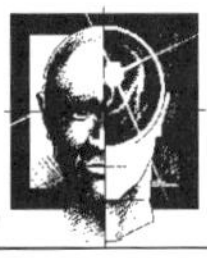

TABLE 9-4 GENERALIZED ANXIETY DISORDER

Discriminating feature:

1. Excessive anxiety and worry

Consistent features

1. Feeling keyed up
2. Feeling easily fatigued
3. Difficulty concentrating
4. Irritability
5. Muscle tension
6. Sleep disturbance
7. Impaired occupational or social functioning

Variable features

1. Onset often in childhood or adolescence
2. Chronic lifelong course
3. Often associated with major depression and substance misuse
4. May run in families

clinical distress (Box 9-6, Table 9-4). GAD co-occurs with several other psychiatric illnesses, including major depression, subtance abuse or dependence, and other anxiety disorders. Case 9-7 describes GAD complicated by asthma.

Differential Diagnosis

GAD is a diagnosis of exclusion. The symptoms are general and may fit into other disorders, such as major depression. GAD often has an insidious onset and an indolent course. After screening for the presence of medical disorders, major depression, substance dependence, or other anxiety disorders as a cause of the symptoms, the diagnosis of GAD is made.

Case 9-8 describes alcohol dependence and withdrawal symptoms that mimic GAD.

Family History

Since GAD is a recently described diagnosis, few family studies exist. However, initial family studies and twin studies support familial transmission in the development of GAD with evidence of a partial genetic predisposition.

CASE 9-7

Ms. C. is a 50-year-old obese woman with asthma who requires treatment with theophylline and inhalers. She experiences anxiety, which she describes as impinging on her relationships. Ms. C. describes herself as a lifelong "worrier." She is on edge all the time, easily fatigued, and irritable. She denies symptoms of major depression, and there is no evidence of substance abuse.

Initially, the anxiety symptoms are attributed to her obesity, asthma, and medications. Initial attempts to manage her asthma without theophylline are unsuccessful. Although theophylline appears to be contributing to the anxiety, there is a history of anxiety independent from the medication. It is thus decided to treat the anxiety symptoms as part of a GAD complex complicated by medical problems and medications.

Ms. C is treated with benzodiazepines, 5 mg of diazepam 3 times per day, and experiences some symptomatic relief. The symptoms of worrying and irritability are diminished, but the fatigue continues. Ms. C. considers this a significant improvement.

CASE 9-8

Mr. B. is a 53-year-old man who came to his physician with anxiety and difficulty sleeping. He had a history of good health, but he reported several recent life stressors, including a change of jobs. Mr. B. complained of increasing stress that disturbed his sleep. He reported feeling keyed up and on edge most of the time, and he had some trouble concentrating. This history is consistent with GAD.

On further examination, Mr. B.'s physician asked about alcohol use. It was revealed that in the past several years, Mr. B. increased the amount that he drank and at the time of the examination was drinking six mixed drinks per night. He had thought about cutting down on his drinking. He had given up social activities with his wife so he could drink, and she was annoyed. It became clear that Mr. B. was suffering from withdrawal symptoms such as shaking and nausea when he was not drinking.

Alcohol use was discussed with Mr. B., and it was strongly recommended that he completely abstain from alcohol since he had signs of alcohol dependence. He was treated for an acute withdrawal with benzodiazepines and referred to Alcoholics Anonymous (AA). He was able to comply with this program, and at a three month followup examination he had a great reduction in his symptoms of anxiety.

Epidemiology

The 1-year and lifetime prevalences of GAD are 3.1% and 5.1%. Women are affected almost 2 times as often as men. The onset of GAD is at a young age, and many patients describe being anxious their whole lives. The course of illness is continuous and chronic.

Treatment

As with other anxiety disorders, standard treatment includes TCAs and benzodiazepines. Additionally, buspirone, a unique anxiolytic agent, is effective in GAD. Since GAD is a chronic illness, psychotherapy is often recommended (see the Pearls & Perils box for GAD).

PEARLS & PERILS

GENERALIZED ANXIETY DISORDER

- Over half of all cases of GAD begin in childhood or adolescence.
- The course of GAD is chronic.
- GAD has a lifetime prevalence of 5.1% (2 times more women than men are affected).
- There is some familial clustering of GAD.
- GAD is commonly associated with major depression and substance misuse.
- Treatment for GAA includes TCAs, benzodiazepines, and buspirone.

Pathophysiology of Anxiety Disorders

An understanding of the biological basis of anxiety is unfolding with pharmacological, animal, and imaging studies. Panic attacks can be reproduced pharmacologically. Infusions of sodium lactate or respiration of 5% carbon dioxide mixtures cause panic attacks in individuals with panic disorder, whereas control subjects without panic disorder are unaffected. This susceptibility to pharmacologically induced panic attacks has led to a "false suffocation alarm" theory of panic disorder, which proposes a brain-stem hypersensitivity to carbon dioxide.

Similarly, benzodiazepine receptors, which are linked to γ-aminobutyric acid (GABA) and are extensively distributed throughout the brain, are hypothesized to be key in the cause of anxiety. Since benzodiazepines can block anxiety, these receptors may be fundamentally involved in the genesis of anxiety.

Animal studies have implicated other areas of the brain that may cause anxiety. The locus caeruleus, which contains more than 50% of all noradrenergic neurons, has extensive projections throughout the brain. Stimulation of this center in animals produces a fear and anxiety response, whereas ablation of this center reduces anxiety responses.

Finally, imaging studies may provide a functional understanding of anxiety disorders. Imaging techniques, such as positron emission tomography (PET), can demonstrate areas of activation in anxiety states. In combination with pharmacological and animal studies, an integrated understanding of the physiology of anxiety in humans is developing.

Special Issues

Anxiety Disorders in Primary Care

Treatment begins with diagnosis. Since one sixth of the population suffers from anxiety disorders, primary care physicians care for the majority of these cases. Patients come to their primary care physicians or to emergency rooms with anxiety masquerading as various physical complaints, such as chest pains or gastrointestinal distress. An awareness of the high prevalence of anxiety disorders aids in its recognition (see the Pearls & Perils box to the right).

Anxiety disorders are diagnosed by clinical history. Thus the signs and symptoms of anxiety disorders must be elicited from patients with a focus on the onset of the symptoms and the triggering events. At the same time, screening for other medical and psychiatric disorders is necessary. Specifically, the presence of major depression and substance abuse must be evaluated.

The diagnosis of an anxiety disorder and co-morbid conditions determine treatment decisions. Antidepressants can treat anxiety and concomitant major depression. Co-morbid substance dependence also points to treatment with antidepressants, since there is abuse potential with benzodiazepine treatment.

The two major tools in the anxiety arsenal are antidepressants and benzodiazepines. Antidepressants are effective anxiolytics. There is evidence of long-term efficacy with no abuse potential. However, it often takes several weeks before there is clinical evidence of a response, and side effects are often troublesome. Benzodiazepines are quickly effective, but they do not adequately treat an accompanying depression and they may be abused.

TCAs (imipramine, amitriptyline, desipramine, nortriptyline, and others) are the most studied medications, and imipramine is the most commonly studied of this group. However, all TCAs are most likely equally effective. These antidepressants need to be prescribed in doses used to treat major depression; for example imipramine is given at 150 mg/day and nortriptyline is prescribed at 75 mg/day. The advantage to the TCAs is that they have been most extensively studied and have been consistently effective. A common side effect is sedation, which may be beneficial for an anxious patient. The major disadvantage of this class of medication is the side-effect profile. There are strong anticholinergic side effects, such as dry mouth, blurred vision, and constipation, along with orthostatic hypotension. These side effects can be minimized by choosing a secondary amine tricyclic (desipramine or nortriptyline), but these side effects can still limit the effective dose. The TCAs are also potentially lethal in overdose.

> **PEARLS & PERILS**
>
> **A CLINICAL APPROACH TO ANXIETY IN PRIMARY CARE**
>
> - One sixth of the population suffers from an anxiety disorder.
> - Diagnosis is made by clinical history. An awareness of the high prevalence of these disorders aids in recognition. An assessment for the presence of co-morbid major depression and substance misuse is necessary.
> - Antidepressants and benzodiazepines are the two major classes of medication used for the treatment of anxiety.
> - Antidepressants can treat co-morbid depression, and there is no abuse potential. However, several weeks of treatment with antidepressants are required before there is an anxiolytic effect. Some antidepressants are lethal in overdose.
> - Benzodiazepines provide immediate relief from anxiety, but they do not adequately treat co-morbid major depression. Benzodiazepines may be misused.

MAOIs (isocarboxazid, phenelzine, and tranylcypromine) are a second classic treatment for many anxiety disorders. Optimal doses are again in the therapeutic range for an antidepressant effect. The advantage of this group is also its consistent efficacy in numerous clinical trials. The disadvantage is that the patient must adhere to a tyramine-free diet (elimination of certain cheeses, wines, and other foods), and hypertensive crises can occur with the ingestion of tyramine or an over-the-counter sympathomimetic such as pseudoephedrine. Since the MAOIs are irreversible inhibitors, and several weeks must pass before this enzyme system returns to functioning. Lethal overdose potential is present. Given these disadvantages, MAOIs are often not a first-line medication.

A newer group of antidepressants, SSRIs (fluoxetine, sertraline, and paroxetine), have recently been shown to be effective in the treatment of some anxiety disorders. Fluoxetine is the medication in this class that has been most often studied, although other SSRIs are likely to have similar effectiveness. The effective dosage again appears in the standard antidepressant range: for example, 20 mg/day of fluoxetine or 20 to 40 mg/day of paroxetine. The advantage of this class of medications is that the side-effect profile is generally minimal and well tolerated by patients. Additionally, it is difficult to successfully commit suicide by overdose. The disadvantages include an increase in anxiety in the initial phase of treatment. This can be minimized by starting at the lowest possible dosage and gradually increasing. These medications have the shortest track record for the long-term treatment of anxiety disorder, since long-term follow-up studies have not been done.

High-potency benzodiazepines (alprazolam and clonazepam), along with many of the other benzodiazepines, are effective in the treatment of anxiety syndromes. The response to this treatment is quick, and patients feel almost immediate relief. However, these medications have abuse potential, which is a significant concern in patients with co-morbid substance dependence. Depression, a common co-morbid condition, cannot be adequately treated with benzodiazepines alone.

Other medications used to treat specific anxiety syndromes include buspirone and beta blockers. Buspirone is the single member of its medication class. It is a specific anxiolytic agent that does not have abuse potential. Similar to the antidepressants, buspirone requires several weeks at a therapeutic dosage before a response is seen. Unfortunately, many patients are unable to tolerate this period of waiting and do not remain compliant with treatment. Beta blockers may suppress some of the autonomic symptoms of anxiety, but they are not considered a first-line choice of treatment.

Treatment-Resistant Anxiety

Anxiety is a treatable disorder, and if a patient does not respond to treatment, the following steps may be taken to evaluate the case.

(1) Reassess the diagnosis. With the increased information from follow-up care, a reassessment of the initial diagnosis of an anxiety disorder is necessary. A medical or psychiatric disorder may now be evident and better explain the clinical picture. The presence of an untreated co-morbid condition such as substance dependence, major depression, or medical illness leads to treatment-resistant anxiety.

(2) Reassess the treatment. Treatment failures are often the result of patient noncompliance, low dose, and time-limited drug trials. Medications are not effective if they are not taken. Patients with anxiety disorders are often sensitive to side effects of medications and therefore discontinue the drug. This may be minimized by starting at the lowest possible dose and gradually increasing the dose. A common mistake with the treatment of anxiety is to underdose the medications, particularly with antidepressant medications. The anxiolytic dose for the antidepressant medications is in the same range as for the antidepressant effect, and treatment must continue at this level for at least 6 weeks before considering it a treatment failure.

(3) Consider referral. If a patient has not responded and a reassessment of diagnosis and treatment does not lead to a reason for treatment resistance, consider referral to a psychiatrist for further treatment.

Conclusions

Anxiety disorders are among the most common psychiatric disorders and result in a significant amount of impairment in social and occupational functioning. Fortunately these disorders are responsive to both pharmacological and psychotherapeutic treatment. Recognition and treatment of these disorders improve the quality of life for many.

CONSIDER CONSULTATION WHEN . . .

- Anxiety is complicated by co-morbid substance dependence or major depression
- The patient has not responded to treatment

Annotated Bibliography

American Psychiatric Association: *Diagnostic and statistical manual of mental disorders,* ed 4, Washington, D.C., 1994, American Psychiatric Press.

This book provides the official nomenclature for psychiatric diagnosis that is a consensus of current formulations in psychiatry. It briefly describes diagnostic features, subtypes, associated features, prevalence, course, and differential diagnosis for each psychiatric diagnosis.

Andreasen NC, Black DW: *Introductory textbook of psychiatry,* Washington, D.C., 1991, American Psychiatric Press.

This is a simple, clear, and factual textbook written primarily for medical students and residents in psychiatry; however, it is also an excellent book for any physician who treats psychiatric patients.

Goodwin DW, Guze SB: *Psychiatric diagnosis,* ed 4, New York, 1989, Oxford University Press.

This book provides a concise, well-written summary of many psychiatric diagnoses, including panic disorder and phobic disorders. There is a richness to this book that is rare in standard medical texts.

Hollander E, Simeon D, Gorman JM: *Anxiety disorders.* In Hales RD, Yudofsky SC, Talbott, JA, editors: *Textbook of psychiatry,* ed 2, Washington, D.C., 1994, American Psychiatric Press.

This chapter is a well-organized up-to-date review of the anxiety disorders.

Winokur G, Clayton P, editors: *The medical basis of psychiatry,* Philadelphia, 1994, W.B. Saunders Company.

This book is organized into groups of syndromes and symptom clusters. The initial chapter about anxiety syndromes, panic disorder, phobic disorders, and generalized anxiety disorders describes these psychiatric illnesses. The following chapter about anxiety symptoms describes medical and other psychiatric illnesses that may mimic anxiety disorders.

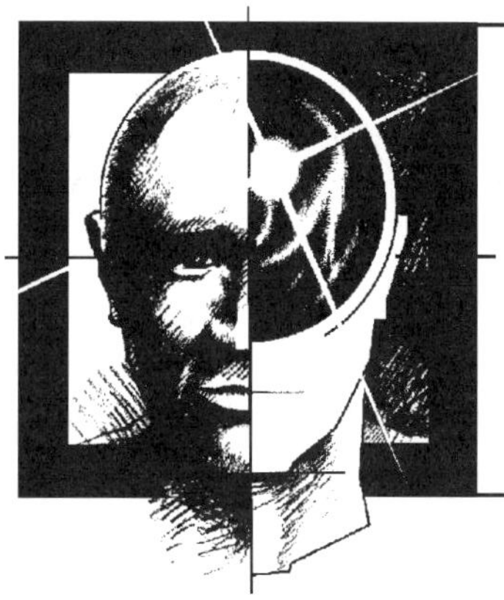

chapter 10

Anxiety Disorders: Obsessive-Compulsive Disorder

Elliot C. Nelson, MD

The ability to voluntarily control one's own thoughts is, understandably, something that virtually everyone takes for granted. In individuals with obsessive-compulsive disorder (OCD), as Case 10-1 illustrates, this ability is unfortunately no longer intact.

Definitions

The DSM-IV criteria for a diagnosis of OCD are displayed in Box 10-1. The most common description of an obsessive thought is, "It just popped into my head." Compulsions are behaviors (including mental acts) that are either performed in response to an obsession or according to stereotyped rules (Table 10-1). Although most individuals with OCD generally consider their symptoms to be excessive or unrealistic, good insight is not always present. Because of this, DSM-IV added the ability to specify "with poor insight."

The most common obsessions involve fears of contamination or fears of harming oneself or others (Table 10-2). The most common compulsions involve checking or washing (Table 10-3). Consistent with strong underlying biological determinants, symptoms of OCD have been observed to be similar across extremely diverse cultures. The severity of any one particular symptom may vary markedly over time or across subjects.

Brief Historical Background

OCD has been well described for many centuries. One early example is Shakespeare's sixteenth-century description of Lady Macbeth. The 15-minute bouts of handwashing that he describes must have been an even rarer occurrence during the author's time, suggesting that Shakespeare was probably acquainted with someone who suffered from OCD. The medical literature of the nineteenth century, particularly that of Germany and France, includes clear depictions of OCD symptoms. One topic vigorously debated in the literature of that period was whether insight should be a criterion for the diagnosis of OCD. Freud's description of OCD displayed a precise understanding of the intrusive nature of obsessive thoughts.

Epidemiology

Until the 1980s, OCD was believed to be a rare psychiatric illness with a lifetime prevalence rate of 0.05% most often quoted. The Epidemiologic Catchment Area (ECA) study was a five-center investigation with the goal of estimating the prevalence rates of a variety of psychiatric disorders in the United States. Trained lay interviewers administered a structured interview to assess the presence or absence of psychiatric illness. One of the most surprising findings of the ECA study was that the lifetime prevalence rate of OCD ranged

BOX 10-1 OBSESSIVE-COMPULSIVE DISORDER

DSM-IV DIAGNOSTIC CRITERIA

A. Either obsessions or compulsions:

Obsessions as defined by (1), (2), (3), and (4):

(1) recurrent and persistent thoughts, impulses, or images that are experienced, at some time during the disturbance, as intrusive and inappropriate and that cause marked anxiety or distress
(2) the thoughts, impulses, or images are not simply excessive worries about real-life problems
(3) the person attempts to ignore or suppress such thoughts, impulses, or images, or to neutralize them with some other thought or action
(4) the person recognizes that the obsessional thoughts, impulses, or images are a product of his or her own mind (not imposed from without as in thought insertion)

Compulsions as defined by (1) and (2):

(1) repetitive behaviors (e.g., hand washing, ordering, checking) or mental acts (e.g., praying, counting, repeating words silently) that the person feels driven to perform in response to an obsession, or according to rules that must be applied rigidly
(2) the behaviors or mental acts are aimed at preventing or reducing distress or preventing some dreaded event or situation; however, these behaviors or mental acts either are not connected in a realistic way with what they are designed to neutralize or prevent or are clearly excessive

B. At some point during the course of the disorder, the person has recognized that the obsessions or compulsions are excessive or unreasonable. **Note:** This does not apply to children.

C. The obsessions or compulsions cause marked distress, are time consuming (take more than 1 hour a day), or significantly interfere with the person's normal routine, occupational (or academic) functioning, or usual social activities or relationships.

D. If another Axis I disorder is present, the content of the obsessions or compulsions is not restricted to it (e.g., preoccupation with food in the presence of an Eating Disorder; hair pulling in the presence of Trichotillomania; concern with appearance in the presence of Body Dysmorphic Disorder; preoccupation with drugs in the presence of a Substance Use Disorder; preoccupation with having a serious illness in the presence of Hypochondriasis; preoccupation with sexual urges or fantasies in the presence of a Paraphilia; or guilty ruminations in the presence of Major Depressive Disorder).

E. The disturbance is not due to the direct physiological effects of a substance (e.g., a drug of abuse, a medication) or a general medical condition.

Specify if:

With Poor Insight: if, for most of the time during the current episode, the person does not recognize that the obsessions and compulsions are excessive or unreasonable

From American Psychiatric Association: *Diagnostic and statistical manual of mental disorders,* ed 4 (DSM-IV), 1994, American Psychiatric *Press.*

CASE 10-1

One day at the age of 22, Mrs. L. was at home caring for her 3-year-old daughter when, ". . .I just saw her and saw the knife. I had this thought and became terribly afraid that I would kill her." Mrs. L. reports that she became almost immobile. "All I did was cry. I didn't know what was the matter with me." She loved her daughter and could not understand why these thoughts were present. They terrified her, and she began to fear that she might act on them. Because of these fears she immediately went to see her gynecologist, who referred her to an outpatient mental health clinic. The 2-week wait for her first appointment seemed endless, since she then began to have thoughts that she might poison someone. When she saw the therapist, he told her that the stress from her problematic marriage caused the thoughts to be directed at her daughter, the object of that marriage. He told her to stay busy. Mrs. L. found the therapy to be somewhat helpful, and over 8 months the thoughts gradually dissipated.

Over the ensuing 2 decades, Mrs. L. had a variety of other obsessions, including fears that she would steal things, that she had cancer and other diseases, and that if something was not in its assigned place, harm would somehow come to her loved ones. She was much less bothered by these obsessions, and because she did not realize that they were symptoms of an illness she never sought treatment for them. The diagnosis of OCD was not made until it was suggested by an internist friend of Mrs. L., whom she told about the homicidal obsessions on their return 27 years later. At that time, Mrs. L. was mailing a condolence card to a friend when she suddenly had the thought that she had killed someone. After mailing the card, she began to worry that she had written a confession on the card. She wondered when the police would arrive. She soon had similar thoughts regarding a bank deposit slip. She stopped serving coffee to her clients at work because of her fear that she might poison them. During trips to the grocery store she was plagued by thoughts that she might have placed poison into someone's milk carton. Thoughts that she had hit someone with her car caused her to go back and check to see that she had not done so, making otherwise short trips take hours. Her brother called to say that he planned to visit her and intended to bring his grandson along. Mrs. L. began to worry that she would kill the child and concluded that she was obligated to kill herself to protect the child. She would wait until her brother actually arrived so as to save him an extra trip for her funeral. Fortunately, at this time she sought help instead.

DIAGNOSIS

TABLE 10-1
OBSESSIVE-COMPULSIVE DISORDER

Discriminating feature

1. Obsessions or compulsions that cause marked distress, interfere with functioning, or are present for more than 1 hour daily

Consistent features

1. Insight preserved
   Thoughts perceived as unwanted
   Behaviors felt to be excessive
2. Both obsessions and compulsions present
3. Not entirely related to another illness
4. Not caused by a substance or general medical condition

Variable features

1. Panic attacks in response to symptom-inducing stimuli
2. Co-morbid affective disorders
3. Substance abuse
4. Other anxiety disorders
5. Tics or Tourette's disorder
6. Eating disorders
7. Family members affected

from 1.9% to 3.3% across sites. Since the publication of these results, similar rates have been reported from numerous countries. Studies in clinical populations have led to estimates of the rate of OCD in psychiatric outpatients varying from 0.6% to 10%. Estimates derived from similar work examining psychiatric inpatients ranged from 0.1% to 4.0%.

The gender ratio of people who suffer from OCD obtained from community samples has typically suggested a mild predominance among women. The gender ratio obtained from adult clinical samples has been near unity, whereas that from children and adolescents has tended to show a small male predominance. The most common age of onset of OCD has been reported to be in the late teens or early 20s, with a somewhat earlier onset seen in males. It is not unusual for symptoms to begin during the first decade of life, and onset after 35 years of age is fairly rare.

Co-Morbidity

The most common co-morbid illness seen among individuals seeking treatment of OCD is major depressive disorder (MDD), for which approximately 30% of all patients meet criteria. When the rates of specific depressive symptoms (for example, low mood) have been examined among people with OCD who are seeking treatment, these range as high as 83%. The life-

TABLE 10-2

PRIMARY OBSESSIONS FROM DSM-IV FIELD TRIALS

Content of obsession	Percentage of subjects reporting symptom as primary obsession across five sites
Contamination	37.8
Fear of harming oneself or others	23.6
Symmetry	10.0
Somatic	7.2
Religious	5.9
Sexual	5.5
Hoarding	4.8
Unacceptable urges	4.3
Miscellaneous	1.0

From Foa et al: *Am J Psychiatry* 152:90-96, 1995.

TABLE 10-3

PRIMARY COMPULSIONS FROM DSM-IV FIELD TRIALS

Type of compulsion	Percentage of subjects reporting symptom as primary compulsion across five sites
Checking	28.2
Cleaning/washing	26.6
Miscellaneous	11.8
Repeating	11.1
Mental rituals	10.9
Ordering	5.7
Hoarding/collecting	3.5
Counting	2.1

From Foa et al: *Am J Psych* 152:90-96, 1995.

time prevalence rate for co-morbid MDD in those with OCD has been reported to be nearly 70%.

Rates of co-morbid social phobia, panic disorder with and without agoraphobia, and simple phobia that are higher than those of the general population have also been reported among patients with OCD. As in other anxiety disorders, increased rates of alcohol and other substance abuse and dependence has been noted. Many of these individuals report self-medicating in this manner in an attempt to control their anxiety and other OCD symptoms.

Individuals with OCD also demonstrate an increased rate of illnesses with symptoms that include preoccupation with their bodies. This group of illnesses include anorexia nervosa, body dysmorphic disorder, and hypochondriasis.

Tourette's disorder and chronic motor tic disorder have been reported to occur at varying rates among patients with OCD. Because Tourette's disorder is a considerably rare illness, the overall rate seen among those with OCD tends to be fairly low. The rate of OCD reported among those with Tourette's disorder has been reported to be as high as 89% or as low as 2%, depending on the criteria used to delineate a complex motor tic from a compulsion.

Rates of personality disorders (illnesses involving a pervasive pattern of impaired interpersonal interactions with onset in adolescence or early adult life) have also been found to be substantially elevated among those with OCD. More recent reports suggest that avoidant and dependent personality disorders are actually more common than obsessive-compulsive personality disorder. Interestingly, treatment of OCD with medication also results in a significant decrease in the rates of these illnesses, which are otherwise thought of as medication nonresponsive and often as requiring long-term psychotherapy.

Differential Diagnosis

Individuals with MDD often manifest repetitive negative thoughts called *ruminations,* which differ from obsessions in that they occur only in the context of low mood and as such rarely seem intrusive. Ruminations often take the form of brooding over past events, as opposed to obsessions, which are more often concerns about the present or future.

Individuals with OCD commonly have panic attacks when they are faced with stimuli or situations related to their fears. This differs from panic disorder, where the attacks are not directly in response to specific stimuli. In social phobia, intrusive thoughts are solely related to particularly feared social situations. In generalized anxiety disorder (GAD), excessive worry about life circumstances is present, but it is not described as being composed of intrusive thoughts and generally involves typical life issues (such as fears of losing a job).

In body dysmorphic disorder, the individual becomes preoccupied with a real or imagined defect in appearance. If the defect is real, the concerns that are present are felt to be grossly excessive. The thoughts driving the individual's absorption are usually described as intrusive and are often accompanied by frequent checking behaviors. Although these thoughts and behaviors are phenomonologically indistinguishable from those of OCD, the presence of other obsessions and compulsions meeting DSM-IV criteria is required for an additional diagnosis of OCD to be made. Similarly, the preoccupation with body habitus seen in anorexia nervosa commonly involves intrusive thoughts that may lead to checking of weight and appearance, but co-morbid OCD is not diagnosed unless other symptoms meeting DSM-IV criteria are also present.

Tics are sudden, rapid, stereotyped movements. They do not occur in response to obsessive thoughts and generally involve only bodily movements rather than goal-directed behaviors. Individuals with Tourette's disorder also have verbal tics that may involve grunting, groaning, or profane utterances. This differs from those with OCD, who may have fears that they will begin to curse at work, school, or in a place of worship but do not actually do so.

Individuals who have difficulty controlling various impulsive behaviors often describe themselves as compulsive, but the behaviors in which they engage (such as gambling, sexual activity, substance abuse, or shoplifting) are initially experienced as pleasure-generating. Compulsions are not enjoyable behaviors, although the relief in anxiety that may result from performing the compulsion may be described as a positive or pleasurable experience.

Individuals with obsessive-compulsive personality disorder tend to be miserly, rigid, cold, perfectionistic, and preoccupied with rules and details. They may hoard worthless or worn-out objects, but not to the degree where the objects are a fire hazard or make travel through the house treacherous. They differ from those with OCD in that neither obsessions nor compulsions comprise a major part of their clinical presentation.

Natural History

Reviews of several studies examining the course of OCD have suggested that patients tended to separate into the following three groups: those with chronic, unremitting illness; those whose illness was partially remitting to the point where social functioning was relatively spared; and those with an episodic course that included periods of complete remission. It is believed that only about 10% of those with OCD demonstrated the chronic deteriorating course.

Family Studies

A review of case reports of OCD in monozygotic twins found that 63% of the monozygotic twins were concordant for OCD. A study that compared the rates of OCD observed no significant difference between groups of monozygotic vs. dizygotic twins. However, when the rates of subclinical OCD (not meeting the severity criterion for OCD) were compared, significantly more subclinical OCD was seen among monozygotic twins. No studies have been performed to date examining the concordance of OCD in monozygotic twins separated at birth.

Early family studies of OCD were limited by a variety of methodological difficulties, but there was a higher than expected rate of OCD typically noted among first-degree relatives. More recently, several groups of investigators have personally interviewed various first-degree relatives of patients with OCD. The parents of children with OCD have consistently been found to display greater rates of both OCD and subclinical OCD than exist in the general population. It is interesting to note that in one study, the primary symptoms of subjects and their ill parents rarely overlapped (with only 13.3% matching), a pattern more consistent with a genetic rather than an environmental or a learning model. One group interviewed the first-degree relatives of adults with OCD and of normal controls matched for age and gender and found no significant intergroup difference in the rate of OCD. However, this group found a significantly higher rate of subclinical OCD in the relatives of patients with OCD. Another group interviewed the first-degree relatives of OCD probands and found a rate of OCD that is higher than exists in the general population and that was observed to be substantially higher among the relatives of subjects whose onset of OCD was before age 14. This tendency to find higher rates of similar illness in the families of patients with childhood onset has been observed across a number of psychiatric disorders.

Several groups have reported evidence of a genetic relationship between Tourette's disorder, chronic motor tic disorder, and OCD. One study compared the rates of OCD, Tourette's disorder, and chronic motor tic among adoptive and biological relatives of patients with Tourette's disorder who had and did not have OCD. None of the adoptive relatives met criteria for these disorders. Among the biological relatives, none of the rates of these illnesses differed between the relatives of patients with Tourette's disorder who had and did not have OCD, and the rates of illness in both groups were increased compared with the general population's rates.

Treatment

Freud provided a cogent description of OCD symptoms and accompanied them with a hypotheses as to the root conflicts from which they were derived and the treatment to which they would respond. Unfortunately, his followers' attempts to apply Freud's views and methods to the treatment of OCD have proven quite fruitless. This led psychiatrists for many years to view OCD as a treatment-resistant psychiatric illness. Consistent with this viewpoint is the relative lack of a placebo response reported across treatment studies of OCD. For example, one group treated 30 patients who had OCD with a 2-week course of placebo in a single-blinded manner. They assessed their subjects with several different scales designed to rate OCD symptoms and noted no significant difference across any scale or subscale with placebo treatment.

Pharmacotherapy

The best-studied agent for the treatment of OCD is clomipramine. Patients' concerns that it has only been available in the United States since 1990 may be relieved by the knowledge of its use in Europe over the previous 2 decades. Clomipramine, a tricyclic antidepressant (TCA), is a potent serotonin reuptake inhibitor (SRI) that also has anticholinergic, antihistaminergic, and anti-alpha$_1$-adrenergic potency, as well as an active metabolite that is a potent norepinephrine uptake inhibitor.

Clomipramine has performed significantly better than placebo across a number of studies. In a large multicenter double-blind comparison with placebo in individuals with OCD who were not depressed, the mean reduction in OCD symptoms after 10 weeks of clomipramine treatment (mean dose of 218.8 mg/day) was 44%, compared with 5% after treatment with placebo. The rate of response, defined as at least a 35% reduction in OCD symptoms, was 60% with clomipramine vs. 7% with placebo. The typical dose range for treating OCD is 100 to 250 mg/day, usually taken as a single bedtime dose. A typical starting dose is 25 to 50 mg at bedtime, and the amount is gradually increased to the above range. Common side effects of clomipramine included dry mouth, dizziness, tremor, somnolence, constipation, and fatigue. As with other TCAs an overdose with clomipramine carries a substantial risk of death, and care must be taken in prescribing it to patients who are potentially suicidal. When clomipramine is used in elderly patients, it is important to be aware that orthostatic hypotension may develop, which carries a substantial risk of dangerous falls. Elderly patients may also metabolize clomipramine more slowly.

Clomipramine has been observed to be superior to desipramine, another TCA that has a different mechanism of action, norepinephrine uptake blockade. The superiority of other SRIs to effective antidepressants with different mechanisms of action has also been established, indicating that SRIs possess specific antiobsessional efficacy as opposed to a nonspecific antidepressant effect. It is important to note that the time required to treat OCD with these drugs is substantially prolonged (with improvement occurring over 10 to 12 weeks or longer) than that typically required to treat depression (commonly 3 to 6 weeks). Therefore it is important to allow more time to pass before making dosage increases. The rate of antiobsessional response is not as high as that observed in studies of the treatment of depression, and patients who do respond often need to remain on the medication for a substantially longer time. When clomipramine was stopped abruptly in one study of 21 responders, 19 had a relapse of OCD symptoms and another became depressed. Gradual reductions in the medication dosage over several months after an adequate response is achieved may allow the patient to maintain a response at a lower overall dose, with complete discontinuation of medication sometimes achievable in this manner.

Treatment with fluoxetine, a serotonin-selective reuptake inhibitor (SSRI) without substantial effects on cholinergic, histaminergic, or alpha$_1$-adrenergic effects, has also been shown to result in significant improvement in symptoms of OCD when compared with placebo. One study compared total daily fluoxetine doses of 20, 40, and 60 mg with placebo and found that when defined as a 35% reduction in OCD symptoms, the response rates were significantly better than that of placebo at each of the three doses. Although a trend towards a better response with the highest dose (60 mg/day) was observed, the response rate of 35.1% vs. 8.5% with placebo was lower than the clomipramine study discussed in the previous paragraph. Fluoxetine at doses of 80 mg/day or more in the treatment of OCD is not unusual. Common side effects of fluoxetine include nausea, diarrhea, decreased appetite, dry mouth, insomnia, somnolence, and anxiety, with some tendency for these to be seen more often at a higher medication dose. Fluoxetine has the longest half-life of the SSRIs, and it may be prolonged in elderly patients. All the SSRIs are metabolized by components of the hepatic cytochrome P-450 system of isoenzymes, and their concomitant use may slow the elimination of other compounds that are similarly metabolized.

Fluvoxamine has also been proven to possess substantial efficacy in the treatment of OCD, and its superiority to placebo and other antidepressants is well established. In a 10-week trial, 53% of patients treated with fluvoxamine responded (here defined as having a 25% reduction in OCD symptoms), vs. 18% of those treated with placebo. Although the primary mechanism of action of these three drugs is believed to be identical, it is interesting to note that 20% of patients with OCD who had an unsatisfactory response to either clomipramine or fluoxetine were observed to respond to fluvoxamine. The range of daily fluvoxamine doses used to treat OCD is commonly 150 to 300 mg. The side-effect profile of fluvoxamine essentially overlaps that of fluoxetine, although nausea and sedation are seen more commonly with the former and restlessness and insomnia occur more often with the latter.

Several reports of the use of sertraline in treating OCD have also been published, but this work is more limited than the literature about the previously discussed medications. Little has been published on the use of paroxetine for OCD treatment, but preliminary evidence suggests that it may offer some benefit.

Two groups have recently performed meta-analyses that suggest that clomipramine may have antiobsessional efficacy superior to the SSRIs, but both tempered their findings by suggesting that direct comparisons are of greater benefit. The major issue here is whether the somewhat greater reduction in OCD symptoms observed with clomipramine vs. the SSRIs is a true reflection of superior efficacy or whether it actually results from a temporal selection bias since the more responsive patients, perhaps with less co-morbid illness, are removed from the pool available for pharmacotherapeutic trials.

Two direct comparisons of clomipramine and an SSRI have been performed. In a randomized, double-blind, crossover study, 10-week trials of fluoxetine and clomipramine treatment were separated by a 4-week washout period. No significant difference was seen between medications in terms of efficacy, although significantly more side effects were observed with clomipramine. Another group completed a 10-week double-blind comparison of fluvoxamine and clomipramine and observed no significant difference in response. It thus remains unclear as to whether clomipramine may confer greater antiobsessional efficacy.

Because for most OCD patients a response to an SRI is limited to a significant reduction in symptoms with improvement in quality of life but not a complete remission, a number of agents have been used in an attempt to augment this response. Studies of augmentation with the addition of either lithium or buspirone have found no significant intergroup differences vs. placebo, but researchers did note that improvement occurred in some individuals. The only agents with documented superiority to placebo in augmentation of an SRI are the antipsychotics haloperidol and pimozide. A closer examination of these data revealed that the patients who benefitted were those with either co-morbid Tourette's disorder or chronic motor tic disorder. Case reports of successful augmentation with clonazepam and fenfluramine have not yet been further evaluated via controlled trials. In one study the response to clonazepam monotherapy was comparable to that seen with clomipramine.

If an inadequate response is obtained to SRIs, treatment with a monoamine oxidase inhibitor (MAOI)—either phenelzine or tranylcypromine—is another alternative. One British study found no significant difference between treatment with phenelzine and treatment with clomipramine. Multiple case reports have suggested that individuals with OCD and co-morbid panic disorder or social phobia may have a preferential response to an MAOI. It is important to remember that MAOIs and SRIs must never be used together, because the interaction may result in serotonin syndrome, a poorly understood but life-threatening cluster of symptoms. This may be avoided by allowing at least 2 weeks after discontinuing clomipramine, fluvoxamine, sertraline, or paroxetine and at least 5 weeks after stopping fluoxetine (because of its substantially longer half-life) before beginning an MAOI. Similarly, after stopping an MAOI, at least 10 days should be allowed to pass before starting treatment with a SRI.

Behavior Therapy

Behavior therapy begins with the therapist obtaining a detailed history not limited to the types of obsessions and compulsions that are being experienced, but also including the specific situations that increase symptoms and the rituals or avoidance behaviors that then occur. A hierarchy is then constructed for each specific type of behavior (for example, checking doorknobs), and the patient is trained in various means of anxiety reduction. The therapist then accompanies the patient in an exposure to a situation that the patient would previously handle by either avoidance behavior or the performance of rituals. The patient is instructed to not perform compulsions and remains in the situation until a reduction in anxiety occurs. The patient may benefit from seeing the therapist perform the exposure at the same time without subsequent ritualizing (participant modeling).

The stimuli of the initial exposures are chosen to cause a tolerable but not extreme degree of anxiety. Situations that the patient finds intolerably anxiety provoking may be first approached via imaginal exposures, in which the patient mentally visualizes the activity rather then directly confronting it. Although the obsessive thoughts typically linger for weeks after the individual stops performing the compulsions, the patient eventually habituates to the involved stimuli with no resulting occurrence of symptoms after successful completion of exposures. Optimally, generalization occurs and the patient also habituates to situations similar but not identical to the exposure. The therapy then proceeds up the patient's hierarchy to more anxiety-producing exposures. Flooding, which involves starting near the top of the sufferer's hierarchy, has been found to be no more effective than starting at more tolerable levels and proceeding more gradually. Flooding may also (understandably) result in a higher dropout rate.

Most studies using behavior therapy to treat OCD have reported success rates at least comparable to pharmacotherapeutic trials. A meta-analysis reported that the rates of much and moderate improvement across studies were 51% and 39%, respectively, and after a follow-up period of months to years, more than 70% had reportedly maintained this level of improvement. It is important to recognize that the direct applicability of the behavior therapy literature to clinical practice is highly dependent on the quality of the therapists who are readily available. Additionally, a not insignificant number of patients either refuse behavior therapy or do not adequately engage in it. Concomitant use of appropriate pharmacotherapeutic agents often allows patients to proceed with behavioral treatment. At the very least, the current standard of care involves making all patients aware of both medication and behavioral treatment options (Case 10-2).

Psychosurgery

A variety of psychosurgical procedures have been performed on patients with OCD, including cingulotomy, orbital undercutting, anterior capsulotomy, bifrontal tractotomy, and bimedial leukotomy. Although generally good success rates have been reported, most prior work has not been limited to individuals with treatment-resistant illness. Because of the reported success of these procedures that share the feature of interrupting connections between frontal lobe and basal ganglia structures, a model implicating involvement of these areas in the pathophysiology of OCD has gained considerable acceptance.

More recently, Swedish researchers evaluated 10 patients with incapacitating treatment-resistant OCD before and 1 year after capsulotomy and noted significant reductions in anxiety and OCD symptoms. Although a recent review of psychosurgical intervention in OCD notes that cingulotomy may actually tend to have a poorer overall outcome than other procedures, it has been the primary procedure performed in the United States. A reevaluation of 33 patients who had undergone at least one cingulotomy within 25 years at the Massachusetts General Hospital was recently completed. An examination of whether these individuals had adequate treatment for OCD before the surgery determined that 85% of the subjects had a record of antidepressant trial and 79% had been treated with a course of ECT; only 9% had been treated with behavior therapy. The most common postoperative complications were found to be easily controlled seizure disorder (9%) and mania (6%). Six patients were found to be deceased at the time of the follow-up studies, including four who had committed suicide. Adequate assessments of symptoms of OCD were made on 14 patients of whom six reported no improvement and eight reported moderate to marked improvement (two of these patients attributed their improvements to other postoperative treatments).

A group at Brown University is planning to conduct a double-blind psychosurgical study in patients with OCD who have not responded to conventional treatment that uses a gamma knife to stereotactically perform an anterior capsulotomy in one half of the subjects. Because the gamma knife allows the procedure to be completed without any incision, the other half of their patients initially receive sham psychosurgery in which no lesions are made. Both groups will then be reevaluated after 6 months, at which time the sham-surgery group will also receive the procedure.

Pathophysiology

Association with Neurological Illness

As physicians' understanding of the functional neuroanatomy underlying the symptoms of OCD has gradually evolved, a relatively clear picture has begun to emerge. As noted, early hints from the relative success of neurosurgical treatments that tended to interrupt cortical connections to basal ganglia structures led researchers to focus some attention on these areas. This attention has led to a realization that higher than expected rates of OCD have been reported among individuals with Sydenham's chorea, an illness involving the formation of autoantibodies to the caudate nucleus after a streptococcal infection. Case reports associating OCD with other diseases involving basal ganglia pathology have included postencephalitic parkinsonism, Huntington's disease, and blepharospasm. Tourette's disorder, in which co-morbid OCD is quite common, is another disorder in which evidence exists suggesting basal ganglia involvement. A number of case reports have also associated OCD with infarct or injury to the caudate nucleus or globus pallidus.

Neuroimaging

A limited number of computed tomography (CT) and magnetic resonance imaging (MRI) studies have been performed to examine brain structures in individuals with OCD, and no specific abnormalities have been consistently reported. Positron emission tomography (PET) has been used to perform functional neuroanatomical examinations in these individuals. A consistent finding across several centers has been increased glucose or oxygen metabolism in the orbital frontal cortex of OCD subjects seen either unilaterally or bilaterally.

When one group restudied subjects after a year of medication therapy, they noted a significant decrease in orbitofrontal glucose metabolism bilaterally with

CASE 10-2

Mrs. T. reported, "I've always been a perfectionist." When she was growing up, she tended to be somewhat territorial around the home. She explained, "I didn't want anyone messing with my stuff." In her late teens she began to worry excessively about hair accumulating on clothing and other household surfaces. The thoughts were intrusive and led to rituals involving having to repeatedly shake the laundry or wipe the surfaces to remove the hair. Other compulsions that involved ordering and arranging household items were soon added. These symptoms continued at a level that the patient found annoying but tolerable until she married at age 32. She then had to incorporate her husband's presence into her routine. She experienced an increase in her obsessions and compulsions that led her to request that her husband restrict their social activities, including time outside the home and having guests visit their house (limiting exposures and allowing more time for rituals).

The amount of time involved in performing the compulsive behaviors gradually increased until it took Mrs. T. an hour to wipe down the kitchen after a meal. This would be continued "until it felt right." Although her husband was supportive, Mrs. T.'s symptoms began to substantially restrict their activities. At his urging, she first sought treatment at age 37. She was seen by a psychiatrist who recommended that she be hospitalized for treatment of depression. She did not have symptoms meeting criteria for depression at that time and sought care elsewhere. She was next evaluated over several sessions by a behavior therapist who forewarned both Mrs. T. and her husband that therapy would be very effortful. She became concerned by his warnings and chose not to proceed at that time.

Mrs. T. next went to a physician for evaluation at age 39. Her symptoms were somewhat worse, causing her to spend more than 3 hours each day engaged in rituals. She was given information on therapeutic alternatives, including medication and behavior therapy. She chose to be treated with a combination of both modalities. She was prescribed 20 mg/day of fluoxetine, and the process of acquiring the detailed history required for behavior therapy was begun. After 1 week, as instructed, she increased her fluoxetine dose to 40 mg/day. With this dose she began to feel less energetic, more depressed, and somewhat jittery. Because of this, fluoxetine was discontinued and she was prescribed clomipramine at a dose of 50 mg/day, which was then increased to 100 mg/day. On the higher dose, she had some complaints of dry mouth, sedation, and orthostatic hypotension, but these were tolerable.

Before formally beginning the behavior therapy, Mrs. T. noted a reduction in her anxiety level and found it considerably easier to delay completing her rituals. She attributed both changes to the medication. Mrs. T.'s behavior therapist established several hierarchies, including one involving the shaking of clothes and others focusing on her wiping surfaces only once and leaving objects out of place. Mrs. T.'s husband was involved with her in the therapy and remained extremely supportive. Mrs. T. began working through each hierarchy with most exposures actually done in her home. She made continuous progress with her behavioral assignments and was able to complete all three hierarchies over 8 months. A clomipramine taper was begun at this time, with the reduction in dose proceeding at 25 mg/day every 2 months. The clomipramine was discontinued, and Mrs. T. has thus far continued to do well without any symptoms of OCD whatsoever.

the right-sided difference correlating significantly with the decrease in OCD symptoms. Similarly, another group reported a decrease in the midfrontal, right anterior frontal, and left caudate glucose metabolism with medication treatment. The UCLA group restudied subjects after 10 weeks of treatment, including a group who received medication and a second group treated with behavior therapy. They noted that responders in both groups demonstrated decreases in glucose metabolism in the head of the right caudate nucleus. Their findings provide the first example in which the successful treatment of a mental illness with two different treatment modalities, either medication or behavior therapy, has been shown to produce similar effects on brain metabolism.

Two somewhat different activation studies have been performed, in which subjects not taking medication were studied in the presence of a stimulus chosen to provoke symptoms of OCD (such as a contaminated glove) after having been studied in the presence of a comparable innocuous stimulus (for example, a sterile glove). One group used a subtraction method in which the control scan was subtracted from the activation scan to create a difference image. They found that significant increases in blood flow had occurred in the left anterior orbital frontal cortex and that these increases positively correlated with the subjects' assessment of change in the degree of their symptoms of OCD. Other regions that lacked this correlation but demonstrated significant increases in blood flow with symptom provocation included the right caudate nucleus and the midline anterior cingulate cortex.

The other group used a somewhat different method of analysis, in which they studied four subjects with OCD across a variety of stimuli designed to provoke symptoms of OCD to varying degrees. They then examined correlations between the degree of symptoms reported and blood flow in various regions. They found changes in blood flow in a variety of structures that were positively correlated with the intensity of symptoms of OCD, including the right inferior frontal cortex, the right caudate nucleus, the right globus pallidus, and the right thalamus.

The PET studies of OCD have generated a great

deal of excitement that may be better understood with an appreciation of the underlying neuroanatomical interconnections. A loop has been described that connects the orbital frontal cortex, caudate nucleus, globus pallidus, and thalamus and then has an additional feedback connection to the orbital frontal cortex. It has been suggested that the excitatory and inhibitory interconnections within the loop may result in increased risk of self-sustained firing. Components of this loop have been implicated in the pathophysiology of OCD by the following converging lines of investigation: (1) PET studies demonstrating increased activity in resting subjects with further increases noted in activation studies involving symptom provocation, (2) the occurrence of symptoms of OCD with neurological illnesses that have pathological changes involving these regions, and (3) the observation that an improvement in symptoms of OCD may result from the psychosurgical interruption of these connections. Researchers hope that these findings lead to the development of improved treatments for people suffering from OCD.

Serotonin

The specific antiobsessional efficacy of the SRIs has led many investigators to suggest that the pathophysiology of OCD must involve serotoninergic dysfunction. Challenge studies with a variety of compounds with serotoninergic mechanisms of action have offered some support for these suggestions. As with other psychiatric disorders, examinations of peripheral serotoninergic markers have not produced consistently replicable results in samples of OCD patients. Patients commonly ask their treating physicians for confirmation that they have a "chemical imbalance involving serotonin." Unfortunately although it appears that serotonergic dysfunction may play a part in the pathophysiology of OCD, it is likely that viewing OCD as a serotoninergic disorder is a gross oversimplification that is comforting to patients and perhaps to physicians but certainly not the entire story. A comprehensive model accounting for basal ganglia and orbital frontal cortex involvement and adequately explaining the specificity of SRIs has yet to be cogently presented.

Obsessive-Compulsive Disorder in a Primary Care Setting

For physicians working in a primary care setting, illnesses like OCD may seem quite far removed from the typical medical practice. Many psychiatrists report that they encounter a limited number of people suffering

CASE 10-3

Mr. V. first appeared for psychiatric evaluation at age 32 during a period of high situational stress. He gave a 3-week history of crying spells; increased anxiety with palpitations; sleep disturbance with terminal insomnia; decreased appetite resulting in a 15-pound weight loss over 1 month; poor concentration; fatigue; lack of enjoyment of activities; and feelings of hopelessness, helplessness, and worthlessness. He was diagnosed with depression and initially treated with imipramine and alprazolam. Because of concerns regarding right bundle branch block on his electrocardiogram (ECG), the imipramine was quickly discontinued and trazodone therapy was started. Mr. V. responded well to this combination, and his depressive symptoms completely remitted. The alprazolam was gradually tapered, and Mr. V. continued to do well.

Several months later Mr. V. began to have increased complaints of throat irritation. He eventually was seen by an otolaryngologist, who recommended a tonsillectomy and adenoidectomy. The surgery was performed without incident, but Mr. V. continued to complain of throat irritation postoperatively. Mr. V. was seen in consultation by another otolaryngologist, who also could find no clear organic cause for Mr. V.'s complaints. Buspirone was added because of anxiety Mr. V. was experiencing, including fears that he would lose his job and be unable to support his wife and their new child because of his throat irritation. Mr. V.'s symptoms improved, but they did not entirely remit. Alprazolam was restarted and further improvement occurred, enabling Mr. V. to return to work. At this time Mr. V. reported that he had been examining his throat often in an attempt to find an explanation of his symptoms. He also reported intrusive thoughts about swallowing, clearing his throat, and blinking his eyes. He spontaneously voiced additional symptoms dating to childhood, including touching compulsions, obsessive thoughts about staring at the sun, and compulsions to repeat certain words. Mr. V. continued to have occasional symptoms that worsened with situational stressors. He was still taking the trazodone and buspirone. A trial of fluoxetine was attempted, but it could not be completed because of sedation. He later developed symptoms that including checking rituals involving doors, appliances, and his son, as well as a resurgence of touching compulsions, which made it necessary for him to touch certain objects up to four times. Mr. V. has remained somewhat symptomatic, but he has not wanted to proceed with a trial of behavior therapy or consider a change in medication. However, he has continued to function fairly well at work and home.

PEARLS & PERILS

TREATMENT OF OBSESSIVE-COMPULSIVE DISORDER

- Patients should be made aware of the relative efficacy and side effects of available agents.
- Higher medication dosages may be needed than those typically used to treat depression.
- Time to respond is longer than in depression, so the medication dose should be increased slowly.
- Risk of relapse may be increased with abrupt discontinuation of medication.
- Lower doses may achieve comparable effects with fewer side effects later in treatment.
- Behavior therapy is beneficial for most people with OCD, but it remains underused.
- The Yale-Brown Obsessive-Compulsive Scale (Y-BOCS) may be used to screen for additional OCD symptoms even when the diagnosis is not in doubt. The patient almost always has other symptoms not appreciated as OCD-related.
- The Y-BOCS may be used to monitor treatment response. Patients with OCD often forget early gains.
- Family members should be educated regarding alternatives to offering the sufferer reassurance.
- Self-help groups allow the patient and family to meet others with similar difficulties and hear how these individuals have coped and progressed.

from OCD. These patients, as epidemiological research confirms, are actually present to a greater extent than is generally appreciated. When a physician does not ask a patient about the specific symptoms of OCD from which he suffers, the information may not be transmitted to the physician. Even a psychiatrist with a strong interest in OCD can be embarrassed to find that a patient has been treated for more than a year before OCD is diagnosed because the psychiatrist failed to screen for symptoms of OCD (Case 10-3).

If a physician has reason to suspect the presence of OCD, it is important to screen for its symptoms. The Yale-Brown Obsessive Compulsive Scale (Y-BOCS) is a useful instrument that is well suited for this purpose. The Y-BOCS contains fairly comprehensive lists of obsessions and compulsions that may be posed to appropriate patients to facilitate the diagnosis of OCD. The reason this is invaluable is that most patients with OCD do have insight into their symptoms, which they often consider embarrassing idiosyncracies until told otherwise. These patients often answer negatively in response to vague questions regarding whether they have ever had intrusive thoughts or repetitive behaviors. Some common scenarios in which the possibility of OCD should be entertained are suggested in Box 10-2.

BOX 10-2

WHEN TO THINK ABOUT OBSESSIVE DISORDER AND RELATED ILLNESSES

- A patient without substantial risk factors requests an HIV test, seems dissatisfied with the negative result, and asks to be retested.
- A patient expresses across time fears of cancer involving multiple sites of origin.
- A patient has chapped or shiny, erythematous hands without a clear explanation.
- A patient requests that a plastic surgeon correct a defect visible only to the patient.
- A patient repeatedly states, "You don't understand."
- A parent repeatedly brings a healthy child in for unnecessary examinations.
- A patient discontinues several medications after 2 to 3 days for vague reasons.
- A patient is constantly asking repetitive questions about a variety of illnesses.
- A patient continually arrives late for appointments without any clear explanation.

With cost containment and other economic issues continuing to drive changes in medical practice in the United States, it is likely that the role of primary care physicians will continue to expand. This trend places on these practitioners an additional burden of functioning as effective gatekeepers making appropriate referrals to a variety of specialty care physicians and other caregivers. Most primary care physicians typically refer individuals with OCD to psychiatrists, but many are being called on to handle the pharmacological aspects of treatment in conjunction with a behavior therapist. It then becomes incumbent on these physicians to possess an improved understanding of the clinical management of OCD, as well as to set a reasonable level of comfort beyond which a referral to a psychiatrist should be made. Some helpful reminders of the basic tenets of OCD treatment are presented in the Pearls & Perils box above.

OCD is a fascinating illness in which each sufferer may have diverse symptoms requiring individualized treatment. Further research will soon provide a clearer understanding of its underlying pathophysiological nature and may even allow for an improved comprehension of normal brain functioning. Although the treatment of patients with OCD may be time consuming, it is extremely satisfying to assist these individuals in their attempts to regain the freedoms we so readily take for granted.

CONSIDER CONSULTATION WHEN . . .

- The patient presents with atypical symptoms (for example, a pervasive lack of insight)
- The patient quickly terminates multiple medication trials secondary to perceived side effects
- Prominent symptoms remain after a trial of an SRI of typically adequate dose and duration
- Symptoms worsen after starting a medication trial
- The patient's symptoms include avoidance behavior or rituals and the treating physician is unfamiliar with behavior therapy

Annotated Bibliography

Baer L: *Getting control: overcoming your obsessions and compulsions,* Boston, 1991, Little, Brown and Co.

This is a do-it-yourself guide to behavior therapy clearly written by a leading behavior therapist.

Jenike MA, Baer L, Minichiello WE, editors: *Obsessive compulsive disorders theory and management,* ed 2, Chicago, 1990, Mosby.

This is a comprehensive textbook that improves with each new edition and contains contributions from the leaders in the field. A copy of the Y-BOCS is also included among its appendices.

Pato MT, Zohar J, editors: *Current treatments of obsessive-compulsive disorder,* Washington, D.C., 1991, American Psychiatric Press.

This text reviews treatment options for the clinician, including pharmacotherapy, behavior therapy, and various family therapy approaches.

Rapoport JL: *The boy who couldn't stop washing: the experiences and treatment of obsessive-compulsive disorder,* New York, 1989, E.P. Dutton.

This is an introductory book for patients and their families that has helped achieve greater public awareness of OCD and its many symptoms.

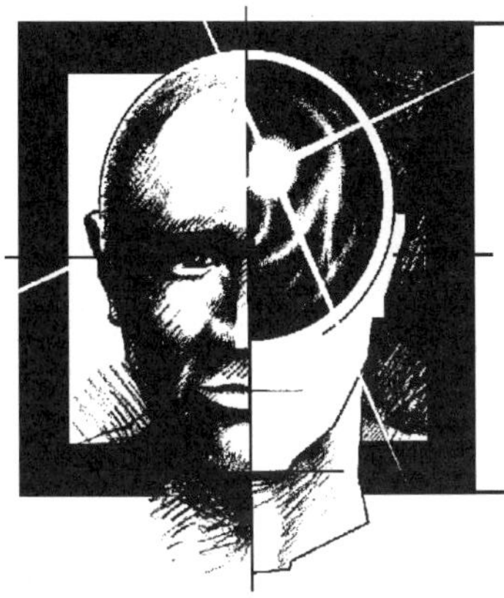

chapter 11

Cognitive Disorders: Delirium and Amnestic Disorder

Keith Eugene Isenberg, MD

The cognitive disorders are impairments of memory and information processing that represent a loss of previous capacity. Diagnostic criteria for delirium, dementia, and amnestic disorder facilitate the recognition of these syndromes of cognitive impairment. Current nosology (DSM-IV) etiologically relates the specific syndromes to nonpsychiatric disorders ("due to a general medical condition") or to a specific substance causing either intoxication or implicated in withdrawal ("substance-induced"). The term *organic mental disorder* was deleted from DSM-IV because the word *organic* was felt to imply that other psychiatric disorders (or "nonorganic" syndromes) were not associated with biological findings. Dementias (chronic brain syndromes associated with memory impairment and other cognitive deficits) are discussed in this chapter primarily as they pertain to the differential diagnosis of delirium and amnestic disorder; further description of dementia is available in Chapter 12.

This chapter focuses on delirium, a disorder characterized by the acute onset of altered consciousness and change in cognition or perception, and amnestic disorder, memory impairment in the absence of other significant cognitive deficits. Classification of delirium and amnestic disorder as caused by drugs or general medical disorders recognizes the importance of extrinsic factors in the causation of both syndromes. In a specific patient, delirium and amnestic disorder may both occur because of the same etiological factor, such as alcohol use. The amnestic disorder associated with alcoholism, Korsakoff's syndrome, is often preceded by a delirium, Wernicke's encephalopathy. Delirium and amnestic disorder are considered separately because delirium, like dementia, is a manifestation of global cognitive dysfunction, whereas amnestic disorder is a relatively specific impairment of memory. The purpose of this chapter is to provide a systematic approach to these disorders that enhances the recognition of the disorders and leads to implementation of proper treatment, minimizing morbidity and mortality.

Delirium

Diagnosis

Delirium is characterized by the rapid onset of impaired consciousness and perceptual changes or altered cognition (Box 11-1); the syndrome typically has

DSM-IV DIAGNOSTIC CRITERIA

BOX 11-1 DELIRIUM

A. Disturbance of consciousness (i.e., reduced clarity of awareness of the environment) with reduced ability to focus, sustain, or shift attention.

B. A change in cognition (such as memory deficit, disorientation, language disturbance) or the development of a perceptual disturbance that is not better accounted for by a preexisting, established, or evolving dementia.

C. The disturbance develops over a short period of time (usually hours to days) and tends to fluctuate during the course of the day.

Delirium due to a general medical condition

D. There is evidence from the history, physical examination, or laboratory findings that the disturbance is caused by the direct physiological consequences of a general medical condition.

Substance intoxication delirium

D. There is evidence from the history, physical examination, or laboratory findings of either (1) or (2):

(1) the symptoms in Criteria A and B developed during Substance Intoxication
(2) medication use is etiologically related to the disturbance

Substance withdrawal delirium

D. There is evidence from the history, physical examination, or laboratory findings that the symptoms in Criteria A and B developed during, or shortly after, a withdrawal syndrome.

Delirium due to multiple etiologies

D. There is evidence from the history, physical examination, or laboratory findings that the delirium has more than one etiology (e.g., more than one etiological general medical condition, a general medical condition plus Substance Intoxication or medication side effect).

Delirium not otherwise specified

This category should be used to diagnose a delirium that does not meet criteria for any of the specific types of delirium described in this section.

Modified from American Psychiatric Association: *Diagnostic and statistical manual of mental disorders,* ed 4 (DSM-IV), Washington, D.C., 1994, American Psychiatric Press.

a fluctuating course. Regardless of the cause of delirium, evidence should exist in each patient to support the presence of DSM-IV Criteria A, B, and C. Etiological specification directs interventions aimed at alleviating delirium. The assignment of Not Otherwise Specified (NOS) should be rare. Physicians have long associated these clinical findings with numerous medical conditions, attaching various names to delirium. The historical lack of uniform terminology and the often subtle onset of delirium probably contribute to underdiagnosis of the syndrome. Timely recognition and treatment of delirium improve the quality of patient care and may reduce the use of services. Consistent features of the syndrome are described in Table 11-1, and suggestions for eliciting these common symptoms can be found in Box 11-2, which outlines an examination to establish the presence of signs of delirium. Although much of the information can be gleaned from direct examination, interview and evaluation of collateral sources may be critical, particularly for the patient who is stuporous or obtunded. Consideration is also given to the variable aspects of the syndrome. Case 11-1 provides an example for further guidance. The symptoms associated with delirium are readily apparent in this case, and appropriate management is described. Although complex, Case 11-1 is illustrative of the most important conditions associated with delirium: drug intoxication, sedative-hypnotic (including alcohol) withdrawal, and metabolic encephalopathy. Each condition probably played a role in the case, which is indicative of multifactorial etiology. Finally, hospital course was prolonged and the postdischarge outcome, placement in a nursing home, was poor; these are unfortunately common results of delirium.

Clinical Features

Patients who are delirious have an impaired awareness of the environment. Although the disturbance of consciousness may be manifested as a "clouding" or somnolence, delirium is more generally associated

DIAGNOSIS

TABLE 11-1
DELIRIUM

Discriminating features

1. Waxing and waning awareness
2. Acute onset of cognitive dysfunction

Consistent features

1. Disorientation, usually to time
2. Memory impairment, particularly recent memory
3. Hallucinations, typically visual, and misperceptions
4. Language dysfunction, such as an impaired ability to name objects
5. Definable cause

Variable features

1. Hyperactivity and/or hypoactivity
2. Mood disturbance
3. Alteration in sleep-wake cycle
4. Delusions
5. Impaired judgment
6. Dream-like experience for patient

with a reduced responsiveness to the surroundings. During an examination, the patient may respond to questions by perseverating with the answer to a previously asked question. It may be necessary to repeat questions because the patient is distracted by irrelevant stimuli. The reduced awareness may be so severe that it is impossible to interview the patient. Interviews of collateral sources (such as family or hospital staff) may be necessary to establish onset of reduced awareness. The patient described in Case 11-1 was usually inattentive and often lethargic.

Disturbances of cognition, a critical aspect of delirium, can affect orientation, memory, and language. Individuals without delirium can respond to name (oriented to name), provide an appropriate name for current location (oriented to place), and know the day, month, season, and year with accuracy for the date within 1 or 2 days (oriented to date). Disorientation may be the first sign of mild delirium. Confusion regarding the date is common, disorientation to place is probably less common, and disorientation to name is rare in delirium. Although disorientation may be observed in other disorders, such as dementia and mental retardation, a recent change in a previously oriented person suggests delirium. The patient in Case 11-1 was, at times, oriented only to name.

Memory impairment usually involves recent events and impairs the quality of the history elicited from the patient. Recall, which is also involved, can be assessed

BOX 11-2

EVALUATION OF DELIRIUM

Disturbance of consciousness

Patient may be difficult to arouse.
Look for excessive sleepiness during examination, in chart, or from collateral sources.
Patient may not attend to a question or task because of a lack of focus.
Patient may not complete an answer to a question or complete a task because he is distractable, showing a failure to sustain attention.
Patient may not be able to shift attention as indicated by perseveration in speech or task.
Patient may have difficulty repeating numbers (digit span) because of inattention.

Change in cognition

Check orientation to person, place and time.
Evaluate memory and patient's ability to recall.
    Recent events (social, personal)
    Remote events (historical, personal)
Evaluate language: have patient name objects such as a watch, pencil, or key.
    Document inappropriate word use or word substitution.
Patient may have altered perception.
    Illusions—mistaken identity
    Hallucinations—no stimuli present

Acute onset and fluctuating course

Observe and obtain information from collateral sources such as the patient's family or chart.

CASE 11-1

Mr. S. was admitted to outpatient surgery for transurethral resection of what proved to be a bladder carcinoma. The patient was premedicated with 100 μg of fentanyl (a narcotic), 1.5 mg of midazolam (a benzodiazepine), and 15 mg of ephedrine (a sympathomimetic, used as a pressor during spinal anesthesia), all given intravenously. The operation was performed without complication while the patient was under spinal anesthesia, which was chosen because of a history of heavy alcohol consumption. After the procedure 1 gm of vancomycin (an antibiotic) was given intravenously. During recovery the patient complained of bladder pain, which was managed with 10 mg of oxybutynin given orally (an anticholinergic). When this did not alleviate the complaints, repeated doses of intravenous meperidine (a narcotic) to a total dose of 190 mg were also given. The patient was agitated, confused, and unable to follow commands, necessitating a prolonged stay in the recovery room and repeated doses of midazolam to a total dose of 8 mg. Vital signs, including oxygen saturation per pulse oximetry, were unremarkable, but as the patient's mental status deteriorated, the blood pressure increased to 190/95 and was managed with 5 mg of labetalol (a selective α_1 and nonselective β adrenergic antagonist) given intravenously.

The patient was transferred from the recovery room to the urology ward, where agitation, diaphoresis, combativeness, orientation only to person and place, and inability to follow commands were noted. These symptoms were worse at night. At times the patient was observed to be lethargic, particularly during the day. The physical examination was not revealing. The patient was afebrile; his electrolytes and complete blood count (CBC) were unremarkable. The internist noted a history of heavy drinking and suggested postoperative delirium caused by alcohol withdrawal. Symptoms were managed with haloperidol (a neuroleptic) and various benzodiazepines.

The patient was transferred from the urology ward to the medicine ward 3 days postoperatively because his mental status had improved only slightly. The patient was initially noted to be tremulous, uncooperative, and oriented to person, month, and year, but he did not know the place. Electrolytes were within normal limits; magnesium was normal. Elevated creatine kinase (peaked at 946 IU/ml 3 days postoperatively), not associated with a cardiac source, was judged to be from agitation. The creatine kinase returned to normal over the next several days. Serum glutamic-oxaloacetic transaminase (SGOT; aspartate aminotransferase [AST]) and lactate dehydrogenase (LDH) were elevated slightly (2 times normal) but decreased to normal; serum glutamate pyruvate transferase (SGPT; alanine aminotransferase [ALT]) and bilirubin were normal. Total protein and albumin were slightly decreased. Orientation and cooperation continued to vary remarkably over the course of a day. A neurology consultant agreed that the patient was suffering from delirium tremens and thought the patient had peripheral neuropathy and chronic cognitive dysfunction secondary to alcohol abuse. He recommended oral and intramuscular vitamin supplementation, including thiamine, as well as continued use of chlordiazepoxide. An ammonia level, recommended by the neurologist, was within normal limits 4 days postoperatively.

Six days postoperatively, a psychiatrist was consulted. He noted a chief complaint of, "Do you have a match?" The patient was oriented to person but not to place; however, he was able to give the day, month, and year, missing the date by 3 days. His fund of knowledge was good; for example, he gave the full names of the President, the Vice-President, and the President's wife. Simple contrasts and comparisons were performed without difficulty. The patient recalled three of three items immediately and two of three items at 5 minutes despite prompting. The family noted concerns about preexisting chronic cognitive impairment, suggestive of alcoholic dementia in addition to delirium. The psychiatrist confirmed the diagnosis of alcohol dependence, concurred with the diagnosis of delirium tremens, and agreed that further evaluation, particularly for central nervous system (CNS) lesions (such as metastatic tumor to the brain) was wise. Computed tomography (CT) of the head with contrast was obtained 1 week postoperatively and showed two small, ill-defined foci of low attenuation consistent with prior ischemic disease but otherwise normal for age. The patient was switched from chlordiazepoxide and diazepam (long half-life benzodiazepines) to lorazepam (a short half-life benzodiazepine), facilitating the intermittent administration of an intramuscular benzodiazepine for severe agitation and minimizing the risk of drug accumulation.

Persistent confusion 10 days after the operation led to a search for causes of delirium other than alcohol withdrawal. The CBC, electrolytes, and other blood chemistries were repeated and were within normal limits or much improved relative to initial evaluations. The patient was afebrile and cultures of blood and urine were negative. Thyroid studies were unremarkable, as were B_{12} and folate levels. An electroencephalogram (EEG) obtained 11 days postoperatively showed background slowing indicative of a mild diffuse encephalopathy. The patient had an elevated ammonia of 44.5 μmole/L (expected range 9 to 33 μmol/L) 12 days postoperatively; the elevated ammonia persisted throughout the remainder of the hospitalization. Consultation between the specialists involved suggested that no further workup was indicated, a recommendation accepted by the patient's family. Benzodiazepines were discontinued; efforts to manage a sleep-wake disturbance and psychosis with haloperidol failed, but the patient slept through the night on 25 mg of thioridazine (a neuroleptic) taken at bedtime every night. The patient was felt to have chronic hepatic encephalopathy and was transferred to a nursing home facility on a 30-gm protein diet.

The patient's cognitive function and ammonia levels were followed up in the nursing home during a 2-month recuperation. Thioridazine was tapered and discontinued. Memory and cognition improved gradually but substantially; ammonia levels slowly returned to normal. At the time of discharge from the nursing home facility, the patient was without clinically obvious signs of delirium or dementia.

by asking the patient to remember several unrelated items or a simple sentence and requesting that the patient repeat the provided information (confirming that the information presented was processed; failure to attend to the task is indicative of impaired attention). After involving the patient in other tasks for several minutes (for example, gathering more history, performing other aspects of the mental status examination), the inquiry is made about the remembered material. Remote memory is relatively spared. Like orientation, the patient's memory in Case 11-1 was impaired. At worst, Mr. S. was unable to give accurate information about his family, (compatible with loss of remote memory); even when he was mildly affected, the patient had difficulty with recall.

Language dysfunction can be manifested as an impaired ability to name objects. Speech may be rambling, perhaps related to the inability to attend to tasks, or incoherent, because of unpredictable switching from topic to topic. The patient described in Case 11-1 was difficult to interview because of rambling speech.

Perceptual disturbances associated with delirium include illusions and hallucinations. Illusions represent the improper labelling of stimuli. Body parts may be perceived as being distorted, shadows may represent real objects, and loud sounds may be interpreted as threatening. Hallucinations represent perceptual experiences in the absence of relevant stimuli. Hallucinations may be simple, such as the visualization of stars or lights, or they may be complex with a patient conversing with nonexistent visitors. When present, illusions and hallucinations can be associated with delusions, or false beliefs that are not shared with others (such as the patient's family). The misinterpretation of a loud sound as a gunshot is elaborated into an execution, and a patient becomes afraid of being the next to be executed. The hallucinated visitors are described as stealing things or as messengers from God. In delirium, illusions and hallucinations tend to be fragmentary, transitory, and visual.

The perceptual disturbances of delirium have been compared with those reported in dreams. Clearly, the experience of illusions and hallucinations has a bizarre aspect that is shared with many dreams. Interestingly, patients afflicted with multiple episodes of delirium may have similar perceptual disturbances during each episode. At times, particularly in the evening, the patient in Case 11-1 attended to nonexistent visual stimuli. When disoriented to place, he substituted locations other than the hospital and acted as if the substitutions were valid, a form of confabulation that is delusional. Management of the patient was complicated by assaultive behavior towards staff that occurred as the result of perceptual symptoms.

Symptoms of delirium develop rapidly, on a time scale measured in hours to days. The patient in Case 1-11 had an acute onset in the immediate postoperative period. Presentation of mild delirium can be subtle because of the fluctuating course. Careful review of patient charting may reveal the notation by hospital staff of "confusion" at night for 1 or 2 days before more obvious manifestations of delirium. The sleep-wake cycle may be disturbed, with somnolence during the day and agitated insomnia at night, as noted for Mr. S. in Case 11-1. The case report describes a patient who was alert and knowledgeable at times, only to decompensate at other times, particularly in the evening. Variation in awareness may further tax a patient's comprehension of events; sleep and dreaming fade into the hallucinations and somnolence of delirium. Mr. S. was observed by numerous medical personnel who documented an acute onset and a fluctuating course. The individual arriving in the office or emergency room with delirium and no collateral source may be a diagnostic problem because the patient may not be able to provide a reliable history.

Symptoms, a critical aspect of diagnosis that are variably present in delirium (see Table 11-1), are discussed before etiology is systematically considered. Many symptoms variably present in delirium were previously regarded as critical components of the syndrome. The simplified criteria codified in DSM-IV should facilitate diagnosis by avoiding variable features of delirium.

Delirium is usually associated with a disturbance of motor activity. Patients may be described as hyperactive compared with their usual selves, hypoactive compared with their usual selves, or suffering from a mixture, with hypoactivity on some occasions and hyperactivity at others. Hyperactivity is made manifest as a purposeless restlessness that may make management particularly difficult. It has been suggested that management difficulties—the patient removing various medical devices, wandering the halls, and entering other patients' rooms—bring the hyperactive variant of delirium to medical attention more often than the hypoactive variant. The patient in Case 11-1 was hyperactive at times, particularly at night. Delirium tremens represents the classical hyperactive delirium. Individuals with delirium who are hypoactive tend to show little spontaneous movement and are more likely to make little effort to assist in self care even if they are apparently awake. The hypoactivity can merge into the inactivity of the patient who is stuporous. Case 11-1 notes daytime lethargy. Solvent exposure can be associated with a quiet delirium that may proceed to respiratory or cardiac arrest and death. Fluctuation in course, a critical component of delirium, may be observed as a variation in motor activity, with the patient being inactive at times (perhaps during the day) and hyperactive at other times (perhaps during the evening), as exemplified by Mr. S. in Case 11-1.

Mood disturbance is an important aspect of delirium that, like motor activity, does not lend itself to simple description and classification. Aberrant mood is apparently fueled to some extent by the perceptual experiences of the patient who is delirious. The patient who experiences hallucinations with an amusing content may be jocular and euphoric. More commonly the patient suffers from depressed mood and morbid perceptual disturbances, which may place the patient at risk of suicide. A fearful mood is probably most common, and even familiar surroundings can be perceived as threatening. For example, the patient who is delirious may find vivid hallucinations of snakes and insects almost unbearable. The individual in Case 1-11 was usually irritable.

Current diagnostic criteria recognize the importance of psychotic symptoms in delirium by specifying the presence of perceptual disturbances or memory impairment. The implication of this approach is that psychotic symptoms such as visual hallucinations need not be invariably present. Language disturbance can be of psychotic proportion, with the disjointed speech suggestive of a formal thought disorder. Although it seems plausible that the presence of psychotic symptoms in delirium would have treatment implications, this has not been demonstrated. Indeed, delirium tremens, a typically psychotic disorder, is probably better treated with benzodiazepines than antipsychotics.

Disturbances of perception and memory leave the individual who is delirious vulnerable to the consequences of impaired judgment. The agitated patient may be particularly difficult to manage because he is less readily redirectable by verbal approaches. An inability to distinguish reality from hallucinations and delusions facilitates behavior that puts the patient at risk of harm to self or others. Impaired judgment, occurring in many psychiatric disorders, is not specific to delirium.

Neurological signs are commonly seen in delirium. Some types of delirium have been classically associated with specific signs, such as asterixis in hepatic encephalopathy, or ataxia and ophthalmoplegia in Wernicke's encephalopathy. The suggestion that these signs are part of specific syndromes of delirium has led some scholars to suggest that classification of delirium ought to be type-specific. However, neurological signs are not invariably present in any etiologically specific syndrome, nor is any sign syndrome-specific. Specifying subsyndromes of delirium based on the presence of particular neurological signs appears unworkable. A general, simplified approach to diagnosing acute cognitive impairment, exemplified by DSM-IV, enhances recognition of delirium.

Classification of delirium as a reversible disorder, as specified by older nosologies, ignores the mortality associated with the condition. Delirium is a common feature of the final stages of disorders such as various cancers and congestive heart failure. Treatment of delirium when death is expected minimizes the distressing impact of psychotic symptoms. The designation of delirium as *reversible* appears to have been intended to facilitate distinguishing delirium from the relatively irreversible dementias. Delirium in patients who are chronically cognitively impaired appears to be associated with persistent residual symptoms, perhaps accelerating the course of dementia but more importantly suggesting irreversible changes induced by delirium. Criteria that emphasize reversibility are likely to exacerbate the failure to recognize delirium in patients who are demented or dying.

Psychometric evaluation of patients who are delirious is not useful clinically. Instruments are available that allow screening for cognitive impairment, such as the Mini-Mental State Examination (MMSE), or help physicians rate the symptoms of delirium, such as the Delirium Rating Scale. The interpretation of instruments that screen for cognitive impairment is known to be confounded by intelligence, educational attainment, and socioeconomic status, which are interrelated variables. The use of screening and rating instruments typically requires that the patient participate systematically in the evaluation. Consciousness is particularly difficult to rate reliably. Furthermore, fluctuating course may permit a mild delirium to go undetected if the patient does not have significant impairment at the time of examination. Lethargy and uncooperativeness, problems noted in Case 11-1, limit the use of screening instruments. Prospective studies of delirium are complicated by the significant number of cases that were probably undetected because patients could not participate in the systematic evaluation required for reliable research. Screening instruments and rating scales are not as specific to delirium as would be desired; the difficulty of employing screening and rating instruments in systematic studies suggests caution in the implementation of such approaches. The physician is advised to incorporate questions about orientation and memory into every examination and make the diagnosis of delirium based on history, physical evaluation, and laboratory tests, minimizing the use of psychometric techniques.

Ascertaining the cause of delirium often leads directly to intervention and appropriate treatment of the cause and ideally to resolution of the delirium. Case 11-1 is illustrative of the process of determining specific causes of delirium. Additionally, Table 11-2 lists causes of delirium as reported in four case series. DSM-IV describes the following four broad etiological diagnostic categories for delirium: (1) substance-induced delirium, either during intoxication or withdrawal; (2) delirium caused by a general medical condition; (3) delirium resulting from multiple etiologies; and (4) delirium NOS (see Box 11-1). Etiology is considered within the framework proposed in DSM-IV and uses the categories outlined in Table 11-2. Categories in Table 11-2 correspond roughly to those employed in the most recent case series, a prospective study of delirium in the elderly (Francis, Martin, and Kapoor, 1990). Adjustments were made to reflect conditions that were found in the other series and relevant to the general practitioner. Categories such as drug intoxication or infection apply to patients who appear to have had delirium as the result of processes related to this category only. One series (Newton and Janati, 1986) does not appear to have considered multiple causes as a category. The relative contribution of each category of condition to the etiology of delirium in each case series is likely to reflect the diagnostic criteria employed for the diagnosis of delirium, the criteria for etiological assignment, and most relevant to the primary care physician, a referral bias. For example, one retrospective series of patients seen by psychiatric consultants (Newton and Janati) notes referral for evaluation of delirium after anesthesia in six instances, a cause of delirium that is likely to be rare in samples generated from hospital admissions (Purdie, Honigman, and Rosen, 1981; Francis, Martin, and Kapoor). A study of elderly patients excluded nursing home admissions and patients with dementia (Francis, Martin, and Kapoor) although poor predelirium functioning is likely to increase the risk of delirium and alter etiological classification (Purdie, Honigman, and Rosen). The geriatric sample (Francis, Martin, and Kapoor) contains the fewest patients, and numbers in parentheses indicate the portion of the sample afflicted with the various causes. The percentages are provided to facilitate direct comparison with the other studies. The elderly, perhaps because of multiple medical problems, may be particularly likely to suffer from a multifactorial disorder. An exhaustive list of diagnostic possibilities is beyond the scope of this presentation; the physician is encouraged to review other sources for a more complete presentation of etiological possibilities (see Annotated Bibliography).

Drug intoxication is arguably the most important etiological category, because in some cases delirium is preventable. Drug-intoxication delirium specifically refers to the direct effect of drugs on the brain rather than an indirect effect mediated by systemic toxicity. Intoxication may arise during the administration of drugs at usually effective doses and is thus a side effect of treatment. Intoxication may also arise when doses of a medication that are larger than those usually recommended are used therapeutically and planned as part of treatment for a patient, when larger-than-usual doses are taken in an intentional or accidental overdose, or when drugs are taken illegally for recreational purposes. Delirium can occur as the result of accidental or intentional exposure to an inducing substance in a work setting. Finally, delirium may occur as the result of intentional poisoning. Recreational drug use, occupational exposure, and intentional poisoning often involve compounds with which most physicians are unlikely to be familiar (such as organic solvents or heavy metals). Consideration of these drugs as etiological agents may benefit from consultation with more knowledgeable specialists (physicians familiar with the effects of drugs of abuse, such as emergency room physicians or psychiatrists, occupational medicine physicians, toxicologists, and forensic specialists). The elderly and the medically ill, particularly those with

TABLE 11-2

CAUSES OF DELIRIUM

	Purdie, Honigman, and Rosen 1981 (n = 100)	Newton and Janati, 1986 (n = 100)	Sirois, 1988 (n = 100)	Francis, Martin, and Kapoor, 1990 (n = 50); %
Drug intoxication	22	17	9	7 (14)
Withdrawal	6	—	13	—
Metabolic	6	43	19	2 (4)
Intracranial	15	10	15	1 (2)
Infection	8	12	6	4 (8)
Fluid and electrolyte imbalance	3	12	4	4 (8)
Functional	16	—	—	—
Postsurgical	—	6	—	—
Multiple	24	—	34	32 (64)

CNS disease are likely to be at greater risk of delirium from drug intoxication than the young and healthy.

Any prescribed drug is a possible cause of delirium, particularly in patients who are at risk for delirium (Box 11-3). After establishing the presence of clinical signs indicative of delirium, a thorough medication history should be obtained. A list of recently prescribed and current medications should be reviewed to note dose, particularly in relation to usually efficacious doses and duration of treatment relative to the onset of symptoms. The initiation of treatment with a medication in the hours or days before the onset of delirium should heighten suspicion that this drug plays a role in the disorder. Consideration should be given to obtaining drug levels; levels are helpful for compounds like lithium and the anticonvulsants. The decision to obtain a drug level should be partly dependent on an estimate of the need for continuing therapy with each specific drug. Drug levels can only serve as a guide because toxicity has been documented in some cases (involving lithium or anticonvulsants, for example) at therapeutic levels. Toxicological screens of blood and urine, as well as screens for drugs of abuse, that employ standard testing batteries may be helpful, particularly for patients without collateral sources. Consultation regarding testing for nonprescribed substances may be helpful if recreational drugs, occupational exposure, or poisoning are suspected.

The task of medication evaluation is more straightforward for the primary care physician than the consultant, given greater patient familiarity. In some cases, drugs are discontinued but because of the recurrence of symptoms for which the drug is indicated need to be added back. The physician with knowledge of the patient's longitudinal course is in the best position to assess benefits, risks, and alternatives in this circumstance. The assessment of pharmacological risks and benefits is a recurring task as long as the patient remains delirious, since drugs administered to manage the patient who is delirious can exacerbate or cause delirium (see Case 11-1 and the following paragraphs). A useful rule of thumb is that CNS-active drugs are more likely culprits in the cause of delirium than compounds with little or no known CNS effect.

Drugs with anticholinergic properties are an especially important cause of delirium (see Box 11-3). The observation that belladonna alkaloids, mixtures of atropine and scopolamine, cause delirium dates to antiquity. Atropine and scopolamine intoxication are associated with dilated pupils, blurred vision, flushed face, dry skin and mucous membranes, tachycardia, diminished or absent bowel sounds, urinary retention, increased blood pressure, and fever. Unfortunately, these signs are usually absent in the case of delirium associated with other potent antimuscarinic drugs, such as tricyclic antidepressants (TCAs), which have many other effects (antihistaminic, for example). The weight of current evidence favors anticholinergic effects as the most likely cause of delirium for the classes of drug listed under the anticholinergic headings. Physostigmine, an inhibitor of acetylcholinesterase, can be given intravenously to reverse anticholinergic delirium and should be used in severe poisoning. However, the increase in cholinergic tone may be associated with

BOX 11-3

THERAPEUTIC AGENTS ASSOCIATED WITH DRUG-INTOXICATION DELIRIUM

These drugs are associated with delirium because of their direct effects on the CNS. General classes of compounds are listed, followed by notation in parentheses of appropriate specific important examples. In some cases, multiple compounds appear to present a similar risk (such as antibiotics and anticonvulsants). In others, a specific drug (cimetidine, for example) appears to pose an increased risk relative to other compounds from that class.

- Anticholinergics
  - Procedure premedicants (atropine)
  - Tricyclic antidepressants and related compounds (amitriptyline, maprotiline)
  - Antiemetics (meclizine)
  - Antipsychotics (chlorpromazine)
  - CNS-active antihistamines (diphenhydramine)
  - Antiparkinsonians (benztropine)
  - Cycloplegics and mydriatics (atropine)
  - Proprietary medications (atropine, scopolamine)
- Sedative-hypnotics (any)
  - Barbiturates
  - Ethanol
  - Benzodiazepines
- Nontricyclic antidepressants (any)
- Anticonvulsants (any)
- Antimicrobials (antibiotics, antifungals, etc.)
- Nonanticholinergic antiparkinsonian agents (levodopa [L-dopa])
- Cardiac compounds (digitalis, lidocaine)
- Antihypertensives (beta blockers such as propranolol or methyldopa)
- Cytotoxic drugs (methotrexate, procarbazine)
- H_2 antagonists (cimetidine)
- Lithium
- Narcotics (meperidine)
- Nonsteroidal antiinflammatory drugs
- Acetaminophen
- Corticosteroids
- Bismuth compounds

side effects that can be severe (such as bradycardia). Physostigmine also has a short half-life, so it should be used judiciously. Anticholinergic drugs have been used to induce delirium in experimental settings, and the apparent importance of cholinergic mechanisms in cognition suggests a more general role for this system in the etiology of delirium. Just before the onset of delirium, the patient described in Case 11-1 received a relatively typical dose of the anticholinergic drug oxybutynin to facilitate bladder emptying. Although this drug is a potent antimuscarinic agent with occasional CNS side effects, delirium appears to be a relatively uncommon problem. Despite the appearance of delirium shortly after the administration of oxybutynin, the drug probably had little to do with the disorder in Mr. S.

Drugs with sedative-hypnotic properties are associated with delirium. Medications of this class, including alcohol, are associated with intoxication, which has symptoms that overlap with delirium. Severe intoxication that is persistent and associated with the need for extensive evaluation and treatment is indicative of delirium. Historically, bromide compounds were associated with a severe and prolonged delirium; these compounds are rarely used at present. Barbiturates are associated with delirium, but indications for the use of drugs from this class have narrowed considerably over the years. Barbiturate-induced delirium may be as likely from illicit use as from therapeutic administration. The benzodiazepines have replaced the barbiturates for many indications and are probably less likely to be the sole agent inducing delirium. The sedative and amnestic effects of the benzodiazepines may contribute to delirium in patients with multiple causes of delirium. For example, benzodiazepines have been implicated as a risk factor for postoperative delirium. Other sedative hypnotics (for example, chloral hydrate) are associated with intoxication delirium. These compounds, like the barbiturates, are probably more likely to cause delirium than the benzodiazepines. The most commonly used drug with sedative properties is ethanol; alcohol intoxication is associated with delirium.

The patient described in Case 11-1 required large doses of a short-acting benzodiazepine in the immediate postoperative period, which, although indicated, may have contributed to the patient's delirium. As the patient's illness persisted, he was switched from benzodiazepines with a long half-life and active metabolites (diazepam and chlordiazepoxide) to benzodiazepines with a shorter half-life and essentially no active metabolites (lorazepam) to minimize the risk of exacerbating his condition. Finally, the benzodiazepines were discontinued when a diagnosis of hepatic encephalopathy was suspected, terminating any possible contribution to the delirium by these compounds. It is probable that withdrawal (see p. 178) from sedative-hypnotic drugs is a more important cause of delirium than sedative-hypnotic intoxication.

Opioids administered in the recovery room may have exacerbated delirium in Mr. S. Meperidine is the opioid most commonly associated with delirium. This old observation is strongly supported by recent work indicating that meperidine is a risk factor for postoperative delirium, unlike other opioid compounds. Perhaps the anticholinergic properties of the meperidine metabolite, normeperidine, are responsible for delirium. Since other opioids may cause delirium, it is prudent to consider as a possible cause any opioid administered to a patient who develops delirium. The suspicion that meperidine played a role in the induction of delirium in Case 11-1 is heightened by the observation that the doses employed are at least twofold to threefold greater than usually effective doses. Premedication with fentanyl is unlikely to have played a role in the induction of delirium in Mr. S. because the drug was used once at a typical dose. Supplementation of opioid analgesia with other approaches (such as acetaminophen or nonsteroidal analgesics) may reduce the risk of opioid delirium.

Multiple other classes of drugs have been implicated in the etiology of delirium (Boxes 11-3, 11-4, and 11-5). The association of delirium with many therapeutic drugs is based on a single case, several case reports, or small case series. Information about symptomatology in these reports tends to be poor, and in some cases systemic drug effects (for example, hyponatremia) may account for delirium rather than direct intoxication. Polypharmacy may be a risk factor for delirium, although the risk may be confounded by concurrent medical illnesses that initiated the polypharmacy. A physician suspecting that a drug is involved in the cause of delirium should consider an estimate of the likelihood that a drug has CNS effects. CNS-active drugs (for example, nontricyclic antidepressants) are probably more likely culprits in the cause of delirium than compounds with little or no known CNS effects (most antibiotics, for example). Nevertheless, it is prudent consider every drug administered to a patient who is delirious as a plausible cause. Mr. S. in Case 11-1 received vancomycin, an antibiotic, and ephedrine, a sympathomimetic. Both compounds, particularly the antibiotic, are somewhat unusual causes of delirium, and although the route of administration would favor effects on the brain, they were used at usual doses on a single occasion. It is unlikely that either vancomycin or ephedrine played a role in the observed delirium.

Illicitly used drugs can cause delirium (see Box 11-4); many of these compounds also have therapeutic applications. Knowledge that the individual under con-

BOX 11-4

ILLEGALLY USED SUBSTANCES ASSOCIATED WITH DRUG-INTOXICATION DELIRIUM

Compounds are listed by class. Some compounds (such as marijuana) may rarely be associated with delirium, whereas others (for example, inhalants) are probably often associated with delirium.

- Amphetamines and related drugs
- Cocaine
- Hallucinogens (such as lysergic acid diethylamide [LSD])
- Inhalants
- Marijuana and related drugs
- Opioids
- Phencyclidine and related drugs
- Sedative-hypnotics (including ethanol)

sideration has a history of illicit drug or alcohol use should suggest strong consideration of illicit drugs as causative of delirium. Finally, some compounds that cause delirium are poisons (see Box 11-5). Detecting delirium from these compounds may require specialized evaluation.

Delirium tremens represents the classic drug-withdrawal delirium. Similar withdrawal deliria have been described for withdrawal from various sedative-hypnotics. Although the benzodiazepines are less likely to be associated with severe withdrawal than other compounds, withdrawal delirium has been reported. Although extremely rare, withdrawal delirium has been described for drugs from other classes of therapeutic compounds. Mr. S. was known to be a heavy drinker, and when he was carefully interviewed it was shown that he fulfilled criteria for alcohol dependence. No alcohol had been consumed by this person in the 24 hours before the onset of delirium, which is somewhat different from the more usual appearance of delirium tremens 72 to 96 hours after the last drink. The rapid onset of delirium in this patient is suggestive of the involvement of other factors in its onset, although alcohol withdrawal was probably the most important aspect of the first phase of the delirium described in Case 11-1. Patients who develop delirium tremens often have other complicating conditions (for example, malnutrition or infection) and need to be thoroughly evaluated for other causes of delirium. Delirium tremens rarely lasts more than 10 days, and when the patient's symptoms of delirium persisted beyond this period, further diagnostic evaluation was performed. Mr. S. developed hepatic encephalopathy, probably during the course of delirium tremens.

So many medical conditions are associated with delirium that it is beyond the scope of this chapter to detail most of them. Types of a disorder are mentioned in Table 11-2. The signs and symptoms of each disorder are better described in other sources. Sometimes, particularly in the elderly, medical disorders co-exist with delirium, with little information from the history or physical examination to provide guidance regarding the cause. Laboratory evaluation may be crucial, and even if a particular cause is clear, it may suggest unsuspected difficulties (such as electrolyte imbalance or drug use). Laboratory tests and procedures to evaluate delirium are listed in Box 11-6 in an order that roughly reflects the complexity, invasiveness, and usefulness of the test. The history and physical examination should suggest a more specific approach, although some patients (most notably the elderly) present their problems in a fashion that merits systematic consideration, including possibly an EEG.

Metabolic encephalopathies such as hepatic encephalopathy are the most important single type of general medical disorder associated with delirium (see Table 11-2). Unfortunately, the term *encephalopathy* has been used in various ways, although many neurologists appear to apply the term in a fashion that is similar to the use of *delirium*. The term *metabolic encephalopathy* is used here to describe delirium resulting from the disruption of the internal milieu caused by the failure of usual compensatory mechanisms. En-

BOX 11-5

POISONS ASSOCIATED WITH DRUG-INTOXICATION DELIRIUM

Classes of toxin are listed and followed by representative examples, when appropriate. Exposure may be accidental (snake or spider venom), occupational (carbon tetrachloride) or the result of intentional poisoning (arsenic). In some cases (organic solvents, refrigerants) exposure may be accidental or part of a pattern of abuse.

- Organic solvents
  - Aliphatic hydrocarbons (propane)
  - Aromatic hydrocarbons (benzene)
  - Halogenated hydrocarbons (carbon tetrachloride)
  - Alcohols (ethylene glycol, methanol)
  - Gasoline and kerosene
- Carbon monoxide
- Carbon disulfide
- Hydrogen sulfide
- Refrigerants (Freon)
- Metals (arsenic, mercury, and lead)
- Organophosphate insecticides
- Biological poisons
  - Animals (snake or spider venom)
  - Plants (jimsonweed, morning glory)
  - Mushrooms (Amanita species)

cephalopathy encompasses organ failure, such as occurs in hepatic encephalopathy as well as vitamin deficiencies, such as the lack of thiamine that is thought to underlie Wernicke's encephalopathy. For largely historical reasons, infection and disturbances of fluids and electrolytes are usually not considered metabolic encephalopathies. Intracranial processes, infection, and possibly fluid and electrolyte disturbances are sufficiently common and require a sufficiently distinct diagnostic process; therefore these classes of etiological factors should be considered separately.

Metabolic encephalopathies are systemic disorders. Failure of vital organs such as the liver, heart, kidney, and lung is associated with delirium; acute failure may rapidly progress to coma and death. Disorders of endocrine organs such as the pancreas and the thyroid are also associated with delirium. The thyroid and pancreas are interesting because too much activity produces symptoms (such as hyperthyroidism or hypoglycemia from an insulinoma) as well as too little activity (for example, hypothyroidism or diabetes mellitus). Cancer of various kinds can cause delirium through multiple systemic effects, although hypercalcemia is one common mechanism. The systemic effects of cancer, which are potentially correctable, should be distinguished from the possibility of metastasis to the brain. In many instances (including hypercapnia and hypercalcemia) it appears that the rapidity with which changes occur is a factor in the development of delirium. The patient who is chronically hypercapnic may tolerate higher levels of CO_2 than the person who develops acute changes.

It is particularly important to distinguish the failure of homeostatic mechanisms, such as that which occurs in hepatic encephalopathy, from the toxicity of drugs used to treat problems caused by the failing organ. For example, efforts were made to minimize drug toxicity in Case 11-1, attempting to separate the effects of benzodiazepines and neuroleptics from symptoms caused by alcohol withdrawal and hepatic encephalopathy. The clinical decision to employ neuroleptics (such as haloperidol) rather than benzodiazepines was made on the presumption that neuroleptics would be less toxic to the CNS than benzodiazepines. The longitudinal course of the patient's illness suggested the possibility of hepatic encephalopathy in addition to delirium tremens; the best available laboratory test for hepatic encephalopathy, a measurement of ammonia levels, supported the diagnosis. Although no signs of Wernicke's encephalopathy were observed in this patient, thiamine supplementation (initially parenteral) was provided to treat this disorder and minimize the risk of Korsakoff's syndrome (see the section on amnestic disorders).

Disturbances of fluid (such as dehydration and water intoxication) and electrolytes (for example, increases or decreases in serum sodium or potassium) have been treated separately from the metabolic encephalopathies in many descriptions of delirium. The ability of patients who are medically ill or elderly to regulate water and electrolyte balance is often impaired. Several prospective studies have identified elevations in BUN, largely reflecting dehydration, to be a predictor of delirium. In many cases, problems with fluids and electrolytes arise from or are exacerbated by medication administration, particularly diuretics. Disturbances of fluid and electrolytes are to some extent iatrogenic complications of drug administration. For example, a physician's awareness that medications such as diuretics can cause delirium via hyponatremia, should lead to systematic evaluation of fluid and electrolyte status in patients who are at risk. Drugs such as lithium and the TCAs, which are associated with delirium via direct CNS effects, can cause systemic fluid and electrolyte disorders. Disturbances of fluids and electrolytes may be more commonly associated with delirium from multiple causes rather than being the sole causes of delirium.

Infection is often associated with delirium, particularly in the elderly. Fever and delirium have been historically associated. Delirium may be the sign of an infection and precede the onset of fever, or delirium may appear at the height of the fever. In some instances, delirium may appear after the fever has resolved. The observation that many elderly people may have an infectious delirium without fever suggests that

BOX 11-6

LABORATORY EVALUATION

- Electrolytes
- CBC, particularly white blood cell count
- Glucose
- Blood urea nitrogen (BUN)/creatinine
- Electrocardiogram (ECG)
- Urinalysis (urine culture)
- Chest x-ray (sputum culture)
- Drug toxicology screen/drug levels
- SGOT/SGPT/LDH, bilirubin, total protein/albumin, ammonia level
- Calcium
- Head scan
- Arterial blood gases
- Venereal Disease Research Laboratory (VDRL)/rapid plasma reagin (RPR), human immunodeficiency virus (HIV)
- Blood cultures
- Thyroid tests
- B_{12}/folate
- EEG
- Lumbar puncture

an infection can produce delirium in the absence of fever. Further consideration was given to infectious disease without a fever as a cause for delirium in Case 11-1 when the delirium did not resolve as expected. Some evidence suggests that host susceptibility plays a role in the likelihood that delirium will develop after an infection.

Infections associated with delirium involve numerous organs and various microorganisms. The brain is considered separately because it seems reasonable that the systemic effects of infection, such as those that produce fever, are distinct from the effects of direct involvement of the brain (see below). The numerous types of infectious disease that can cause delirium cannot be adequately considered here, but some general guidance based on available literature can be provided. Given the increased risk of delirium from afebrile infection in the elderly, infection of commonly affected organs (such as the lungs or bladder) should be given priority consideration at presentation. Clear signs of systemic toxicity from a bacteremia should be addressed with cultures, treatment, and consideration of the source.

Infections of the nervous system cause delirium. Viruses such as herpes simplex and influenza cause an encephalitis that is associated with delirium; distinguishing the systemic effects of influenza from the direct effects of the virus on the brain may be difficult. Acquired immunodeficiency syndrome (AIDS) causes a dementia that may be preceded by delirium; equally important, the immunocompromised status of these patients predisposes them to other intracranial infectious processes such as cytomegalovirus encephalitis, cryptococcosis, and *Toxoplasma gondii* infection. Delirium is probably a sufficiently unusual symptom of AIDS dementia that consideration of other intracranial processes, such as the noted infections, is wise. Delirium has been associated with various types of meningitis, most notably the pneumococcal and tuberculous types. Bacteria can cause an abscess, which may be seen with delirium and is probably the result of processes similar to other intracranial masses. The presence of infection outside the CNS, particularly in areas of the head near the brain (such as the sinuses or the ear), suggests the diagnosis of abscess. Neurosyphilis can have the symptom of delirium. Various fungal and parasitic conditions may feature delirium as an important aspect of the course. Finally, some individuals develop a postinfectious encephalomyelitis after an infectious illness (usually viral) or after immunization. Delirium is an important part of the course of this illness and is thought to be the result of cell-mediated immunity.

Other intracranial processes are associated with delirium. These heterogeneous disorders represent direct insults to the brain, with acute global impairment as one possible result. Mass lesions, either benign (subdural hematoma) or cancerous (glioblastoma) may have delirium as a presenting symptom. Although bladder cancer usually spreads locally, the unusual presentation and course in Case 11-1 suggested consideration of metastases to the head; an imaging study was obtained despite the minimal evidence of other neurological signs.

Head trauma is commonly associated with delirium. The typical case of head trauma involves a young adult who has been drinking ethanol and is subsequently involved in an accident, suggesting a multifactorial cause for many cases of delirium from head trauma. Loss of consciousness is often followed by delirium. Finally, head trauma can be associated with multiple other injuries, some of which have systemic effects that can cause delirium. The immobility necessary to manage many orthopedic injuries aggravates the course and management of the delirium associated with head trauma.

Epilepsy is associated with delirium, either as an ictal phenomenon, a postictal phenomenon, or an interictal phenomenon. Ictal deliria are associated with generalized absence (petit mal) status and complex partial status, situations that constitute medical emergencies. Postictal and interictal deliria must be distinguished from the toxicity of anticonvulsants.

Several pathological processes involving the vasculature of the CNS are associated with delirium. Infarction, embolism, and hemorrhage can cause delirium. Hypertensive encephalopathy and, less commonly, migraine are associated with delirium. Inflammation and necrosis of CNS vasculature occurs in several vasculitides, most notably systemic lupus erythematosus, and can produce a delirium. All these disorders appear to cause delirium as a direct consequence of CNS involvement.

Inspection of Table 11-2 suggests that the most important cause of delirium is multifactorial. This observation should not be surprising, since serious medical illness predisposes a patient to delirium. Furthermore, the patient series with the largest portion of delirium caused by multiple factors is composed of elderly patients who were admitted to a general medical ward, suggesting that age is also a risk factor for delirium from multiple factors. Dementia and other types of preexisting CNS pathologic conditions are thought to predispose a patient to delirium. It seems reasonable to suspect polypharmacy as a risk factor for multifactorial delirium, although underlying medical illnesses may explain much of the increased risk. Regardless of risk factors, many deliria are the result of more than one etiological factor.

One type of typically multifactorial delirium, that

which occurs after surgery, is particularly interesting since delirium may be the first manifestation of complications. Delirium has been associated with virtually every type of medical procedure. Cardiovascular surgery, particularly postcardiotomy, is a risk factor for the development of delirium. Independent of surgical repair, fractures seem to be a risk factor for delirium, particularly in the elderly. Similarly, burns may predispose a patient to a multifactorial type of delirium. The onset of agitated postoperative delirium in the recovery room, as occurred with Mr. S of Case 11-1, is thought to develop in about 2% of surgical cases. Other patients become delirious in the days after the procedure. Risk factors associated with delirium after elective surgery include poor preoperative cognitive status, poor preoperative function, and abnormal preoperative serum sodium, potassium, or glucose. The risk associated with abnormal preoperative laboratory test results is particularly important since corrective action before surgery may diminish the risk of delirium. Preoperative evaluation of electrolytes should be part of the preparation for invasive procedures. Drugs associated with an increased risk of postsurgical delirium include ethanol, benzodiazepines, and meperidine; other narcotics are not so clearly associated with increased risk of delirium. Consideration should be given to a period of abstinence or perhaps even specific treatment when elective surgery is planned for a patient suffering from drug or alcohol problems. Mr. S. apparently represents an example of a delirium caused by multiple factors, with onset in the immediate postoperative period.

Not all cases of delirium have an identifiable cause. Although the rate at which delirium occurs is unknown, it should not be surprising, given the enormous number of possible causes, that it is not always possible to identify the etiological agent or agents with certainty during a brief episode of delirium. The diagnosis of delirium NOS is appropriate in these rare circumstances. This designation may be appropriate for deliria thought to arise from sensory deprivation. Although sensory deprivation may predispose an individual to delirium, attributing delirium to sensory deprivation as the sole etiological agent is controversial. If phenomena such as sensory deprivation, immobilization, and sleep deprivation cause delirium, they probably do so in patients who are already at risk, such as the elderly, patients with dementia, and patients who have suffered an insult to the CNS.

Natural History

The natural history of delirium is poorly understood, in part because the syndrome has received many different labels in the past and in part because the disorder is underrecognized. Delirium may be the presenting manifestation of numerous disorders, as exemplified by the onset of hepatic encephalopathy in Case 11-1. Although its onset is acute, by definition and according to current literature, initial symptoms of mild delirium can be subtle. An insidious onset appears possible when symptoms are present most prominently at night. Furthermore, the fluctuating course of delirium may allow a patient to appear relatively normal during a single interview. Careful review of charting by other physicians and hospital staff is a necessary component of the evaluation for delirium.

Some types of delirium are limited in duration. For example, delirium tremens has a relatively typical onset and duration. Postoperative delirium that occurs outside of the recovery suite is said to be often preceded by a lucid interval of 1 or 2 days. In both cases the duration of delirium is typically 4 to 7 days, with more complicated and severe cases lasting slightly longer.

Death can be a result of delirium. Studies of delirium have demonstrated that death occurs more often in patients who are delirious than in matched controls, although the portion of cases with this outcome varies remarkably from series to series. Presumably the risk of death is largely attributable to the risk associated with the severity of the causative illness (or illnesses). Similarly, dementia is said to be an outcome of delirium. The process that converts delirium into dementia is unknown. Chronic exposure to organic solvents appears to produce an irreversible syndrome of cognitive impairment, suggesting that sustained exposure to a noxious agent is one pathway from delirium to dementia. Dementia is usually associated with neuronal loss; perhaps prolonged deliria produce dementia through cell death. Additional cell death would explain the irreversible deficits that are thought to occur when delirium is superimposed on dementia. Finally, the process by which Wernicke's encephalopathy (a form of delirium) merges into Korsakoff's syndrome (a type of amnestic disorder) is unknown. What is unequivocal is the observation that patients who are delirious have more complicated courses, longer hospital stays, and poorer outcomes than matched patients without delirium.

Differential Diagnosis

The key issue in the diagnosis of delirium is recognition. Distinguishing the disorder from other psychiatric disorders is relatively straightforward once consideration is given to delirium. Physicians who care for patients in hospitals who are acutely ill should recognize that at least 1 of 10 patients (higher in the elderly) is delirious at some point during hospitalization. Questions about memory and orientation should be incorporated into the examination of all patients (see

Box 11-2). The clinician doing a chart review should consider the possibility of delirium by looking for signs of a fluctuating course and altered consciousness. Finally, appearance of complications such as infection should immediately alert the physician to the possibility of delirium and stimulate an examination that considers signs of delirium and a search for additional causes of delirium. The payoff for the patient and the doctor is a less complicated course of illness and possibly a reduced length of stay. Appropriate recognition and treatment of delirium is good medical practice, even in terminally ill patients, if the management of symptoms results in an amelioration of symptoms (for example, hallucinations).

Delirium can be readily distinguished from dementia, although both may occur concurrently (Table 11-3). The most important distinction is the acuteness of onset. Rapid deterioration (hours to days) in the mental functioning of any patient, regardless of prior cognitive status, should suggest delirium. Fluctuation in the course of dementia is possible but is rarely as dramatic as is typical of delirium. Patients who are demented should have a clear consciousness. Hallucinations at the time of presentation are probably unusual in dementia. Patients who are delirious are more likely to have disorganized thought than the impoverished thought seen in dementia. Current diagnostic criteria for dementia emphasize neurological signs such as apraxias and agnosias; these are presumably rare signs during delirium in the absence of another CNS process associated with these findings.

Depression and mania rarely present with a picture typical of delirium. Nevertheless, one series notes a substantial number of patients with a psychiatric disorder who had signs and symptoms suggestive of delirium (see Table 11-2). The distinction between delirium and mood disorder is made by ascertaining the presence of sufficient symptoms of depression or mania to meet criteria for an affective episode. A prior history of affective illness supports the diagnosis of mood disorder. Distinguishing delirium from schizophrenia and schizophrenia-like illnesses is performed similarly. Catatonia is associated with affective disorders, schizophrenia, or delirium; a careful history, physical examination, and laboratory evaluation will suggest the underlying disorder. As is the case with dementia, delirium can be superimposed on any other psychiatric condition. Acute onset and a rapidly fluctuating course of cognitive impairment strongly suggest the presence of delirium; hopefully the simplified criteria of DSM-IV will facilitate recognition.

Genetics and Family History

Delirium is the psychiatric disorder most clearly caused by extrinsic influences and as such has been little studied from a family-history perspective. Studying the effects of experimental infection on the performance of healthy volunteers suggests that individual variation in cognitive impairment is large, even in the face of clinically similar infections. This observation suggests a limited role for intrinsic, possibly genetic, factors in the risk of developing delirium. Other risk factors, such as severe medical illness, presence of known brain disease, age, and possibly polypharmacy seem more important than any genetic contribution.

Epidemiology

Delirium is a common psychiatric disorder among patients who are medically ill. Accurate estimates are difficult to obtain and sensitive to patient referral sources in addition to the variable presence in any clinical sample of the risk factors mentioned above. A reasonable estimate is that about 10% to 15% of inpatients who are medically ill suffer from delirium; this

TABLE 11-3

CLINICAL FEATURES THAT DISTINGUISH DELIRIUM FROM DEMENTIA

Feature	Delirium	Dementia
Onset	Acute: hours to days	Insidious: months to a year or more
Course	Fluctuating, generally lasts days to weeks	Chronic with stable or, in the case of presumptive dementia of the Alzheimer's type, gradually worsening function
Consciousness	Decreased awareness and alertness, sometimes with stupor	Usually clear
Perception	Hallucinations, typically visual, often part of the syndrome	Hallucinations, typically visual, and delusions often a feature of midphase dementia of the Alzheimer's type and may be absent in others
Thought	Disorganized	Impoverished

The features are arranged in order of importance. None of these items unequivocally distinguishes dementia from delirium. Furthermore, since dementia appears to be a risk factor for delirium, patients may have features of delirium and dementia.

estimate is increased to 15% to 20% if the patient population is over age 65. Postoperative delirium occurs at a similar rate, excepting patients who undergo open heart surgery, in whom the incidence of delirium is likely to be doubled. Only about 1 in 10 patients suffering from delirium is likely to receive the diagnosis.

Pathophysiology

The final common pathway that produces the cognitive impairment characteristic of delirium is unknown. Signs and symptoms of delirium are sufficiently characteristic that a common pathway presumably exists. The disturbance of consciousness that has been so difficult to define, at least historically, is relatively uncommon in many other neuropsychiatric disorders. Any pathophysiological mechanism should be sufficiently general to apply to most cases of delirium, regardless of cause. A theory of delirium must also accommodate the vulnerability conferred by age, dementia, other types of structural brain disease, systemic illness, and polypharmacy. An adequate pathophysiological understanding of delirium is likely to illuminate the understanding of mental mechanisms relevant to phenomena such as consciousness and hallucinations. A review of current hypotheses about pathophysiological mechanisms of delirium provides a helpful framework for considering the disorder. Theories can be described as fitting into the following four general and not mutually exclusive categories: (1) disturbance of cortical metabolism, (2) disturbances of electrical excitability, (3) dysfunction in a neurotransmitter system or systems, and (4) neurohumoral hypotheses.

One of the oldest hypotheses is that delirium represents cerebral insufficiency because of a generalized lack of a critical CNS metabolic need. This notion is derived from the observation that delirium is associated with a decrease in brain electrical activity, reflected in the appearance of slow waves (delta and theta) in the EEG. Furthermore, deficits in the availability of critical cerebral metabolites—O_2 in hypoxia and glucose in hypoglycemia—are known to be associated with delirium. Oxygen and glucose are critical to the function of all neurons, an attractive aspect to a theory that would explain the global dysfunction of delirium. Functional imaging studies, such as positron emission tomography (PET) and single photon emission computed tomography (SPECT), of patients suffering from chronic exposure to organic solvents suggest global decreases in cerebral metabolism that are particularly striking in the frontal and temporal lobes. These findings were generally not associated with structural lesions as detected by typical static imaging methods (CT and magnetic resonance imaging [MRI]). Unfortunately, it is unclear to what extent these findings generalize to the acute pathology of delirium, as well as to other causes of delirium. Specific facets of delirium, such as disorientation and visual hallucinations, would presumably reflect the relatively greater sensitivity of neurons associated with these cognitive impairments to deprivation of critical metabolic needs than other nerve cells.

The function of the nervous system is dependent on the ability of nerve cells to generate and efficiently transmit electrical signals. Neurons have the capacity to rapidly move ions in and out of the cell, generating action potentials, a process that is sensitive to the ionic milieu. Alterations in fluid and electrolyte status disrupt this process and are clearly causes of delirium, whether because of a decrease (for example, hyponatremia or hypoosmolality) or because of an increase (such as in hypernatremia or hyperosmolality). Disturbances of critical metabolic needs, such as those that occur in decreased cerebral blood flow, hypoxia, or hypoglycemia, would affect ionic transmission indirectly by impairing the ability of nerve cells to appropriately pump ions. As would have to be the case with the hypothesis that delirium is caused by a decrement in critical metabolic components, certain populations of nerve cells would presumably be more sensitive to ionic disturbance than others.

The hypothesis that dysfunction of a specific population of neurons causes the symptoms of delirium is attractive when considering the role of a particular neurotransmitter system in delirium. Involvement of the CNS cholinergic system in delirium is an especially robust concept. Antimuscarinic drugs and drugs with antimuscarinic properties are known and common causes of delirium. Furthermore, overcoming cholinergic blockage by treating patients with the acetylcholinesterase inhibitor physostigmine reverses the symptoms of delirium, at least temporarily. Numerous lines of evidence implicate the cholinergic system in memory impairment, a key aspect of delirium. However, the specificity of the cholinergic hypothesis to delirium is open to question. Physostigmine may reverse delirium when it appears in situations that are not the result of obvious anticholinergic effects. Equally important, cholinergic mechanisms have been implicated in dementia, particularly in dementia of the Alzheimer's type (DAT). Although this may explain the somewhat similar defects in memory noted for delirium and dementia, it is unclear how cholinergic mechanisms can cause the acute change of consciousness seen in delirium yet not cause similar symptoms in dementia.

Various other neurotransmitter systems have been implicated in delirium. The signs of autonomic instability characteristic of delirium tremens and some other deliria suggest the involvement of central catecholaminergic neurons in delirium. Sedative hypnotics, such as ethanol, appear to exert CNS effect partly through the γ-aminobutyric $acid_A$ ($GABA_A$) receptor; some evidence in animals suggests dysregulation of receptor expression during withdrawal. Hypotheses to explain the CNS dysfunction seen in hepatic encephalopathy invoke dysregulation of GABAergic and glutamatergic systems. The GABAergic and glutamatergic systems are widely distributed yet appear to have regional specificity by virtue of subtype-specific receptor expression. It may be possible to study the role of the various neurotransmitter systems in delirium by employing system-specific ligands in functional imaging studies.

Neurohumoral hypotheses of delirium have been advanced. The notion that stress facilitates the appearance of delirium suggests involvement of stress hormones, such as corticosteroids. Whereas stress from sleep deprivation, immobility, and extreme alteration of the sensory environment (either overload or deprivation) may predispose to delirium, it appears unlikely that these factors are sole etiological agents. Equally important, treatment with corticosteroids is not always associated with a psychiatric disorder. Corticosteroids are probably as likely to cause mania or depression as delirium. A corticosteroid hypothesis is interesting because of the capacity of this and other hormones (and perhaps vitamins such as thiamine) to exert an effect on most neurons, resulting in global dysfunction. The relatively greater impact of a hormone on specific populations of neurons would account for specific symptoms (for example, impaired consciousness).

These hypotheses are not mutually exclusive. For example, it is possible to imagine that cholinergic neurons are more sensitive to metabolic deprivation, ionic disturbance, and neurohumoral factors than serotoninergic neurons. Furthermore, acute disruption of the function of cholinergic neurons could disturb consciousness through an effect mediated by the reticular system, producing dysfunction of many other nerve cells because cholinergic cells have a wide distribution in the brain. The point to this line of reasoning is merely to illustrate the concept that the hypotheses outlined above do not necessarily exclude each other. However, an approach to the pathophysiology of delirium such as outlined here produces hypotheses that are testable at the systems, cellular, and molecular levels.

Management and Treatment

Establishing the cause of delirium is the most critical aspect of treatment, since treatment of the causative disorders usually reverses most symptoms of delirium. The treatment of the numerous disorders listed on pp. 175-181 and in Table 11-2 constitutes much of the practice of medicine and involves topics beyond the scope of this chapter; physicians should review the treatment of various medical disorders for interventions specific to a cause of delirium. As Case 11-1 and the list of causes illustrate (see Table 11-2), the existence of delirium in many patients involves multiple possible causes.

General observations about the process of evaluation provide guidance for treatment. The history and physical examination are the starting point for most diagnoses and are thus critical to the etiology of delirium. A systematic approach to laboratory tests guided by the history and physical examination is appropriate (see Box 11-6). Laboratory tests may be critical for the patient who is incoherent or obtunded and without readily available collateral sources. Consultants may be helpful in sorting out etiology, particularly for the individual with multiple possible causes. Patients who abuse alcohol or drugs and patients with malnutrition should receive parenteral vitamins, particularly thiamine, to prevent delirium caused by vitamin deficiency, such as Wernicke's encephalopathy.

The section describing the role that drugs play in delirium suggests an approach to considering the role each compound plays in a case of delirium (Figure 11-1). Drugs should be discontinued if the indication is uncertain or the repercussions of discontinuation are minimal. Doses, in conjunction with appropriate drug levels, should be carefully considered for pharmacological agents deemed necessary and should be lowered if at all possible. Many times another agent with a lower risk of inducing delirium or a nonpharmacological treatment may be substituted. If a single agent is deemed to be the probable cause of delirium, cessation of administration is likely to be followed by relatively rapid improvement, although exceptions are known (for example, lithium and bromide compounds). Observation of improvement supports the hypothesis that the selected drug was the cause. Given that serious medical illness is a risk factor for delirium, the more typical approach to consideration of drug intoxication is to make multiple changes in a regimen that involves many compounds.

Identification of individuals who are at risk for delirium facilitates a preventive approach. Several studies have considered risk factors as indicators for preventive measures. Although these preventive intervention studies lack the rigor of double-blind placebo-controlled studies, they demonstrate an improved outcome, particularly a reduction in length of stay and number of complications. Anticipation of delirium, especially in elderly patients undergoing elective surgery, and aggressively managing risk factors such as hypoxemia and concurrent medications seem to be prudent even in the absence of controlled studies.

An important aspect of delirium management is manipulation of the patient's environment to enhance

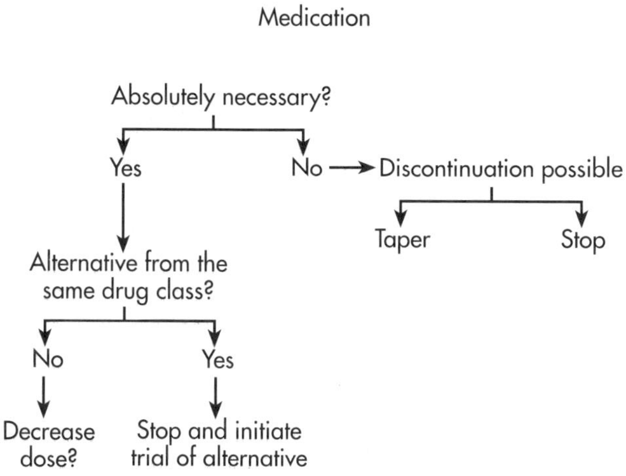

FIGURE 11-1 Managing possible drug intoxication delirium. Evaluation of many critical drugs (for example, digoxin) can be difficult, since the condition for which the compound is indicated (such as congestive heart failure) may also be associated with delirium. Determining drug levels may be helpful under these circumstances. Measuring drug concentrations can also be useful if elevations in drug level are clearly associated with delirium (for example, carbamazepine, TCAs). In some cases, indications for "absolutely necessary" drugs may be unclear and diagnostic evaluation may suggest that a drug can be discontinued. Initiation of trials with alternatives should give some consideration to the half-lives of both compounds, since the alternative also poses some risk of inducing delirium and concurrent administration of both drugs would presumably increase the risk. Discontinuation by tapering may be useful for drugs associated with withdrawal symptoms (such as sedative-hypnotics) and permit the selection of a lower, presumably more appropriate, dose at which delirium is not a problem. Application of the algorithm in cases of polypharmacy (probably the typical situation) is best accomplished if drugs are considered from most important to least important.

cognitive status. Many of these interventions date to antiquity. The physician can readily conceptualize these interventions as part of good nursing care. Sensory stimulation is modulated to match the patient's apparent state of awareness and, if possible, expressed wishes. Patients who are lethargic are provided with modest amounts of sensory stimulus, and patients who are hyperactive are placed in an environment that minimizes stimulation. The hospital routine is modified to emphasize daytime activity and nighttime sleep. Explanations of events as they unfold are provided (typically repeatedly) in a direct and simple fashion. Family members are involved in reassuring the patient and making the environment more like home. Finally, the use of restraints is minimized and targeted to the situation. Nevertheless, the need to protect the integrity of life-sustaining medical devices (such as endotracheal tubes and central lines) necessitates the use of restraints, as do life-threatening behaviors directed toward others (assaultive behavior towards staff) and self (for example, a suicide attempt or wandering away). Although good nursing management is critical to the care of delirious patients, effects on course are modest at best.

Antipsychotic medication plays a role in the management of delirium. Many patients suffer from hallucinations, and some have delusions that impair the patient's understanding. Because the experiences are real to the patient, they can lead to dangerous behavior. The compounds from this class of drugs also have sedative properties that are likely to contribute to effectiveness. Haloperidol is the drug of choice because it has minimal anticholinergic (and thereby presumably deliriogenic) and cardiovascular effects. The medication can be given intravenously (a common method, although it is not a route of administration that has been approved by the Food and Drug Administration [FDA]), intramuscularly, or orally. Therapy may be initiated parenterally with modest doses (0.5 to 5 mg), and as the patient is stabilized administration may be switched to the oral route. As the patient's mental status improves, the drug is tapered and discontinued. Much larger doses can be employed if the clinical situation poses sufficient risk to the patient. Haloperidol is associated with various neuromuscular syndromes, the most important during short-term use being an acute dystonia or dystonias. Other antipsychotic compounds may be useful, as Case 11-1 illustrates, although the risks of serious medical problems, particularly cardiovascular problems, and exacerbation of delirium are probably increased.

Benzodiazepines are the drug of choice for sedative-hypnotic withdrawal delirium, including delirium tremens. Members of this class of compounds may also be useful adjuncts to pharmacotherapy with haloperidol, presumably by potentiating the sedative properties of haloperidol. Lorazepam is the agent of choice because it is effective when administered via various routes (intravenously, intramuscularly, and orally), thus facilitating emergency management and permitting the switch to an oral formulation for subsequent treatment. The drug does not have any active metabolites and has a modest half-life, which minimizes accumulation of active drug yet provides coverage for a number of hours. Other commonly used short-acting benzodiazepines include midazolam and oxazepam. Drawbacks of the benzodiazepines include amnestic effects, which probably contribute to the propensity of these compounds to cause delirium. The benzodiazepines also cause ataxia and can be oversedating. Acute benzodiazepine toxicity is reversible with flumazenil. However, since this drug with a short half-life induces withdrawal and causes seizures (at higher doses), its use should be reserved for emergent toxicity. Chlordiazepoxide, a long-acting compound, is used in sedative-hypnotic withdrawal because the long half-life facilitates management by titration to the desired effect and discontinuation. Cessation of administration is followed by a gradual fall in drug levels, ameliorating the subsequent withdrawal symptoms. This and other long-acting sedative-hypnotics (such as clonazepam and phenobarbital) may be useful in some cases of sedative-hypnotic delirium. However, these compounds are not necessarily more effective; they may have a narrower therapeutic index (barbiturates); and because of drug accumulation, they may be more deliriogenic.

Special Topics

The importance of delirium as a clinical entity has sometimes been diminished. The argument is that delirium is really a proxy for an underlying cause or causes. Addressing the etiological condition (or conditions) presumably makes the presence or absence of delirium a moot point. Unfortunately, the argument ignores the fact that delirium can be the presentation for virtually any condition, particularly in patients who are at risk of delirium. Controlled observation has repeatedly demonstrated that patients who are delirious suffer greater morbidity and probably greater mortality than matched patients without delirium. Physicians should be particularly concerned about the iatrogenic aspects of delirium. Downplaying the importance of delirium reduces the quality of patient care.

Similar arguments about quality of life underlie the suggestion that delirium should be recognized and addressed in the terminally ill. For instance, most patients dying of cancer develop a delirium during their last days. The cause is likely to be multifactorial, since multiple organs fail. The goal of recognition is to provide treatment that is palliative and ameliorates the disturbing hallucinations and delusions, as well as providing more restful sleep.

Psychiatrists are commonly consulted to establish the diagnosis of delirium and advise about management. Other specialists (for example, neurologists, internists, and physicians with various subspecialties) are perhaps more likely to be consulted to evaluate and treat causative disorders. Case 11-1, which involves an obviously complicated patient, exemplifies a coordinated approach to evaluation and treatment. It is reasonable to expect the consulting psychiatrist to examine any hospital-based referral with the diagnosis of delirium in mind. Probably the most common diagnostic issue after failure to consider delirium is the inability of the referring physician to distinguish delirium from other psychiatric disorders. Patients with preexisting psychiatric disorders can be particularly difficult to evaluate. The widespread use of compounds such as haloperidol and lorazepam makes physicians in acute care settings aware that psychotropics can be used to manage delirium. Psychiatrists can be helpful when considering alternative choices, evaluating patients for side effects, and suggesting a reasonable approach to tapering medications.

Psychiatric consultation may be particularly useful when drugs are thought to play an etiological role. Psychotropic drugs are often implicated as causes. Probably the best-studied example is the risk of delirium from TCAs. About 5% of patients hospitalized

PEARLS & PERILS

DELIRIUM

- Delirium afflicts at least 1 in 10 hospitalized patients.
- Most cases of delirium are not recognized.
- Delirium is associated with death, longer hospital stay, and disability.
- Age, dementia, other types of coarse brain disease, severe systemic illness, and dehydration put patients at risk for developing delirium.
- Acute onset and fluctuating course of a disturbance of consciousness strongly suggest the diagnosis of delirium.
- Abnormalities of orientation, memory, language ability, and perception (for example, visual hallucinations) establish the diagnosis.
- Evaluation of drug therapy and current medical conditions suggest diagnostic evaluation to find causes.
- Many patients have multiple possible causes of delirium.
- Treatment of delirium is directed at the cause or causes.
- Patient safety and comfort should be sustained by judicious use of neuroleptics (for example, haloperidol) and benzodiazepines (for example, lorazepam).
- Nursing interventions enhance the quality of patient care.
- Restraints may be required in life-threatening circumstances.
- Individuals with dementia who develop delirium may not return to predelirium cognitive functioning after resolution of delirium.
- Delirium is a common aspect of terminal illnesses.
- Most patients with delirium who are not terminally ill recover.

for psychiatric reasons develop delirium when treated with TCAs. TCA-induced delirium is correlated with drug level, age, and female gender. A psychiatrist is the appropriate consultant to evaluate patients who are delirious and receiving any psychotropic drug, not only to consider the etiological role of the drugs a patient is receiving but also to advise regarding alternative management. During a follow-up visit the physician evaluates the effectiveness of alternative therapies. Patients who experience delirium as the result of illicit drug use may need further psychiatric treatment and should be advised to cease using illicit substances.

In summary, delirium is a common complication of drug treatment (particularly when CNS-active compounds are used) and many medical conditions. Useful criteria exist for establishing the diagnosis. Patients can be systematically evaluated, the diagnosis can be established, and treatment can be initiated in a straightforward fashion (see the Pearls & Perils box on p. 186). Treatment is largely directed at the underlying cause; neuroleptics (such as haloperidol) and benzodiazepines (such as lorazepam) may be an important part of patient management. Prevention and early recognition are likely to diminish morbidity and mortality.

Amnestic Disorders

Amnestic disorders represent cognitive disorders that are largely, if not solely, a disturbance of memory (Box 11-7). As is the case with the more global cognitive disorders of delirium and dementia, amnestic disorders are classified on an etiological basis as either the result of a general medical condition or induced by a specific substance. DSM-IV diagnostic criteria A, B, and C must be met for every case of suspected amnestic disorder. Etiological specification should focus on general medical conditions, since amnestic disorder caused by drugs and toxins independent of malnutrition and apart from intoxication or withdrawal is rare. The clinical description of patients with amnesia over the past 40 years has contributed significantly to the understanding of the mechanisms responsible for memory, providing knowledge useful to clinicians and basic scientists (Table 11-4). Amnestic disorders are important to the primary care physician because the recognition of individuals at risk for amnestic disorders should diminish the probability that they will experience the devastating and often irreversible effects of chronic amnestic disorder. A case report of Korsakoff's syndrome is provided (Case 11-2).

BOX 11-7 AMNESTIC DISORDER

DSM-IV DIAGNOSTIC CRITERIA

A. The development of memory impairment as manifested by impairment in the ability to learn new information or the inability to recall previously learned information.

B. The memory disturbance causes significant impairment in social or occupational functioning and represents a significant decline from a previous level of functioning.

C. The memory disturbance does not occur exclusively during the course of a delirium or a dementia and persists beyond the usual duration of Substance Intoxication or Withdrawal.

Amnestic disorder due to a general medical condition

D. There is evidence from the history, physical examination, or laboratory findings that the disturbance is the direct physiological consequence of a general medical condition (including physical trauma).

Specify if:

Transient: if memory impairment lasts for 1 month or less
Chronic: if memory impairment lasts for more than 1 month

Substance-induced persisting amnestic disorder

D. There is evidence from the history, physical examination, or laboratory findings that the memory disturbance is etiologically related to the persisting effects of substance use (e.g., a drug of abuse, a medication).

Amnestic disorder not otherwise specified

This category should be used to diagnose an amnestic disorder that does not meet criteria for any of the specific types described in this section.

Modified from American Psychiatric Association: *Diagnostic and statistical manual of mental disorders,* ed 4 (DSM-IV), Washington, D.C., 1994, American Psychiatric Press.

DIAGNOSIS

TABLE 11-4
AMNESTIC DISORDER

Discriminating features

1) Difficulty remembering the past, particularly recent events
2) Impaired ability to learn new information
3) Absence of other clinically significant cognitive dysfunction, particularly that seen in delirium and dementia
4) Substantial change from previous function

Consistent features

1) Social or occupational dysfunction of variable severity
2) Clear consciousness
3) Definable cause

Variable features

1) Confabulation
2) Poor insight
3) Bad judgment
4) Inability to perform activities of daily living outside of an institution
5) Disorientation
6) Indifference to memory problems

Diagnosis

Amnestic disorders are characterized by memory failure (see Box 11-7). Patients afflicted with these disorders suffer from an impaired ability to learn new material (anterograde amnesia), as well as a significant deficit in the recall of previously learned information (retrograde amnesia). The ability to remember the distant past, material learned long before the onset of the amnestic disorder, is conserved. The ability to immediately repeat information (such as a digit span) is also preserved. A profound amnesia can produce disorientation to time and place with sustained orientation to person, although this is not an essential feature. Mr. W. in Case 11-2 had impaired recall and an inability to learn new material, although his immediate repetition ability and remote memory were good.

The memory disturbance results in substantial impairment of social and occupational functioning and represents a significant decline from previous status. Severe amnesia can impair the affected individual to the extent that custodial care is required to sustain the activities of daily life. Chronic amnesia is often complicated by an indifference to the memory deficits, although this is a variable feature of the disorder. The potentially profound effects of amnesia on the ability of an affected individual to lead a normal life are the impetus for prevention and recognition. The patient in Case 11-2 required assistance with all activities of daily living because amnesia made it impossible for him to run a household; he lived with his son, who managed his affairs. The patient was unable to return to his job as a laborer; he was indifferent to this turn of events.

Other features of amnestic disorders are not invariant (see Table 11-4) but occur at such a sufficient rate that they are important. Many patients with memory problems respond to questions with incorrect answers as the result of mixing remembered events that occurred at different times, of using completely fabricated material, or a mixture of both. It may be difficult to discern that this is occurring without reliable collateral sources. In the extreme case, fantastic information is offered voluntarily; this form of confabulation tends to occur early in the course of chronic amnestic disorders. Fantastic confabulation appears to be similar to a delusion, although the patient is unlikely to sustain the content because of memory problems.

Severe amnestic disorder is commonly associated with a lack of insight into the condition, which further complicates the course of chronic profound amnesia. Patients may become agitated when poor memory leads to disagreements with others. The associated features of amnestic disorder obviously contribute to the disability seen from the disorder.

Current criteria emphasize the exclusion of delirium and dementia as part of the diagnosis of amnestic disorder. Dementia and delirium must be distinguished from amnestic disorders because these global disorders include a significant component of memory impairment. Examination of patients along the lines suggested in Box 11-2 facilitates the distinction between amnestic disorder and more global cognitive impairment. The distinction of amnestic disorders from dementia hinges on the absence of other signs of clinically significant cognitive impairment in amnestic disorders. Delirium and dementia typically involve impaired perception with disturbances such as visual hallucinations, which are rare, unrelated occurrences in amnestic disorder. Delirium characteristically involves a disturbance of consciousness that is not part of amnestic disorder. The patient described in Case 11-2 was significantly impaired by poor memory without clear signs and symptoms of either delirium or dementia.

Amnestic disorders are classified as the result of a general medical condition (Box 11-8) or as substance induced (Box 11-9). Transient forms of amnestic disorder are seen in transient global amnesia, as a manifestation of a seizure, and after head injury. Recovery from the amnestic disorder after head injury can take considerably longer than recovery from the other dis-

CASE 11-2

Mr. W. is a 55-year-old black man who was referred for evaluation and treatment of memory problems. He had long been described as acting strange but was brought to the emergency room when he was found wandering about at work with no idea as to what he was supposed to be doing. He had been sent home from work 2 days before but returned to work with the same problem. He had a long history of alcohol dependence complicated by withdrawal, seizures, and a right frontal hematoma; he was not intoxicated when he arrived at the hospital, nor did he show any signs of withdrawal during the hospitalization. No evidence was obtained from collateral sources to suggest recent head trauma or recent seizures. A brother carried the diagnosis of mental retardation. Mr. W. had only an eighth grade education, which complicated the evaluation of his intellect, although he had worked as a laborer for the same employer for several years. The patient did not have any focal or lateralizing neurological signs. At the time of initial evaluation he was alert and oriented in all three spheres. No psychotic symptoms were elicited, although the patient did not feel he had a problem. He recalled three of three items at 1 minute but only one of three items at 5 minutes. Simple arithmetic was not a problem (subtraction from 20 by 3s), and he could perform simple comparisons (apple and orange). He could not perform more difficult arithmetic or make more complicated comparisons, difficulties that were attributed to his lack of education. The patient could repeat six digits forward and four in reverse, although he had a great deal of difficulty learning the task of reversing the digits. An emergent CT scan of the head showed mild cerebellar vermian atrophy and a tiny low density lesion of uncertain origin lateral to the left frontal horn. He was advised to stop drinking and was given thiamine. He was without impairment of consciousness throughout the hospitalization. Mr. W. left the hospital against medical advice but returned for an EEG 2 weeks later; his EEG was normal.

When evaluated by a psychiatrist in an office visit 1 week after his hospitalization, his recall and other tests of cognitive function were unchanged. His chief complaint concerned physical symptoms such as swollen feet and shortness of breath, which were not obvious on examination. The patient had no memory of the hospitalization. Consideration was given to neuropsychological testing, particularly a comparison of intelligence quotient (IQ) as measured by a standardized test such as the Wechsler Adult Intelligence Scale (WAIS) with memory as measured by a standardized test such as the Wechsler Memory Scale-Revised (WMS-R). Poor compliance and an inability to accurately determine baseline intellectual function (the patient's rural school district was no longer in existence because of consolidation) suggested that testing would not be useful. This decision was discussed with the patient's son and the primary care physician; they agreed. Mr. W. had symptoms of depression that included low mood, poor energy, poor sleep, a history of poor appetite, and thoughts of death. He was treated with an antidepressant. He was also treated with thiamine throughout the follow-up period. Mr. W.'s symptoms of depression improved, but he showed consistent difficulty with recall over the next 9 months. He was oriented and eventually able to learn the name of the current President. The patient read the paper, but his reporting of content events was inaccurate; he mixed events from the remote past with current events. He lived with his son, who provided for his needs and monitored his environment. The patient was felt to be disabled by his memory problems. The patient was repeatedly advised to avoid alcohol use but was known to be drinking intermittently when he was lost to follow-up evaluation.

orders associated with transient amnestic disorder. Next to head injury, transient global amnesia is the second most common type of transient amnestic disorder. A benign disorder of acute onset and short duration (24 hours or less), transient global amnesia is not associated with focal neurological signs or symptoms. Amnestic disorder as a manifestation of epilepsy can be distinguished from transient global amnesia by the brief duration (less than 1 hour) and recurrent nature of epileptic amnesia. Partial complex seizures are a relatively rare cause of a brief amnestic disorder; most patients with epilepsy have other obvious signs and symptoms of nervous system involvement as part of the seizure. An amnestic disorder as the result of electroconvulsive therapy (ECT) is uncommon. Rarely patients relate remote memory loss, a problem unlike amnestic disorder, to ECT. Most patients who receive ECT have some memory loss that is partly attributable to the induced seizure but also probably related to the electricity used to induce the seizure and the anesthetic agents that are part of the procedure (see Chapter 22). Cerebrovascular disease can cause a short period of amnesia, but these episodes of transient ischemic amnesia are usually associated with focal neurological signs.

The most common medical condition associated with chronic amnestic disorder is thiamine deficiency as the result of malnutrition. In Western societies the preceding delirium (Wernicke's encephalopathy) and resulting memory problems (Korsakoff's syndrome) are almost always seen in people who are addicted to alcohol. Amnestic disorder as the result of a cerebral infection reverses slowly or not at all. Anoxia can produce irreversible amnestic disorder. Bilateral surgical removal of temporal lobe structures, usually performed to control intractable seizures, produces an amnestic disorder. Neoplasm and cerebral vascular disease can cause an amnestic disorder but are unlikely to be the sole cause; usually other signs and symptoms of CNS involvement are present.

BOX 11-8

MEDICAL CONDITIONS ASSOCIATED WITH AMNESTIC DISORDER

Transient global amnesia
Head injury
Seizures
  Epilepsy/partial complex seizures
  ECT
Malnutrition
  Thiamine deficiency (Wernicke-Korsakoff syndrome)
Cerebral infection (e.g., herpes encephalitis)
Anoxia
Surgical intervention
  Removal of all or a significant portion of the temporal lobe
Neoplasm
Cerebral vascular disease
  Posterior cerebral artery

Some of the listed conditions (such as seizures or cerebral vascular disease) do not usually cause amnesia without other clinically significant neurological signs or symptoms and are thus unusual causes of amnestic disorder.

The use of ethanol, the most important substance associated with amnestic disorder, appears to produce persisting amnestic disorder in an indirect manner involving thiamine deficiency. Other sedative-hypnotic compounds also may cause a persistent amnestic disorder, although these drugs are more commonly associated with amnesia during intoxication or withdrawal, conditions distinct from amnestic disorder. Compounds listed in Box 11-9 are rare causes of amnestic disorder.

Neuropsychological testing is an important adjunct to the evaluation and diagnosis of chronic amnestic disorder; the brevity of transient global amnesia and amnestic disorder associated with epilepsy severely limits the usefulness of testing in brief episodes of amnesia. The most widely used memory instrument is the WMS-R. Psychological instruments are useful for documenting the absence of more generalized cognitive impairment and providing an estimate of the rate of recovery in generally reversible amnestic disorders (for example, after head injury). Unfortunately, testing may reveal abnormalities of doubtful or unknown clinical relevance.

Natural History

The natural history of amnestic disorders reflects the etiological condition. The duration of amnestic disorder should be specified as either transient or chronic. By definition, transient amnestic disorders last no more than 1 month. The natural history of amnestic disorder is presented based on a distinction between transient and chronic disorders.

BOX 11-9

SUBSTANCES ASSOCIATED WITH SUBSTANCE-INDUCED PERSISTING AMNESTIC DISORDER

Sedative-hypnotics
  Alcohol
  Barbiturates
Anticonvulsants
Methotrexate (intrathecal)
Heavy metals
  Lead
  Mercury
Organophosphate insecticides
Carbon monoxide
Industrial solvents

Caution should be used in attributing amnestic disorder to any of these substances. For example, thiamine deficiency is a far more common cause of chronic amnestic disorder.

Transient global amnesia is a benign transient amnestic disorder. Patients, typically in late middle age, experience a relatively sudden onset of memory failure; many cases are preceded by some type of emotional or physical stress (such as running and swimming, sexual relations, or medical procedures). Men and women are probably equally affected. The patients are alert and have at most only minor neurological signs; laboratory studies are generally uninformative, although recent functional imaging studies suggest the presence of a bilateral decrease in temporal lobe perfusion. Symptoms resolve gradually over hours to a day or perhaps a bit longer; as noted previously, epileptic amnestic disorder generally is of even briefer duration. The affected individual is left with amnesia for the period of the disturbance (anterograde amnesia) and for about an hour before the onset of amnesia (retrograde amnesia). No greater impediment than the amnesia is observed in patients who experience a single episode of transient global amnesia; only about 10% of patients experience repeated episodes. Transient amnestic disorder as the result of seizures is associated with a greater risk of recurrence; consideration of partial complex seizures should be given patients with apparently recurrent transient global amnesia.

Head trauma is associated with amnesia of variable duration. Even in the absence of loss of consciousness or other neurological findings, mild head injury can produce amnesia that lasts an hour or so. The more severe the injury, the more prolonged the amnesia. Interestingly, the duration of amnesia predicts a significant portion of the disability that results from head trauma. The longer the amnesia, the greater the resulting disability. Amnestic disorder from head trauma will probably be associated with neuropsychological findings, although the presence of other clinically significant cognitive difficulties should suggest either delirium or dementia. Head trauma and presumably the associated amnestic disorder are usually seen in young patients, particularly those who use alcohol or drugs. Older age is probably associated with a worse prognosis, based on what is known about the outcome of head injury.

Bilateral lesions involving temporal lobe structures (such as surgical removal or anoxia) typically produce irreversible chronic amnestic disorder. The most famous patient with amnestic disorder suffered anterograde and retrograde memory loss after bilateral removal of the medial temporal lobe in 1953 to alleviate intractable epilepsy. This individual is of above average intelligence but because of the profound memory impairment is unable to live independently.

Patients with Korsakoff's syndrome tend to be men in their 50s and 60s who have alcohol addiction; females may have an earlier onset of the disorder. Most have additional complications of alcoholism, as did the patient in Case 11-2. Although many patients with Korsakoff's syndrome have Wernicke's encephalopathy, some have a more insidious onset of Korsakoff's syndrome without a clear preceding delirium, as was the case for Mr. W. Some individuals such as Mr. W. show modest recovery with the passage of time, particularly if they abstain from alcohol. Abstinence and proper diet may lead to a better outcome. Nevertheless, these older malnourished individuals are likely to require custodial care until death occurs; death is commonly the result of the medical complications of alcoholism.

Differential Diagnosis

The separation of amnestic disorder from the more generalized cognitive dysfunction characteristic of delirium and dementia is sufficiently important that the criteria for amnestic disorder insist that delirium and dementia be excluded to meet criteria. Many of the medical conditions associated with amnestic disorder are also associated with delirium and dementia. Dementia is characterized by the presence of memory dysfunction and clear evidence of at least two kinds of additional cognitive impairment, including aphasia (disturbance of language), agnosia (failure to identify objects despite intact sensory function), apraxia (inability to perform motor tasks despite intact motor function), or disturbance of executive function (skills involved in planning, sequencing, organizing, and abstracting). Amnestic disorder is largely a disorder of memory without clinically significant impairment of other cognitive function. Although patients with amnestic disorder may provide imaginary events to fill in missing memory, they do not suffer from the visual hallucinations and persecutory delusions so commonly seen in many patients with dementia of the Alzheimer's type (DAT). Finally, the course of amnestic disorder is variable, depending on its cause (see the discussion on pp. 188-190), whereas the dementias tend to be static or, in the case of DAT, progressive.

Delirium is a disorder of impaired consciousness, a cognitive function that is preserved in amnestic disorder. Patients who are amnestic should do well on tasks that reflect attention, such as digit span, whereas patients who are delirious typically suffer from impairment. Patients with delirium, like many patients afflicted with dementia, tend to have perceptual disturbances such as illusions or visual and auditory hallucinations. Language dysfunction, such as an inability to name objects or rambling incoherent speech, is common in delirium. The course of delirium fluctuates on a time span that is measured in hours, which is unusual in amnestic disorder.

Drugs with sedative-hypnotic properties, most notably alcohol, can cause transitory memory disturbances during intoxication or withdrawal. Interestingly, the alcoholic blackout is commonly associated with an inability to retrieve learned material in the absence of alcohol; reexposure may bring back memories of material learned during previous blackouts. This characteristic, a form of state-dependent learning, distinguishes the blackout from the inability of the person who is amnestic to learn new material. Amnestic symptoms that develop during intoxication or withdrawal are classified as part of a particular type of substance-induced intoxication or withdrawal.

Epilepsy and cerebrovascular disease cause amnesia but rarely cause amnestic disorder. Patients experiencing amnestic disorder attributed either to seizures or cerebrovascular disease should be carefully evaluated to elicit clinically significant neurological signs and symptoms. Individuals suffering from seizures are likely to benefit from anticonvulsant therapy, whereas no treatment is indicated for transient global amnesia. Furthermore, patients who suffer from transient amnestic episodes caused by ictal phenomena without initial evidence of epilepsy will probably develop clear seizures. Cerebrovascular disease is associated with a relatively poor outcome because of an increased risk of myocardial infarction and stroke.

Amnestic disorders must be distinguished from the poorly understood dissociative states (see Chapter 17). The primary care physician also needs to be aware that apparent memory problems can be the result of malingering or factitious (self-induced) disorder. A key to the distinction between malingering, factitious disorder, and the dissociative states on the one hand, and amnestic disorder on the other, lies in the ability to ascertain a cause for the amnestic disorders. Etiological conditions should be temporally related to the onset of amnestic disorder. A great deal of information is available about etiological factors associated with amnestic disorder, many of which are common disorders (for example, alcoholism and head trauma) that are likely to occur in patients with dissociative states. Historically, the so-called psychogenic amnesias have been separated from amnestic disorder on the basis of lost personal memories in the face of adequate function on formal memory testing observed in psychogenic amnesia. Several case reports suggesting that autobiographical memories may be lost as a result of lesions in the CNS advise caution in the application of this distinction. The primary care provider would probably be wise to refer any cases of suspected dissociative state, malingering, or factitious disorder to a specialist with an interest in these controversial and probably rare disorders.

Most other psychiatric disorders are readily distinguished from amnestic disorder. Patients with other psychiatric disorders (such as depression, anxiety disorders, or mania) may complain of poor memory and in some cases exhibit poor performance on formal testing. However, most patients with amnestic disorder are unaware of the extent of the memory problems. The presence of symptoms suggestive of a psychiatric disorder (for example, suicidal ideation and poor appetite suggest depression) other than amnestic disorder in a patient who complains of poor memory should lead to a diligent effort to evaluate the patient to estimate the possibility that an individual complaining of poor memory meets criteria for a disorder other than amnestic disorder. The individual in Case 11-2 exhibited a significant number of depressive symptoms and appears to have benefited from treatment. Perhaps some of the apparent reversal of memory difficulties in this person is attributable to appropriate antidepressant treatment.

Genetics and Family History

Like delirium, amnestic disorder is likely to be almost entirely the product of environmental insults on the brain, with little familiality or evidence for genetic effects. Transient global amnesia has been rarely noted to be familial. Interestingly, the disorder most closely associated with transient global amnesia, migraine, shows significant family loading. Further study of transient global amnesia will help researchers estimate the extent of familiality and perhaps relate it to migraine in some instances.

Korsakoff's syndrome was postulated to be the result of a genetic defect in an enzyme called *transketolase* that requires thiamine pyrophosphate as a cofactor. At present, no variation in the transketolase gene of patients with Wernicke-Korsakoff syndrome has been described. Patients who develop thiamine deficiency as the result of malnutrition from other causes have been described; amnestic disorder in these cases is virtually indistinguishable from that seen in people with alcoholism. The enduring puzzle is that only a fraction of people with alcoholism develop amnestic disorder. Whereas a significant underestimate of clinical cases is probable (see the following section), the familiality (if any) of Korsakoff's syndrome in people with alcoholism needs to be separated from the familiality of alcoholism and related medical conditions.

Epidemiology

The epidemiology of amnestic disorder is closely related to the epidemiology of the causative disorders. The occurrences of transient global amnesia, a brief benign disorder, and Wernicke-Korsakoff syndrome, typically a chronic state, are relatively well understood. At least four population-based studies provide an estimate of the annual incidence of transient global amnesia, with numbers ranging from 3 to 10 cases per 100,000 people. Patients who suffer from transient global amnesia are at little risk of suffering from epilepsy and cerebrovascular disease, although there seems to be increased risk of migraine.

Korsakoff's syndrome is much more common than transient global amnesia. Estimates of prevalence based on postmortem series suggest a prevalence of 0.8% to 2.8%. The higher estimates are derived from Australia, where an epidemic of Korsakoff's syndrome appeared to occur in the 1970s and early 1980s. A community-based study from The Hague, The Netherlands, suggests a prevalence of about five cases per 10,000 people, an order of magnitude lower than the postmortem estimates. These findings suggest that although prevalences based on postmortem series may overestimate the occurrence of Wernicke-Korsakoff syndrome, a substantial number of cases are not recognized as long as the patients are alive. Furthermore, the Australian experience suggests that rates are tied to environmental factors such as per capita alcohol consumption and dietary thiamine supplementation. Primary preventive measures, such as thiamine supplementation and education about the consequences of excessive alcohol intake, may have the desirable effect of reducing the prevalence of Korsakoff's syndrome.

Pathophysiology

To understand what is known about the pathophysiology of amnestic disorder, it is necessary to develop some general principles about learning and memory. First and foremost, memory is an integral aspect of thinking and is thus involved in most cognitive processes. Clinically, this observation is substantiated most obviously by noting that memory is impaired in other global disorders of cognitive functioning, such as dementia and delirium. Memory consists of multiple processes, many of which are difficult to define and poorly understood. In amnestic disorder, patients can repeat digits or words immediately after presentation but are unable to retain the information much beyond this brief period; patients who are delirious have difficulty performing both tasks. Patients with amnestic disorder also have variable problems retrieving information learned before the onset of the causative disorder (for example, after head trauma or surgery). These observations, supported by much additional data reviewed in the annotated bibliography, suggest that the process of learning involves acquisition (indicated by the ability to repeat information immediately after presentation), retention (storing the data), and retrieval (repetition of some or all of the information when desired). The processes are bounded by an element of time in the sense that the process of learning takes some time to occur (minutes to hours). Time, as marked by the pathological event responsible for the impaired memory of amnestic disorder, delineates the difficulties in learning new items (anterograde amnesia) and retrieving older memories (retrograde amnesia) from memories of the distant past (remote memory), which are more likely to be spared.

The study of patients with amnesia has shown that these individuals do not lack the capability of learning new material. In particular, they can learn and retain complex procedural skills (such as reading words as they appear in a mirror) despite an inability to remember the content or nature of the task. Observations such as this suggest that amnestic disorder typically involves a type of memory that requires some conscious effort, unlike more automatic memory that is associated with many motor tasks, for example. The memory impaired in amnestic disorder is heavily but not solely related to verbal output. A more general observation is that memory is distributed with specific networks serving different functions; some of these functions, such as those involved in execution of the mirror-reading task, are spared in amnestic disorder. Finally, the observation that patients develop amnestic disorder as the result of lesions in different parts of the brain suggests that the memory systems involved in amnestic disorder are distributed and interconnected (Figure 11-2).

The exploration of clinical cases of amnestic disorder provides a great deal of information about the anatomical basis of amnestic disorder. The surprising memory deficits of the most famous patient with amnestic disorder (see p. 191) were initially interpreted as the failure of all memory, because no learning could be demonstrated despite the preservation of intellect. Subsequent research has demonstrated the ability of this patient and other similarly affected individuals to learn and preserve the ability to execute various tasks (such as the mirror-reading test) even though they were unaware of having previously practiced such tasks. Since the site of surgical intervention was known, it was surmised that the hippocampus and associated structures performed critical learning and memory functions (see Figure 11-2). Unilateral lesions

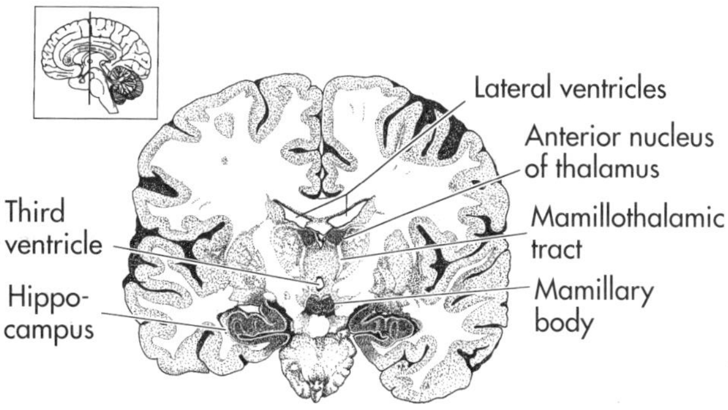

FIGURE 11-2 Neuroanatomical structures implicated in amnestic disorder. Two separate but interconnected systems have been implicated in amnestic disorder and are readily visualized in this line drawing of a brain slice taken at the level indicated in the inset. Externally, this slice would be in front of the ear. The ventricles are indicated; clear areas otherwise correspond to white matter, lightly stippled areas to gray matter and dark areas to sulci. Neuroanatomical regions thought to be involved in amnestic disorder are heavily stippled. The hippocampus and related structures implicated in amnestic disorder are indicated on the left; the mammillary body, mammillothalamic tract, and thalamic regions involved in Korsakoff's syndrome are on the right. This slice shows neuroanatomical structures in two dimensions; all structures extend in anterior and posterior directions, with the hippocampus and related structures occupying an extensive portion of the temporal lobe. Bilateral lesions of either region are usually required for amnestic disorder. The dorsal medial thalamic nucleus is not shown, and the involvement of this structure in amnestic disorder is controversial.

are generally not associated with amnestic disorder. Mapping pathologically affected regions of the brain with scanning techniques (CT and MRI) in this individual and others with chronic amnestic disorder confirmed the original hypothesis. Chronic amnestic disorder associated with anoxia and carbon monoxide poisoning is presumably the result of hippocampal neuronal loss, which can be seen at autopsy. Functional scanning data (from PET and SPECT images) support the belief that temporal lobe structures such as the hippocampus and associated subcortical regions are involved in the pathophysiology of amnesia that is associated with disorders without clear pathology, such as transient global amnesia and epilepsy.

The neuroanatomical basis of Korsakoff's syndrome has been a more controversial subject although it is quite clear that the sites do not include the hippocampus and related structures (see Figure 11-2). Acute pathological changes associated with Wernicke-Korsakoff syndrome have been described in the mammillary bodies and associated structures. Microscopic hemorrhages, hyperplasia of blood vessel walls with proliferation of capillaries, and glial proliferation with initial sparing of neurons but later development of neuronal chromatolysis are observed in Wernicke's encephalopathy; the affected regions in Korsakoff's syndrome show atrophy as a result of neuronal loss and discoloration. Involvement of thalamic nuclei has been unequivocal, although disagreement exists as to which regions of the thalamus are included. The best available information suggests that the anterior thalamus and possibly the medial dorsal nucleus of the thalamus, in addition to the mammillary bodies, are affected in Korsakoff's syndrome. Regardless of the status of the medial dorsal nucleus in Korsakoff's syndrome, this region appears to have played a key role in the amnestic disorder that followed unilateral trauma of the brain in one individual. Korsakoff's syndrome is also likely to involve the interconnection between the mammillary bodies and the thalamus, the mammillothalamic tract.

Additional controversy regarding the pathophysiology of Korsakoff's syndrome surrounds the role of the frontal lobes in the resulting disability. Cortical atrophy, particularly in the frontal lobes, is seen in many autopsies and on neuroimaging studies. The distinction between Korsakoff's syndrome and a dementia related to chronic ethanol consumption would be difficult if some patients with Korsakoff's syndrome show additional chronic cognitive impairment, perhaps because of frontal lobe pathological changes. It is unclear why some regions of the brain are selectively affected by thiamine deficiency when it appears that all brain cells require a continuous supply of thiamine. A related issue is the importance of ethanol in causing the pathological condition. Ethanol may have direct neuronal toxicity, although this has been hard to demonstrate in animals, largely because most animals have the good sense to avoid ethanol. In humans who are alcoholic, this has been hard to demonstrate because the interpretation of postmortem lesions is confounded at least to some extent by the complex premortem pathologic state associated with death in people with alcoholism. People addicted to alcohol probably develop thiamine deficiency as the result of reduced dietary intake, decreased intestinal absorption, and depletion of thiamine stores. Although the mechanism by which thiamine deficiency causes Korsakoff's syndrome is unknown, thiamine is critically involved in glucose metabolism; perhaps deficiency of thiamine produces a relative deficiency in the function of a neurotransmitter system such as acetylcholine involved in memory.

Management and Treatment

The treatment of amnestic disorder is the treatment of the associated conditions. Enhancing memory by teaching patients mnemonic devices is of no proven benefit. Addressing the various conditions requires distinguishing one condition from the other, including the separation of transient conditions from chronic amnestic disorder. Transient global amnesia does not need to be treated except to keep the patient safe. Epileptic amnestic disorder should be addressed by treating the underlying partial complex seizures with an appropriate anticonvulsant; information on the use of these drugs can be found in various sources. Transient ischemic amnesia and amnestic stroke need to be distinguished from amnestic disorders largely for prognostic reasons at present.

Treatment of head injury is a complex issue commonly complicated by other injuries. Recovery from even minor head injury can be prolonged by the presence of symptoms described under the rubric of "postconcussive syndrome," although the boundaries of this entity are poorly defined. Hopefully, further study of patients who have suffered varying degrees of brain trauma will further define the relationship between amnestic disorder, other trauma, and the postconcussive syndrome.

As noted previously, supplementation of dietary sources with thiamine may decrease the prevalence of Wernicke-Korsakoff syndrome. Public education about the consequences of excessive alcohol consumption may also reduce the prevalence of Korsakoff's syndrome. Patients who come to a physician with malnutrition, especially patients who are alcoholic or suspected of being alcoholic, should receive additional vitamin supplementation, particularly thiamine. The management of delirium ought to include the administration of parenteral thiamine, hopefully preventing Korsakoff's syndrome. The continued administration of thiamine to patients with Korsakoff's syndrome is of unknown benefit but of little harm and probably makes good sense, since these individuals are likely to have other pathologic disorders and to continue to

PEARLS & PERILS

AMNESTIC DISORDER

- Amnestic disorder is restricted to memory dysfunction.
- Other disorders associated with amnesia (dementia and delirium) need to be considered and excluded.
- Amnestic disorder may be brief in duration (for example, transient global amnesia) or chronic (such as Korsakoff's syndrome).
- Prognosis reflects underlying condition and duration.
- Chronic amnestic disorder may require custodial care to sustain life.
- Korsakoff's syndrome (thiamine deficiency), usually seen in people who are alcoholic, is a common but preventable disorder.

drink. Most vitamin preparations are adequate. Patients with chronic amnestic disorder, regardless of the cause, probably require custodial care, usually in an institution such as a nursing home. These individuals can survive a long time, with prognosis likely to reflect the associated medical conditions.

Amnestic disorder is cognitive impairment limited to the most obvious type of memory in humans (see the Pearls & Perils box on p. 194). The disorder should be classified according to the signs and symptoms indicative of an etiological condition and further characterized on the basis of amnesia duration. The presence of clinically significant cognitive impairment suggests other disorders, particularly delirium and dementia, even if amnesia is present. Chronic amnestic disorder often results in profound disability requiring custodial care.

CONSIDER CONSULTATION WHEN . . .

- The diagnosis of delirium is uncertain, particularly if history and symptoms suggest another or an additional psychiatric disorder (such as depression or dementia)
- Management with usually effective approaches (for example, haloperidol or restraints) is not sufficient to allow treatment of concurrent medical conditions, particularly if behavior is a danger to self or others
- Symptoms of delirium fail to resolve despite apparent resolution of causative/contributive medical conditions
- The diagnosis of amnestic disorder is unclear, particularly if the patient has features of dementia, delirium, dissociative states, or malingering
- The apparent etiological condition is treatable (for example, alcohol dependence or epilepsy) or may benefit from rehabilitation (such as a head injury)

Acknowledgments

The author acknowledges the helpful input of Dr. Barry Hong and Dr. Thomas Woolsey, in addition to the efforts of the editors.

Annotated Bibliography

American Psychiatric Association: *Diagnostic and statistical manual of mental disorders,* ed 4 (DSM-IV), Washington, D.C., 1994, American Psychiatric Press.

This book supports diagnostic criteria for delirium and amnestic disorder with a presentation of essential information that allows the busy physician to rapidly develop a diagnosis.

Benson DF: *The neurology of thinking,* New York, 1994, Oxford University Press.

The book is organized around types of cognitive function, emphasizing clinical aspects, to develop a theory about thinking. It presents the material discussed in this chapter from the perspective of a neurologist (for example, *acute confusion* appears to be the same as delirium) with many excellent case reports.

Dudai Y: *The neurobiology of memory: concepts, findings, trends,* Oxford, England, 1989, Oxford University Press.

This is a readable introduction to the exploration of memory from molecules to man; a good start for the inquisitive, although events since publication have altered a few of the details.

Kopelman MD: The Korsakoff syndrome, *Br J Psych* 166:154, 1995.

This article provides an excellent review of this form of amnestic disorder; it also presents related memory concepts in a succinct and thorough fashion.

Lipowski ZJ: *Delirium: acute confusional states,* New York, 1990, Oxford University Press.

This is a complete review of delirium; the bibliography to this chapter largely adds more recent work than appears in this book.

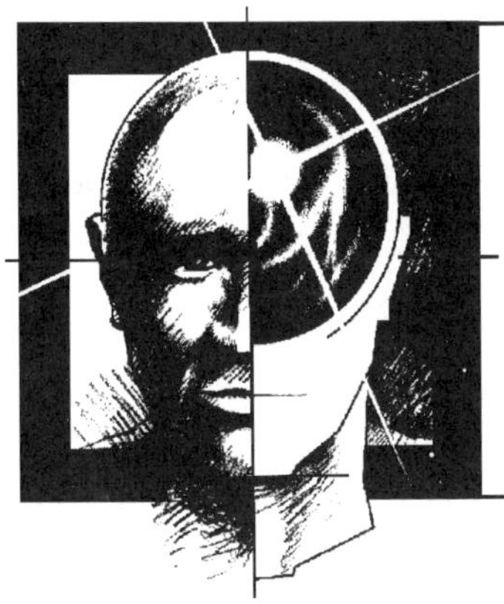

chapter 12

Cognitive Disorders: Dementias

Eugene H. Rubin, MD, PhD

Dementia is a syndrome characterized by deterioration in memory and multiple cognitive functions that interferes with a person's ability to manage everyday activities. Functions involving complex cortical processing—including general intellect; abilities to plan, organize, and reason; orientation; speech; mathematical skills; visuospatial abilities; and motor planning—are often involved. Changes in personality are common. Psychotic symptoms, including delusions and hallucinations, often appear as the illness progresses. Although there are many illnesses leading to the syndrome of dementia, dementia of the Alzheimer type (DAT) is by far the most common cause in North America. Only a small percentage of dementias are the result of processes that can be interrupted, stabilized, or reversed. DAT and most other dementias are progressive disorders that rob a person of what it is to be human. Over a period of years, a highly successful and productive person is reduced to an individual who no longer recognizes her spouse or children and who requires full-time nursing care because of incontinence, agitation, and the inability to take care of basic everyday functions. A person may live for a decade or more in this frightening and heart-rending state.

Compromised brain function that interferes with daily activities is not normal and should not be dismissed with, "What do you expect for someone who is 80 years old?" When such changes occur, it is imperative to evaluate and diagnose the illness responsible for the breakdown of brain function. As increasingly effective treatments become available, early diagnosis is becoming even more important. Diagnosis is also the first step in long-term planning for both the patient and her family.

DAT is common, occurring in 5% to 10% of people age 65 and older. Its prevalence increases dramatically with advancing age; perhaps over one third of people age 85 and older suffer from DAT. Major progress in elucidating the pathophysiological mechanisms responsible for this disorder is occurring. It is becoming increasingly apparent that several pathways lead to the symptoms of DAT. Treatments with improved efficacy and specificity will be available when more is understood about the pathophysiological nature of DAT. It is essential to be able to diagnose DAT and to understand the different mechanisms involved as targeted therapies come on the market.

This chapter focuses on DAT. The term *DAT* refers to the clinical syndrome; the term *Alzheimer's disease* refers to this clinical syndrome when it is further confirmed by characteristic neuropathological changes as determined from brain autopsy or biopsy. Other causes of dementia are briefly discussed in the section on differential diagnosis. Case 12-1 demonstrates a typical natural history of DAT. When treatments are discovered that delay the biochemical and neuropathologic changes, it will be important to initiate such treatment early in the course of illness. Increased clinical skills at diagnosis are imperative until physiological markers are discovered that may aid in diagnosis early in the course or before the appearance of clinical symptoms.

CASE 12-1

Mr. A., a 68-year-old corporate president, has been the patient of a primary care physician for 25 years and has enjoyed excellent health other than periodic upper respiratory infections and mild arthritis. During an annual checkup, Mrs. A. pulls the physician aside and relates that Mr. A. has become more absent-minded over the last year. He is still working full time, apparently without difficulties, but she has become aware that he misplaces keys and forgets where he parks when he is shopping. These behaviors are new. She states that he still remembers everyday messages and would remember the details of dinner at a restaurant the previous night. He would remember a wedding from several weeks ago, but he might not be as accurate with details of that event as he would have been 10 years ago. It has become harder for him to organize documents for tax preparation. Occasionally he forgets an appointment, which he never did before. He has become a little more socially withdrawn. When the physician evaluates Mr. A., he states that he feels fine and that he is doing well in terms of his memory and thinking skills. Routine tests, including tests for thyroid and liver function, electrolytes, creatinine, blood urea nitrogen (BUN), sedimentation rate, and venereal disease are all normal. A neurological examination reveals no abnormalities. On several brief cognitive batteries, such as the Mini-Mental State Examination (MMSE), Mr. A. scores perfectly. The physician reassures Mrs. A. that everything seems fine.

The next year Mrs. A. reports that there has been definite slow progressive slippage. Mr. A. still works full time, but their son who works with him reports that his father is starting to forget earlier business decisions and to mix up accounts. This has not occurred often, but it is often enough that other company executives are concerned. Mrs. A. reports that Mr. A. seemed more confused during a vacation to Europe 3 months before his examination. He usually enjoys planning such trips, but this year he asked Mrs. A. to take over. She has noticed that he not only was having difficulties remembering names, but that he was also repeating stories without realizing it. He would forget to tell her that someone called, and forgot appointments more often. She also has noticed that he was less able to recall certain words and that she has been completing sentences for him. He had always been accurate in leaving an 18% to 20% tip at restaurants, but lately he leaves from 10% to 30% without apparent intent.

When the physician interviews Mr. A., he states that everything is fine other than forgetting a name occasionally. Everything is okay at work, and he is beginning to think about retirement. His performance on cognitive testing is still within normal limits, but he does not fully remember a name and address that are part of a brief cognitive battery. The physician orders magnetic resonance imaging (MRI), which shows mild global atrophy. The physician then talks with the couple and indicates that he is not sure what these subtle cognitive changes may represent, but that it is possible that an illness such as DAT might be beginning. He also states that he wants to see them more often.

Over the next 2 years, the illness declares itself. Mr. A. has increasing difficulty with memory, orientation, judgment, visuospatial skills, speech, and behavior. He has trouble remembering the details of an event from several days ago. If he forgets to write down a phone message, it is likely to be forgotten. He still drives but has lost his car at malls on several occasions. He forgot his wife's birthday for the first time. He thought that a visit 2 weeks ago from a son occurred several months ago. He is no longer able to program his VCR. He reads much less and has trouble with finding words, which is noticeable during casual conversation. He can no longer mentally manipulate figures. In an attempt to draw a clock indicating 2:45, he sketches three hands—one pointing to each number. On testing, his short-term memory is obviously compromised.

Within 2 more years, Mr. A. becomes irritable and at times, physically threatening. He is more secluded and spends much of his time sitting and watching TV. He is certain that his family is stealing from him. On occasion, he believes that the people on TV are actually in his house. He imagines people in his yard and hears their conversations. Eventually, the agitation coupled with increasing incontinence necessitates nursing home admission.

Diagnosis

DAT is a slowly progressive dementia that eventually involves many cortical brain functions (Box 12-1, Table 12-1). It is important to emphasize that symptoms represent change from a person's baseline, are gradually progressive, and interfere with general ability to function. If an individual always has had trouble with misplacing glasses or keys, then such a complaint is not a symptom of a progressive dementia. Objective memory testing is useful in documenting changes over time. Some age-related cognitive changes occur normally. Name recall may become more difficult. Performance on memory tasks involving visuospatial relations declines. Performance on tasks requiring speed and memory may decrease with age. Complex tasks requiring attention to many events simultaneously become more difficult. However, these changes are subtle and rarely interfere with everyday social or occupational function.

As noted, Case 12-1 is typical of DAT. The earliest clinical symptoms involve subtle memory changes that are noted by an observant collateral source. Another common early symptom is increasing passivity and withdrawal. Collateral source observations of these earliest symptoms are usually more accurate than reports from the patient. It is not rare for patients to deny symptoms, even when cognitive failure is evident to all who are close to them. It is important to integrate the history from both the collateral source and the patient.

Natural History

DAT is a progressive disorder that over several years leads to deterioration in most brain functions, including memory, orientation, judgment, intellect, language, social behavior, personality, and activities of daily living (including self care). The presenting symptoms usually include subtle changes in memory and personality. More focal presentations are not rare (see p. 201). These early changes usually progress slowly over several years, although rapid progression over several months can occur.

The progression of illness can be monitored by several different approaches. Some physicians use a series of questions that are asked at each visit to check cognitive functioning. These questions coupled with neurological and mental status examinations can be sufficient. Other physicians have an assistant in the office administer brief cognitive batteries such as the MMSE every 6 to 12 months. More detailed global staging instruments are also available and helpful for clinical research. The group from the Alzheimer's Disease Research Center at Washington University has developed and refined the Clinical Dementia Rating Scale (CDR). This scale has been shown to be reliable and useful for staging illness as very mild, mild, moderate, or severe, based on the six individually rated domains of memory, orientation, judgment and problem solving, home and hobbies, community affairs, and personal care. By using such scales in longitudinal studies, an accurate description of the rate and nature of progression has been elucidated.

DAT in its earliest clinical stages can be difficult to diagnose because the symptoms can remain subtle for several years. Follow-up examinations and monitoring of function are useful for determining whether a gradually progressive decline is taking place. When suspicion of DAT arises, differential diagnosis is important to rule out other dementing disorders that may have a different prognosis and treatment.

Eventually, perhaps over several years, symptoms become consistent and progressive enough to allow a diagnosis of very mild or mild DAT. Memory changes start to interfere with everyday functioning. If the patient is still working, performance most likely deteriorates and co-workers become aware that something is wrong. If the person is retired, the collateral source may acknowledge that their loved one's memory and thinking have deteriorated to a point that would prohibit her from returning to a preretirement level of functioning. Stories are repeated; messages are forgotten. It is common that affected people who are involved in volunteer organizations are encouraged to give up positions of leadership because of poorer performance. Money management abilities deteriorate. At the very mild or mild stage of illness, the person still can be active with family and friends. A patient may not be able to organize vacations, but she may often still enjoy travelling with family members. However, overseas travel may prove quite disorienting. Hobbies are still maintained, although they are performed less well. Bowling or golf partners may report that their friend has trouble calculating the score or becomes mixed up with the number of strokes already played. Activities around the home are usually maintained, although perhaps they are performed at a less intense level; self care in terms of grooming, toileting, and eating is not yet influenced.

Once this mild stage of illness is reached, over half of all patients progress to a moderate or severe stage of disease over the next 15 months. Within 3 years, 80% of people with mild DAT progress beyond the mild stage and more than half are either severely demented or dead.

The moderate stage of dementia is characterized by substantial memory loss. Patients retain little from events or conversations. They may forget that their caregivers are their spouses; they may not recognize

DSM-IV DIAGNOSTIC CRITERIA

BOX 12-1 DEMENTIA OF THE ALZHEIMER'S TYPE

A. The development of multiple cognitive deficits manifested by both

(1) memory impairment (impaired ability to learn new information or to recall previously learned information)
(2) one (or more) of the following cognitive disturbances:

(a) aphasia (language disturbance)
(b) apraxia (impaired ability to carry out motor activities despite intact motor function)
(c) agnosia (failure to recognize or identify objects despite intact sensory function)
(d) disturbance in executive functioning (i.e., planning, organizing, sequencing, abstracting)

B. The cognitive deficits in Criteria A1 and A2 each cause significant impairment in social or occupational functioning and represent a significant decline from a previous level of functioning.

C. The course is characterized by gradual onset and continuing cognitive decline.

D. The cognitive deficits in Criteria A1 and A2 are not due to any of the following:

(1) other central nervous system conditions that cause progressive deficits in memory and cognition (e.g., cerebrovascular disease, Parkinson's disease, Huntington's disease, subdural hematoma, normal-pressure hydrocephalus, brain tumor)
(2) systemic conditions that are known to cause dementia (e.g., hypothyroidism, vitamin B_{12} or folic acid deficiency, niacin deficiency, hypercalcemia, neurosyphilis, HIV infection)
(3) substance-induced conditions

E. The deficits do not occur exclusively during the course of a delirium.

F. The disturbance is not better accounted for by another Axis I disorder (e.g., Major Depressive Disorder, Schizophrenia).

Code based on type of onset and predominant features:

With Early Onset: if onset is at age 65 years or below
- **With Delirium:** if delirium is superimposed on the dementia
- **With Delusions:** if delusions are the predominant feature
- **With Depressed Mood:** if depressed mood (including presentations that meet full symptom criteria for a Major Depressive Episode) is the predominant feature. A separate diagnosis of Mood Disorder Due to a General Medical Condition is not given.
- **Uncomplicated:** if none of the above predominates in the current clinical presentation

With Late Onset: if onset is after age 65 years
- **With Delirium:** if delirium is superimposed on the dementia
- **With Delusions:** if delusions are the predominant feature
- **With Depressed Mood:** if depressed mood (including presentations that meet full symptom criteria for a Major Depressive Episode) is the predominant feature. A separate diagnosis of Mood Disorder Due to a General Medical Condition is not given.
- **Uncomplicated:** if none of the above predominates in the current clinical presentation

Specify if:

With Behavioral Disturbance

Coding note: Also code Alzheimer's disease on Axis III.

From American Psychiatric Association: *Diagnostic and statistical manual of mental disorders,* ed 4 (DSM-IV), Washington, D.C., 1994, American Psychiatric Press.

DIAGNOSIS

TABLE 12-1

DEMENTIA OF THE ALZHEIMER TYPE

Discriminating features

1. Gradual, progressive deterioration involving multiple cognitive functions, including memory, that eventually interferes with ability to function; speech, learning, reasoning, mathematical skills, visuospatial abilities, and complex motor skills may be involved

Consistent features

1. Personality changes, (for example, the person becomes more passive and less interested) are common early in the illness
2. Agitation, delusions, and hallucinations may occur with illness progression
3. Complete inability to perform basic activities of daily living eventually occurs

Variable features

1. Major depression
2. Progressive aphasia preceding cognitive deterioration
3. Marked social inappropriateness and unusual behaviors preceding cognitive deterioration

their children. It becomes difficult to take them to gatherings or restaurants because their social judgment is compromised. They are unable to help with chores. They require help with dressing, bathing, and eating. Wandering and agitation occur often. Such people may become increasingly withdrawn. They may sit in front of the television all day with little evidence of attentiveness. In mild stages of DAT, suspicious patients may believe that people are stealing from them. These suspicions can increase in intensity and rate during moderate stages. Hallucinations and delusions are most common during this moderate stage of illness. Behavioral disturbances such as wandering, agitation, and psychotic symptoms are difficult to manage without help. Education and support groups for caregivers and knowledge about community resources are essential and are provided by the Alzheimer's Association and its local chapters.

During the severe stage of illness, memory abilities are almost totally destroyed. Patients may not recognize themselves or their loved ones. Incontinence is usual, and nursing home admission is commonly necessary. Persons with severe DAT may be either mobile or bedridden. When mobile, they do not participate in activities even though they may be brought into the room where such activities are occurring.

Although the progression from the mild to the severe stage of illness usually occurs over 1 to 5 years, death may not occur for many more years. About one half of all otherwise healthy people with mild DAT are still alive after 8 years; however, almost all of them are in the severely demented stage of illness. Therefore once this illness clearly declares itself and reaches a mild stage, it will rob a person of his most important brain functions over the next few years, leaving a severely incapacitated, totally dependent individual for many more years until death ends the ordeal.

Focal Presentations

On occasion, DAT can begin with symptoms suggestive of more focal brain pathological conditions. Most cortical and subcortical regions are involved in advanced DAT; however, early illness may involve discrete brain regions before the pathological changes become more general. When frontal lobe regions are involved early in the illness, characteristic behavioral symptoms occur that can be mistaken for other psychiatric disorders. Similarly, if areas involving language are more selectively involved early in the illness, aphasia is prominent.

DAT can have early focal involvement in the frontal lobe or in the frontal lobe and the anterior temporal lobe. Clinically, such patients demonstrate marked personality changes that can be troublesome. Careful evaluation usually reveals memory and other cognitive deficits, but such deficits initially are mild compared with the marked changes in behavior. Patients exhibit behavioral disinhibition and poor social judgment. A conservative college professor may relate increasingly inappropriate sexual jokes. A patient may make fun of a stranger who is overweight or tell inappropriate ethnic jokes. Insight and judgment are usually markedly impaired; these patients may have little understanding that they are acting in a socially embarrassing manner. Their abilities to plan are compromised. Eating habits may change, with periods of marked overeating. Obsessional behaviors are exhibited at times. A hypomanic picture may develop, with grandiosity, hyperactivity, euphoria, and inappropriate jocularity. Language abilities may gradually deteriorate. It is critical to talk with knowledgeable collateral sources about symptom onset. Careful questioning about memory and cognitive changes other than these behaviors is important. Over time, memory and speech changes progress, and after a few years the patient clinically resembles the more typical patient with moderate or severe DAT. This syndrome has been referred to as dementia of the frontal lobe type. Several dementias can demonstrate this clinical picture, including Pick's disease, vascular dementia, and frontal lobe degeneration of the non-Alzheimer type; however, Alzheimer's disease accounts for a substantial proportion of such cases.

DAT can also begin with focal involvement of the areas of the dominant temporal and parietal lobes subserving language. Such patients may have several years of progressive difficulty with finding words, and it becomes increasingly difficult for them to convey meaning verbally. They may substitute the wrong word or demonstrate thought blockage. Over years, such a patient may become completely mute. Early in the course of this aphasic syndrome, memory, judgment, intelligence, functioning, hobbies, and activities may be preserved, but eventually such patients begin to demonstrate memory deficits and other symptoms of dementia appear. These patients eventually resemble the more typical patient with DAT. This clinical presentation may occur in rare non-Alzheimer dementing processes; however, more often this syndrome represents a more focal presentation of Alzheimer's disease.

Differential Diagnosis

Many illnesses can cause the syndrome of dementia; however, DAT, either alone or with other dementing disorders, is the most common cause of dementia among the elderly in North America. Accurate diagnosis of the specific type of dementia is becoming increasingly important as treatments become more specific. Drugs that interfere with amyloid deposition may prove effective in slowing the progression of DAT, but they are unlikely to influence the natural history of vascular dementia.

Some causes of dementia are listed in Box 12-2. A major purpose of evaluating patients with dementia is to determine whether diseases other than DAT are causing or contributing to the dementia. If so, treating the primary disorder may halt the progression of the dementia or possibly reverse it. Unfortunately, few patients have truly reversible dementias. Two of the more common causes of reversible dementia are medications and major depression.

The evaluation of a patient with dementia requires a careful history from knowledgeable collateral sources and the patient. This history gathering may require multiple visits and examinations over time. A complete workup that includes a physical examination is important. In addition to psychiatric and neurological examinations, brief or more formal cognitive testing is often valuable to establish a baseline for comparison as the illness progresses.

The extent of laboratory and imaging workup remains controversial. Examining electrolytes, BUN, creatinine, liver function tests, calcium, vitamin B_{12}, sedimentation rate, complete blood count (CBC), syphilis screening, thyroid function, and urine is often recommended. Human immunodeficiency virus (HIV) testing might be considered. Measuring plasma levels of currently used medications can be helpful. Many physicians believe that computerized tomography (CT) or MRI of the brain is useful and worth the expense. Lumbar puncture is usually not required or helpful if the illness has a typical course that has been present for 1 year or more. Special tests may be important if a physician suspects rare genetic causes of dementias, such as Huntington's disease, but this is likely to require consultation with physicians who are experts in genetic illnesses.

The non-Alzheimer brain degenerative disorders that cause dementia consist of a group of interesting diseases. Patients with Parkinson's disease are at high risk for both depression and dementia. Approximately 50% of people with Parkinson's disease have had or will subsequently develop major depression. Approximately 30% of patients with Parkinson's disease de-

BOX 12-2

EXAMPLES OF DEMENTIAS OTHER THAN DEMENTIA OF THE ALZHEIMER TYPE

Non-Alzheimer primary central nervous system (CNS) degenerative disorders

Parkinson's disease with dementia
Lewy body dementia
Pick's disease
Huntington's disease
Non-Alzheimer frontal lobe dementia

Other CNS disorders

Vascular dementias
Major depression
Brain injury
CNS infections
Neoplasms involving CNS
Hydrocephalus
Subdural hematoma

Disorders related to exogenous substances

Medication-induced disorders
Substance-abuse-induced disorders

Systemic disorders

Endocrine disorders: thyroid, parathyroid disorders
Cardiovascular disorders
Immune system disorders
Hepatic disorders
Renal disorders
Nutritional deficits: vitamin B_{12} deficiency

velop a dementia. The relationship between dementia and Parkinson's disease is complex. People with DAT are at increased risk for developing extrapyramidal symptoms such as bradykinesia, tremor, gait disturbance, and rigidity, and they may have anatomical changes in the substantia nigra consistent with Parkinson's disease. Patients who develop Parkinson's disease without initial symptoms of cognitive impairment have an increased risk of developing a dementia; however, the pathological changes related to dementia are varied. In addition to evidence of Parkinson's disease involving the substantia nigra, typical pathological findings of Alzheimer's disease with widely distributed senile plaques and neurofibrillary tangles may be present. Other patients may have evidence of Parkinson's disease together with cortical Lewy bodies but be without evidence of Alzheimer's disease. Further research is necessary to elucidate and clinically identify the multiple mechanisms responsible for dementia in Parkinson's disease.

A syndrome referred to as Lewy body dementia has been described, and recent work suggests that this disorder may be one of the more common dementias after DAT. The brains of people with this illness demonstrate intraneuronal cortical Lewy bodies with or without the presence of amyloid plaques, especially in areas such as the anterior cingulate cortex. Neurofibrillary tangles are commonly absent. (Even at the microscopic level, there is likely to be overlap in the pathological diagnoses of Alzheimer's disease with plaques, tangles, and occasional Lewy bodies, and "primary" Lewy body dementia.) Although the clinical presentation can overlap with that of DAT, several clinical features may increase the likelihood of pathologically defined Lewy body dementia. These clinical features include substantial fluctuation in cognitive abilities, visual or auditory hallucinations at an early stage of illness when cognitive abilities are relatively intact, extrapyramidal symptoms, and repeated falls. Distinguishing Lewy body disease from DAT plus a delirium can be difficult. Careful longitudinal evaluation may be necessary. This distinction will become increasingly important as medications are developed that target the abnormal pathophysiological processes of DAT.

Vascular dementia is defined as dementia as a consequence of cerebrovascular disease. Risk factors are those that predispose patients to cerebrovascular disease, including hypertension, heart disease, and disorders leading to cerebral emboli. The precise relationship of cerebral infarcts to dementia requires further research. The number, location, and size of infarcts necessary for symptoms of dementia are not well characterized. Most agree that multiple strokes involving large areas of the brain compromise CNS cognitive function. However, the role of single discrete lesions or multiple clinically silent lesions demonstrated by brain imaging studies is uncertain. Evidence of strokes from clinical history, clinical examination, and imaging coupled with cognitive changes linked to the cerebrovascular event suggest the diagnosis of vascular dementia. The course of symptoms fluctuates substantially, depending on the nature of the infarct. Cerebrovascular disease is common, and people who die without clinical evidence of dementia can have significant numbers of small infarcts. Patients dying with Alzheimer's disease but with no clinical evidence of cerebrovascular disease similarly can have multiple, small, scattered infarcts. Patients with DAT can also have clinically evident infarcts. Infarcts can worsen the symptoms of DAT (see the Pearls & Perils box below). Pure vascular dementia in the absence of Alzheimer's disease occurs, but separating such cases from patients with mixed vascular dementia and DAT is difficult. Vascular dementias have a fluctuating course but can progress rapidly. Minimizing the risk of future cerebrovascular events may slow the progression of pure vascular dementia if the reason for progression is recurrent infarcts.

Epidemiology

Alzheimer's disease can be caused by different mechanisms (Box 12-3). A small percentage of patients have one of several rare genetic forms of the disease that clearly follow autosomal dominant inheritance. Recently, an important relationship between apolipoprotein E (apoE) subtype and the risk of DAT has been reported. A person can inherit zero, one, or two copies of the apoE4 allele. The greater the number of

PEARLS & PERILS

ISSUES PERTAINING TO DIFFERENTIAL DIAGNOSIS OF DEMENTIA OF THE ALZHEIMER TYPE

- Although DAT often initially presents with subtle changes in memory and personality, presentations suggesting initial focal pathological conditions can occur.
- Contrary to earlier beliefs, truly reversible dementias in the elderly are not common. Medication-induced dementia and dementia of depression are two types of potentially reversible dementias.
- Patients with DAT can also have symptomatic or silent cerebral infarcts.
- Pure vascular dementia in the absence of Alzheimer's disease may be difficult to differentiate from a mixed dementia caused by Alzheimer's disease and cerebral infarcts.

apoE4 alleles, the greater the risk for DAT. A substantial percentage of patients who develop DAT do not have known genetic, biochemical, or environmental risk factors. Little is known about the epidemiology of these different subtypes, and the epidemiological information discussed in this section pertains to clinically defined DAT without regard to subtypes.

The major risk factor for DAT is age. The illness is rare in people younger than age 50. Dementias occur in 5% to 10% of those age 65 and older and in one third or more of people who are 85 and older. Over one half of people with dementia have DAT. The incidence doubles every 5 years from age 65 to 85, but the incidence over age 90 is not clear. About 1% to 2% of people age 70 to 79 develop dementia annually; this percentage increases to about 3% to 3.5% in people age 80 to 84 and to about 8% in people age 85 and older. Any intervention that delays the illness onset by 5 years can eventually decrease the prevalence by one half. The lifetime risk of developing DAT is estimated at 6% for men and 16% for women.

An estimate of the number of people with dementia is influenced by how the illness is defined in the epidemiological survey. Some survey instruments define dementia in terms of performance on brief cognitive batteries. Using these instruments, a large number of people in the very mild stage of illness are not counted. Conservative estimates suggest that there are over 2.5 million people with dementia; 1.5 million of these have DAT. As the baby-boom generation ages, this number is likely to triple over the next 40 to 50 years. The cost in dollars is staggering; the emotional cost is devastating.

In addition to increasing age, a family history of DAT in a first-degree relative increases risk. Although the risk to an identical twin of a proband is high, concordance is not near 100%, suggesting that environmental factors are also involved. DAT is more common in women than in men, even after correcting for the increased proportion of elderly women. There is increasing evidence that educational achievement or early intellectual abilities may influence the risk of DAT; the higher the achievement, the lower the risk. The mechanism for this relationship is not well defined.

Down syndrome is a major risk factor for the development of DAT. Approximately one half of all people with Down syndrome who reach their 40s develop a progressive dementing disorder consistent with DAT that is superimposed on their baseline cognitive abilities. At autopsy, such people with Down syndrome have the neuropathological changes of Alzheimer's disease. It is likely that the extra copy of chromosome 21 carrying the gene for amyloid precursor protein is responsible for this relationship between Down syndrome and Alzheimer's disease.

BOX 12-3

ALZHEIMER'S DISEASES

Autosomal dominant genetic disorders

Chromosome 21: amyloid precursor protein mutations
Chromosome 14: mutation in S182 (presenilin 1)
Chromosome 1: mutation in STM2 (presenilin 2)

Associated with other genetic disorders

Down syndrome: trisomy 21

Genetic risk factors

ApoE4 associated
Family history in first-degree relative

Environmental factors

Head trauma

Boxers may develop a dementia (dementia pugilistica), and it is likely that major recurrent head trauma may increase the risk of DAT. Additionally, major depressive disorder (MDD) might be a risk factor for developing DAT. The risk from aluminum remains poorly defined and controversial.

Pathophysiology

Alzheimer's disease is defined by clinical course coupled with characteristic pathological findings in the brain. Characterizing the CNS pathology associated with Alzheimer's disease is important for determining the pathophysiology. At the level of the whole brain, atrophy can be evident; however, there is great variability in its degree and location. Usually primary motor and sensory areas are affected less than association regions. In some cases, disproportionate focal atrophy can be substantial. Such atrophy can be seen with brain imaging studies.

At the microscopic level, neuronal loss can be dramatic. Senile plaques, consisting of β-amyloid together with many other substances, occur in large numbers throughout many cortical regions. Some plaques are diffuse in appearance; others have dense central cores. Some plaques have components of deteriorating intracellular neuronal material referred to as *neuritic changes;* some do not. It is possible but not proven that plaques age from younger, diffuse forms to the dense core appearance. There is great heterogeneity in plaque type, burden, and location in the brains of people who died during similar stages of illness. Although neocortical plaques can occur in small clumps in a few areas of the cortex in people without dementia, the presence of multiple plaques in several regions of the cortex is highly suggestive of Alzheimer's disease.

Intraneuronal neurofibrillary tangles are another neuropathological feature of most patients with Alzheimer's disease. A major component of tangles is an abnormally phosphorylated cytoskeletal protein called *tau*. The number and location of tangles is also quite variable in persons with DAT. With age, tangles can accumulate in areas in and near the hippocampus in the absence of Alzheimer's disease. With DAT, tangles increase in and near the hippocampus, and they occur in many neocortical regions. The presence of neocortical (but not hippocampal) tangles is usually indicative of a pathological condition.

DAT is almost always associated with both amyloid plaques and neurofibrillary tangles. The relationship between plaque formation and the development of neurofibrillary tangles is unclear. Relationships between the various markers of the illness and the mechanisms linking structural and functional changes in neurons will be greatly aided by study of animal models.

Other neuropathological abnormalities can be seen in the brains of people affected by Alzheimer's disease. These include Hirano bodies, granulovacuolar degeneration, and Lewy bodies. Little is known about the relationship of these changes to neuronal loss, plaques, and tangles.

Over the last several years, substantial progress has been made in understanding the molecular biology and genetics of Alzheimer's disease. The brains of people with Down syndrome who live beyond 40 years invariably have the neuropathological lesions of Alzheimer's disease. These patients have three copies of chromosome 21. The gene for amyloid precursor protein is located on chromosome 21. One of the main chemical constituents of amyloid plaques is β-amyloid, a 39 to 42 amino acid fragment of amyloid precursor protein. The association of Down syndrome with DAT suggests that excess amyloid precursor protein from an extra copy of chromosome 21 leads to the production of excess β-amyloid. Such accumulation may eventually cause DAT.

As noted, several families have a history of early-onset DAT with an autosomal dominant pattern of inheritance. Recently, genetic defects on chromosome 21 in such families have been described as leading to single amino acid substitutions in amyloid precursor protein. When the mutated form of amyloid precursor protein is inherited, the individual develops Alzheimer's disease.

Amyloid precursor protein is a transmembrane protein. Its function is unknown. Amyloid precursor protein is processed by multiple proteases into smaller fragments, most of which appear to be soluble and eliminated, and varying amounts of less soluble β-amyloid. This β-amyloid can accumulate, aggregate, and form plaques. Some of the single amino acid mutations found in families with autosomal dominant Alzheimer's disease lead to abnormal processing of amyloid precursor protein and increased production of the less soluble β-amyloid.

Another group of families has autosomal dominant early-onset DAT but the location of the genetic abnormality is on chromosome 14. The specific location on chromosome 14 and its associated gene product have recently been identified. Similarly, another familial form of DAT associated with Volga German kindreds has recently been localized to a defect on chromosome 1. The predicted gene product of the candidate gene on chromosome 1 demonstrates intriguing similarities with the chromosome 14 gene product. Knowledge concerning the pathophysiology of Alzheimer's disease continues to advance as more is learned about the relationship of these gene products and symptoms of the illness.

The hypothesis that β-amyloid may be directly involved in the pathogenesis of Alzheimer's disease has been further strengthened by the recent work with transgenic mice who produce either excess or mutated forms of amyloid precursor protein. These animals develop senile plaques with age.

To summarize, increasing evidence strongly suggests that one pathway leading to Alzheimer's disease involves abnormalities in the amyloid precursor protein gene, leading to the accumulation of β-amyloid, which in turn may lead to further pathological changes and clinical symptoms.

Components of the complement system, microglia, and cytokines also accumulate in senile plaques along with amyloid. It is possible that plaque formation and maturation trigger several events, including an immune response. Other compounds such as excitotoxins (excess excitatory amino acid transmitters) may be released by injured cells, leading to further damage. It is not difficult to envision several cascades of destructive events. The recent development of transgenic animal models of Alzheimer's disease should help elucidate some of these events.

Another important recent finding involves apolipoproteins. ApoE2, E3, and E4 are involved in the body's handling of triglycerides and cholesterol. They are produced in the brain, but their specific functions have not been elucidated. ApoE2, E3, and E4 differ from each other by a single amino acid substitution. Every person inherits an apoE allele from each parent. As mentioned, a strong correlation has recently been demonstrated between the number of copies of E4 and risk of developing DAT. In people who have dementia, those with apoE4 alleles have an earlier onset of illness than those without E4 alleles. Furthermore, apoE2 appears to decrease the risk of developing DAT. It needs to be emphasized that many elderly individuals with apoE4 alleles do not have symptoms of DAT. Additionally, people without apoE4 alleles develop Alzheimer's disease.

The mechanisms responsible for the relationship of E4 burden and increased risk for DAT are not known. The relationship of DAT and apolipoprotein genotype may be stronger in whites than in blacks. Much more epidemiological research is necessary to clarify the cultural and biological diversity of the relationship between DAT and the apoE system.

It is possible that the pathophysiological changes responsible for the clinical presentation of DAT occur for decades before the appearance of symptoms. Extracellular amyloid might accumulate until a critical threshold is reached and biophysical changes that lead to the formation of less soluble amyloid occur. Once precipitation into diffuse and then hard core plaques occurs, further damage to neurons can be initiated. Dying neurons may release other toxins (Figure 12-1). If this amyloid cascade hypothesis is correct, factors that increase the production or decrease the removal of amyloid should increase the risk of disease. People who remain below a critical amyloid burden should be spared the illness. If there is some truth to the above hypothesis, determination of amyloid burden could lead to early detection and early intervention. Delaying onset or slowing progression in illnesses that clinically begin late in life can decrease the prevalence substantially.

Treatment

Over the next several years, better treatments will become available for DAT. Existing treatments act by replacing or increasing neurotransmitters, such as acetylcholine, that are lost as a result of cellular destruction. The efficacy of treatments that block processes involved in CNS destruction, such as inflammatory responses, are actively being investigated. Future treatments may attempt to block or reverse the formation of abnormal CNS substances such as amyloid plaques. Reversal of damage, although unlikely in the near future, remains an eventual possibility as the science and clinical utility of growth factors and genetic manipulations advance. The focus of this section is a discussion of the treatment approaches currently available.

DAT is an illness that involves patients together with their families and loved ones. Without good caregiver support, the person with DAT suffers. Current treatment strategies include biopsychosocial approaches (see the Pearls & Perils box on p. 207). Biological treatment includes pharmacotherapy for cognitive and other psychiatric symptoms of the illness. Psychosocial intervention involves educational programs, resource referrals, and psychological support systems for patients and caregivers. The Alzheimer's Association provides groups and expertise in resource referrals.

An early phase of treatment involves teaching the patient and the family about Alzheimer's disease. Emphasizing to the caregiver that changes in behavior are not the patient's fault but a result of gradual CNS deterioration helps minimize blame and stress. The abilities of patients and their families to accept and understand the implications of a diagnosis of DAT vary greatly, and it is important to individualize the manner in which this information is conveyed. Discussions may require several visits. Appropriate referrals to reading material, the Alzheimer's Association, and social services should be done in a timely but sensitive manner. Several visits are often necessary to confirm initial diagnostic impressions in people with very mild symptoms, and it is important to be convinced of the likelihood of the diagnosis before beginning the full educational process. Many elderly people are appropriately fearful of the diagnosis of DAT, and words need to be chosen carefully.

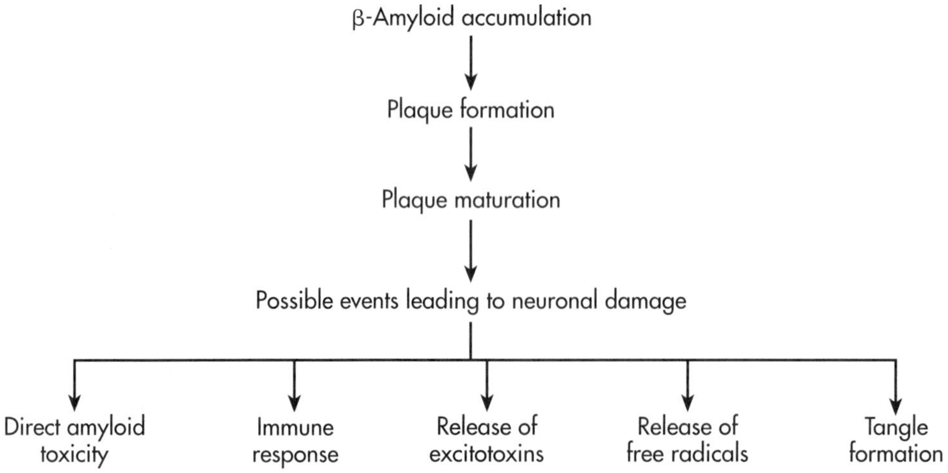

FIGURE 12-1 Possible mechanisms involving amyloid and Alzheimer's disease.

If the diagnosis is likely but uncertain, it is important to indicate that there is uncertainty and explain that time will be necessary to clarify the diagnosis. Once the illness has declared itself, patients and their families need to know so planning can begin. If a patient and his family have not yet formalized an advanced directive regarding health care, this should be addressed. The course of the illness is gradual but progressive, and medical, financial, and legal plans need to be made with patients' full input. People's reactions to learning about the illness vary from fear to relief. Insight may be compromised even early in the illness. The disclosure of the diagnosis and education can be the most difficult phase of treatment for the physician. Patients and families are usually appreciative of a direct but caring approach.

General principles of pharmacological management in the elderly are reviewed in Chapter 25. Patients with DAT are often sensitive to cognition-impairing side effects of medications, and therefore simplifying pharmacological regimens and minimizing doses of necessary medications can help improve cognitive function.

PEARLS & PERILS

TREATMENT OF DEMENTIA OF THE ALZHEIMER TYPE

- Pharmacological treatments for DAT are under active investigation, and it is likely that a variety of agents that work via different mechanisms will become available over the next several years.
- Education of caregivers as well as patients about DAT is crucial.
- Depressive symptoms are common in DAT and should be carefully evaluated and treated.
- Psychotic symptoms should be evaluated in light of how disruptive and uncomfortable they are for the patient and caregivers. A brief course of antipsychotic medication may be beneficial. Side effects should be monitored carefully. Attempts should often be made to decrease the dose and discontinue these medications while evaluating the presence and severity of target symptoms.
- Agitation can be precipitated by medical illness, pain, or delirium in patients with DAT. Therefore these conditions should be addressed in the agitated patient.

Cognitive Symptoms

Specific pharmacological management of the progressive cognitive dysfunction is evolving. As CNS destruction occurs, various neurotransmitter systems are compromised. The central acetylcholinergic system is involved in memory and learning. It has been thought that the cholinergic system is selectively involved in DAT, and initial pharmacological strategies involving acetylcholine were proposed to be analogous to dopaminergic strategies in treating Parkinson's disease. Although it has become apparent that multiple other CNS transmitter systems are involved in DAT, cholinergic replacement strategies have been the most aggressively investigated. Increasing acetylcholinergic function by inhibiting metabolism via acetylcholinesterase has been successful in producing an agent that is more effective than placebo in temporarily improving cognitive symptoms. Tacrine became available for treatment of DAT in 1993. It is helpful in only a minority of patients. The higher doses that are associated with the best response are difficult to tolerate because of gastrointestinal side effects and elevations in liver enzymes. Responses are rarely dramatic. Tacrine is started at low doses and gradually increased, with careful monitoring of liver enzymes. Little is known about the utility of this agent in the patient who is medically frail and requires other medications. Increasing reports of pharmacokinetic and pharmacodynamic interactions are likely to accumulate, as is true with any new medication. Tacrine represents the beginning of an era of pharmacotherapies that are more effective than placebo. It is not a cure but a beginning. Other cholinergic agents are likely to become available and eventually may provide better efficacy with fewer side effects.

Studies of a large variety of agents that interact with neurotransmitter receptors are underway. These studies include drugs that interact with transmitters other than acetylcholine. Such trials will provide alternative treatments in the not too distant future. In addition to transmitter system replacement therapies, work investigating antiinflammatory agents is in progress. The basis for these trials involves data suggesting that an inflammatory response is involved in the CNS damage. There is evidence suggesting that estrogens exert a protective effect from DAT in women, and studies are being conducted or planned to explore this possibility.

Recent knowledge about the possible pathophysiology of DAT involving amyloid processing, as well as the relationship of apoE4 and DAT, suggests possibilities for designing specific agents to interfere with amyloid production or to block the role of apoE4. The recent development of transgenic mouse models of Alzheimer's disease should aid in the development of pharmacotherapies to target these processes. Eventually, a variety of therapies may be used in combination to aid in the treatment of specific subtypes of DAT.

Depressive Symptoms

Depressive symptoms are common in DAT, as discussed in Chapter 25. It may be difficult to determine whether such symptoms represent a concurrent major depressive episode. However, if depressive symptoms include dysphoria, marked decreased interest, guilt, low self-esteem, or suicidal thoughts, they should be addressed. Treatment depends on the nature and number of symptoms and the degree of discomfort they create. Suicidal ideations require careful evaluation. Patients who become severely dysphoric and apathetic may stop eating and become withdrawn. Their sleep becomes disrupted, and they may develop delusions of sin or guilt, as well as hallucinations. Untreated, such patients can die from suicide or self-neglect. They may lack insight, and their symptoms of dementia may be confounded by additional cognitive decline as a result of depression. Although there is not a great deal of research on the responsivity of depressive symptoms to treatment in patients with DAT, major depression generally responds to treatment in patients with other medical illnesses. Treatment options include pharmacotherapies, psychotherapies, and electroconvulsive therapy (ECT), depending on the severity of symptoms, the nature of family support, and the patient's cognitive ability. These patients often have a gratifying response to ECT. During treatment they may become confused; however, shortly after the course of ECT their cognition returns to baseline and their mood, appetite, activities, and self-care return to levels present before the depression began. Once such depressive symptoms are successfully treated, maintaining remission may require either maintenance ECT (see Chapter 22) or maintenance pharmacotherapy.

If a patient in the very mild stages of dementia has depressive symptoms that are not life threatening (that is, suicidal ideations or plans are absent and adequate self-care is maintained), psychotherapeutic therapy or pharmacotherapy can be helpful. Patients and their families benefit from supportive therapy. Behavioral approaches may help with mild symptoms. Frequent office visits where mood is assessed and practical information exchanged can lead to symptomatic improvement. Specific psychotherapies may be helpful, depending on the patient's ability to understand and actively participate in such approaches. Antidepressant medications can be effective, especially when they are coupled with support and advice. Tricyclic antidepressants (TCAs) with high anticholinergic properties such as amitriptyline are not good choices for the elderly patient who is cognitively impaired. In addition to interfering with cognition and having peripheral anticholinergic side effects, these agents can cause orthostatic hypotension and sedation. Recently, a number of effective and relatively safe antidepressants have become available, although little is specifically known concerning their safety and efficacy in individuals who are depressed and demented. Serotonin-selective reuptake inhibitors (SSRIs) such as fluoxetine, paroxetine, and sertraline are often prescribed. The SSRIs are powerful inhibitors of the P-450 enzymes in the liver, and therefore the physician needs to be aware of the potential for pharmacokinetic interactions. Starting with low doses, building gradually to therapeutic levels, and being aware of the potential for drug interactions and long half-lives are important principles. Newer agents, such as venlafaxine and nefazodone, have potential to be useful in this population. Monoamine oxidase inhibitors (MAOIs) have been reported to be excellent antidepressants in the elderly; however, concerns exist about dietary complications, potentially severe drug interactions, and compliance. Excellent books are available to address specifics of antidepressant pharmacotherapies. Especially during early stages of treatment, patients should be closely monitored. Once depressive symptoms are stable, treatment should be maintained for about 6 months before considering a gradual withdrawal of the antidepressant. Side effects need to be assessed often to determine whether benefits of treatment outweigh risks. When tapering patients off medications, follow-up visits are important to evaluate whether symptoms are returning. If symptoms reappear, increasing the dose of medication can minimize morbidity. The natural history of depressive symptoms in dementia is unknown, and therefore attention to reoccurrence over the years is necessary.

Psychotic Symptoms

Psychotic symptoms commonly occur during the middle stages of DAT. The natural history of such symptoms in dementia has not been well characterized. Such symptoms may not become chronic. Although hallucinations and delusions respond to judicious use of low doses of antipsychotic medication, antipsychotic medications have potentially severe side effects in the elderly patient with dementia, including parkinsonian symptoms, orthostatic hypotension, falls, sedation, confusion, and tardive dyskinesia. Before initiating treatment, it is important to evaluate how disruptive and uncomfortable the symptoms are to the patient and their caregivers. If the symptoms do not seem overly distressing, explaining that such symptoms are common and teaching simple behavioral approaches may adequately alleviate the discomfort. If symptoms become overwhelming or interfere with function, a course of antipsychotic medication such as haloperidol can be helpful. Frequent, brief visits to the physician are recommended to monitor efficacy and side effects. In some patients, agitation and irritability may be triggered by psychotic symptoms, and substantial improvement in these behaviors is possible with antipsychotic medication. The risk of tardive dyskinesia increases with length of treatment and can occur within months in elderly patients who have compromised brain function. After psychotic symptoms have remitted for a few weeks, dose reduction should be attempted. Medications can sometimes be gradually stopped, and psychotic symptoms remain in remission. If symptoms reappear, another decision based on risk vs. benefit needs to be made regarding resuming pharmacotherapy.

Agitation

Patients in the moderate or late stages of dementia can develop severe irritability and agitation. These behaviors are difficult for a caregiver either at home or in a nursing home. A careful history and observation may reveal precipitating factors in the environment, and behavioral interventions can be initiated. Additionally, concomitant medical illnesses, pain, or a delirium can precipitate agitation. If a delirium is caused by a urinary tract infection, an antibiotic might be the treatment of choice for the accompanying agitation. If agitation is primarily related to DAT, and if behavioral approaches have been ineffective, pharmacotherapy together with behavioral management may be required. Antipsychotic medications can be effective at alleviating agitation; however, the cautions concerning side effects that have already been discussed still apply. If an antipsychotic is required, the need to continue treatment should be reevaluated frequently, since the underlying symptoms may spontaneously resolve. Too often a patient in a nursing home is kept on antipsychotic medication for months or years. Once the behavior has subsided for several weeks, a slow tapering of antipsychotic medication should begin. Removal of the antipsychotic drug and increased attention to behavioral and supportive approaches can be successful in maintaining remission of the agitation. Some patients require long-term pharmacotherapy, but this should be empirically determined by repeated attempts at dose reduction of these agents. New antipsychotic medications with fewer serious side effects are likely to become available in the near future and should allow for safer effective treatment.

Since antipsychotic medications have substantial side effects, other agents have been tried for treating agitation or aggressiveness. Agents as diverse as trazodone, beta blockers, anticonvulsants, lithium, and buspirone have been reported to help specific patients. Large-scale controlled studies are necessary to define which agents are more effective than placebo or antipsychotics.

There are a variety of other behaviors that can be disabling and disruptive. Patients can have hypomanic behaviors. Little is known about efficacy of treatment of these behaviors with antimanic agents such as lithium or valproic acid. Some patients with moderate to severe illness exhibit loud and repetitive screaming behavior. These patients may not even realize that they are the ones who are screaming. These patients may respond to behavioral or to low-dose pharmacological interventions, but some do not improve and are difficult management challenges.

Conclusion

In the past, when an elderly person became extremely forgetful, it was labelled *senility* and considered a part of the aging process. Few physicians were interested in treating these frail elderly people. Over the last 15 years, increased attention has been devoted to diagnosis, staging, and elucidation of the natural history of dementia. The majority of people who reach their mid-80s can enjoy cognitive health. Severe cognitive deterioration is not inevitable. Advances in molecular genetics and neurobiology coupled with careful diagnostic and descriptive clinical research have led to major advances in the understanding of dementing disorders. Therapeutic nihilism is being replaced by excitement about the therapeutic possibilities that are in the near future. This chapter has attempted to review some of the advances and reflect the excitement that exists in the field of dementia research. The primary care practitioner is the front line physician in treating dementia. Although geriatricians, geriatric psychiatrists, and geriatric neurologists can help provide consultation, there are too few such specialists to provide the primary care for the millions of patients affected. The more the primary care physician becomes interested in evaluating mental status, including cognition, mood, and psychosis, the better equipped he will be to help these patients and their families. Whether new pharmacological treatments will be only minimally, moderately, or very effective is unknown. However, there is little doubt that a large number of treatments will become available; staying current with this rapidly advancing field will be an exciting challenge for all physicians.

CONSIDER CONSULTATION WHEN . . .

- There is diagnostic confusion
- The patient's behavior becomes dangerous to himself or others
- Psychiatric symptoms are not responding to behavioral intervention or standard use of psychotropic medications
- Psychotropic management becomes complicated as a result of side effects or interactions with other medications

Acknowledgment

I would like to acknowledge the support of the Washington University Alzheimer's Disease Research Center (grant no. P50 AGO 5681). I would also like to thank Dr. Leonard Berg for his leadership and for his critical review of this chapter.

Annotated Bibliography

Coffey CE, Cummings JL, editors: *Textbook of geriatric neuropsychiatry,* Washington, D.C., 1994, American Psychiatric Press.
This is a superb book that contains excellent chapters addressing geriatric psychiatric disorders, as well as reviews of CNS structure and function.

Morris JC, editor: *Handbook of dementing illnesses,* New York, 1994, Marcel Dekker.
This book contains excellent reviews of Alzheimer's disease and other dementias.

Salzman C, editor: *Clinical geriatric psychopharmacology,* ed 2, Baltimore, 1992, Williams and Wilkins.
This is a good review of the principles and practice of geriatric psychopharmacology.

Schatzberg AF, Nemeroff CB, editors: *Textbook of psychopharmacology,* Washington, D.C., 1995, American Psychiatric Press.
This is an excellent, up-to-date general psychopharmacological text.

Terry RD, Katzman R, Bick KL, editors: *Alzheimer's disease,* New York, 1994, Raven Press.
This is another source for excellent reviews of Alzheimer's disease and other dementias.

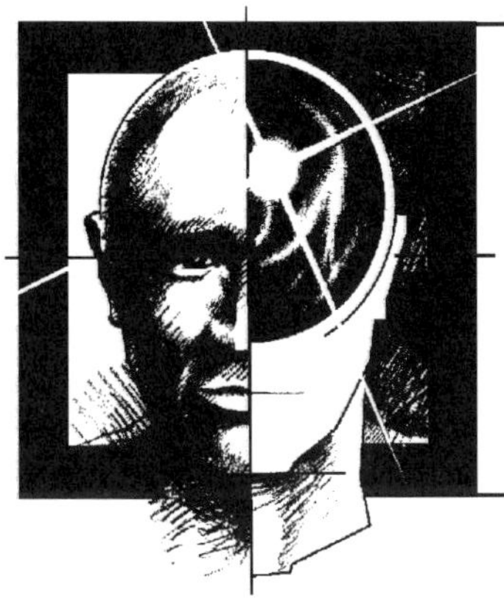

chapter 13

Schizophrenia and Delusional Disorders

John W. Newcomer, MD

This chapter will provide an overview of the psychotic disorders, schizophrenia and delusional disorders. As a group, psychotic disorders present an array of some of the most striking, and disabling, behavioral signs and symptoms to be found in clinical practice. The results of the recent National Comorbidity Survey suggested that 0.7% of the general population has a "nonaffective psychosis" (that is, schizophrenia, schizophreniform disorder, schizoaffective disorder, delusional disorder, or atypical psychosis) at some point in their lifetime. The Epidemiologic Catchment Area (ECA) survey, sponsored by the National Institute of Mental Health (NIMH), suggested that 1% to 1.5% of the general population is afflicted with schizophrenia over the course of their life. It has been estimated that more than 1 million individuals in the United States currently suffer from schizophrenia. These studies suggest that every primary care physician is likely to be involved in the care of some patients with schizophrenia. In fact, many primary care physicians are the only people responsible for the psychiatric management of some patients with schizophrenia or delusional disorders. The elevated mortality rate (estimated at 8 times the base rate for the general population), the high rate of suicide attempts and successful suicides (10% of all patients with schizophrenia die by suicide), and the adverse effect of the illness on general medical compliance all contribute to the problems that physicians face in treating these patients. Patients with these disorders can have symptoms that are a source of enormous subjective distress and disturb various aspects of physical, psychological, cognitive, occupational, and social functioning. These disorders also can be devastating to families and create a chronic stress and psychological burden that falls especially hard on the principal caregiver, as well as a financial burden that can

TABLE 13-1

PERCENTAGES OF U.S. ADULTS WITH SEVERE MENTAL DISORDERS*

Diagnosis	Percentage of adults (ages 18 years and above)
Schizophrenia	1.5
Manic-depressive illness (bipolar disorder)	1.0
Major depressive disorder	1.1
Panic disorder	0.4
Obsessive-compulsive disorder	0.6
Any of these diagnoses	2.8†

*Unpublished ECA data from the National Institute of Mental Health.
†A person may have more than one diagnosis at the same time. In this table these persons are counted once for each diagnosis and are included in more than one row. The percentages for each individual diagnosis cannot be added together to obtain the total percentage of the study population with any disorder.
From National Advisory Mental Health Council: Health care reform for Americans with severe mental illnesses: report of the National Advisory Mental Health Council, *Am J Psychiatry* 150:1450, 1993.

TABLE 13-2

COSTS OF RESPIRATORY DISEASE, CARDIOVASCULAR DISEASE, AND MENTAL ILLNESS IN 1990

	Amount (billions of dollars)		
Type of cost	Respiratory disease*	Cardiovascular disease*	Mental illness†
Direct	57	85	67
Indirect	42	75	75
Other, related	0	0	6
Total	99	160	148

*Unpublished data from the National Heart, Lung, and Blood Institute.
†Unpublished 1992 paper by DP Rice and LS Miller.
Modified from National Advisory Mental Health Council: Health care reform for Americans with severe mental illnesses: report of the National Advisory Mental Health Council, *Am J Psychiatry* 150:1460, 1993.

have long-lasting effects. The central primary care issue involves how to minimize morbidity, mortality, and the adverse effects of these disorders.

Schizophrenia is not rare. It is among the most common of the "severe mental illnesses" (Table 13-1), a grouping defined by the Senate Committee on Appropriations in relation to their 1993 appropriations bill for the Department of Health and Human Services. The Committee requested a report from the National Advisory Mental Health Council (NAMHC) concerning the costs and efficacy of treatment for severe mental illnesses in relation to other medical illnesses. This report was based on the wealth of data available through NIMH-supported research. The report underscores that, despite persistent myth, severe mental illnesses such as schizophrenia and delusional disorders are now readily definable and treatable. In fact, recent research advances in diagnosis and treatment permit many of those with severe mental illnesses to be treated as outpatients and have allowed millions of individuals to return to productive lives. Research from numerous well-controlled clinical trials has established the efficacy of specific treatments and the scientific basis for making clinical decisions, which has put the management of severe mental illnesses on par with other medical or surgical conditions (Figure 13-1). Unfortunately, schizophrenia and delusional disorders are typical of the severe mental illnesses in their chronicity and costs to society and closely match the overall costs of medical conditions such as respiratory and cardiovascular disease (Table 13-2). The NAMHC report also includes a more illustrative and detailed cost comparison of diabetes and schizophrenia (Table 13-3), which demonstrates comparable direct treatment costs but a greater potential for reducing morbidity and mortality costs through the treatment of schizophrenia.

This chapter will summarize the latest information on the epidemiology, course, symptom definitions, differential diagnoses, etiology, pathophysiology, and treatment for schizophrenia and delusional disorders. This chapter is organized by sections devoted to each general area, which can be read together or referred to separately for ease of use. The purpose of this chapter is to provide the primary care physician and the psychiatrist with a readable, succinct, state-of-the-art summary of information that bears on the evaluation, diagnosis, and management of patients with schizophrenia and delusional disorders. Schizophrenia is selected for review because of its higher prevalence and costs to society relative to other psychotic disorders and the correspondingly larger amount of research and clinical experience available for this disorder. Delusional disorders are selected for review principally to highlight the varied presentation of this entity, the central role of delusions in the presentation, and the illustrative differences in presentation and course relative to schizophrenia. A discussion of other nonaffective psychoses (such as schizoaffective disorder and brief psychotic disorder) is available from references in the annotated bibliography at the end of this chapter.

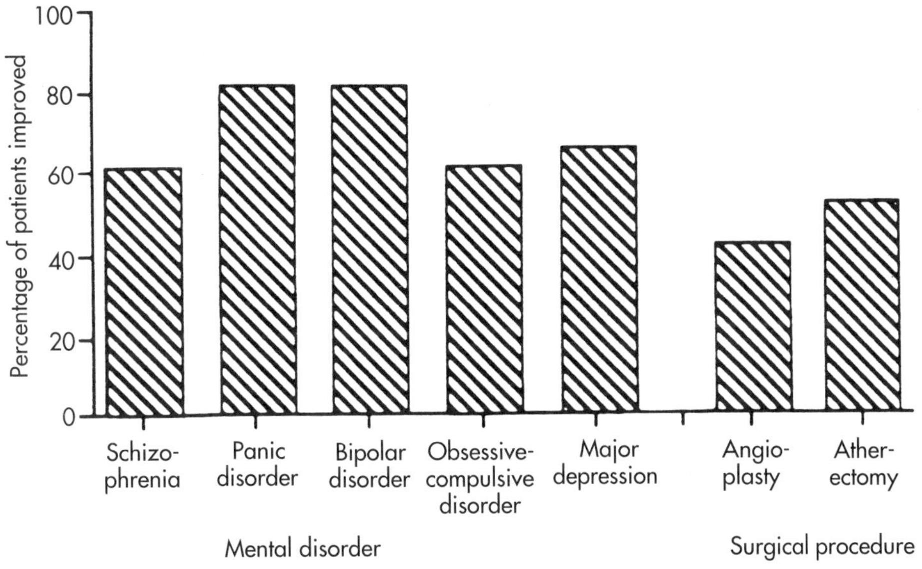

FIGURE 13-1 Treatment efficacy (early treatment outcome) for five severe mental disorders and two cardiovascular surgical procedures. Unpublished data from scientific reports on treatment efficacy commissioned by the National Institute of Mental Health. (From *Am J Psychiatry* 150:1447-1465, 1993.)

TABLE 13-3

COMPARATIVE COSTS OF SCHIZOPHRENIA AND DIABETES

Type of cost	Amount (billions of dollars)
Cost of schizophrenia (1990 estimates)*	
Direct	18
Patient care	17
Related	1
Indirect	15
Morbidity	11
Mortality	1
Other	3
Total	33
Cost of diabetes in 1990†	
Direct	17
Hospitalization	4
Nursing home	3
Related medical conditions	7
Other	3
Indirect	10
Disability	3
Mortality	7
Total	27

*Unpublished 1992 paper by DP Rice and LS Miller
†Data from Huse MA et al: The economic costs of non-insulin-dependent diabetes mellitus, *JAMA* 262:2708, 1989.
Modified from National Advisory Mental Health Council: Health care reform for Americans with severe mental illnesses: report of the National Advisory Mental Health Council, *Am J Psychiatry* 150:1461, 1993.

Epidemiology, Risk Factors, and Age of Onset

The most commonly cited lifetime prevalence of schizophrenia (how many people are diagnosed over the course of their lives) is 1.0% of the general population. The recent National Comorbidity Survey (NCS) suggests that 0.7% of the general population has a "nonaffective psychosis" at some point in their lifetime. This survey was based on a stratified multistage area probability sample of individuals between the ages of 15 and 54 in the noninstitutionalized civilian population of the 48 contiguous states. The NCS represents the state-of-the-art survey for epidemiology surveys of psychiatric disorder prevalence. Surveying samples of more than 3000 subjects at each of several sites in the United States, the ECA survey found that, overall, between 1.0% and 1.5% of the general population is afflicted with schizophrenia over the course of their life. This survey used careful controls for differences in age, sex, and ethnicity across the different sites and found no consistent confounding relationship between any demographic variable and the prevalence of schizophrenia. Remarkably, this prevalence figure of approximately 1% has generally been confirmed across large numbers of studies that cover most of the globe. There are specific reports that appear to describe a prevalence for schizophrenia that ranges more than tenfold across samples. However, this broad range of prevalence values is not generally believed to reflect true differences in the prevalence of schizophrenia across different countries, regions, or times but has instead been interpreted to reflect differences in the "strictness" of the diagnostic criteria used in the specific studies, the method of finding "cases," and other study-specific methodological issues. The true exceptions come from well-designed studies that use structured diagnostic interviews and that find a higher prevalence of schizophrenia in parts of Sweden and Croatia and a lower prevalence in parts of Micronesia and Papua-New Guinea.

The lifetime prevalence of delusional disorders is harder to estimate because of (1) changing diagnostic criteria for this entity over the past several decades, (2) the smaller number of studies addressing the prevalence of these disorders, and (3) most importantly, the relative infrequency of delusional disorders. Kendler and colleagues estimated the prevalence of delusional disorders to be between 0.024% and 0.030% and the prevalence of "other nonaffective psychoses" (inclusive of delusional disorders, schizophreniform disorders, and atypical psychoses) to be between 0.7% and 0.8% in the well-described Roscommon Family Study sample, a case-controlled epidemiologic family study based in a rural county in western Ireland. This result suggested that delusional disorders may be uncommon but not rare in the general population. Overall, these results emphasize that the group of all nonaffective psychoses occurs with sufficient frequency in an unscreened population (1.9% in the Roscommon sample) so that all physicians in primary practice will encounter such patients. In addition, the prevalence of all nonaffective psychoses in the first-degree relatives of patients with schizophrenia was found to be fivefold higher than in the relatives of unscreened controls.

TABLE 13-4

AGE-DISTRIBUTED RISK OF FIRST HOSPITALIZATION (BY SEX) FOR SCHIZOPHRENIA IN THE BRITISH POPULATION

	Cumulative % of total risk	
By age	**Men**	**Women**
15	1	1
20	11	11
25	31	25
30	51	44
35	70	60
40	81	72
45	91	83
50	96	92
55	100	100

Modified from Gottesman II: *Schizophrenia genesis: the origins of madness,* New York, 1991, W.H. Freeman and Company.

Risk factors (such as genetic factors, substance abuse, perinatal injuries) for the development of schizophrenia have been difficult to identify, with associations or risk factors sometimes found in one study but not in others. This inconsistency is in part a result of study-related methodological problems and in part may be the consequence of studying a heterogeneous disorder with different risk factors across different individuals. There is strong evidence that schizophrenia and other nonaffective psychoses have a genetic component. Several lines of converging evidence suggest that schizophrenia may be best conceptualized as a neurodevelopmental disorder related to genetic susceptibility and early brain insults that subsequently lead to progressive endogenous excitotoxic injury in critical brain regions. The role of genetic factors, environmental insults, and excitotoxic injury in the development of schizophrenia is discussed in the section on etiology and pathophysiology.

Although the lifetime risk of developing schizophrenia is not different for men and women, men have an earlier age of illness onset (Table 13-4). Additionally, men may have a more chronic course, but this is less clear. Delusional disorders have been reported to have a generally later age of illness onset (between 35 and 45 years) and to occur in both men and women, with conflicting data regarding a more common occurrence in either one gender or the other. When studies carefully and appropriately control for numerous potentially confounding factors, there is no convincing evidence for differences in relative rates of schizophrenia across different racial or ethnic groups or in urban vs. rural settings. Lower socioeconomic status, certainly a consequence of the disorders and perhaps a nonspecific contributing risk or stressor, is associated with both schizophrenia and delusional disorders. Similarly, substance abuse and adverse life events have been described as either causally related to the onset time for schizophrenia or, alternatively, as a psychosocial consequence of illness onset with its disruptions of multiple aspects of normal functioning. Sorting out these issues of cause vs. consequence requires careful and often prospective (that is, expensive) studies with large sample sizes. Despite their importance to primary prevention, these issues remain unsettled for schizophrenia and relatively unstudied for delusional disorders.

Recent investigations have addressed the special features of those patients with schizophrenia who have an uncharacteristic age of illness onset. Although early investigators recognized presentations with a late age of onset, some American diagnostic systems initially excluded patients with an age of onset over 40 or 45 years. The principal diagnostic system in use today (see Box 13-2, p. 221) has corrected this exclusion and now permits a diagnosis of schizophrenia independent of the age of the individual. Careful investigations have suggested that late-onset schizophrenia is more often of the paranoid subtype and has better social and occupational premorbid functioning in adolescence and early adulthood. In contrast, childhood or juvenile onset cases of schizophrenia have been reported to show greater prepsychotic impairments in social, developmental, and cognitive functioning.

Prognosis, Course, and Co-Morbidity

The prognosis for individual patients with schizophrenia or delusional disorders is a complex function of (1) the specific illness-related impairments suffered by the individual (some impairments have long-lasting consequences such as school failure or job and insurance loss); (2) their remission, persistence, or worsening over time (that is, the illness course); (3) treatment factors (such as antipsychotic medications); and (4) harmful prognosis-altering factors (Box 13-1). Overall, the course of illness in patients with schizophrenia is often chronic with a highly variable range of different patterns of exacerbation and remission (Figure 13-2). The variable clinical courses associated with schizophrenia have led to some debate about overall rates of remission or deterioration. There is some evidence that the frequency of progressively deteriorating outcomes may have diminished in recent decades. Since the advent of neuroleptic treatment in the late 1950s, treatment with antipsychotic medication may partly explain the apparent reduction in very poor outcomes. Recent work with an important model for schizophre-

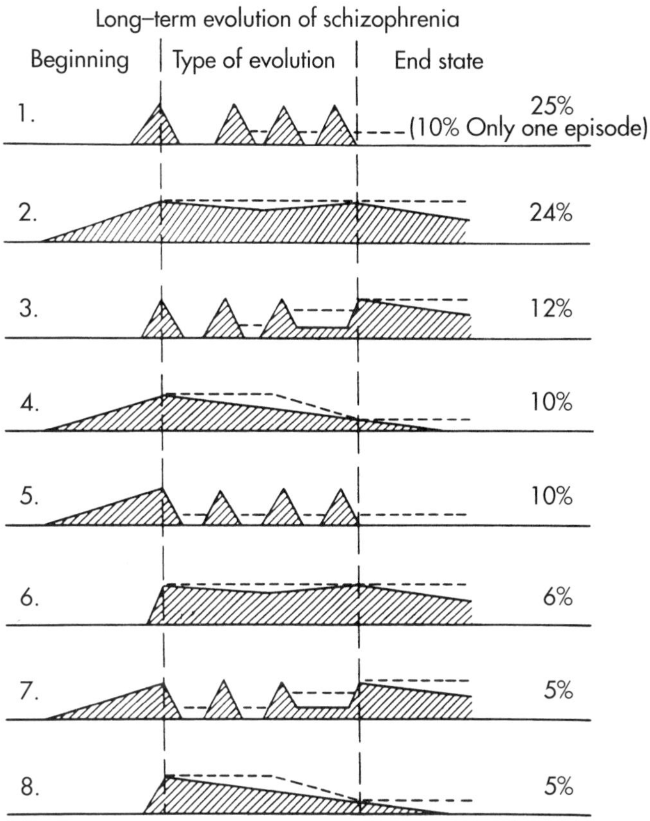

FIGURE 13-2 Schematic representations of the different types of long-term courses of schizophrenia (average follow-up 36.9 years, n = 228; *Dotted line* alternative forms of evolution within the same type). (From Ciompi L, Miller NE, Cohen GD, editors: *Schizophrenia and aging,* New York 1987, Guilford Press.

BOX 13-1

FEATURES ASSOCIATED WITH BETTER AND WORSE OUTCOMES IN SCHIZOPHRENIA

Better	Worse
Early, effective, and continuous antipsychotic medication treatment	No antipsychotic medication treatment, extended periods of untreated psychosis, or poor medication compliance
Relatively preserved cognitive function	Cognitive impairment, especially decreased memory and learning performance
Few relapses	Numerous relapses
No neurological examination findings	Neurological examination findings, including soft signs
Acute onset and course	Insidious onset and chronic course
Better premorbid social adjustment (e.g. married), sexual history, and work history	Worse premorbid social adjustment, sexual history, and work history
Late onset	Early onset
Predominantly positive symptoms	Predominantly negative symptoms
Affective symptoms	No affective symptoms
Family history of mood disorders	Family history of schizophrenia
Good support system	Poor support system (possibly including highly involved but highly critical systems)
No marked ventricular enlargement	Marked ventricular enlargement
No history of perinatal trauma	History of perinatal trauma

nia (see the section related to etiology and pathophysiology) suggests that antipsychotic medications may protect against a progressive endogenous neurotoxicity that could explain the deteriorating course of some patients.

Multiple hospitalizations have a profoundly disruptive and long-lasting effect on the social and occupational functioning of patients. The risk of exacerbation and repeated hospitalizations for patients with schizophrenia is principally reduced by adequate treatment with antipsychotic medications (Table 13-5). Morbidity is further enhanced by the loss of medical benefits and poor self-care that often accompany psychosis. Patients with schizophrenia also have a high rate of depression that adds to overall morbidity. The lifetime risk of a major depressive episode occurring secondary to schizophrenia has been estimated to be approximately 60%. Furthermore, it has been suggested that patients with negative symptoms may be at an even greater risk for depression. Beyond increased morbidity, schizophrenia has been found to be associated with an increased mortality rate that is largely explained by increased rates of completed suicide (as many as 10% of these patients die by suicide) and increased rates of violent deaths and cardiovascular disorders. Although the prediction of suicide is impossible, a number of factors confer increased risk (as they can also do in the general population): (1) male gender, (2) white race, (3) social isolation, (4) depression, (5) sense of hopelessness, (6) past history of suicide attempts, (7) family history of suicide, (8) unmarried status, (9) unemployed status, (10) deteriorating health with a high level of premorbid functioning, (11) recent loss or rejection, (12) parental loss during childhood, (13) limited external support, (14) family stress or instability.

Another important factor in the prediction of the illness course is substance abuse and dependence. The lifetime risk of comorbidity for alcohol and/or drug abuse and dependence in patients with schizophrenia is approximately 50%. Substance abuse and dependence has been associated with increased rates of violence and suicide, noncompliance with treatment, psychotic exacerbation, antipsychotic treatment refractoriness, hospitalization, tardive dyskinesia (TD), and homelessness. Treatment of the substance use disorder can reverse the adverse effects on overall prognosis. In general, violence and homicide do not appear to be more common in schizophrenia. The risk factors for violence in the hospital are low (subtherapeutic) plasma levels of antipsychotic medication, higher levels of overall psychosis, and a past history of violence. Contrary to persistent myth, psychotic patients are probably more likely to be the victims rather than the perpetrators of violence.

TABLE 13-5

CUMULATIVE RELAPSE RISK IN SCHIZOPHRENIA AFTER CONTINUED VS. DISCONTINUED NEUROLEPTIC TREATMENT*

Time at risk (mo)	Continued treatment	Discontinued treatment	Ratio
0-3	3.8 ± 2.7 (26)	49.5 ± 1.2 (173)	12.9
3-6	17.4 ± 4.0 (402)	55.8 ± 7.4 (1254)	3.2
6.5-12	22.6 ± 3.5 (450)	62.1 ± 4.5 (639)	2.7
18-24	28.5 ± 3.6 (247)	54.0 ± 6.1 (281)	1.9

*Data are given as relapse risk ± SD (total number of subjects studied) weighted by the number of subjects per study on the basis of data of Gilbert PL, Harris MJ, Jeste DV: Neuroleptic withdrawal in schizophrenic patients, *Arch Gen Psychiatry* 52:173-188, 1995. The overall weighted mean ratio of the within-study difference in relapse risk was 5.78 ± 7.12.

Modified from Baldessarini RJ, Viguera AC: Neuroleptic withdrawal in schizophrenic patients, *Arch Gen Psychiatry* 52:189-191, 1995.

Clinical Syndromes, Symptom Descriptions, and Diagnoses

Clinical Syndromes

The symptoms of schizophrenia have received extensive study, originally in the process of simply describing and characterizing the various individual presentations of psychotic patients. Beginning in the late nineteenth century, German psychiatrists sought to reproduce the success of Koch, who had identified the infectious etiology of tuberculosis in relation to the clinical lesions found in patients with the disorder. Like other investigators in many fields of medicine at the time, the German psychiatrists sought to identify specific clinical presentations in larger patient populations that would, they hoped, correspond to specific underlying organic disease etiologies. Increasingly restrictive criteria are required to move from the description of a clinical syndrome to that of a discrete clinical disorder and from there to a pathophysiologic (that is, disease) entity (Table 13-6). The development of formal diagnostic criteria for schizophrenia and delusional disorders continues to date; the latest iteration of criteria are reviewed in Boxes 13-2 and 13-3. These criteria have evolved on the basis of the results of a century of clinical investigations of symptoms and syndromes in patients with psychotic disorders.

In 1898 Emil Kraepelin incorporated earlier symptom descriptions into a unified description of symptoms, course, and outcome called *dementia praecox,* which is closely related to what would be called

TABLE 13-6

LEVELS IN THE VALIDATION OF A DISEASE

Levels of disease concept	Criteria for validation
Clinical syndrome	1. Characteristics distinguishable from other syndromes
	2. Intercorrelated group of symptoms
	3. Consistent clinical picture (stable and homogenous correlational structure of symptoms)
Discrete clinical disorder	4. Explicit inclusion and exclusion rules
	5. Predictable progression of interrelated syndromes as a unit
	6. Rarity of intermediate or combined cases (discrete boundaries from other disorders)
Pathophysiological entity	7. Identification of biosocial risk factors
	8. Pathophysiologic explanation of symptoms, syndromes, and course
	9. Specific pathway from risk factors to disturbed pathophysiology

Modified from Cloninger CR et al: Diagnosis and prognosis in schizophrenia, *Arch Gen Psychiatry:* 42:15-25, 1985.

schizophrenia today. He recognized the typical early onset and asserted the distinguishing characteristic of a progressive deteriorating or dementing course. He considered dementia praecox to be an "organic" brain disorder. Kraepelin also described three different "paranoid" or delusional disorders: (1) paranoia, a very uncommon chronic illness with an insidious onset of fixed delusions (not restricted to paranoid delusions) and an absence of hallucinations or progressive deterioration or dementia; (2) paraphrenia, a mild form of dementia praecox, with delusions and hallucinations but no progressive deterioration; and (3) dementia paranoides, a form of dementia praecox that was similar to paranoia but had an earlier onset and progressive deterioration. Kraepelin's writings were based on careful prospective and longitudinal studies of patient outcomes, and they included excellent descriptions of delusions, hallucinations, certain negative symptoms (which refer to the absence of normal functions), and interesting abnormal and stereotyped movements. The latter occur in never-medicated patients and have become important because they confound the interpretation of neuroleptic-induced abnormal movements (such as TD). First coining the term schizophrenia in 1911 in reference to a splitting of mental functions, Eugen Bleuler also described hallucinations, delusions, and other psychotic symptoms. However, he deemphasized course and outcome and described four symptoms as central to the schizophrenic condition (the 4 *As*): a disturbance or loosening of *associations, autistic* behavior and thought, a disturbance of *affect,* and *ambivalence.* Despite his belief that schizophrenia has an organic basis, he maintained a more psychodynamic view of the disorder and used Freudian theory to explain several psychotic symptoms.

In 1939 Kurt Schneider described a set of "first rank symptoms" that he viewed as pathognomonic for the diagnosis of schizophrenia: (1) audible thoughts, or a patient's experience of auditory hallucinations of voices speaking his thoughts; (2) voices arguing, which refers to hallucinatory voices that usually discuss the patient in the third person; (3) voices commenting on the patient's actions or activities as they occur; (4) influence playing on the body, in which the patient describes being a passive or reluctant recipient of sensations imposed on him by an external agent; (5) thought withdrawal, or the patient's experience of having his thoughts taken from his mind by some external force; (6) thought insertion, or the patient's experience of having thoughts which are not his own; (7) diffusion or broadcasting of thoughts, in which the patient experiences his thoughts leaving his mind where they might be perceived by others; (8) made feelings, in which the patient experiences feelings that do not seem to belong to him; (9) made impulses, in which the patient experiences an impulse to do something; the impulse is imposed by some external agent, but acting on the impulse (if carried out) is not; (10) made volitional acts, in which the patient experiences his actions as being under the control of some external force; (11) delusional perception, a two-stage phenomenon in which the patient first experiences what he acknowledges as an ordinary perception (such as someone dropping a pencil) that almost immediately takes on delusional importance (such as meaning that the patient has been selected for a special mission by the CIA). Although first-rank symptoms have been recognized to have inadequate sensitivity and specificity to serve as diagnostic criteria for schizophrenia, they have been reported to occur in as many as 80% of those patients otherwise diagnosed with schizophrenia.

Following this early period, a proliferation of descriptions and diagnostic criteria arose for schizophrenia and paranoia (an early variant of what was to become a delusional disorder) that began to offer explicit inclusion and exclusion rules—the first elements of a clinical disorder. However, as recently as two decades ago, psychiatric diagnosis was generally an object of derision. A series of reports demonstrated that physicians and researchers typically were unable to achieve even a reasonable level of agreement in diagnosing disorders. The assessment of schizophrenia was especially problematic and was studied intensively through the U.S.-U.K. Cross National Project. A direct comparison of diagnoses made by staff members of several British and American hospitals showed that the diagnoses made in the United States were considerably broader, with significantly more patients whose consensus project diagnosis was an affective disorder being diagnosed as schizophrenic. This difference suggested that clinicians were using inconsistent criteria for making diagnoses or, more worrisome, that clinicians were unable to apply the same criteria consistently, which would obscure, among other things, any ability to detect real differences in the prevalence of schizophrenia from one location to another.

Concerns about the reliability and validity of existing definitions of schizophrenia led to the World Health Organization (WHO) International Pilot Study of Schizophrenia (IPSS). This international project sought to identify a standardized and reliable means of diagnosing schizophrenia using the Present State Examination (PSE), a standardized interview, as the principal source of diagnostic data for the study. The development and application of explicit diagnostic criteria over the last 20 years, such as the St. Louis Criteria, Taylor and Abrams' Criteria, the Research Diagnostic Criteria, and the DSM-IV, as well as the use of semistructured interview schedules, has led to a dramatic improvement in the reliability of classification of schizophrenia and delusional disorders. The DSM-IV serves as the official set of diagnostic guidelines and is used by the American Psychiatric Association; it continues a focus on objectively verified data concerning the presence or absence of particular symptoms, the duration of illness, the use of specific exclusions for biological confounds to an accurate diagnosis (that is, schizophrenia remains an idiopathic diagnosis of exclusion), and the requirement for evidence of functional impairment or clinical deterioration secondary to the disorder.

The distinct advantage of standardized operational diagnostic criteria is that they allow high levels of agreement, which are essential if studies of pathophysiologic and etiologic mechanisms are to be replicated. The incorporation (or removal) of specific symptoms from psychiatric diagnostic criteria such as the DSM has continued to revolve around concerns for both reliability and validity. In the past several decades, investigators have also focused on the study of reliable and validated groups of symptoms within the confusing array of overall schizophrenic psychopathology. The two principal senses of *reliability* are (1) interrater reliability, or the ability of independent clinicians to agree on the presence and severity of a symptom (it is very easy to get agreement on symptoms such as "orientation," whereas others such as "emotional withdrawal" are more difficult); and (2) test-retest reliability, or the ability of a single clinician to confirm the presence and same severity of a given symptom at two different points in time. The two principal senses of *validity* are (1) construct validity, or the confirmation that specific groups of symptoms correspond to specific underlying pathophysiologies or neural mechanisms (such as confirmation that the group of symptoms really should be thought of as a group because the symptoms in this group are all caused by *Mycobacterium tuberculosis*); and (2) predictive validity, or the confirmation that the presence or severity of a group of symptoms predicts the course or outcome of the illness. The use of standardized operational diagnostic criteria has led to some predictive validity for schizophrenia and less for delusional disorders. However, construct validity, or the objective verification that the diagnostic groupings are related to distinct underlying pathophysiological or disease processes, remains to be established.

Investigators have, over time, contributed to a long list of symptoms that may be seen in patients with schizophrenia and delusional disorders. The symptoms of these disorders are remarkably diverse and reflect the range of mind and brain function. The specific symptoms are remarkable for reflecting disturbances in behavioral, emotional, perceptual, physical, and cognitive domains. These domains are in contrast to the more common two domains—perceptual (such as pain, nausea, blurred vision) and physical (such as rashes, fractures, tachypnea)—spanned by most medical illnesses. The symptoms that may accompany schizophrenia and/or delusional disorders are outlined in the next section. Although individual symptoms are categorized into different domains, this categorization is to some extent arbitrary because many of these symptoms are complex and multidimensional phenomena. The DSM-IV definitions of those symptoms that constitute the current diagnostic criteria for schizophrenia and delusional disorders are also included for some of the symptoms described in the next section.

Symptom Descriptions

The behavioral symptoms that can accompany schizophrenia include bizarre or stereotyped behaviors (such as strange hand signals while speaking or repetitive odd speech); motor hyperactivity or hypoactivity, including catatonia, reductions in facial or bodily (such as hand) expressiveness and gesturing; poor hygiene; unusual dress; reductions in impulse control (such as suicidality); and reduced occupational and social performance. The DSM-IV defines and uses as a diagnostic criterion "grossly disorganized behavior," which "may manifest itself in a variety of ways, ranging from childlike silliness to unpredictable agitation . . . [and] may be noted in any form of goal-directed behavior, leading to difficulties in performing activities of daily living such as organizing meals or maintaining hygiene." Catatonic motor behaviors in the DSM-IV can "include a marked decrease in reactivity to the environment, sometimes reaching an extreme degree of complete unawareness (catatonic stupor), maintaining a rigid posture and resisting efforts to be moved (catatonic rigidity), active resistance to instructions or attempts to be moved (catatonic negativism), the assumption of inappropriate or bizarre postures (catatonic posturing), or purposeless and unstimulated excessive motor activity (catatonic excitement) . . . [but these] are nonspecific and may occur in other mental conditions [e.g., mood disorders], in general medical conditions [e.g., hypercalcemia], and medication-induced movement disorders [e.g., neuroleptic-induced parkinsonism]." The DSM-IV identifies three key negative symptoms that are manifested behaviorally: (1) affective flattening, "characterized by the person's face appearing immobile and unresponsive, with poor eye contact and reduced body language"; (2) alogia or poverty of speech, "manifested by brief, laconic, empty replies . . . [in which the] individual . . . appears to have a diminution of thoughts that is reflected in decreased fluency and productivity of speech"; and (3) avolition, one of the characteristic symptoms identified by Kraepelin and described as "an inability to initiate and persist in goal-directed activities."

A variety of emotional disturbances can occur in patients with schizophrenia and to some extent in patients with delusional disorders. Patients with schizophrenia can experience a reduction in emotional tone, feeling, or responsiveness, which may, as previously described, be manifested behaviorally as a blunting or flattening of affect. The internal, subjective emotional state of patients may become impoverished, with a loss of ability to experience pleasure (anhedonia) and loss of drive or will (avolition). Patients with schizophrenia can also experience inappropriate emotions (such as glee or sadness without evident environmental cues). Although not generally considered to be part of schizophrenia per se, a depressed mood and other symptoms of depression often occur in patients with schizophrenia. As previously noted, as many as 60% of all patients with schizophrenia have been estimated to experience an episode of depression at some time during the course of their illness. Together with evidence that depression clusters in the families of patients with schizophrenia, it is important for the primary care physician to remain alert for the manifestations of this disturbance in the overall management of patients.

The perceptual symptoms of schizophrenia consist of illusions and hallucinations; the latter figure prominently in most diagnostic systems. Hallucinations can occur in any sensory domain but are most commonly auditory and/or visual. Auditory hallucinations can consist of "voices" that are single or multiple, intelligible or unintelligible, and either subjectively perceived as coming from inside the patient's head or from the outside. These voices can speak to each other or to the patient and can range (within and between subjects) from being the patient's helpful allies to being the patient's harshest critics and dreaded enemies. Auditory hallucinations of a voice or voices can also include so-called command hallucinations that may instruct the patient to act in various ways, including injuring themselves. Patients may have more or less capacity to resist these commands at different times in their illness. Because of the personification of such voices, patients may feel that they are locked alone in a struggle with a powerful adversary. It is always important to inquire in detail about hallucinations and any related commands both because of the obvious risks and because many patients welcome the offer of an alliance that may (with treatment) reduce the strength and authority of their "adversary."

The physical findings associated with schizophrenia are largely relevant only to studies of the pathophysiology of the disorder, with little well-defined clinical relevance. So-called soft neurological signs (such as abnormal right-left discrimination, astereognosis, and abnormal finger-thumb opposition) have been reported in some patients with schizophrenia. These patients may be more sensitive to the adverse effects of neuroleptic treatment and may have a poorer antipsychotic treatment response. Neuroimaging has shown patients with schizophrenia to have an enlarged brain ventricular system (which may also be associated with poorer treatment response) and a reduced volume of specific brain structures. A disturbance in normal eye-tracking function and its central regulation has been well-studied in patients with schizophrenia and their relatives, which suggests a promising genetic marker for the disorder. Some of these findings may also have relevance to specific symptoms (such as memory deficits, hallucinations) and to generalized hypotheses concerning the pathophysiology of the disorder. Unfortunately, these findings show considerable intersubject variability, and none of these findings are diagnostic for the disorder. Delusional disorders offer no physical findings to aid in their assessment.

The cognitive symptoms of schizophrenia and delusional disorders represent a broad group of disturbances. To be precise, there are two senses of the term *cognitive* used here; one is a psychiatric reference to "disorders of thought" and the other is a more formal cognitive neuropsychology reference to specific mental abilities such as memory and attention. The psychiatric meaning can be further divided into so-called disorders of form vs. disorders of content. Disorders of content include delusional thinking, lack of insight, and impoverishment of thought content. A thought disorder of form, or "formal thought disorder," includes disruptions in the associations between ideas (loosening of associations) and thought blocking (that is, the sudden interruption of a patient's train of thought). A loosening of associations can range from mild circumstantiality in which the patient deviates from the usual line of association but eventually returns to the point, all the way to a loss of the normal associations between words within even a single sentence, which results in a so-called "word salad." In the neuropsychology domain, schizophrenia is characterized by a variety of specific cognitive deficits. Memory and learning deficits appear to be quantitatively large compared with deficits in other differentiated elements of cognitive performance. A series of well-reviewed studies suggest that the memory and learning deficits in schizophrenia are related to ineffective organization and encoding of information. The association between various attentional dysfunctions and schizophrenia has also been widely reported. Investigators have reported attentional deficits in acute, chronic, and residual schizophrenic patients, as well as in the clinically unaffected children of schizophrenic parents. Selective attention and processing speed have also been reported to be impaired in patients with schizophrenia and in their relatives. Patients with schizophrenia have demonstrated an impaired ability to utilize abstract concepts, shift between concepts or mental sets, and perform working memory tasks (involving the capacity to hold information "on-line" during brief intervals).

Both schizophrenia and delusional disorders can present with delusions. With schizophrenia these delusions can be either bizarre or nonbizarre in nature; in delusional disorders, the delusions must by definition be nonbizarre. The DSM-IV defines delusions as "erroneous beliefs that usually involve a misinterpretation of perceptions or experiences . . . [and whose] content may include a variety of themes (e.g., persecutory, referential, somatic, religious, or grandiose) . . . [which] are deemed bizarre if they are clearly implausible and not understandable and do not derive from ordinary life experiences." The DSM-IV defines hallucinations as phenomena that "may occur in any sensory modality (e.g., auditory, visual, olfactory, gustatory, and tactile), [with] auditory hallucinations . . . by far the most common" and that "must occur in the context of a clear sensorium." The DSM-IV defines the core schizophrenic symptom of disorganized thinking (that is, formal thought disorder or loosening of associations) in terms of disorganized speech, recognizing that "because mildly disorganized speech is common and nonspecific, the symptom must be severe enough to substantially impair effective communication . . . [with] less severe disorganized thinking or speech . . . occur[ing] during the prodromal and residual periods of schizophrenia."

In addition to the importance of individual symptoms, specific groups of symptoms have been defined with attention to both reliability and validity. Considerable effort has been devoted over the course of this century to classify the symptoms and signs of psychotic illness into groups or diagnoses that represent specific disease processes. Unfortunately, the principal psychotic illness, schizophrenia, is still widely believed to be a group of schizophrenias. In the face of changing and uncertain diagnostic boundaries for schizophrenia, clinical researchers have long had an interest in establishing valid groupings of symptoms within the disorder. The work to link different symptom groups to different underlying dimensions of disease remains active and fruitful in the effort to better understand schizophrenia. A negative vs. positive symptom construct was first articulated by nineteenth-century neurologists and has been refined and extended to define positive, disorganized, and negative symptom groupings. Positive symptoms are exemplified by hallucinations and delusions. Disorganized symptoms are exemplified by disturbances in the associations between ideas. Negative symptoms are exemplified by blunted affect, emotional withdrawal, and social and occupational deficits. These groups of symptoms are defined as those that tend to cluster together statistically in large patient samples and in which all of the symptoms can be more prominent or less prominent but tend to occur together as a group. A symptom group may sometimes cluster within individual patients who might, for example, have predominantly negative symptoms at a particular point in time. However, patients typically have a mixture of different symptom groups. This mixed and varying clinical presentation has confounded efforts to subtype schizophrenia into different disorders with distinct etiologies. Some investigators have hypothesized that different underlying pathophysiologic mechanisms may operate simultaneously in the same patient to produce this varied symptom presentation.

Current Diagnostic Criteria and Clinical Vignettes

The precursors of the DSM in the United States first arose out of the need to classify mental disorders for statistical purposes, which was first attempted in the 1840 census with the single category of "idiocy/insanity." Further development of a nomenclature for severe, usually inpatient, psychiatric disorders involved collaborations between the American Medico-Psychological Association (later the American Psychiatric Association [APA]) and the National Commission on Mental Hygiene for use by the Bureau of the Census in 1917, and later between the APA and the New York Academy of Medicine for use in the first edition of the American Medical Association's Standard Classified Nomenclature of Disease. The U.S. Army and the Veterans Administration expanded the scope of this psychiatric nomenclature to accommodate the presentations of World War II servicemen and veterans; the WHO, influenced by the development of this nomenclature, included 10 categories for psychosis in its new section on mental disorders for the sixth edition of the International Classification of Diseases (ICD). Beginning with the DSM-I in 1952, the APA has published an evolving series of more descriptively explicit classification schemes for principal use by physicians and researchers rather than census workers. The evolution of the DSM classification system to the current DSM-IV has in principle aimed for an atheoretical descriptive approach and requires that any changes to criteria be substantiated by

DSM-IV DIAGNOSTIC CRITERIA

BOX 13-2 SCHIZOPHRENIA

A. *Characteristic symptoms:* Two (or more) of the following, each present for a significant portion of time during a 1-month period (or less if successfully treated):

(1) delusions
(2) hallucinations
(3) disorganized speech (e.g., frequent derailment or incoherence)
(4) grossly disorganized or catatonic behavior
(5) negative symptoms (i.e., affective flattening, alogia, or avolition)

Note: Only one Criterion A symptom is required if delusions are bizarre or hallucinations consist of a voice keeping up a running commentary on the person's behavior or thoughts, or two or more voices conversing with each other.

B. *Social/occupational dysfunction:* For a significant portion of the time since the onset of the disturbance, one or more major areas of functioning such as work, interpersonal relations, or self-care are markedly below the level achieved prior to the onset (or when the onset is in childhood or adolescence, failure to achieve expected level of interpersonal, academic, or occupational achievement).

C. *Duration:* Continuous signs of the disturbance persist for at least 6 months. This 6-month period must include at least 1 month of symptoms (or less if successfully treated) that meet Criterion A (i.e., active-phase symptoms) and may include periods of prodromal or residual symptoms. During these prodromal or residual periods, the signs of the disturbance may be manifested by only negative symptoms or two or more symptoms listed in Criterion A present in an attenuated form (e.g., odd beliefs, unusual perceptual experiences).

D. *Schizoaffective and Mood Disorder exclusion:* Schizoaffective Disorder and Mood Disorder With Psychotic Features have been ruled out because either (1) no Major Depressive, Manic, or Mixed Episodes have occurred concurrently with the active-phase symptoms; or (2) if mood episodes have occurred during active-phase symptoms, their total duration has been brief relative to the duration of the active and residual periods.

E. *Substance/general medical condition exclusion:* The disturbance is not due to the direct physiological effects of a substance (e.g., a drug of abuse, a medication) or a general medical condition.

F. *Relationship to a Pervasive Developmental Disorder:* If there is a history of Autistic Disorder or another Pervasive Developmental Disorder, the additional diagnosis of Schizophrenia is made only if prominent delusions or hallucinations are also present for at least a month (or less if successfully treated).

Classification of longitudinal course (can be applied only after at least 1 year has elapsed since the initial onset of active-phase symptoms):

Episodic With Interepisode Residual Symptoms (episodes are defined by the reemergence of prominent psychotic symptoms); *also specify if:* **With Prominent Negative Symptoms**
Episodic With No Interepisode Residual Symptoms
Continuous (prominent psychotic symptoms are present throughout the period of observation); *also specify if:* **With Prominent Negative Symptoms**
Single Episode In Partial Remission; *also specify if:* **With Prominent Negative Symptoms**
Single Episode In Full Remission
Other or Unspecified Pattern

From American Psychiatric Association: *Diagnostic and statistical manual of mental disorders,* ed 4 (DSM-IV), Washington, D.C., 1994, American Psychiatric Press.

DIAGNOSIS

TABLE 13-7
SCHIZOPHRENIA

Discriminating features

1. Two (or more) of the following, each present for a significant portion of time during a 1-month period (or less if successfully treated):
   a. delusions
   b. hallucinations
   c. disorganized speech (e.g., frequent derailment or incoherence)
   d. grossly disorganized or catatonic behavior
   e. negative symptoms (i.e., affective flattening, alogia, or avolition)
2. One or more major areas of functioning are markedly below the level achieved before the onset
3. Continuous signs of the disturbance persist for at least 6 months

Consistent features

1. Not due to the effects of substances or general medical conditions
2. If there is a history of Autistic Disorder or another Pervasive Developmental Disorder, the diagnosis of Schizophrenia is made only if prominent delusions or hallucinations are also present
3. Not accounted for by Major Affective Disorder

Variable Features

1. Inappropriate affect (e.g., smiling, laughing, or a silly facial expression in the absence of an appropriate stimulus)
2. Anhedonia
3. Dysphoric mood
4. Disturbances in sleep pattern
5. Abnormalities of psychomotor activity (e.g., pacing, rocking, or apathetic immobility)
6. Difficulty concentrating
7. Cognitive dysfunction
8. Confused or disoriented
9. Lack of insight
10. Depersonalization, derealization, and somatic concerns
11. Motor abnormalities (e.g., grimacing, posturing, odd mannerisms, ritualistic or stereotyped behavior)

empirical data, field trials of new criteria, and a "consensus of the field."

The DSM-IV definition for schizophrenia is listed in Box 13-2 with associated features listed in Table 13-7. Cases 13-1 and 13-2 are provided as an example of the application of DSM-IV diagnostic criteria to clinical situations.

A recent change in the diagnostic criteria for schizophrenia involves the age of onset for the disorder. The DSM-III did not permit the diagnosis of schizophrenia when the onset of the disorder was at or after the age of 45 years. This restriction was removed beginning with DSM-III-R and continues to be absent from the DSM-IV. The inclusion of late-onset patients in the diagnosis of schizophrenia is based on recent careful investigations in this country, which find more similarities than differences between patients with younger vs. later onsets in comparison to healthy normal controls. Specifically, younger and later onset patients have similar overall levels of positive- and negative-symptom psychopathology, similar levels of neuropsychological impairment, similar levels of impaired childhood adjustment, and a similar family history of schizophrenia. Late-onset patients function better in adolescence and young adulthood (when younger onset patients are typically beginning to get ill), are more often of the paranoid subtype, and more often women; this later point remains less established. The most important issue with late-onset patients with schizophrenia is the need to scrupulously address the differential diagnosis because of the increased possibility that the presenting symptoms may, in fact, be accounted for by increasingly prevalent medical or neurological conditions in this older population. Case 13-3 shows an example of a case of late-onset schizophrenia.

The DSM-IV definition for delusional disorders is listed in Box 13-3, and specific features of delusional disorders are shown in Table 13-8. Case 13-4 discusses the case of a patient with a delusional disorder.

Differential Diagnoses

Schizophrenia and delusional disorders remain essentially diagnoses of exclusion. The serious prognostic and treatment implications of assigning patients diagnoses such as schizophrenia or delusional disorders make the differential diagnosis for these disorders assume added importance. Although many students in psychiatry, psychology, and related fields tend to focus on the negative consequences of making a diagnosis of schizophrenia, it cannot be overlooked that failing to make this diagnosis when it is appropriate can undermine proper treatment decisions. The symptoms of these disorders reflect a profound disruption of nor-

CASE 13-1

Mr. S. is a 44-year-old, single, unemployed, white man brought to the emergency room by the police for striking an elderly woman in his apartment building. His chief complaint is, "That damn bitch. She and the rest of them deserved more than that for what they put me through."

History of present illness: Mr. S. maintains that his apartment is the center of a large communication system that involves all three major television networks, his neighbors, and apparently hundreds of "actors" in his neighborhood. There are secret cameras in his apartment that carefully monitor all his activities. When he is watching television, many of his minor actions (e.g., going to the bathroom) are soon directly commented on by the announcer. Whenever he goes outside, everyone on the street watches him. His neighbors operate two different "machines"; one is responsible for all of his voices, which he hears many times each day. He sometimes thinks this machine is directly run by the neighbor whom he attacked. The other machine he calls "the dream machine." Mr. S. recently went to a shoe store 30 miles from his house in the hope of getting some shoes that wouldn't be "altered." However, he soon found out that, like the rest of the shoes he buys, special nails had been put into the bottom of the shoes to annoy him. He realizes that great effort and "millions of dollars" are involved in keeping him under surveillance. He sometimes thinks this is all part of a large experiment to discover the secret of his "superior intelligence."

Past psychiatric history: The patient has been continuously ill since age 22. During his first year of law school, he gradually became more and more convinced that his classmates were making fun of him. He noticed that they would snort and sneeze whenever he entered the classroom. When a girl he was dating broke off the relationship with him, he believed that she had been "replaced" by a look-alike. He called the police and asked for their help to solve the "kidnapping." His academic performance in school declined dramatically, and he was asked to leave and seek psychiatric care. Mr. S. then got a job as an investment counselor at a bank, which he held for 7 months. However, he was getting an increasing number of distracting "signals" from co-workers, and he became more and more suspicious and withdrawn. It was at this time that he first reported hearing voices. He was eventually fired and soon thereafter was hospitalized for the first time at age 24. He has not worked since. Mr. S. has been hospitalized 12 times; the longest stay was 8 months. However, in the last 5 years he has been hospitalized only once, for 3 weeks. During the hospitalizations he has received various antipsychotic drugs. Although outpatient medication has been prescribed, he usually stops taking it shortly after leaving the hospital. Aside from twice-yearly lunch meetings with his uncle and his contacts with mental health workers, he is totally isolated socially. He lives on his own and manages his own financial affairs, including a modest inheritance. He reads the *Wall Street Journal* daily. He cooks and cleans for himself.

Pertinent findings from the mental status examination: At the interview, Mr. S. is well-groomed, and his speech is coherent and goal-directed. His affect is, at most, only mildly blunted. He was initially very angry at being brought in by the police. His thought content is significant for the paranoid, bizarre, and grandiose delusions previously noted.

Discussion: Mr. S.'s long illness apparently began with delusions of reference (his classmates making fun of him by snorting and sneezing when he entered the classroom). Over the years his delusions have become increasingly complex and bizarre (his neighbors are actually actors, his thoughts are monitored, a machine puts voices and dreams into his head). In addition, he has prominent hallucinations of different voices that harass him. Bizarre delusions and prominent hallucinations are the characteristic psychotic symptoms of schizophrenia. The diagnosis is confirmed by the marked disturbance in his work and social functioning and by the absence of a sustained mood disturbance or a general medical condition or use of a substance that can account for the disturbance. All of Mr. S.'s delusions and hallucinations seem to involve the single theme of a conspiracy to harass him. This preoccupation with a delusion, in the absence of disorganized speech, flat or inappropriate affect, or catatonic or grossly disorganized behavior, indicates the paranoid type, further specified as continuous, because he has not been free of psychotic symptoms for many years. The prognosis for someone like Mr. S. with the paranoid type of schizophrenia is expected to be better than the prognosis for disorganized and undifferentiated types. Mr. S. has, in fact, done remarkably well despite a chronic psychotic illness because during the past 5 years he has been able to take care of himself.

Modified from American Psychiatric Association: *DSM-IV case book* Washington, D.C., 1994.

mal functioning in behavioral, emotional, perceptual, physical, and cognitive domains. The range of symptoms found in schizophrenia implicates a broad array of brain functions that can, in turn, be altered by a variety of abnormal processes within the central nervous system (CNS) and the periphery. Many of the pathological processes that can produce secondary symptoms resembling schizophrenia and delusional disorders are also treatable medical or neurological conditions. It is critical to perform a complete medical and neurological evaluation on any patient with schizophrenia-like symptoms (see Pearls & Perils on p. 228). An abbreviated list of differential diagnostic entities is provided in Box 13-4. This list of possible explanations for psychotic symptoms is difficult to review in the abstract because factors such as an acute versus

CASE 13-2

Ms. L. is a pale, stooped woman of 39 years, whose childlike face is surrounded by scraggly blond braids tied with pink ribbons. She was referred for a psychiatric evaluation for possible hospitalization by her family doctor, who was concerned about her low level of functioning. Her only complaint to him was, "I have a decline in self-care and a low life level."

History of present/past illness: The patient's mother reports that there has indeed been a decline but that it has been over many years. In the last few months Ms. L. has remained in her room, mute and still. Twelve years ago Ms. L. was a supervisor in the occupational therapy department of a large hospital, living in her own apartment, and engaged to a young man. He broke the engagement, and she became increasingly disorganized, wandering aimlessly in the street, wearing mismatched clothing. She was fired from her job, and eventually the police were called to hospitalize her. They broke into her apartment, which was filled with papers, food, and broken objects. No information is available from this hospitalization, which lasted 3 months and from which she was discharged to her mother's house with a prescription for an unknown medication that she never had filled. After her discharge, Ms. L.'s family hoped that she would gather herself together and embark again on a real life, but over the years she became more withdrawn and less functional. Most of her time was spent watching television and cooking. Her cooking consisted of mixing bizarre combinations of ingredients such as broccoli and cake mix, cooking them, and then eating them alone because no one else in the family would eat her meals. Often when her mother entered her room, she would quickly grab a magazine and pretend to be reading when in fact she had apparently just been sitting and staring into space. She stopped bathing and brushing her hair or teeth. She ate less and less, although she denied a loss of appetite, and over a period of several years she lost 20 pounds. She would sleep at odd hours. Eventually she became enuretic, wetting her bed frequently and filling the room with the pungent odor of urine.

Pertinent findings from the mental status examination: On admission to the psychiatric hospital, Ms. L. sat with her hands tightly clasped in her lap and avoided looking at the doctor who interviewed her. She answered questions readily and did not appear suspicious or guarded, but her affect was shallow. She denied having a depressed mood, delusions, or hallucinations. However, her answers became increasingly idiosyncratic and irrelevant as the interview progressed. In response to a question about her strange cooking habits, she replied that she did not wish to discuss recent events in Russia. When discussing her decline in functioning, she said, "There's more of a take-off mechanism when you're younger." Asked about ideas of reference, she said, "I doubt it's true, but if one knows the writers involved, it could be an element that would be directed in a comical way." Her answers were interspersed with the mantra, "I'm safe, I'm safe."

Discussion: Several features of this case suggest the diagnosis of schizophrenia. There are Ms. L.'s extreme decline in functioning over a period of several years and her many oddities of behavior and speech. In addition, there is no evidence of a mood disorder or of a general medical condition or substance that could account for this disturbance. What makes the diagnosis more problematic is the apparent absence of delusions or hallucinations, which are usually present during the active phase of schizophrenia. Ms. L.'s speech is at times incoherent, but her affect, although described as shallow, is not flat or grossly inappropriate, and she has no catatonic symptoms. The criteria for the diagnosis of schizophrenia in DSM-IV includes additional negative symptoms: alogia (poverty of amount of content of speech) and avolition (a pervasive inability to persist in goal-directed activities). Because her speech is at times incoherent and she is unable to work or cope with more than minimal self-care (avolition), the DSM-IV diagnosis would be schizophrenia.

Modified from American Psychiatric Association: *DSM-IV case book,* Washington, D.C., 1994.

insidious onset, the relationship to other symptoms, and the presence or absence of physical and/or laboratory findings can sharply narrow the list. A more detailed discussion of the psychiatric presentations of medical and neurological conditions is provided in Chapter 26.

Some entities in the differential diagnosis can be detected by history or examination, whereas others require laboratory assessment. Some physicians may argue that expensive laboratory tests should not be performed for the detection of entities that are less common than schizophrenia itself and that are eventually detected through the history and examination. However, most of these entities are treatable conditions that, without early detection, can produce significant morbidity and possible mortality; therefore early assessment is necessary. The general work-up for a patient with new-onset psychosis should include a complete history (including family history); physical and neurological examination; a blood sample for laboratory assessment of electrolyte, glucose, albumin, blood urea nitrogen (BUN), and calcium levels; human immunodeficiency virus (HIV) and Venereal Disease Research Laboratories/fluorescein treponema antibody (VDRL/FTA) testing (in patients who may be at risk); erythrocyte sedimentation level (to inexpensively provide a crude screen for inflammatory processes); and thyroid function tests. Physicians should consider obtaining either a ceruloplasmin plasma level or a slit-lamp examination (looking for Kayser-Fleischer rings)

CASE 13-3

Mr. A. was a 67-year-old man with 8 years of education who had worked as an apartment manager. His behavior reportedly was unremarkable until 1½ years before presentation, when his wife noted increased angry outbursts and a tendency to become increasingly guarded and overprotective of his family. This initial behavior change gradually progressed to bizarre and more overt paranoid behavior, with a diminished capacity to attend to his managerial duties. Mr. A. reportedly put tin foil on all the windows of his home, the ceiling, over his right eye, and on the top of his head. He removed all brass knobs and fixtures and covered all shiny objects; he also rearranged furniture and took all the drapes off the windows. By his own report, all this was designed to decrease the penetration of laser beams and gamma rays into the home. His wife also stated that he looked for "bugs" on all the telephones, cut wires in the apartment, and heard "bugging" occurring from an apartment upstairs. He subsequently called the F.B.I. and reported his suspicions. Mr. A. believed that an implant from previous cataract surgery on his right eye was a "receiver" for the laser beams and gamma rays. The symptoms were present for approximately 9 months before the current (his first) psychiatric hospitalization.

Past psychiatric history: Mr. A. and his wife denied a history of alcohol or other substance abuse. They also denied any past history of the DSM-III-R symptoms of mania (grandiosity, reduced need for sleep, pressure of speech, flight of ideas, distractibility, psychomotor agitation, or activities such as spending sprees) or depression (a depressed mood almost daily), anhedonia, significant weight loss or weight gain, sleep disturbance, psychomotor retardation, loss of energy, guilt, inability to concentrate, or suicidal ideation). The past history was significant for one visit to a mental health clinic 3 years earlier for complaints of insomnia and anxiety caused by a lawsuit concerning a motor vehicle accident in which his son was involved. No psychotic symptoms were noted at that time.

Past medical history: The history was significant for right ear tympanoplasty 10 years before presentation (ear damage caused by an explosion at a previous job). Mr. A. also had a cataract removal and lens implantation performed 1½ years before admission.

Pertinent findings from the mental status examination: The findings included a constricted affect, some looseness of association, and poor insight.

Physical examination: The examination was unremarkable except for an enlarged prostate and a decreased vibratory sense in the lower extremities. On clinical examination, the patient had no visual or hearing loss. Laboratory evaluations, including a complete blood count, serum chemistry, thyroid function tests, and vitamin B_{12} and folate levels were within normal limits. A magnetic resonance imaging (MRI) scan of the brain showed a mild prominence of the ventricles and subarachnoid space, which was interpreted by a neuroradiologist as being commensurate with age.

Neuropsychological performance: Mr. A. scored 29 (perfect is 30) on the Mini-Mental State Examination and 97 on the Wechsler Adult Intelligence Scale-Revised (WAIS-R) Full-Scale IQ test. His verbal IQ was 94, and his performance IQ was 103. Other than a mild inefficiency in verbal learning, Mr. A.'s performance on the expanded Halstead-Reitan Battery was entirely within normal limits.

Hospital course: During the course of hospitalization, Mr. A. experienced gradual improvement in psychotic symptoms without antipsychotic medication. On his first pass home, Mr. A. became paranoid and agitated. He improved again after returning to the hospital. Several days later, he went home without developing a recurrence of his symptoms. Apart from irritability and an excessive concern for world affairs, Mr. A. remained essentially symptom-free without antipsychotic medication for approximately 6 months. After that time, he began staring for hours at the sun under a "command." He also became socially withdrawn and noncommunicative. He was treated with haloperidol, 5 mg daily, and improvement in symptoms occurred after about 1 week. The dose of haloperidol was reduced, and he was monitored on 2 mg a day.

Discussion: The presentation of this case is consistent with a diagnosis of schizophrenia. Bizarre delusions, paranoid delusions, possible auditory hallucinations (hearing "bugging" going on upstairs) and a decreased occupational function together suggest the diagnosis. However, a number of medical and neurological conditions that are more common in older individuals needed to be ruled out before arriving at this conclusion. The principal conditions to be ruled out in the differential diagnosis are (1) psychosis secondary to a general medical condition or the use of a substance, including but not limited to intracranial masses, cerebrovascular accidents, endocrinopathies, B_{12} deficiency (such as peripheral decreased vibratory sensation), and the use of alcohol and over-the-counter medications; (2) mood disorders; (3) delusional disorders; and (4) dementia. This case also provides a good example of a therapeutic response to relatively low doses of antipsychotic medication in an older individual (see the section on treatment).

Modified from Harris MJ, Cullum CM, Jeste DV: Clinical presentation of late-onset schizophrenia, *J Clin Psychiatry* 49:356-360, 1988.

DSM-IV DIAGNOSTIC CRITERIA

BOX 13-3 DELUSIONAL DISORDER

A. Nonbizarre delusions (i.e., involving situations that occur in real life, such as being followed, poisoned, infected, loved at a distance, or deceived by spouse or lover, or having a disease) of at least 1 month's duration.

B. Criterion A for Schizophrenia has never been met. **Note:** Tactile and olfactory hallucinations may be present in Delusional Disorder if they are related to the delusional theme.

C. Apart from the impact of the delusion(s) or its ramifications, functioning is not markedly impaired and behavior is not obviously odd or bizarre.

D. If mood episodes have occurred concurrently with delusions, their total duration has been brief relative to the duration of the delusional periods.

E. The disturbance is not due to the direct physiological effects of a substance (e.g., a drug of abuse, a medication) or a general medical condition.

Specify type (the following types are assigned based on the predominant delusional theme):

Erotomanic Type: delusions that another person, usually of higher status, is in love with the individual
Grandiose Type: delusions of inflated worth, power, knowledge, identity, or special relationship to a deity or famous person
Jealous Type: delusions that the individual's sexual partner is unfaithful
Persecutory Type: delusions that the person (or someone to whom the person is close) is being malevolently treated in some way
Somatic Type: delusions that the person has some physical defect or general medical condition
Mixed Type: delusions characteristic of more than one of the above types but no one theme predominates
Unspecified Type

From American Psychiatric Association: *Diagnostic and statistical manual of mental disorders,* ed 4 (DSM-IV), Washington, D.C., 1994, American Psychiatric Press.

to address the relatively low probability of early (that is, highly treatable) Wilson's disease, which may present with or without early evidence of the characteristic movement disorder. Urine should be collected for routine analysis and a toxicology screen. A computed tomography (CT) scan of the head should be obtained, principally for the evaluation of otherwise "silent" mass lesions of the frontal and temporal lobe. Specific historical or physical examination findings may lead to additional tests such as serum B_{12} and folate levels, heavy metal levels, a lumbar puncture, or an electroencephalogram (EEG).

Etiology and Pathophysiology

The etiology of schizophrenia and delusional disorders remains uncertain. Several promising lines of evidence suggest that schizophrenia may be best conceptualized as a neurodevelopmental disorder related to genetic susceptibility and early brain insults that subsequently render the brain vulnerable to progressive, endogenous, neurotoxic injury. Relevant findings have emerged from basic neuroscience research, genetic studies, and clinical schizophrenia research that may explain key increases in risk for the disorder, key changes in neurotransmitter function, and key mechanisms underlying neuronal injury. However, schizophrenia and delusional disorders are heterogeneous disorders with a variety of clinical presentations, both within and between subjects, and highly variable biological characteristics that have complicated the search for etiology. The most promising etiological explanations may all work together to produce schizophrenia or, alternatively, make variable contributions in different individuals to produce variable forms of the disorder. The latter prospect is widely believed to be the likely state of affairs, which makes variable patient characteristics (that is, diagnostic heterogeneity) an important factor that undermines the ability to detect changes (such as reductions in specific receptor concentrations or specific neuronal changes) predicted by a particular hypothesis.

The belief that different factors may operate to different degrees to produce somewhat different presentations of the disorder in different individuals, of course, reflects the limitations of diagnostic criteria that are set, as with many medical disorders, without knowledge about etiology. The advantage of standardized operational diagnostic criteria (as in the DSM system) is that they at least allow the high levels of agreement that are essential to replicating studies of pathophysiological and etiological mechanisms. However,

DIAGNOSIS

TABLE 13-8
DELUSIONAL DISORDER

Discriminating features

1. Nonbizarre delusions of at least 1 month's duration
2. Apart from the impact of the delusion(s), functioning is not markedly impaired and behavior is not obviously odd or bizarre

Consistent features

1. If tactile and olfactory hallucinations are present in delusional disorder, they are related to the delusional theme
2. If mood episodes have occurred concurrently, their total duration has been brief relative to the duration of the delusional periods
3. The disturbance is not a result of the effects of a substance or medical condition

Variable features

1. Delusions that another person, usually of higher status, is in love with the individual
2. Delusions of inflated worth, power, knowledge, identity, or special relationship to a deity or famous person
3. Delusions that the individual's sexual partner is unfaithful
4. Delusions that the person (or someone to whom the person is close) is being malevolently treated in some way
5. Delusions that the person has some physical defect or general medical condition

given the bottom-line limitation that it is difficult to say whether one definition of schizophrenia has greater validity than any other, some investigators have suggested that a flexible polydiagnostic approach be adopted for biological research paradigms. Using this approach, diagnoses and analyses can be made using multiple criterion systems. A new structured interview, the Diagnostic Interview for Genetic Studies (DIGS), recently was constructed to offer a state-of-the-art diagnostic assessment for schizophrenia on the basis of several diagnostic systems (such as DSM, ICD, and Research Diagnostic Criteria [RDC]).

This section reviews several important lines of research on the etiology and pathophysiology of schizophrenia and, to a lesser extent, delusional disorders. A wealth of important findings from structural neuroimaging (such as enlarged cerebral ventricles, reduced gray matter volumes), functional neuroimaging (such as reduced frontal activation during demand conditions, so-called hypofrontality), neuropsychology (such as prominent impairments in medial temporal lobe functions, attentional impairments), eye-tracking studies (such as abnormalities that suggest frontal lobe impairments), and postmortem studies (such as injury to the cingulate cortex, hippocampus, parahippocampal gyrus, and entorhinal cortex) are not reviewed here, but the interested reader is referred to references associated with this chapter.

Genetic Factors

A series of findings that confirm a higher risk for psychotic disorders in families in which another member has already been affected have provided strong support for the idea that schizophrenia and delusional disorders cluster in families. The pattern of familial transmission, especially for schizophrenia, strongly supports a genetic component in the risk of developing the illness. Key observations come from studies of monozygotic twins (which show an approximately 50% concordance rate for schizophrenia in the second twin when the first has been diagnosed with the disorder), from adoption studies in which the influence of genetic and at least some environmental factors can be distinguished, and from family studies (which show higher rates of schizophrenia in the first-degree vs. the second-degree relatives of those diagnosed with the disorder). Family studies demonstrate an increased risk of developing schizophrenia when raised by parents who have the disorder. However, this *familial* risk could be related to either genetic factors or to psychosocial or intrauterine environmental effects. Adoption or foster-rearing studies provide a way to separate the psychosocial effects of being raised by a parent(s) with schizophrenia vs. the genetic effects on the risk of developing the disorder. The results of the first study of this type (conducted in Oregon by Heston and colleagues), a group of important adoption studies in Denmark (a collaboration between American [Kety, Rosenthal, and Wender] and Danish investigators [Schulsinger, Welner, and Jacobsen]) that used national registers for both psychiatric illness and adoption, and a Finnish adoption study all support the important role of congenital factors (genetic or intrauterine). The work by Kety and colleagues included a comparison of maternal and paternal half-siblings, which provided evidence that genetic factors were stronger contributors to the risk of developing schizophrenia than was the intrauterine environment. Gottesman has articulated the concept of increasing genetic risk as individuals share increasing amounts of genetic material with the affected relative(s) (Figure 13-3). Kendler and colleagues have interpreted the results of their careful family studies of psychiatric illness to suggest that what is transmitted in families is not the schizophrenic

CASE 13-4

Mr. P., a 42-year-old married African-American postal worker and father of two, is brought to the emergency room by his wife because he has been insisting that "there is a contract out on my life."

History of present illness: According to Mr. P., his problems began 4 months ago when his supervisor at work accused him of tampering with a package. Mr. P. denied that this was true and, because his job was in jeopardy, filed a protest. At a formal hearing, he was exonerated and, according to him, "This made my boss furious. He felt he had been publicly humiliated." About 2 weeks later, Mr. P. noticed that his co-workers were avoiding him. He said, "When I'd walk toward them, they'd just turn away like they didn't want to see me." Shortly thereafter, he began to feel that they were talking about him at work. He never could make out clearly what they were saying, but he gradually became convinced that they were avoiding him because his boss had taken out a contract on his life. This state of affairs was stable for about 2 months, until Mr. P. began noticing several "large white cars," new to his neighborhood, driving up and down the street on which he lived. He became increasingly frightened and was convinced that the "hit men" were in these cars. He refused to go out of his apartment without an escort. Several times when he saw the white cars he would panic and run home. After one such incident, his wife finally insisted that he accompany her to the emergency room.

Past Psychiatric History: Mr. P. was described by his wife and brother as a basically well-adjusted, outgoing man who enjoyed being with his family. He had served with distinction in Vietnam. He saw little combat there, but was pulled from a burning truck by a buddy seconds before the truck blew up.

Pertinent Findings from Mental Status Examination: When interviewed, Mr. P. was obviously frightened. Aside from his belief that he was in danger of being killed, his speech, behavior, and demeanor were in no way odd or strange. His predominant mood was anxious. He denied having hallucinations and all other psychotic symptoms except those previously noted. He claimed not to be depressed, and although he noted that he had recently had some difficulty falling asleep, he said there had been no change in his appetite, sex drive, energy level, or concentration.

Discussion: Mr. P. believes that his boss has taken a contract out on his life, but because the clinician finds no reason to believe this, he must conclude that Mr. P. has a delusion. Because contract killers are sometimes hired in real life, the delusion is nonbizarre. Mr. P. has no auditory or visual hallucinations, no manic or depressive syndrome, and no evidence of a general medical condition or the use of a substance that might have caused the disturbance. His behavior, apart from the delusion and its ramifications, is not odd or bizarre. These signs are the characteristics of delusional disorders. Because the content of his delusion involves the theme of being malevolently treated in some way, the disorder is specified as the persecutory type. Individuals with the persecutory type of delusional disorder are often reluctant to seek help.

Follow-up: Mr. P. was hospitalized and received treatment with an antipsychotic medication. He remained delusional, however, and in fact became convinced that several of the other patients on the ward with Italian names were part of the "hit team" sent to kill him. Over the ensuing 3 weeks, with continued treatment, these beliefs faded. At discharge, 1 month after admission, he stated, "I guess my boss has called off the contract. He couldn't get away with it now without publicity." Mr. P. was followed up over a period of 18 months, during which time he had two relapses into more active delusions, all with the same content and each occurring after he stopped taking his medication. Both episodes resolved relatively rapidly with outpatient treatment and antipsychotic medication.

Modified from American Psychiatric Association: *DSM-IV case book,* Washington, D.C., 1994.

PEARLS & PERILS

IMPORTANCE OF DIFFERENTIAL DIAGNOSIS

- Schizophrenia and delusional disorders remain essentially diagnoses of exclusion.
- The serious prognostic and treatment implications of assigning patients diagnoses such as schizophrenia or delusional disorders make the differential diagnosis for these disorders assume added importance.
- Although many students in psychiatry, psychology, and related fields tend to focus on the negative consequences of making a diagnosis of schizophrenia, it cannot be overlooked that failing to make this diagnosis when it is appropriate can undermine proper treatment decisions.
- The symptoms of these disorders reflect a profound disruption of normal functioning in behavioral, emotional, perceptual, physical, and cognitive domains.
- The range of symptoms found in schizophrenia implicates a broad array of brain functions that can, in turn, be altered by a variety of abnormal processes within the CNS and the periphery.
- Many of the pathological processes that can produce secondary symptoms resembling schizophrenia and delusional disorders are also treatable medical or neurological conditions.
- It is critical to perform a complete medical and neurological evaluation on any patient with schizophrenia-like symptoms.

BOX 13-4

DIFFERENTIAL DIAGNOSIS OF SCHIZOPHRENIA-LIKE SYMPTOMS

Medical or neurological*

Drug-induced intoxications: especially phencyclidine (PCP), ketamine, also amphetamines, cocaine, hallucinogens, levodopa (L-dopa), alcohol (e.g., hallucinosis); less commonly agents such as anticholinergic medications, belladonna alkaloids, cimetidine, digitalis, disulfiram

Drug-related withdrawal syndromes: such as alcohol, benzodiazepines, barbiturates, other sedative-hypnotic agents

CNS infections: such as human immunodeficiency virus (HIV), herpes encephalitis, Creutzfeldt-Jakob disease, neurosyphilis

Epilepsy: especially temporal lobe foci

Mass lesions: including frontal or temporal tumors, subdural/epidural hematoma, normal-pressure hydrocephalus

Metabolic abnormalities: such as acute intermittent porphyria, carbon monoxide poisoning, metachromatic leukodystrophy, heavy metal poisoning (arsenic, manganese, mercury, thallium), homocystinuria, Wilson's disease, Hallervorden-Spatz disease

Endocrinopathies: especially adrenal and thyroid

Progressive neurological disorders: such as Alzheimer's disease, Huntington's disease, Pick's disease

Autoimmune disorders: such as systemic lupus erythematosus, CNS vasculitis

Nutritional: such as B_{12} deficiency, pellagra

Psychiatric: including schizophreniform disorder, brief reactive psychosis, schizoaffective disorder, atypical psychosis, delusional disorder, major depressive disorder with psychotic features, bipolar affective disorder with psychotic features, personality disorders (especially schizotypal, schizoid, borderline, paranoid types), autism, mental retardation, malingering, factitious disorder with psychological symptoms

*Categories are defined for convenience of review and organization; some entities could be assigned to multiple categories (such as Wilson's disease to metabolic, progressive neurological, and psychiatric disorders)

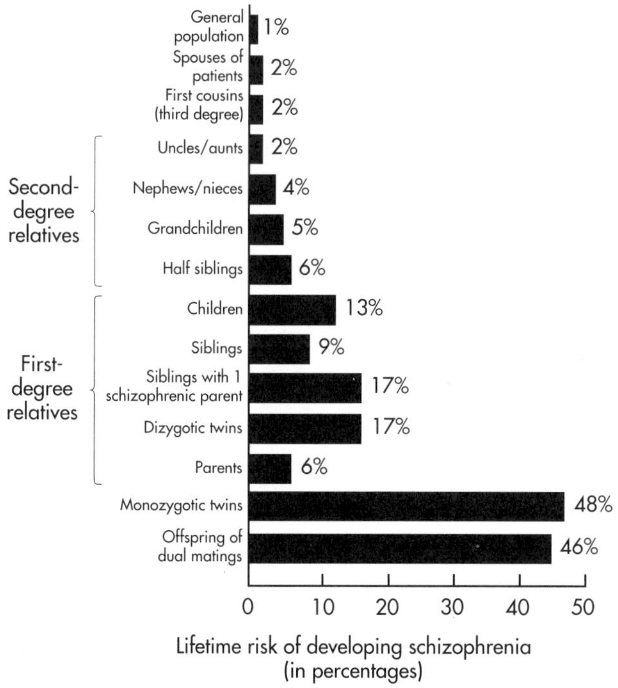

FIGURE 13-3 Grand average risks for developing schizophrenia show that the degree of risk is strongly associated with the degree of genetic relatedness (compiled from family and twin studies conducted in European populations between 1920 and 1987). (From Gottesman II: *Schizophrenia genesis,* New York 1991, W.H. Freeman and Co.)

syndrome per se but instead a more general vulnerability to the entire group of nonaffective psychoses, including schizophrenia, delusional disorders, schizophreniform disorder, schizoaffective disorder, and atypical psychosis.

The significant but variable risk for the transmission of schizophrenia within families is important information for couples who plan to have children and who have a family history of psychosis. For some time, physicians and genetic counselors have been trained to provide couples with important information about the familial transmission of medical disorders such as sickle cell anemia, which allows adequate planning and preparation preceding the birth of an affected child. More recently, researchers and genetic counselors have applied the additional knowledge gleaned from studies of the familial transmission of psychiatric disorders to the field of genetic counseling. As discussed in detail in Chapter 23, psychiatric genetic counseling presents unique challenges but offers families important information from a wealth of well-designed genetic studies.

In line with the high risk of co-morbid depression in patients with schizophrenia, genetic studies have also found that depression (and not mania) clusters in families with schizophrenia. Conversely, patients with depression do not have familial clustering of schizophrenia. This difference may be a function of the more heterogeneous nature of depression, which is capable of being caused by multiple biological and environmental factors, some of which occur in schizophrenia. It is worth noting that twin studies have strongly supported the diagnostic and familial separation of schizophrenia and bipolar disorder; however, there is less data available regarding delusional disorders and the other nonaffective psychoses.

Early Brain Injury

A growing understanding of normal maturational processes in the brain has led to important hypotheses regarding specific disruptions in the normal brain cell migration and organization that occurs during the second trimester in utero. A disruption in these normal developmental events has been proposed to explain post mortem findings of abnormal patterns of cellular orientation, abnormal cell counts, other abnormal morphological features, and reduced gray matter (cell body) volume as found by an MRI of the brain in patients with schizophrenia. Several studies have reported that patients with schizophrenia have a higher probability of having been born to mothers who were exposed to influenza in the second trimester, which suggests that a maternal-infant second-trimester viral infection may contribute to the risk for the development of the disorder. However, this association has not always been replicated. Other developmental events in the second trimester include the migration and organization of those cells that form the ridges of permanent fingertip patterns. Although these patterns are normally almost identical in monozygotic twins, researchers have found that twins who are discordant for schizophrenia show significant differences in these patterns. In line with neurodevelopmental hypotheses, other studies have suggested that patients with schizophrenia may have been subjected to a higher rate of perinatal complications than matched controls. Such obstetric complications seem to be more common in patients who do not have a family history for the disorder. However, these findings remain only nonspecific associations (that is no causality has been established). Whether such early developmental insults produce a higher risk for the development of schizophrenia alone or only in association with concomitant genetic risk remains to be established. Similar studies for delusional disorders have yet to be performed.

Combined Dysfunction of Dopamine and Glutamate Neurotransmitter Systems

The important early hypothesis for a primary disturbance in dopamine neurotransmitter systems in the brains of patients with schizophrenia was supported by several key observations, including the following: (1) effective antipsychotic medications block dopamine receptors, and their clinical potency is related to their ability to block those receptors; (2) indirect measures of dopamine activity in the brain are related to levels of psychosis before, during, and after withdrawal of treatment; (3) drugs that increase dopamine transmission increase psychosis; and (4) investigators have reported increased dopamine receptor concentrations in never-treated patients with schizophrenia. However, the dopamine hypothesis fails to explain the structural changes that occur in specific brain regions, the reason for a dissociation between the temporal onset of those changes and symptom onset, the progressive deteriorating course that afflicts some patients (and characterized the disorder before the availability of antipsychotic medications), and the ability of early and effective treatment to beneficially alter long-term course.

Considerable efforts have recently gone into the formulation of several competing hypotheses (with more or less in common) that propose a combined dysfunction of dopamine and glutamate neurotransmitter systems. For example, an important version of such a combined system dysfunction model and one that has substantial preclinical and clinical supporting data is the *N*-methyl-D-aspartate (NMDA) glutamate receptor hypofunction (NRH) hypothesis. The NRH hypothesis focuses on the NMDA subtype of the glutamate receptor, which can be effectively blocked to produce NRH by a number of agents, including ketamine and phencyclidine (PCP). These drugs also produce a relatively complete clinical model of schizophrenia-like symptoms when administered to humans, including positive, negative, disorganized and cognitive symptoms (in comparison to drugs such as amphetamine and lysergic acid diethylamide [LSD]). NRH that is sufficiently prolonged and/or pronounced is now known to produce excitotoxic brain injury in an anatomical distribution that has some overlap with the distribution of brain injury found in schizophrenia. However, this mechanism for neurotoxicity is not active until puberty, which is consistent with the observation that the psychotomimetic effects of NMDA antagonists are relatively absent in children and begin to occur in adolescents, and consistent with the young-adult age-of-onset of schizophrenia. Further, NRH-induced neurotoxicity seems to require simultaneous activation of several neurotransmitter systems, which contributes to the well-developed hypothesis of a complex circuit involving glutamatergic, GABAergic, noradrenergic, and various other excitatory pathways. Incorporating the dopamine hypothesis, the known interaction of dopamine receptors with this circuit suggests that dopaminergic hyperactivity can result in reduced glutamate release at NMDA receptors and a state of NRH with psychosis.

In-utero damage to the brain that leads to schizophrenia might be produced by a viral infection and a variety of other mechanisms, some of which are known to target NMDA-receptor–bearing GABAergic neurons. The NRH hypothesis predicts that in-utero damage to NMDA receptors and/or GABAergic neurons would lead to an NRH-equivalent condition with latent psychotogenic potential that would not manifest itself until adolescence. Interestingly, investigators have reported just such a lesion of GABAergic neurons in patients with schizophrenia. Subsequent activation of NRH-induced neurotoxic mechanisms could produce the pattern of structural brain changes found in neuroimaging and postmortem studies and involve neuronal damage in the cingulate cortex, hippocampus, parahippocampal gyrus, and entorhinal cortex. A number of specific pharmacologic agents can block the NRH-related circuit required for both psychosis and neurotoxicity. These include typical and atypical (see the section on treatment) antipsychotic medications, which provides an expanded explanation for their acute antipsychotic effects and a new and powerful explanation for the observation that early treatment with these medications can prevent long-term clinical deterioration. The NRH hypothesis also has implications for previous work that suggests that a relative failure of those brain circuits providing a gate or filter for sensorimotor pathways leads to a flood of unmodulated input (such as hallucinations). The NRH hypothesis increases the complexity of this gating hypothesis by suggesting a mechanism whereby several different cortical input paths could be disinhibited by the state of NRH. Overall, the NRH hypothesis is an important version of several more complex circuitry models that incorporate and extend the dopamine hypothesis. The NRH hypothesis sets an important standard with a substantial amount of preclinical and clinical supporting data, as well as a powerful explanatory capacity to incorporate previous work on early viral injury, the dopamine hypothesis, gating models, and findings from postmortem and structural neuroimaging studies.

Treatment

Few points are certain about the premodern history of treatments for conditions such as schizophrenia and delusional disorders except that this history probably extends back as far as humans have attempted to care for others with disease and dysfunction. Treatments have included an often bizarre array of physical and pharmacological approaches. This century has witnessed a revolution in the treatment of these disorders with the advent of relatively effective pharmacologic therapies for psychosis, which are now the principal mode of treatment. The use of surgical procedures on the brain has transformed from trephining to more modern procedures involving relatively specific brain structures and has been recently guided by sophisticated structural and/or functional neuroimaging procedures. So-called psychosurgery is currently used only very rarely and as a last resort in psychiatric cases, with a high degree of appropriate regulation. This century has also seen the evolution of insulin coma and early convulsive therapy into current techniques for the safe and effective application of electroconvulsive therapy (ECT) (see Chapter 22). Schizophrenia and delusional disorders are currently considered among the group of potential indications for the use of ECT in the American Psychiatric Association's ECT Task Force Report, particularly in the setting of catatonia, prominent affective symptoms, a prior ECT response, or a poor response to medication. However, further research in this area is needed to more clearly define indications and the relative efficacy of ECT with respect to drug therapy.

The mainstay of effective treatment for schizophrenia and delusional disorders is antipsychotic medication. Such medication is the principal factor accounting for therapeutic improvement during acute treatment and for relapse prevention during maintenance treatment. The efficacy of antipsychotic medications for the treatment of psychotic symptoms during acute exacerbations of illness is firmly established by a large number of placebo-controlled randomized clinical trials. This has secured a critical role for antipsychotic medications in the treatment of hospitalized patients and in the often effective outpatient treatment of acutely ill patients. Antipsychotic medications appear to effectively treat as many as 80% of the patients with schizophrenia, primarily targeting the positive symptoms found in schizophrenia and delusional disorders and the disorganization that can be prominent in schizophrenia. Most antipsychotic medications, with the exception of "atypical" drugs (discussed later in this section), are less helpful or even ineffective for the negative and cognitive symptoms of schizophrenia. Lithium, valproic acid, and carbamazepine all have been used adjunctively to treat schizophrenia, with little convincing and controlled data about the efficacy of these medications for this indication.

The efficacy of antipsychotic medications for the prevention of a psychotic relapse following acute treatment is also clearly established. The prescription of and compliance with effective maintenance doses of antipsychotic medications are the most important determinants of a patient's relative risk of relapse following successful acute treatment (see Table 13-5). Although individual variations in illness course suggest that some patients may not require continuous prophylactic treatment, there is still no clinical means of predicting who will or will not relapse after treatment discontinuation. The average rate of psychotic relapse in placebo-treated patients in remission or partial remission appears to be approximately 60% within 1 year, with no evidence that overall rates of relapse change appreciably in the second or third year. Unfortunately, medication side effects, a lack of knowledge about the long-term adverse consequences of undertreatment, and an illness-related loss of insight into the need for treatment can all undermine compliance. Long-acting depot antipsychotic medications can address some compliance issues, but attention to the unpleasant subjective effects and neurologic side effects of these medications is critical to maintaining an effective relationship with the patient. Clinical research has helped define the primary importance of forming a strong treatment alliance with patients and their families to ensure medication compliance and treatment follow-up.

Even with medication compliance and excellent follow-up, some patients experience a psychotic relapse or symptom exacerbations that may be most safely treated in the hospital, usually on a well-staffed and locked psychiatric unit. The major indications for hospitalization are usually disorder-related episodes of dangerousness to self or others or a temporary state of severe disability that compromises the patient's capacity to provide food, shelter, or adequate clothing. The decision to hospitalize a patient is best made in consultation with a psychiatrist who has expertise in the hospital management of patients with psychotic disorders (optimally the treating psychiatrist). This individual can also assist with decisions regarding the capacity of the patient to be treated on a voluntary (vs. involuntary) basis and can provide expertise on the safest and most expeditious means of getting the patient out of any danger and into a safer setting. Most patients can be treated and stabilized during a relatively brief hospitalization, usually 1 or more weeks as a direct function of the time needed for the onset of antipsychotic medication effects.

The Treatment Alliance

The treatment alliance is based on the patient's fundamental belief that the physician is there to provide help. To achieve a strong treatment alliance, physicians must build rapport with their patients through a commitment to educating patients about their condition and its treatment. Busy primary care physicians can receive some assistance with this goal through the use of written materials from sources such as the NIMH, the National Alliance for the Mentally Ill, and the local/state department of mental health offices. This treatment alliance should be explained to patients and conducted as a cooperative relationship in which the physician brings expertise about the disorder and its treatment to the patient and in which the patient brings to the physician expertise on his own experiences and treatment responses. Patients should be provided with as much information as they can understand on the basis of their clinical condition. The important point is that patients may be psychotic, but they are not "crazy" (that is, necessarily incompetent, unreasonable, incomprehensible, or irrational), and an effective working relationship with them cannot be excluded from an effective treatment plan. Simply prescribing medications, monitoring side effects, and leaving the relationship to someone else (that is, the nurse, psychologist, social worker, or other ancillary staff) provides a less effective level of care and is analogous to prescribing insulin to a patient with diabetes without personally providing instructions about the role of insulin in their illness and its overall management (see the Pearls & Perils box on p. 233).

Specific impediments to the treatment alliance and an understanding of the illness and its treatment can be found within each symptom grouping. An initial approach to such problems is outlined below, but their management is ultimately guided by the physician's judgment about how best to strengthen the alliance with individual patients. Although some patients may appear to engage only slowly or minimally in the alliance, and although setbacks may be encountered during periods of illness exacerbation, steady and unpressured effort from a physician who remains comfortable with the patient is usually rewarded. Families should also be included in this process of education and alliance to the greatest extent possible. (Meeting with the family may be problematic when chronic paranoid delusions regarding them could jeopardize the alliance with the patient.) Including families provides support to the patient and family, brings valuable data and extra partners into the physician's care of the patient, and can further ensure medication compliance.

Patients with positive psychotic symptoms may have delusions or hallucinations with content that impinges on an effective relationship with the physician or others (such as a delusion that the physician aims to harm them). This issue should be directly addressed in an interview and, if found, directly and matter-of-factly countered. Most helpful are simple statements indicating the physician's belief that these ideas, although very real for the patient, are part of a brain illness that interferes with the patient's otherwise accurate perceptions. When it is likely to be accepted, the physician should offer to work together with the patient to help distinguish those perceptions that are distorted by the illness from those that are accurate, stu-

PEARLS & PERILS

TREATMENT ALLIANCE

- The treatment alliance should be explained to patients and conducted as a cooperative relationship in which the physician brings expertise regarding the disorder and its treatment to the patients and in which the patients bring to the physician expertise about their own experiences and treatment responses.
- Patients should be provided with as much information as they can understand on the basis of their clinical condition.
- The important point is that patients may be psychotic, but they are not "crazy" (that is, necessarily incompetent, unreasonable, incomprehensible, or irrational), and an effective working relationship with them can not be excluded from an effective treatment plan.
- Simply prescribing medication, monitoring the side effects, and leaving the relationship to someone else (that is, the nurse, psychologist, social worker, or other ancillary staff) provides a less effective level of care that is analogous to prescribing insulin to patients with diabetes without personally providing instructions about the role of insulin in their illness and its overall management.

diously avoiding the impression that the patient's experience is being belittled or devalued. Avolition and ambivalence can be equally devastating to the therapeutic alliance. A persistent effort to engage and educate the patient combined with gentle encouragement is the best approach. Disorganization and cognitive impairment can also seriously undermine an educational program but should not be considered a justification not to make the effort to provide it. Such patients instead require extra time from the clinical staff, who should provide straightforward, clear explanations in plain language and ensure that the patient understands each step of the conversation. A large number of patients can be helped to understand even difficult issues such as the risk-benefit balance concerning TD and antipsychotic medications, to make reasonable decisions, and to give well-informed consent when provided with the facts. These discussions can occur initially over several visits and should be repeated over multiple visits, which reinforces the initial information and adds additional information as understanding permits.

Rational Choice of Medication and Medication Doses

The principal medication choices for the treatment of schizophrenia and delusional disorders currently center on the selection of so-called typical vs. atypical agents and the selection of appropriate doses. On a practical level, these choices are identical for schizophrenia and delusional disorders. Few controlled clinical trials are available for delusional disorders, but clinical wisdom suggests that no specific agents or dose ranges selectively target one group of psychotic disorders over another. Since their introduction into practice in the 1950s, typical antipsychotic medications—also referred to as neuroleptics or major tranquilizers—have been essentially the only available choice for the pharmacological treatment of these disorders. Despite their capacity to produce a number of important adverse effects (see Chapter 21), including the important extrapyramidal symptoms that define their "typicality," the clear efficacy of these agents for the treatment of positive symptoms and disorganization was rapidly recognized, and widespread treatment was instituted.

Individual typical antipsychotic medications are generally considered to be equally effective when given at equipotent doses. Clinical experience suggests that individual patients may preferentially respond to another typical medication, particularly one from a distinct class (such as aliphatic phenothiazine vs. butyrophenone), when they fail to respond adequately to one agent. However, there is little data to support this point, and some evidence suggests that patients fare just as well by continuing an optimal dose of whatever typical antipsychotic medication they are currently receiving. There is no rational reason for concomitant therapy with more than a single typical antipsychotic medication, and the potential for additional problematic side effects (discussed in the next paragraph) suggests a relative contraindication. An exception occurs during the transition from one antipsychotic to another and rarely for the brief management of psychotic exacerbations in which the single agent may lack sufficient sedation. Individual medications have been characterized as "low potency" vs. "high potency," with an inverse relationship to the effective acute treatment dose. Significant interindividual differences in absorption, metabolism, and effects on sites of action produce substantial interindividual differences in clinically effective doses, which underscores the importance of individual dose titration. Important ethnic/racial differences in drug metabolism have been identified (such as a higher rate of adverse effects and relatively higher plasma antipsychotic levels for a given dose in Asian patients, specifically those of Chinese and Japanese ethnicity). Another important example is found in the growing elderly population of patients, in which age-related declines in the capacity to metabolize drugs lead to lower effective doses and a lower dose threshold for the development of problematic side-effects.

The important differences among individual typical antipsychotic agents are with respect to adverse effects, mainly varying levels of sedation, autonomic, and neurological side effects. In general, typical lower potency antipsychotic agents (such as substituted phenothiazines) tend to be associated with more sedative, more autonomic, and other unwanted side effects than higher potency agents (such as the butyrophenone, haloperidol). On the other hand, the higher potency agents are more likely than low-potency agents to cause extrapyramidal and other neurological symptoms at clinically effective doses. Although sedation is sometimes tolerated during acute treatment (less often during maintenance), autonomic effects are generally problematic and unwanted (such as a dry mouth and accommodation disturbance), and poorly tolerated or even contraindicated in the elderly (such as constipation, tachycardia, hypotension). Further, the CNS consequences of anticholinergic effects, which are prominent with lower potency agents, include an impairment in memory and learning that is detectable in young subjects and becomes even more pronounced in the elderly. Anticholinergic effects are an important reason to avoid low-potency agents in the elderly, if not in all patients, many of whom already suffer some degree of disorder-related cognitive impairment. The general rule that a past therapeutic response to a specific agent suggests using it again is a good rule except when applied to aging patients or to those with impaired metabolic capacity (such as competing drugs and hepatic injury) who may have previously tolerated a particular agent or combination but are now less equipped to do so (see the Pearls & Perils box below).

Typical high-potency antipsychotic medications have seen increasing use because they have certain clinical advantages over lower potency agents. As previously stated, these agents generally have less sedative, autonomic, and other adverse effects than their lower potency counterparts. Haloperidol and fluphenazine are available as long-acting depot injections (generally 2- to 4-week dosing intervals) and can improve relapse prevention. This is mostly but perhaps not entirely explained by improved treatment compliance. Haloperidol and fluphenazine have also had the greatest amount of investigation on the relationship between their plasma levels and clinical response. When appropriate assays and expert consultants are available, plasma levels can be used to help guide dose selection in patients who fail to respond adequately to conventional dose titration. However, high-potency agents are more likely to produce neurological side effects, particularly extrapyramidal effects, which are unpleasant and can have a deleterious effect on the overall treatment response. Neurological side effects of antipsychotic medications that have been termed extrapyramidal symptoms include parkinsonism, akathisia, dyskinesias (acute and tardive), and dystonias (acute and tardive). None of these symptoms are desirable to the patient and all can adversely affect compliance

PEARLS & PERILS

SELECTION OF "TYPICAL" ANTIPSYCHOTIC AGENTS

- The important differences among individual typical antipsychotic agents are with respect to side effects, mainly varying levels of sedative, autonomic, and neurological side-effects.
- In general, lower potency typical antipsychotic agents (such as substituted phenothiazines) tend to be associated with more sedative, more autonomic, and other unwanted side effects than higher potency agents (such as the butyrophenone, haloperidol).
- The higher potency agents are more likely than low-potency agents to cause extrapyramidal and other neurological symptoms at clinically effective doses.
- Although sedation is sometimes tolerated during acute treatment (less often during maintenance), autonomic side effects are generally problematic and unwanted (such as a dry mouth and accommodation disturbance) and poorly tolerated or even contraindicated in the elderly (such as constipation, tachycardia, hypotension).
- The CNS consequences of anticholinergic effects are prominent with lower potency agents and include an impairment in memory and learning that is detectable in young subjects and becomes even more pronounced in the elderly.
- Anticholinergic effects are an important reason to avoid low-potency agents in the elderly, if not in all patients, many of whom already suffer some degree of disorder-related cognitive impairment.
- The general rule that a past therapeutic response to a specific agent suggests using it again is a good rule except when applied to aging patients or to those with an impaired metabolic capacity (such as competing drugs and hepatic injury) and who may have previously tolerated a particular agent or combination but are now less equipped to do so.

and overall functioning and can "mark" or stigmatize patients. The tardive (that is, late-onset) variant of dyskinesia is relatively common (that is, approximately 15% to 20% average prevalence, and 4% to 5% average annual incidence), with variable degrees of resolution and persistence.

Although the desired antipsychotic effects, along with some degree of sedation, are usually considered to be the only behavioral or psychological effects of antipsychotic medications, both parkinsonism and akathisia are associated with important behavioral and/or psychological effects. Considerable research has found that both of these side effects can mimic the primary symptoms of these disorders and can adversely affect therapeutic outcome in a generally dose-dependent manner. For example, even experts trained to make such discriminations cannot separate some negative symptoms from parkinsonism, which means, in short, that treatment-induced parkinsonism associated with higher doses of antipsychotic medications appears to worsen some negative symptoms. Akathisia is defined as a subjective desire to move with or without objective motor signs and is a common and unpleasant side effect of typical antipsychotic medications, with an average prevalence estimate of 20%. Akathisia is also associated with higher doses of antipsychotic medications and may have a major impact on treatment compliance and treatment outcome. Some investigators have found that patients with akathisia have more positive psychotic symptoms and a poor positive psychotic symptom response during acute treatment that is independent of the success or failure of akathisia treatment with benztropine mesylate. Akathisia has been more consistently related to anxiety and depression during both acute and maintenance haloperidol treatment, which is consistent with subjective descriptions of akathisia and with an early observation that akathisia may be mistaken for agitated depression. Parkinsonism and akathisia remain underrecognized side effects of antipsychotic therapy that, either directly or as a stress or cue for additional symptoms, account for higher levels of psychopathology in affected patients (see the Pearls & Perils box below).

An important goal, therefore, of antipsychotic medication treatment is to achieve a clinically effective dose without producing adverse effects, especially extrapyramidal side effects such as parkinsonism and/or akathisia. One approach to this goal has been simply to treat any extrapyramidal side effects with anticholinergic medications. Alternatively, some physicians choose to start prophylactic anticholinergic medications along with the neuroleptic medications, especially in younger, muscular individuals (who may be at higher risk), to avoid the adverse effects of an acute dystonic reaction on long-term medication compliance. However, these strategies expose patients to the adverse effects of anticholinergic therapy and may not completely resolve either the extrapyramidal symptom or its behavioral consequences. In addition, the prophylactic approach prevents an initial dose titration against side effects (described in the next paragraph) and might be reserved for patients with a history of prior acute dystonias. A rational approach to the emergence of extrapyramidal side effects during maintenance treatment is to attempt to lower the dose of the antipsychotic medication without adding anticholinergics, carefully monitoring for any reductions in therapeutic effect while titrating against improvement in side effects. Studies have suggested that the minimum effective dosages for the depot antipsychotics fluphenazine decanoate and haloperidol decanoate are in the range of 5 to 10 mg/2 weeks and 50 mg/4

PEARLS & PERILS

ADVERSE NEUROLOGICAL (EXTRAPYRAMIDAL) EFFECTS OF ANTIPSYCHOTIC MEDICATION

- Some negative symptoms cannot be separated from parkinsonism, even by experts trained to make such discriminations, which means, in short, that treatment-induced parkinsonism associated with higher doses of antipsychotic medications appears to worsen some negative symptoms.
- Akathisia is defined as a subjective desire to move with or without objective motor signs and is a common and unpleasant side effect of typical antipsychotic medications, with an average prevalence estimate of 20%.
- Akathisia is also associated with higher doses of antipsychotic medications and may have a major impact on treatment compliance and treatment outcome.
- Some investigators have found that patients with akathisia have more positive psychotic symptoms and a poor positive psychotic symptom response during acute treatment that is independent of the success or failure of akathisia treatment with benztropine mesylate.
- Akathisia has been more consistently related to anxiety and depression during both acute and maintenance haloperidol treatment, which is consistent with subjective descriptions of akathisia and with an early observation that akathisia may be mistaken for agitated depression.
- Parkinsonism and akathisia remain underrecognized side effects of antipsychotic therapy that, either directly or as a stress or cue for additional symptoms, account for higher levels of psychopathology in affected patients.

weeks, respectively. These dosages have efficacy for the prevention of relapse in many patients that is comparable with higher dosages, with beneficial reductions in neurological side effects and a subjectively improved sense of well-being. Investigators recently reported the results of a multicenter, double-blind evaluation of haloperidol decanoate, with patients randomly assigned to one of four fixed monthly dosages for 48 weeks: 25 mg, 50 mg, 100 mg, or 200 mg. The rates of psychotic relapse for the four treatment groups were 63%, 25%, 23%, and 15% respectively, which suggests comparable efficacy for the 50 mg and 100 mg doses and only a small increase in relapse protection for patients treated with the 200 mg dose. These studies suggest that lower doses of maintenance antipsychotics could benefit many patients with schizophrenia. However, attempts to lower the dose of maintenance antipsychotic medications may result in the reappearance of psychotic symptoms in some patients. Careful clinical monitoring should be used whenever dose adjustments are made.

The use of lower doses of typical antipsychotic medications during acute treatment in an effort to prevent extrapyramidal side effects such as parkinsonism and/or akathisia has been the subject of considerable research. In general, (1) acute treatment studies have suggested that dosages equivalent to oral haloperidol at more than 15 to 20 mg/day offer no additional benefits and an increased incidence of side effects, (2) dosages in the 15- to 20-mg/day range offer a slight advantage over lower dosages during the first weeks of acute treatment but are subsequently associated with higher dropout rates as a result of adverse effects, (3) dosages equivalent to haloperidol at 10 mg/day are efficacious and can be superior to lower dosages in many patients but may still produce adverse effects and could offer no advantages over lower dosages in patients who experience extrapyramidal effects, and (4) even lower dosages may be optimally effective when extrapyramidal side effects emerge at higher dosages, an observation that may be more common in patients who are naive to previous antipsychotic treatment. A promising and rational (so-called neuroleptic threshold) approach to dosage escalation is to gradually increase the dosage while monitoring for the emergence of parkinsonism or akathisia (such as starting at 2 mg/day of haloperidol and increasing by 2 mg every other day), aiming to maximize the dosage while maintaining minimal side-effect levels. This strategy depends on the idea that the onset of side effects occurs at dosages above those required for clinical efficacy, which produces a "therapeutic window" (Figure 13-4). In general, there is good evidence from clinical studies and positron emission tomography (PET) studies to support this approach to optimizing the therapeutic

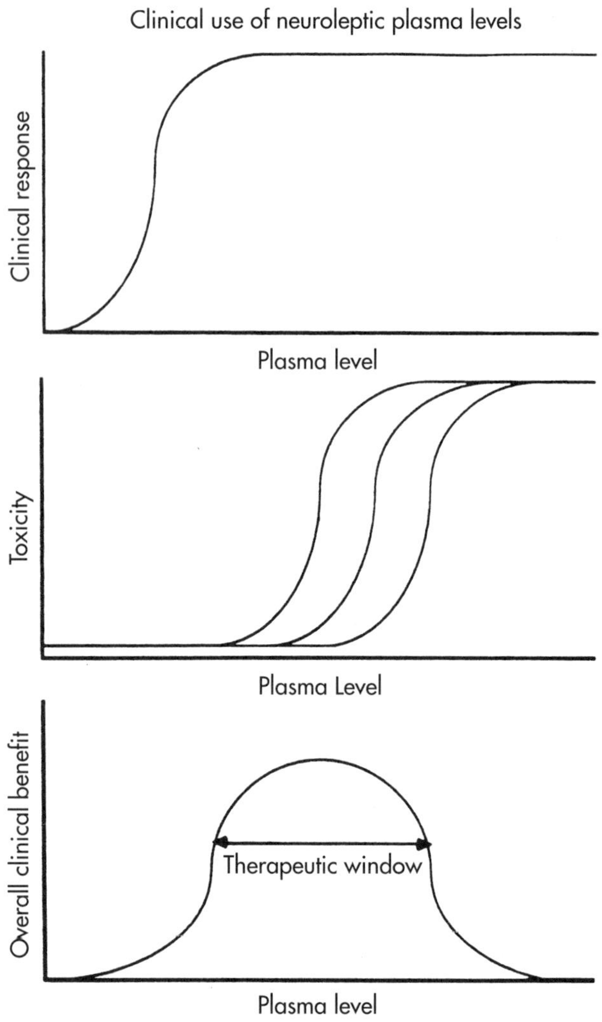

FIGURE 13-4 Theoretical concept of the therapeutic window produced by the difference between plasma level producing clinical effect and plasma level producing toxic side effects. (From Marder SR, Davis JM, Janicak PG, editors: *Clinical use of neuroleptic plasma levels,* Washington, D.C., 1993, American Psychiatric Press.)

response. However, some evidence suggests that akathisia may be more difficult to avoid than parkinsonism during treatment with typical antipsychotics.

One of the more difficult clinical dilemmas involves how long to wait for a desired response before making a change and then whether to increase or decrease the dosage of the current agent or to switch to a different (for example, atypical) antipsychotic agent. In general, the acute therapeutic effects of antipsychotic drugs require 2 to 4 weeks to manifest, a fact that remains underappreciated by third-party payers anxious to reduce inpatient length of stay. Although some therapeutic response can occur within the first hours and days of initiating treatment, some clinically relevant improvements can take as long as 6 to 8 weeks to occur, and further clinical improvement can continue to accrue for months. For these reasons, it is impossible for a physician to determine whether an improvement in symptoms following a switch to a different typical agent would have occurred anyway with additional time on the previous agent. Furthermore, the efficacy of a typical antipsychotic medication is thought to involve dopamine (D_2) receptor blockade, which may be maximized at dosages equivalent to, or even below, approximately 15 mg/day of haloperidol. Similarly, most efforts to increase treatment response or decrease response onset time by using significantly higher dosages have been ineffective and have produced higher levels of adverse effects.

The other approach to achieving therapeutic effects without extrapyramidal side effects is through the use of so-called atypical antipsychotic medications. No single agreed-on definition of "atypicality" is available, but on a practical clinical level, atypical medications share the characteristic of being relatively free of extrapyramidal side effects at clinically effective dosages. The currently marketed atypical antipsychotic medications are risperidone and clozapine. Risperidone was recently approved by the Food and Drug Administration for the first-line treatment of psychotic disorders and—supported by large-scale, well-controlled, randomized clinical trials in patients with schizophrenia—offers clinically significant advantages over typical drugs. The average clinically optimal acute treatment dosage for risperidone is 4 to 6 mg/day, except in older patients or those with impaired hepatic metabolism, in whom lower doses are appropriate. In a multicenter US/Canadian study, 6 mg/day of risperidone was more effective than haloperidol (20 mg/day), both overall as well as for the treatment of positive and negative symptoms. This improved effectiveness included a more rapid onset of action, with significant effects at 1 to 2 weeks vs. 4 weeks for haloperidol. In general, at dosages less than 10 mg/day, risperidone produces significantly less extrapyramidal side effects than the typical antipsychotic haloperidol at dosages of 10 to 20 mg/day. However, more is not better, and at higher dosages risperidone appears to lose its "atypicality" and produces extrapyramidal effects at levels more comparable to haloperidol. The relative risk of tardive dyskinesia while taking risperidone is unknown at this time. In contrast to typical medications, risperidone also importantly offers efficacy for the treatment of negative symptoms, which provides physicians and patients with the first front-line agent to effectively treat this symptom grouping. Risperidone also appears to have a lower propensity to produce other subjectively bothersome side effects, including less sedation than haloperidol at clinically effective dosages. Despite the favorable data for the 6 mg/day dosage, some patients may not tolerate this dosage and still others may require a higher dosage, which underscores the need for clinical titration in each patient and the utility of postmarketing data collection. Preliminary reports suggest the following: (1) the long half-life (22 hours) of the clinically active metabolite of risperidone, 9-hydroxy-risperidone, may permit once-a-day dosing (vs. initially recommended twice-a-day dosing), and (2) risperidone may be effective for patients who are unresponsive to other antipsychotic medications, with efficacy for some patients comparable to clozapine.

Clozapine is the other currently marketed atypical antipsychotic medication and is primarily indicated (and approved by the FDA) for the treatment of so-called treatment-resistant patients with schizophrenia. There is some consensus that these patients can be defined as having an inadequate response to two previous trials of typical antipsychotic medications of adequate dose and duration. It is reasonable to expect that clozapine will be tested for similarly refractory patients with delusional disorders, but such data do not currently exist. Clozapine has been demonstrated to produce improvements in symptoms in approximately 30% of all treatment-resistant patients, with as many as 60% improving when treatment is continued for 12 months, which offers an important and well-established option for those patients who fail previous therapy. Clozapine provides improvements in positive, disorganized, and some negative symptoms, as well as in social and occupational functioning. There is important evidence that clozapine can also improve some cognitive symptoms in patients with schizophrenia. Optimal clozapine dosages are in the range of 400 to 600 mg/day, which is achieved by very slow titration that generally starts at 12.5 mg/day (lower in elderly or debilitated individuals), but dosages up to 900 mg/day may be needed in some patients. Again, lower dosages are effective in older patients, usually 200 to 300 mg/day or less. Unfortunately, clozapine is not a first-line treatment because of the occurrence of agranulocytosis in 1% to 2% of the patients treated with this agent (in contrast to 1 out of every 2000 patients who are treated with typical antipsychotics). This occurrence has resulted in mandatory weekly monitoring of complete blood counts (CBCs) for the duration of treatment. Clozapine also carries a dose-dependent risk of inducing seizures, orthostatic hypotension, tachycardia, and sedation. Approximately 30% of all clozapine-treated patients develop hypersalivation, but this condition is usually easily treated with anticholinergic agents or dosage reduction. Clozapine itself is highly anticholinergic, accounting for some specific concerns previously noted for cognitive function especially in older patients, and for the important risk of cholinergic rebound (such as insomnia, agitation, abdominal cramping, and loose stool) if high dosages of clozapine are abruptly discontinued. When patients are not lost to follow-up, this risk is easily addressed by instituting an anticholinergic treatment such as benztropine mesylate, which can then be gradually tapered. Clozapine can have a delayed onset of therapeutic action, perhaps partly as a function of the population usually treated with this drug, with responses sometimes occurring after 6 months or even later. This delayed response has led to some controversy about the length of an adequate clozapine trial, ranging from 2 to 4 months to 6 to 9 months, before the risks and costs of treatment are thought to outweigh potential benefits. On a practical level, clozapine is currently the only clearly established treatment for otherwise long-suffering treatment-resistant patients. Until an alternative exists, there is a compelling logic to pursue extended trials that seek improvements in the quality of patients' lives.

General considerations for both clozapine and risperidone include the issue of concomitant antipsychotic medication use, the initiation of treatment, the order of use, and cost-effectiveness. There is no data to support the addition of a second antipsychotic medication to ongoing treatment with clozapine or risperidone, and the proposed mechanisms of action for these drugs suggest that concomitant treatment may compromise the "atypical" pharmacological profile of the therapeutic regimen. However, it remains prudent to continue the previous antipsychotic therapy for a brief period (for example, several weeks in outpatients) during the initial titration onto either clozapine or risperidone. Conversely, the gradual addition of the next agent is prudent during the gradual discontinuation of either clozapine or risperidone, but there is little data available for guidance about when to start and the optimal length of such overlapping titrations. Clinical vigilance and judgment should be applied to any periods of medication change.

A group of promising atypical antipsychotic medications are currently working their way through clinical trials (e.g., seroquel, ziprasidone, olanzapine, sertindole) and may become available sometime in the near future. These medications may also offer additional first-line treatments and yet-to-be-established effects for treatment-resistant patients. The addition of new atypical choices that may, like risperidone, offer advantages over typical agents for both efficacy and side effects, is likely to bring important and dramatic changes to clinical practice. The issue of which medications to use first in which patient populations and what continuing role should be played by typical agents will need to be established by controlled comparative trials in appropriate populations. For the present, risperidone is the only atypical medication for first-line use and is a relatively safer initial alternative to clozapine for treatment-resistant patients. However, the relative efficacy of risperidone for treatment-resistant patients has yet to be established, and clozapine remains the proven standard for this population. The development and expansion of atypical medication options is likely, in the long run, to change the recommended first-line approach to the treatment of these disorders, much as the addition of new medication classes has altered the management of cardiac disease over the past two decades. However, the new atypical medications are coming of age at a difficult time in terms of the economics of psychiatric care. Pressure to hold down public sector costs for the psychiatric care of the seriously mentally ill has led some groups to a simplistic comparison of medication costs for clozapine or risperidone vs. typical treatment, with the conclusion that access to the more expensive newer medications should be limited. Recent reports have countered such conclusions with more comprehensive analyses of the costs associated with the treatment and care of patients on both risperidone and clozapine, including factors such as hospital, outpatient, housing, family burden (such as lost wages by caretakers), and other illness-related expenses. In these analyses, risperidone reduces physician visits and the number of days in the hospital, and clozapine treatment significantly lowers costs associated with hospitalization, strongly supporting cost effectiveness in patients who use the hospital.

Constant vs. Intermittent Treatment

The rate of psychotic relapse in placebo-treated patients suggests that 40% of patients might avoid relapse for as long as 1 year without receiving any antipsychotic medication. This point suggests, at least in principle, that treatment could be used on an as-needed basis, which would limit exposure to side-effects. Since the strategy of identifying early signs of psychotic exacerbation to target time-limited treatment with antipsychotic medications was first suggested, several groups have demonstrated the feasibility of this approach. In these studies, intermittent dosing strategies have been associated with higher rates of relapse or rehospitalization, lower total doses over the period of study, and a lower incidence of side effects, with either no differences or modest disadvantages for intermittently dosed patients on measures of psychopathology and social functioning. The intermittent-dosing strategy might offer advantages but only for carefully selected, particularly insightful, and cooperative patients.

An important comparison of lower dose (2.5 to 10 mg fluphenazine decanoate every 2 weeks) and targeted intermittent treatment with standard continuous treatment (12.5 to 50 mg fluphenazine decanoate every 2 weeks) was recently completed. Investigators have reported preliminary results of this study that compare the three medication treatment conditions in combination with different family management interventions. A preliminary analysis of these data found an advantage for standard treatment over lower dose treatment and for lower dose over targeted intermittent treatment on measures of psychotic relapse. Standard treatment did not differ from lower dose treatment in either the time it took for patients to be rehospitalized or the percentage of patients rehospitalized during the 2 years of study. Importantly, both treatments were better than targeted intermittent treatment on these measures. In keeping with the previously mentioned discussions, negative symptom measures appeared to favor targeted and lower dose treatment over standard doses. Further analyses of the data from this definitive study of maintenance drug treatment in schizophrenia should yield further recommendations for achieving the optimal risk-to-benefit ratio.

Use of Adjunctive Medications

For specific indications, an adjunctive psychotropic medication can be very useful for treating symptoms that are not responsive to, or perhaps caused by, the primary antipsychotic medication. It is important to always consider the possibility that the primary agent may be contributing in some way to the problematic symptoms. Symptoms such as agitation or insomnia may be related to inadequate dosing or may reflect higher akathisia-producing doses. It is generally preferable to optimize treatment with the primary antipsychotic medication and to even consider a change in the primary agent (such as to an atypical agent) before adding second (or third) agents. The common indications for adding adjunctive medications are listed in Box 13-5.

Conclusion

This chapter has reviewed current information on the epidemiology, course, symptom definitions, diagnoses, etiology, pathophysiology, and treatment for schizophrenia and delusional disorders. The purpose was to provide the primary care physician, psychiatrists, and others with practical information bearing on the evaluation, diagnosis, and treatment of patients with these disorders. Such information is particularly important for schizophrenia, a relatively common psychiatric disorder that physicians are likely to encounter in their practice. Although schizophrenia remains a devastating and generally chronic disorder, it is important that physicians have up-to-date information to counter the perception and/or practice approach that assumes that patients will necessarily have a "bad" outcome. The information provided is aimed to be helpful to physicians practicing with and without ready access to psychiatric referral and consultation. This review was not intended as a "how-to" manual or as a statement that primary care physicians should take on a greater role as the sole providers of care for these patients. Rather, this chapter acknowledges the important role that is now and will be played in the future by primary care physicians in the management of patients with these disorders. An increased understanding of current clinical perspectives and research on schizophrenia and delusional disorders can be used to

BOX 13-5

COMMON INDICATIONS FOR ADDING ADJUNCTIVE MEDICATIONS

1. For the treatment of drug-induced parkinsonism, anticholinergic medications can be used (with attention to additional unwanted effects), but an antipsychotic dose decrease, when feasible, is preferred.
2. For the treatment of akathisia, β-blockers (e.g., propranolol 20 to 80 mg/day) and anticholinergics are often effective, but again an antipsychotic dose decrease, when feasible, may produce the desired effect.
3. The treatment of agitation and/or insomnia is less straightforward because such symptoms may reflect an overall exacerbation that suggests the utility of a dose increase and/or the temporary addition of a benzodiazepine. Such symptoms may also reflect akathisia related to treatment with a high potency agent or higher doses in general.
4. For the treatment of persistent or emergent depression, tricyclic antidepressants and serotonin-selective reuptake inhibitors have been used effectively. However, overall response rates may be lower in schizophrenia than in primary affective disorders.
5. For the treatment of acute dystonic reactions, anticholinergic agents are highly effective first choices and may not be needed chronically as dystonias seem to be more common early in the treatment course.
6. For the treatment of mood instability or the appearance of "manic" symptoms in patients with schizophrenia, lithium, valproic acid, and carbamazepine have been used adjunctively with an antipsychotic medication. However, there remains relatively little well-controlled data to guide clinical practice in this indication.

sharpen diagnostic and symptom recognition skills, to recognize problems early, and to clarify the approach to solving clinical management problems. The overall goal is to strengthen the working relationship between primary care physicians and psychiatrists in the management of patients with psychotic disorders.

CONSIDER CONSULTATION WHEN...

- Initial evaluation, diagnosis, and treatment plan is needed for first onset of illness or initial clinical presentation in the treatment setting
- Patient presents with new onset suicidal or dangerous ideation or behavior.
- Patient is not responding adequately to first-line treatment plans
- Patient requires hospitalization

Acknowledgment

Supported by a Scientist Development Award to JWN (MH 01045) from the National Institute of Mental Health.

Annotated Bibliography

American Psychiatric Association: *Diagnostic and statistical manual of mental disorders,* ed 4 (DSM-IV), Washington, D.C., 1994, American Psychiatric Press.

This book provides the currently used diagnostic criteria for schizophrenia and delusional disorders, including a general description of the disorders, their symptoms, course, associated features, and differential diagnosis.

Andreasen NC: Diagnosis and classification of schizophrenia, *Schizophr Bull* 19:199-214, 1993.

This article provides background concerning the diagnostic and classification systems applied to schizophrenia.

Gottesman II: *Schizophrenia genesis: the origins of madness,* New York, 1991, W.H. Freeman.

This book is a very readable text, is aimed at a sophisticated lay reader, and covers the history of the disorder called schizophrenia. There is a detailed discussion of genetic and some environmental insults, moving clinical anecdotes, and a discussion of some of the important social policy issues related to the disorder.

Manschreck TC: Delusional (paranoid) disorders. In Kaplan HI, Sadock BJ, editors: *Comprehensive textbook of psychiatry/V,* 1989, Williams and Wilkins.

This chapter provides a more in-depth discussion of delusional disorders, with interesting historical detail.

Wyatt RJ: Schizophrenia: biochemical, endocrine, and immunological studies. In Kaplan HI, Sadock BJ, editors: *Comprehensive textbook of psychiatry/V,* Baltimore, 1989, Williams and Wilkins.

This chapter provides a comprehensive discussion of the long list of biochemical, endocrine, and immunological hypotheses that have been studied in the search for causes of schizophrenia.

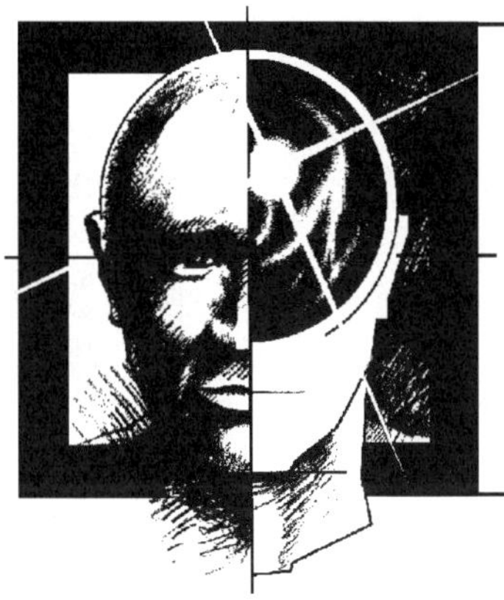

chapter 14

Alcoholism and Other Substance Use Disorders

Wilson M. Compton, MD

Extreme, end-stage cases of alcoholism and other addictions are unfortunately common (Case 14-1). They are readily diagnosed by all clinicians. On the other hand, milder cases of alcoholism and other addictions are some of the most commonly overlooked medical disorders. Even the most competent physician may miss these cases because the chief complaint is apparently unrelated to substance use. The chief complaint to the primary care physician is usually a nonspecific medical complication of the substance use. Headaches, gastrointestinal complaints, and accidents are some of the most common reasons for consultation. Each may be a symptom of a substance abuse problem.

Why is it so difficult to diagnose substance abuse problems in the primary care setting? Often the answer is that the presenting physical symptom is easily treated and responds to short-term care. By focusing on the immediate issues and ignoring the underlying addiction the physician avoids confrontation with the patient, and indeed, substance abuse disorders are often subtle and difficult to detect in their earliest forms. Nevertheless, if substance abuse is not recognized and addressed, the chances for further complications are high.

The lack of insight that many substance abusers have concerning their own substance use patterns contributes to the underdiagnosis of addiction. Perhaps the most difficult aspect of recognizing and treating these disorders is the baffling and complex presenting symptoms in the face of massive denial by the patient; that is, patients in the earlier stages of addiction rarely recognize the impact of the disease on their own lives and on those around them. Statements often include: "I'm still working—it hasn't hurt my job. I can't be an addict," or, "I can quit any time. I just don't want to right now." How do competent physicians diagnose these disorders, and what can a primary care physician do about them? Patients often minimize or ignore altogether the early warning signs; thus the primary care physician's role is most important for such people. Developing techniques to evaluate and treat patients with substance use disorders represents a challenging (and rewarding) clinical task.

CASE 14-1

Mrs. C. consumes at least a fifth of vodka each day, starting early in the morning and continuing throughout the day. She wakes every day with tremors, nausea and diarrhea, and has been hospitalized for pancreatitis and alcoholic hepatitis. Mrs. C. feels unable to function without alcohol and has lost all contact with her children because they have "given up" on her. She has been unable to quit drinking for longer than a few weeks despite multiple attempts. This inability to control her drinking is in spite of the fact that she has been in several alcohol treatment programs both for detoxification and for rehabilitation. Mrs. C.'s physicians are frustrated with her care, and she seems destined for an early alcohol-related demise.

PEARLS & PERILS

EVALUATION AND MANAGEMENT OF SUBSTANCE ABUSE

- Routine questioning about substance use patterns should be incorporated into every new patient evaluation.
- Current diagnostic practice is to diagnose dependence or abuse for each appropriate substance separately.
- Common illicit substances vary from community to community, so clinicians need to keep up with local drug use patterns.
- Patients with medical conditions such as diabetes mellitus or hypertension unresponsive to typical therapies or who are noncompliant may be substance abusers.
- Community support such as Alcoholics Anonymous (AA) is important for short- and long-term sobriety for many patients.
- New medications for addiction include naltrexone for alcoholism.
- Relapses are common, although not universal, especially in the first few months of sobriety.
- Self-administered and clinical screening questionnaires for alcoholism and drug abuse are easy to use and can be incorporated into usual practices.
- Screening instruments do not take the place of careful and thorough history and physical examination of patients with substance abuse.
- Avoiding anger in dealing with substance abusing patients is sometimes difficult.
- Overlap of substance abuse with psychiatric symptoms is common, and patients with psychiatric symptoms may have an underlying addiction.
- For patients with substance abuse and psychiatric symptoms (dual diagnosis), substance abuse problems should almost always be addressed first, since many psychiatric symptoms will improve markedly if substance use is eliminated.
- The human immunodeficiency virus (HIV)-risk behaviors of substance abusers include increased sexually risky behaviors, as well as needle-use behaviors.

The goal of this chapter is to provide ways to recognize and treat alcoholism and other addictions in their early forms, where intervention and treatment are most critical (see the Pearls & Perils box above).

Diagnosis

Alcoholism and other substance use disorders are behavioral diseases with the (obvious) necessary component of substance consumption. In addition, for a substance use disorder to be diagnosable, there must be evidence of problems caused by the consumption (see Table 14-1). The types of problems vary considerably, but it is important to keep in mind several concepts: (1) the progressive nature of substance dependence; (2) the stereotyped and consistent manifestations of the severe forms of substance dependence; (3) how substance dependence can affect all aspects of human existence (physical, psychological, emotional, familial, legal, employment, or spiritual), and (4) how the pharmacology of different substances explains some of the variation in addictive potential and withdrawal severity.

The term *alcoholism* originated in the mid-nineteenth century, but descriptions of problems from alcohol consumption date from antiquity. The first writings to describe alcoholism as a disease were from the early nineteenth century, and by the end of that century several facilities had been established for the treatment of alcoholism. In fact, the *Journal of Inebriety* was established in 1876, based on the explicit idea that drunkenness was a mental disease. In the modern era perhaps the best known descriptions of alcoholism as a disease were written by Jellinek, whose writings helped convince the medical community of the usefulness of the disease model of alcoholism. He described the symptoms and signs of alcoholism and emphasized the chronic, progressive course of the syndrome. His detailed analyses of the differences between men's and women's symptoms and courses remain a major contribution to the clinical understanding of these difficult conditions.

In the mid-1970s, Edwards and Gross described the "dependence syndrome," which emphasized symptoms of loss of control over alcohol in addition to tolerance and withdrawal. This approach to the diagnosis of alcoholism was adopted in the International Classification of Diseases-Tenth Edition (ICD-10) and the American Psychiatric Association's Diagnostic and Statistical Manual for Mental Disorders, Third Edition-Revised and the recently released Fourth Edition (DSM-III-R and DSM-IV), although the precise criteria vary between each of these systems. The approach has been applied to other substance dependence syndromes as well so that a single set of criteria is used for all substances in DSM-IV and ICD-10. As mentioned, the exact symptoms vary from one nomenclature to another, but the basic concepts include:

- Loss of control over substance use, seen in the inability to quit or cut down; excessive time spent in activities surrounding substance use; the way non-substance-related activities are reduced; continued substance use despite significant problems; and use of more of a substance than intended.
- Physiological symptoms of dependence, such as tolerance (needing more or responding less to the same doses); typical withdrawal symptoms, which vary depending on the substance; and use of a substance to avoid withdrawal.
- Significant problems from substance use, including problems with physical health, psychological health, the legal system, employment, and social relationships.
- Feeling dependent on a substance, including cravings or urges to use and inability to function without substance use.

DSM-IV defines substance dependence as three or more symptoms (from a list of seven) occurring within a 1-year period (Box 14-1 and Table 14-1). Substance abuse is defined as a residual category for people with certain social or legal problems from substance use but not enough of the dependence symptoms to meet criteria for that disorder (see Box 14-1). People can abuse or be dependent on several substances at the same time, and according to DSM-IV, each of these diagnoses would be made separately. Because each particular substance has unique associated problems, it is important to list all of the individual diagnoses. That way, communication with other physicians is facilitated, and the physician's own charts become a clearer record of all clinical symptoms.

As mentioned, despite the common approach to the diagnosis of addiction, each substance has distinct characteristics. In nearly all communities, alcohol and nicotine addiction are the disorders that cause the greatest morbidity. However, with illicit substances, particular communities may face unique challenges. For example, amphetamines are not commonly abused in most parts of the United States today except for parts of southern California and a few other localities.

Which substances should the primary care physician know about? The list of abusable substances is long, and new substances are added all the time, such as the recently developed methylenedioxymethamphetamine (MDMA) (produced illicitly as one of the famous "designer" drugs) and fentanyl (produced by a pharmaceutical company) (Box 14-2). Pharmacological principles are important in understanding the abuse potential of various substances: (1) rapid onset is generally associated with abuse potential; thus injectable and smokable forms of a drug are generally more addictive than an oral form and (2) a short half-life is generally associated with abuse potential.

In focusing on those substances that have the greatest "public health concern," five main categories are covered: nicotine, alcohol, opiates, cocaine, and cannabinoids. Other categories of substances may also be important for certain groups of patients but are mentioned only briefly in this chapter.

Nicotine is the most common and most destructive single substance of abuse. It is the main psychoactive substance in tobacco products. The physical destructiveness of these agents is well-known to physicians. They include mouth, larynx, and lung carcinomas; emphysema; cardiovascular diseases; and a variety of other conditions. The addictive potential of these agents is also familiar to physicians who have become frustrated in attempts to get their patients to quit smoking. The addictive potential of nicotine has been shown conclusively in animal and clinical models; it is ranked with heroin and cocaine in terms of addictive potential, which is well above alcohol, sedatives, and cannabis. No diagnosis of tobacco abuse is made, but the usual criteria for tobacco dependence are used.

Alcohol is responsible for thousands of injuries and deaths in every region of the country each year. Symptoms of alcoholism (alcohol dependence), in addition to those that are part of the general substance dependence syndrome described above, include blackouts (anterograde amnesia), benders, and drinking of nonbeverage alcohol. Alcohol withdrawal is a typical reason for medical consultation and is discussed in some detail in the following.

Opiates include an important group of analgesic agents derived from the sap of the opium poppy and chemically related synthetic compounds. The routes of administration include by mouth, injection, or smoking. Opiate use disorders include abuse, dependence, withdrawal, and overdose. These conditions have been recognized and studied for decades. Opiate dependence usually involves significant tolerance and withdrawal symptoms, but all of the other symptoms of dependence may also be present. People who become

DSM-IV DIAGNOSTIC CRITERIA

BOX 14-1 SUBSTANCE DEPENDENCE

A maladaptive pattern of substance use, leading to clinically significant impairment or distress, as manifested by three (or more) of the following, occurring at any time in the same 12-month period:

(1) tolerance, as defined by either of the following:

- (a) a need for markedly increased amounts of the substance to achieve intoxication or desired effect
- (b) markedly diminished effect with continued use of the same amount of the substance

(2) withdrawal, as manifested by either of the following:

- (a) the characteristic withdrawal syndrome for the substance (refer to Criteria A and B of the criteria sets for Withdrawal from the specific substances)
- (b) the same (or a closely related) substance is taken to relieve or avoid withdrawal symptoms

(3) the substance is often taken in larger amounts or over a longer period than was intended

(4) there is a persistent desire or unsuccessful efforts to cut down or control substance use

(5) a great deal of time is spent in activities necessary to obtain the substance (e.g., visiting multiple doctors or driving long distances), use the substance (e.g., chain-smoking), or recover from its effects

(6) important social, occupational, or recreational activities are given up or reduced because of substance use

(7) the substance use is continued despite knowledge of having a persistent or recurrent physical or psychological problem that is likely to have been caused or exacerbated by the substance (e.g., current cocaine use despite recognition of cocaine-induced depression, or continued drinking despite recognition that an ulcer was made worse by alcohol consumption)

Specify if:

With Physiological Dependence: evidence of tolerance or withdrawal (i.e., either Item 1 or 2 is present)

Without Physiological Dependence: no evidence of tolerance or withdrawal (i.e., neither Item 1 nor 2 is present)

Course specifiers (see DSM-IV for definitions):

Early Full Remission
Early Partial Remission
Sustained Full Remission
Sustained Partial Remission
On Agonist Therapy
In a Controlled Environment

SUBSTANCE ABUSE

A. A maladaptive pattern of substance use leading to clinically significant impairment or distress, as manifested by one (or more) of the following, occurring within a 12-month period:

- (1) recurrent substance use resulting in a failure to fulfill major role obligations at work, school, or home (e.g., repeated absences or poor work performance related to substance use; substance-related absences, suspensions, or expulsions from school: neglect of children or household)
- (2) recurrent substance use in situations in which it is physically hazardous (e.g., driving an automobile or operating a machine when impaired by substance use)
- (3) recurrent substance-related legal problems (e.g., arrests for substance-related disorderly conduct)
- (4) continued substance use despite having persistent or recurrent social or interpersonal problems caused or exacerbated by the effects of the substance (e.g., arguments with spouse about consequences of intoxication, physical fights)

B. The symptoms have never met the criteria for Substance Dependence for this class of substance.

Modified from American Psychiatric Association: *Diagnostic and statistical manual of mental disorders,* ed 4 (DSM-IV), Washington, D.C., 1994, American Psychiatric Press.

DIAGNOSIS

TABLE 14-1

SUBSTANCE DEPENDENCE

Discriminating features

1. Continued use of a substance despite significant problems
2. Repeated self-administration of a substance
3. Evidence of loss of control over substance use

Consistent features

1. Chronic relapsing course
2. Multiple social, psychological, and physical complications
3. Craving for the substance is common

Variable features

1. Physiological signs and symptoms (tolerance and withdrawal)
2. Psychiatric comorbidity, especially antisocial personality disorder and mood disorders
3. Family history of substance-related problems.

dependent on heroin (the classic street opiate) generally begin use in their late teens or early 20s but do not seek treatment for many years. Such progression of symptoms may be dependent on the context of opiate use, as shown by Robins in her study of opiate dependence among Vietnam veterans returning to the United States.

Cocaine has become one of the most significant drugs of abuse in the past decade with the dissemination of the crack (smokable base) form of the drug. Because of its quick absorption, this form has as rapid an onset as injected cocaine. Cocaine dependence has the usual symptoms, except that the withdrawal syndrome is mild and has quite nonspecific symptoms of poor concentration, disrupted sleep pattern, depression, appetite change, craving, and restlessness. The progression of the dependence syndrome seems to be more rapid for cocaine than for alcohol or opiates in that the time from first use to treatment entry is shorter for cocaine than for these other substances.

Cannabis is generally administered by smoking but can be taken orally. Cannabis use is quite common, but abuse and dependence are seen less often. Thus the addictive liability for cannabis seems to be less than for nicotine, alcohol, opiates, and cocaine. Withdrawal symptoms from cannabis, if any, are generally mild; they include sleep disturbance, impaired concentration, irritability or anxiety, and craving for the drug. Psychosis has also been described as a rare complication of cannabis use.

BOX 14-2

ABUSABLE SUBSTANCES

Cannabinoids: marijuana, hashish
Stimulants: amphetamines, MDMA
Sedatives: barbiturates, Quaalude, benzodiazepines
Opioids: codeine, Demerol, morphine, Percodan, methadone, Darvon, Dilaudid, Talwin, fentanyl, heroin
Cocaine, crack
Phencylidine (PCP)
Hallucinogens: LSD, mescaline, peyote, psilocybin
Inhalants: glue, toluene, gasoline, paint
Other: nitrous oxide, amyl nitrite

There are many other psychoactive substances, and as new therapeutic agents are introduced and the drug users develop tastes for different substances, the profile of substances abused in a given community may change. Thus it is important that physicians remain up-to-date concerning substances commonly used in their own communities. This can be accomplished by asking colleagues which substances are identified in emergency room admissions and through local or national sources of data, such as the Drug Use Forecasting Survey of the National Institute of Justice, publications of state public health agencies, and the Drug Abuse Warning Network Survey, all of which present early indications of newly prevalent substances. At present, other substances include the following:

- Other stimulants (amphetamines) are very similar to cocaine in their action and side effects. The amphetamines used to be prescribed quite liberally until the abuse potential was recognized approximately 20 years ago. Presently, the main indication for prescription of amphetamines is attention deficit disorder.
- Sedative/hypnotics (benzodiazepines and barbiturates primarily) are commonly prescribed and are usually taken without significant symptoms of abuse or dependence. Barbiturates historically were the prototype for these agents, but prescriptions for barbiturates have been replaced with benzodiazepines, which have a much wider margin of safety in overdose and have less potential for abuse. Withdrawal symptoms are identical to those of alcohol and can be fatal in the most extreme cases. Agents with short half-lives are the most likely to produce significant withdrawal. It should also be noted that abuse potential varies among the benzodiazepines, with diazepam being the most popular among substance abusers.
- Hallucinogens (lysergic acid diethylamide [LSD], psilocybin, etc.) are usually taken orally, but

some preparations may be taken intranasally, injected, or absorbed through mucous membranes. Tolerance to the effects of hallucinogens develops very quickly, so daily use is uncommon. Dependence is unusual, but overdose or intoxication is marked by agitation, perceptual distortions, frank hallucinations (especially visual), and severe anxiety. Flashbacks may occur chronically.
- Phencyclidine has been gaining in popularity in certain areas again. The usual route of administration is by smoking, but it is sometimes taken orally, intranasally, or by injection. Acute effects include nystagmus, especially vertical nystagmus; disinhibition; analgesia; flushing; diaphoresis; disorientation; and disorganized violent attacks. It has been reported to precipitate chronic psychosis.
- Hydrocarbon inhalants include toluene, gasoline, paint thinner, and others. The effects of these substances are short-lived (about 30 minutes) with ataxia, euphoria, and sometimes hallucinations. Significant neurological damage is seen in chronic abusers. A full dependence syndrome is unusual, but progression to other substances is common. An association of inhalant use with future injection drug use has also been hypothesized.
- Other agents (steroids, amyl nitrite). The bottom line is "if it has a significant acute effect on the central nervous system (CNS), someone will abuse it." Most of these other agents would not be expected to lead to a dependence syndrome.

Natural History

The course of alcoholism and other addictions has been described by many different authors from retrospective analysis, but only a few have examined these conditions prospectively; most of these have focused primarily on alcoholism and not on other substances. Published longitudinal studies have included samples from a variety of settings: prisons, outpatients, inpatients, and college students. Despite different samples, different definitions of alcoholism and addiction, and different lengths of follow-up, several important characteristics emerge from these studies: a small but significant percentage of addicts remit each year, regardless of the sample's origin. Return to controlled substance use (mostly shown for drinking) seems to be rare and primarily limited to mild cases at baseline. The onset of addiction is generally insidious, and the course and symptoms vary between men and women. Women seem to begin substance use at a later age, have more varied courses, and may have a more rapid progression of symptoms. In general, alcoholism and other addictions fit the pattern of chronic, relapsing disorders. Periods of remission may last for varying times, and outcome can be expected to include relapse in the majority of cases.

Differential Diagnosis

Substance use disorders are fairly straightforward and have clearly operationalized criteria, thus the differential is not difficult. Screening for primary and secondary psychiatric conditions is important, that is, patients with other psychiatric symptoms are at particularly high risk of having substance abuse problems. When substance abuse is suspected, it is reasonable to consider carefully whether other psychiatric conditions such as depression, anxiety, or personality disorders are present. Similarly, when psychiatric symptoms are detected, it is critical that substance abuse be considered as part of the differential diagnosis. Screening for additional substance use problems is also important when one disorder is suspected.

Case Identification

What tools can help the primary care physician screen for alcoholism and other addictions? Several have been described in the literature and have been used extensively during the past 2 decades. Commonly used screening instruments include the Michigan Alcohol Screening Test (MAST), a related drug abuse instrument called the Drug Abuse Screening Test (DAST), and the Alcohol Use Disorders Identification Test (AUDIT). The MAST and DAST are similar to each other in that they are self-administered by respondents and have been shown to identify most people with substance problems. People scoring positive on three or more items on either of these tests need further evaluation for possible substance abuse problems, and people scoring positive on five or more items have a strong likelihood of having a substance use disorder.

The AUDIT, a newer instrument developed by the World Health Organization (WHO), is a short screening test for alcoholism that has very good sensitivity and specificity. As shown in Box 14-3, the AUDIT consists of 10 items. A score of eight means there is a possible alcohol disorder; a score of 10 or greater is indicative of a probable disorder. A complementary clinical screening evaluation can also be used. This clinical scale includes gamma glutamyl transferase (GGT), history of head injury and accidents, and coded results of a physical examination. These screening instruments can be used in a variety of inpatient and outpatient settings. They may be particularly appropriate for new evaluations of outpatients.

To incorporate questions concerning substance abuse into clinical evaluations, it is important to keep

BOX 14-3

WORLD HEALTH ORGANIZATION ALCOHOL USE DISORDERS IDENTIFICATION TEST

1. How often do you have a drink containing alcohol?
   (0) Never
   (1) Monthly or less
   (2) 2 to 4 times a month
   (3) 2 to 3 times a week
   (4) 4 or more times a week
2. How many drinks containing alcohol do you have on a typical day when you are drinking?
   (0) 1 or 2
   (1) 3 or 4
   (2) 5 or 6
   (3) 7, 8, or 9
   (4) 10 or more
3. How often do you have six or more drinks on one occasion?
   (0) Never
   (1) < monthly
   (2) Monthly
   (3) Weekly
   (4) Daily or almost daily
4. How often during the last year have you found that you were not able to stop drinking once you had started?
   (0) Never
   (1) < monthly
   (2) Monthly
   (3) Weekly
   (4) Daily or almost daily
5. How often during the last year have you failed to do what was normally expected of you because of drinking?
   (0) Never
   (1) < monthly
   (2) Monthly
   (3) Weekly
   (4) Daily or almost daily
6. How often during the last year have you needed a first drink in the morning to get yourself going after a heavy drinking session?
   (0) Never
   (1) < monthly
   (2) Monthly
   (3) Weekly
   (4) Daily or almost daily
7. How often during the last year have you had a feeling of guilt or remorse after drinking?
   (0) Never
   (1) < monthly
   (2) Monthly
   (3) Weekly
   (4) Daily or almost daily
8. How often during the last year have you been unable to remember what happened the night before because you had been drinking?
   (0) Never
   (1) < monthly
   (2) Monthly
   (3) Weekly
   (4) Daily or almost daily
9. Have you or someone else been injured as a result of your drinking?
   (0) Never
   (1) < monthly
   (2) Monthly
   (3) Weekly
   (4) Daily or almost daily
10. Has a relative or friend or a doctor or another health worker been concerned about your drinking or suggested you cut down?
   (0) No
   (2) Yes, but not in the last year
   (4) Yes, during the last year

From Babor TF et al: *AUDIT—the Alcohol Use Disorders Identification Test: guidelines for use in primary health care,* Geneva, 1992 World Health Organization Programme on Substance Abuse.

in mind the communication techniques that help improve accurate reporting of substance use and substance-related symptoms (Box 14-4), that is, ways to reduce "denial." First and foremost is asking detailed and direct questions. Other techniques must be considered in the context of particular clinical settings. In general it is appropriate to assume the behavior will be present and to avoid undue confrontation (balanced with the need to clarify responses). Assuming the behavior means to ask, "What drugs have you ever taken to feel better, more alert, or high?" instead of, "Have you ever used drugs to feel better, more alert, or high?" Using these techniques, many "unexpected" cases will be discovered.

BOX 14-4

CLINICAL INTERVIEWING TECHNIQUES TO IMPROVE ACCURACY OF REPORTING OF SUBSTANCE ABUSE

Communicate expectation for accurate information.
Show empathy.
Assume behavior, but ask for details.
Suggest behavior is common.
Avoid undue confrontation but clarify responses.
Avoid moralistic or threatening overtones.
Integrate information from different sources.

Epidemiology and Pathophysiology

Understanding the rates of alcoholism and other addictions among different groups gives an important glimpse of the places where prevention (both primary and secondary) is most needed. Although the rates of alcoholism and illicit substance abuse vary across studies (perhaps based on different samples, diagnostic instruments, and different diagnostic criteria), the association with certain "risk factors" remains consistent. For example, in a large number of epidemiological samples, strong associations have been found between male gender and substance abuse and between antisocial personality disorder and substance abuse. According to recent studies of the general population, nicotine dependence is the most common of all substance use disorders. Up to 25% of the adult population is currently addicted to nicotine. Recently the rate among women has nearly equalled that of men (seen indirectly in the increasing rates of lung cancer among women). Alcohol dependence (alcoholism) is the next most common substance use disorder; approximately 25% have had alcohol dependence at some time in their lives, and 10% have had symptoms within the past year. This means that currently there are more than 10 million alcoholics in the United States. Alcoholism is more common among men than women and tends to run in families (although the hereditary pattern is somewhat uncertain). Other substance abuse and dependence is less common; about 12% of the adult population has been dependent on another substance (that is, any substance except tobacco or alcohol) at some time in their lives, and 4% have had symptoms in the past year. Like alcohol, other substance abuse and dependence is more common among younger age groups and men.

The association of substance use disorders and other psychiatric conditions (such as antisocial personality disorder, depression, anxiety, and schizophrenia) is complex. Overlap is extremely common; it is well-documented that an excess of substance use disorders is found among people with other psychiatric conditions and an excess of other psychiatric conditions is found in people diagnosed with substance use disorders.

HIV-risk behaviors are more common among people with substance abuse and dependence. These include both the obvious injection behaviors as well as sexual risk behaviors. Substance abusers may trade sex for drugs or may engage in prostitution in order to make money to support a drug habit. Use of safer sex techniques unfortunately is not the norm. In addition, use of psychoactive substances reduces inhibitions and impairs judgment. Heavy alcohol users and other substance abusers engage in more risky sexual behaviors than other people. Furthermore, Compton and colleagues have shown that increased HIV-risk behaviors may be even more common among substance abusers with comorbid psychiatric conditions such as antisocial personality disorder.

Genetic Epidemiology

Family, twin, and adoption studies have provided evidence for a genetic component to alcoholism. Virtually all family studies have shown much higher than expected rates of alcoholism among the relatives of alcoholics. Of course familial clustering does not prove a genetic component to the inheritance of alcoholism. For such evidence, adoption and twin studies are examined. Adoption studies have generally shown that alcoholism in offspring is predicted by alcoholism among biological, not adoptive, relatives. One study showed some evidence that drug misuse also was associated with alcoholism in biological relatives, and another showed a tendency for antisocial behavior to be inherited by a subgroup of adoptees of alcoholics. However, no other psychiatric conditions were consistently seen to coexist with the alcoholism.

Twin studies have consistently shown an excess of alcoholism in the co-twins of monozygotic (MZ) twins compared with dizygotic (DZ) twins. Most recently, twin studies from Minnesota and Virginia have provided more evidence of the heredity of alcoholism by showing that MZ twins have higher concordance than DZ twins among both male and female twin pairs. These studies, from the general family studies to the most specific twin projects, clearly indicate a genetic predisposition to alcoholism.

Currently, a major project supported by the National Institute on Alcoholism and Alcohol Abuse (NIAAA) is underway to determine the genetic basis for alcoholism through the molecular genetic study of high-risk families. This project is based on the longstanding observation that alcoholism runs in families and has a strong genetic component. Thus the acceptance of the familial/genetic nature of alcoholism has led to a study that may be able to uncover a specific cause of these devastating conditions.

For other addictions, less work in the genetic/family study area has been completed. This is partly because of the complications of studying illicit substance use across generations when the exposure to substances in the social environment has changed dramatically over the past decades. Since the exposure to various substances has changed so much over time, specific study of parental rates of illicit substance abuse may be confounded with differential environments. This problem may be solved by the sib-pair method of genetic studies (where pairs of siblings are studied) or by twin methods. In fact, one twin study has demonstrated preliminary evidence for heritability of drug dependence. Nevertheless, the family/twin/adoption study of illicit substance abuse has lagged significantly behind alcoholism projects.

Pathophysiology

Animal and behavioral models of addiction have begun to unravel the underlying brain mechanisms of reward and reinforcement, which are key components of addiction, and thus may provide evidence about the etiologic factors of addictive behavior. The circuitry and neurochemistry of the brain reward system is complex and primarily involves the mesolimbic and mesocortical dopamine pathways. Investigation of the brain mechanisms of reward is based on demonstration of animals' addiction to various substances and has provided some of the strongest evidence of the external validity of addiction. No longer can simple morality be invoked to explain addictive behavior. Furthermore, as major strides have been made to unravel the brain reward systems, these studies have allowed us to begin to integrate basic science and clinical medicine in a way that has not been possible in other areas of psychiatry.

Why is pathophysiology important when the precise mechanisms of action have not yet been determined? The cause of substance dependence is unknown, but examples of compulsive administration of abusable substances by animals has allowed extensive laboratory manipulation and evaluation of brain structures thought to be important in addictive behavior. New treatments are likely to be based on this understanding of the pathophysiology of addiction. The most important pathways in animal models of the brain's reward and reinforcement circuitry are the ventral tegmental area—nucleus accumbens dopamine pathways. A consistent body of evidence has indicated these pathways to be at the core of the brain reward system and to be affected by all the common substances of abuse. In addition, receptors for most abused substances have been identified and represent an important area of investigation in psychiatric research.

Treatment Issues

When evaluating the results of any treatment of addiction, consider that alcoholism and other addictions fit the pattern of chronic, relapsing disorders. Many factors such as comorbid psychiatric illness, environmentally limited substance use, severity of symptoms, age of onset of symptoms, and duration of dependence influence the prognosis. Thus a successful but hardly ideal outcome may include extending the time to next relapse, reducing the severity of the dependence syndrome, or reducing complications. The clinical goal is total abstinence because there is little evidence showing that return to controlled substance use is feasible and that progression of symptoms with continued use is the rule. However, knowing that relapse is common, especially in the first few months of sobriety, helps clinicians avoid becoming upset when patients do relapse. The trick is to remain empathetic but firm with patients who have relapsed. Thus one of the goals for physicians caring for patients struggling with addiction is to remain consistent about treatment goals while communicating an understanding of the difficulties inherent in changing behaviors.

The primary care physician's role in the treatment of patients with substance abuse depends on where the patient is identified. For example, a comatose patient with an opiate overdose has a medical emergency that requires immediate assistance; a chronic alcoholic with long-standing, severe drinking patterns needs prompt (24 to 48 hours) evaluation, and a nicotine addict with no current medical emergencies who requests help to quit smoking requires an outpatient appointment, preferably within 1 week. To perform appropriate triage of patients, it is useful to consider when and how to interact with treatment programs, hospitals, and community support systems such as AA.

When to consider referral to specialists is outlined in the Consider Consultation When box at the end of the chapter. Remember that interactions with community support do not involve referral. For complex patients, however, referral will be needed. Medical emergencies directly attributable to substance use itself include overdose, severe alcohol or sedative/hypnotic withdrawal, and idiosyncratic reactions. Medical complications of substance use represent the other main category of medical care; this includes such conditions as intracranial bleed or myocardial infarction (MI) from cocaine, chronic obstructive pulmonary disease (COPD) or lung cancer from tobacco, cirrhosis of the liver or cardiomyopathy from alcohol, or HIV infection from intravenous (IV) drug use. The treatment and evaluation of these conditions is beyond the scope of this chapter. Interested readers are referred to Lowinson's textbook.

Overdose/Intoxication

Most substances can be dangerous when consumed in large quantities. Symptoms of alcohol (and other sedative/hypnotic) overdose and intoxication include agitation, nystagmus, uncoordinated speech and ambulation, and impairment on tests of cognitive functioning. In extreme cases, overdose can be fatal. Opiate overdose can be a medical emergency. Symptoms include small pupils, somnolence, uncoordinated gait, coma, and poor respiration. Death usually occurs from respiratory depression. Overdose is easily treated with

BOX 14-5

ADDICTION RESEARCH FOUNDATION—CLINICAL INSTITUTE WITHDRAWAL ASSESSMENT FOR ALCOHOL

NAUSEA AND VOMITING—Ask "Do you feel sick to your stomach? Have you vomited?" and observe.

0 no nausea and no vomiting
1 mild nausea with no vomiting
2
3
4 intermittent nausea with dry heaves
5
6
7 constant nausea, frequent dry heaves and vomiting

TREMOR—Observe arms extended and fingers spread apart.

0 no tremor
1 not visible, but can be felt fingertip to fingertip
2
3
4 moderate, with patient's arms extended
5
6
7 severe, even with arms not extended

PAROXYSMAL SWEATS—Observe.

0 no sweat visible
1 barely perceptible sweating, palms moist
2
3
4 beads of sweat obvious on forehead
5
6
7 drenching sweats

ANXIETY—Ask "Do you feel nervous?" and observe.

0 no anxiety
1 mildly anxious
2
3
4 moderately anxious, or guarded, so anxiety is inferred
5
6
7 equivalent to acute panic states as seen in severe delirium or acute schizophrenic reactions

AGITATION—Observe.

0 normal activity
1 somewhat more than normal activity
2
3
4 moderately fidgety and restless
5
6
7 paces back and forth during most of the interview, or constantly thrashes about

naloxone (a potent opiate receptor antagonist). Cocaine (and other stimulant) overdose and intoxication include tachycardia, arrhythmias, hypertension, tremor, paranoid psychosis, overactivity, and mood elevation (or sometimes irritability). Overdose can be fatal.

Withdrawal Treatment/Detoxification

Detoxification from addictive substances is one of the foremost areas in which physicians are expected to care for substance abusers. The assessment and treatment of alcohol, opiate, and other withdrawal syndromes are therefore discussed in some detail. When considering treatment options, the first step is careful physical and mental assessment of the patient's condition. Once the severity of the withdrawal syndrome is assessed, treatment options need to be considered. In general for mild cases with few symptoms, observation is all that is needed. Perhaps the most important question to ask when assessing withdrawal potential is when a substance was last used. If more than 4 half-lives have passed since the last consumption without significant symptoms, no severe withdrawal is anticipated. On the other hand, if the last dose was only a few hours before evaluation, the prognosis is much more uncertain. When considering medications for withdrawal, it is important to consider cross-tolerance with the substance being detoxified and the relative half-life of the medication. It is thus generally recommended that long-acting agents be used, that they be gradually tapered, and that careful clinical monitoring and judgment be used in all cases in which medications are required for acute detoxification.

Alcohol withdrawal symptoms include four major types: acute withdrawal symptoms begin 4 to 8 hours after the last drink and peak within 48 to 72 hours. Symptoms include tremor, diaphoresis, nausea, head-

BOX 14-5

ADDICTION RESEARCH FOUNDATION—CLINICAL INSTITUTE WITHDRAWAL ASSESSMENT FOR ALCOHOL—CONT'D

TACTILE DISTURBANCES—Ask "Have you any itching, pins and needles sensations, any burning, any numbness or do you feel bugs crawling on or under your skin?" and observe.

0 none
1 very mild itching, pins and needles, burning or numbness
2 mild itching, pins and needles, burning or numbness
3 moderate itching, pins and needles, burning or numbness
4 moderately severe hallucinations
5 severe hallucinations
6 extremely severe hallucinations
7 continuous hallucinations

AUDITORY DISTURBANCES—Ask "Are you more aware of sounds around you? Are they harsh? Do they frighten you? Are you hearing anything that is disturbing to you? Are you hearing things you know are not there?" Observation.

0 not present
1 very mild harshness or ability to frighten
2 mild harshness or ability to frighten
3 moderate harshness or ability to frighten
4 moderately severe hallucinations
5 severe hallucinations
6 extremely severe hallucinations
7 continuous hallucinations

VISUAL DISTURBANCES—Ask "Does the light appear to be too bright? Is its color different? Does it hurt your eyes? Are you seeing anything that is disturbing to you? Are you seeing things you know are not there?" and observe.

0 not present
1 very mild sensitivity
2 mild sensitivity
3 moderate sensitivity
4 moderately severe hallucinations
5 severe hallucinations
6 extremely severe hallucinations
7 continuous hallucinations

HEADACHE, FULLNESS IN HEAD—Ask "Does your head feel different? Does it feel like there is a band around your head?" Do not rate for dizziness or lightheadedness. Otherwise, rate severity.

0 not present
1 very mild
2 mild
3 moderate
4 moderately severe
5 severe
6 very severe
7 extremely severe

ORIENTATION AND CLOUDING OF SENSORIUM—Ask "What day is this? Where are you? Who are you?"

0 oriented and can do serial additions
1 cannot do serial additions or is uncertain about date
2 disoriented for date by no more than 2 calendar days
3 disoriented for date by more than 2 calendar days
4 disoriented for place and/or person

ache, and diarrhea. Alcoholic hallucinosis, which includes auditory and/or visual hallucinations but no disorientation, starts 4 to 24 hours after the last drink. Generally, the hallucinations subside within a few days but rarely will persist for weeks or months. Alcohol withdrawal seizures, which are generalized tonic-clonic seizures, occur 12 to 48 hours after the last drink. They seem to be more common among people with any history of prior seizures and people who have had multiple detoxifications in the past. Thus treatment recommendations include consideration of a brief course of antiseizure medications such as carbamazepine in high-risk patients. Delirium tremens (DTs) are rare and usually follow the other withdrawal symptoms. More likely to occur in seriously debilitated patients and those with an intercurrent medical condition, DTs usually begin 24 to 72 hours after the last drink. The syndrome is characterized by delirium (waxing and waning level of consciousness, disorientation, hallucinations, or delusions) with severe tremors and autonomic instability (elevated temperature, blood pressure, pulse, and respirations). The mortality rate is up to 15%.

One easy way to evaluate patients with alcohol withdrawal is to administer the Clinical Institute Withdrawal Assessment for Alcohol, Revised (CIWA-AR). As shown in Box 14-5, this instrument gives a score of 0 to 67 from clinical items rated to assess the severity of alcohol withdrawal.

As shown in the flow sheet in Box 14-6, the triage of patients at risk for alcohol withdrawal can be standardized. For patients with significant withdrawal symptoms who are not at particularly high risk of seizures (based on the lack of a clinical history of sei-

BOX 14-6

ALCOHOL WITHDRAWAL TREATMENT ALGORITHM

1. Treat all patients with withdrawal symptoms with high doses of B vitamins and especially thiamine.
2. Is there a history of any past seizures or has the patient had four or more medical detoxifications?
   - Yes: Give carbamazepine for 3 to 5 days
   - No: Is the CIWA-AR score greater than 10?
     - Yes: Does the patient have significant liver pathology?
       - Yes: Use benzodiazepines, which are not oxidatively metabolized, such as oxazepam or lorazepam for detoxification.
       - No: Use benzodiazepines with a long half-life, such as diazepam or chlordiazepoxide, for detoxification.
     - No: Observe without sedative medications.

From Anton RF: *Pharmacology of alcohol withdrawal: an update,* Miami, 1995, Annual Meeting of the American Psychiatric Association.

zures and fewer than four previous medical detoxifications), benzodiazepines are the treatment of choice because of the high therapeutic safety index of these agents. Long-acting benzodiazepines are usually used because they are cross-tolerant with the alcohol and have a good safety profile. In patients with significantly impaired liver function, use of lorazepam or oxazepam is recommended to avoid risk of oversedation. These benzodiazepines do not undergo oxidative metabolism, which is reduced in the face of impaired liver function. Treatment usually begins with an "as needed" dosing, based on clinical rating of withdrawal symptoms. Doses of medication are increased until withdrawal symptoms are controlled. If a patient becomes somnolent, the dose is reduced. After the first 24 hours, the dose is reduced by 25% to 50% each day. With this rapid taper, detoxification can be completed in 2 to 5 days. It is important to note that this rapid taper does not necessarily prevent development of DTs. If such a severe withdrawal syndrome develops, high-dose IV benzodiazepines are often required and monitoring in an intensive care unit (ICU) is indicated because supportive measures (IV fluids, cardiac monitoring, etc.) are needed. High doses of B vitamins, especially thiamine, should be administered to reduce the risk of peripheral neuropathy and the Wernicke-Korsakoff syndrome.

Nicotine withdrawal follows quickly after the last use of tobacco because of the brief half-life of nicotine (2 to 4 hours). Symptoms include irritability, restlessness, poor concentration, increased appetite, depression, anxiety, poor sleep, and craving for tobacco. These symptoms are not medically serious but can lead to relapse. Most symptoms resolve within several days but some, such as appetite increase, depression, and craving, may last for months or years. Use of topical nicotine transdermal patches has been shown to reduce symptoms of withdrawal and to reduce relapse to tobacco among patients in behavioral treatment programs.

Opiate withdrawal has a well-described course and symptom profile. The first symptoms generally begin within 8 to 12 hours after the last dose of a short-acting opiate (longer if a long-acting agent) with restlessness, pupil dilation, yawning, lacrimation, rhinorrhea, diaphoresis, and poor sleep. Within 24 to 48 hours nausea, vomiting, chills, muscle pain, abdominal cramps, diarrhea, tremor, mild tachycardia, and increased blood pressure develop. Rarely, unstable blood pressure and pulse become clinically significant. Untreated, symptoms will subside within 4 to 7 days. Opiate detoxification can most easily be accomplished with a long-acting opiate agent such as methadone, although use of methadone for detoxification is highly regulated and may not be feasible in many settings. The initial dose is based on severity of withdrawal symptoms and is reduced over a 7-to-10-day period. Alternatively, clonidine (an α-2 agonist) has been shown to be effective in ameliorating some of the symptoms of opiate withdrawal. Clonidine's usefulness may be a result of the presence of increased adrenergic stimulation in opiate withdrawal. If clonidine is used, monitoring of blood pressure is warranted and additional medications for specific symptoms may be needed, such as a benzodiazepine for agitation, poor sleep, and restlessness, and an antiemetic for nausea.

Cocaine (and other stimulants) generally have nonspecific withdrawal symptoms that do not require medical intervention. Withdrawal from chronic cannabis consumption is not clearly associated with specific withdrawal symptoms, although some patients report craving, changes in sleep pattern and appetite, irritability, and impaired concentration. For hallucinogens, phencyclidine, and inhalants no particular withdrawal syndromes have been noted.

Urine Drug Testing

Urine drug screening is considered for many treatment modalities, and physicians often ask when such testing is useful. For patients admitted to an emergency room after accidents or injuries, drug testing should always be considered. The evaluation of unconscious patients or those with new onset psychiatric symptoms also must include drug testing. In the outpatient setting, for the initial assessment of patients with a "history of" illicit substance abuse, urine drug testing can be useful in uncovering recent substance use that may be otherwise denied by the patient. Letting patients know that urine drug testing will be obtained should be done before asking about substance use to enhance the self-report of such use. Routinely obtaining urine specimens from recently sober patients is also advised to detect early substance use, which may otherwise be denied. That way, such use can be discussed before a long-term pattern is established. On the other hand, there are severe limitations to urine drug screening. All abusable substances (with the exception of cannabinoids) can only be detected for 24 to 72 hours after last ingestion. Even cannabinoids are routinely detected for only 1 to 2 weeks unless particularly sensitive tests are used or if the use has been particularly heavy and chronic. Thus only very recent substance use is detected.

Treatment of Addiction

The mainstay of substance abuse and dependence treatment is psychosocial rehabilitation. This general label includes community support treatments (AA and other 12-step groups), specific relapse prevention behavioral therapies, psychoeducation, and supportive individual therapies. AA is by far the most common treatment approach to alcoholism (and probably to other addictions as well), but little data support, or disavow, the effectiveness of AA. What is certainly true is that these support groups for people with addictions offer fellowship in times of need and have been lifesaving for many people. Physicians need to be aware of where and when meetings are held in their communities so that referral of appropriate individuals will be made. What remains uncertain is for which patients these referrals are "appropriate." Many clinicians refer all addicted patients to AA groups, although additional treatment referral to professional programs may be warranted in more severe cases, especially those with intercurrent medical or psychiatric disorders.

Medications for Addictions

Psychological treatments are often combined with pharmacological therapies. For some alcoholic patients, disulfiram (Antabuse) is recommended, although evidence indicates that the effects of this agent are primarily psychological in that the dose does not matter much and only the most motivated patients do well on disulfiram—the same patients who would likely do well on no medication. Recently, O'Malley and Volpicelli showed naltrexone, which is an orally active opiate receptor blocker, to be helpful in the treatment of alcoholism when used in combination with traditional alcohol rehabilitation treatment. Because naltrexone has only been shown to be useful when combined with psychosocial treatment, some caution in the primary care setting is advised. Other medications for alcoholism are less certain. No antidepressants have been shown to be helpful in reducing alcohol consumption, although they may be helpful in treating concurrent depressive syndromes. On the other hand, recent reports have indicated that buspirone may be helpful in the treatment of alcoholism, particularly among anxious alcoholics.

Nicotine dependence is often treated with transdermal nicotine replacement. Such treatment, combined with behavioral psychotherapies, is more useful than placebo, but the relapse rate remains high even in the best prognostic groups. Treatment of co-occurring depression or anxiety may improve the outcome of nicotine dependence.

Opiate dependence has been treated most successfully with long-term methadone substitution therapy. With such treatment, the psychosocial and medical complications of illicit opiate addiction are ameliorated. Unfortunately, it is not clear how long patients should be maintained on methadone. Some long-term studies have indicated significant relapse rates on discontinuation of methadone, even after many years of treatment. If methadone maintenance is requested, it is important that the clinic that administers the methadone does so appropriately. For the most part, this means using adequately high doses of methadone to produce significant tolerance to the effects of opiates. Programs that use lower doses have much higher rates of illicit opiate use in their patients compared with programs administering high doses. The purported mechanism of this improved outcome for high-dose programs is that additional doses of opiates, that is, those ingested illicitly, do not produce any euphoria because of the significant tolerance. Thus patients quickly learn not to use opiates illicitly. In contrast, low methadone doses block withdrawal symptoms but do not prevent euphoria with additional doses of opiates. Patients will continue to use opiates illicitly.

Naltrexone, a potent and orally active opiate receptor antagonist, has been helpful in the treatment of many narcotic addicts. Naltrexone has a long half-life, so it can be administered three times per week in a supervised setting. Such dosing will completely block effects of opiates; therefore illicit use is curtailed because no euphoria is obtained even with high doses. This medication has been most widely used in the treatment of addicted physicians who are exposed to opiates in the workplace and are at risk of job loss if they do not follow treatment recommendations. Otherwise, most opiate addicts do not volunteer for naltrexone treatment.

No medications have proven consistently helpful in the treatment of cocaine or other addictions not discussed above. Although several agents such as desipramine, fluoxetine, and amantadine appeared promising after initial trials, larger and more comprehensive studies have failed to demonstrate consistent treatment effects. Trials of antidepressants, dopamine agonists, and antagonists have all been disappointing. Despite these results, ongoing studies of other agents continue.

Treatment of Dual Diagnosis

Psychiatric illnesses such as depression, anxiety, and personality disorder often coexist with substance abuse. When such "dual diagnosis" patients show symptoms, several questions confront the treating physician: (1) How should these difficult patients be evaluated?, (2) Which condition should be addressed first?, and (3) When is it appropriate to institute medications for the nonsubstance abuse disorder?

In general, most such complicated patients require treatment by addiction psychiatrists (that is, specialists); however, this need not always be the case. It is important to keep in mind that most patients with psychiatric symptoms improve markedly if substance use is eliminated. Thus the substance abuse problems should almost always be addressed first. The main exceptions to this rule are patients with acute psychosis and those with acute suicidal symptoms. In both of these urgent situations, the psychiatric symptoms must be addressed before treatment of the substance abuse would be appropriate or safe. On the other hand, for patients with depressive or anxiety symptoms, focusing on eliminating substance use often leads to an amelioration of the psychiatric symptoms without specific intervention. For patients whose anxiety or depressive symptoms persist despite at least several weeks of sobriety, treatment with nonaddictive medications is generally indicated. Particularly to be avoided are the benzodiazepines, whose long-term use would be relatively contraindicated in substance abusers because of their addictive potential. Buspirone can be considered for anxiety symptoms, and selective serotonin reuptake inhibitors (SSRIs) such as fluoxetine or other nontricyclic antidepressants would generally be the first-line antidepressants. Tricyclics can also be considered, but the potential for lethal overdose usually would make these agents a second choice.

Conclusion

The epitome of the medical approach to any disorder is to diagnose the illness, plan treatment, and predict outcome. In 1992 Guze wrote that applying the medical model to addiction psychiatry implies that the "concepts, strategies, and jargon of general medicine are applied to psychiatric disorders: diagnosis, differential diagnosis, etiologic factors, pathogenesis, treatment, natural history, epidemiology, complications, and so on." As in all other medical specialties, evidence about treatment does not necessarily have to go hand-in-hand with knowledge of pathophysiology, and novel approaches are always acceptable if based on available evidence. Differential diagnosis is a key component in the medical approach because it forces the clinician to weigh the possible explanations for a given patient's symptoms or signs and is based on a general understanding that variability of presentation is usual for virtually all illnesses.

Alcoholism and other addictions have been recognized as the underlying cause of severe medical conditions for centuries. Although the precise pathophysiology of addiction has not been elucidated, significant clues to the brain mechanisms involved in reward and reinforcement have allowed significant insight into the connection between basic brain mechanisms and pathological behavior. Similarly, the commonality of these conditions and their familial nature have been demonstrated through many studies. Yet in subtle forms, these conditions are often unrecognized by competent clinicians. Using appropriate screening instruments such as the MAST, DAST, and AUDIT, clinicians can increase the identification of these patients. In fact, perhaps the most important way to improve recognition of these disorders is to routinely ask all patients about their substance use in ways which enhance reporting of substance-related problems.

Case 14-2 is typical in many ways of what most primary care physicians confront. Little direct evidence is presented to indicate that alcoholism was the underlying condition, although several clues might have been recognized. These clues include unresponsive hypertension, history of injuries, attending a physician's appointment smelling of alcohol, and mild elevation of GGT. The physician's first question about consuming a lot of alcohol was structured in such a way that the patient could easily deny having any problems because of the lack of precision and the nonobjective approach. Use of collateral informants was most helpful in eliciting the history, and a "happy ending" has been posited.

Once identified, substance use disorders need to be managed forthrightly and nonjudgmentally, keeping in mind their chronic relapsing nature. Certain substance-related conditions such as overdoses, head injury and delirium represent medical emergencies. Medical complications of chronic substance use need careful con-

CASE 14-2

Mr. I. has been treated for hypertension for many years by his primary care physician. He has required multiple medications and has had only a moderate reduction in blood pressure, despite "triple therapy." Mr. I. is divorced but has had consistent employment. He has had several injuries requiring sutures, and once came to a doctor's appointment with alcohol on his breath. Physical examination was unremarkable except for obesity, which made evaluation of liver size impossible. Routine laboratory evaluation was unremarkable, except that GGT was at the upper end of the normal range. When asked if he "drank a lot," Mr. I. said "no." Yet on further evaluation, including interviews with Mr. I.'s children, a 20-year history of heavy alcohol consumption was revealed, along with evidence of continued use despite family problems, two arrests for driving while intoxicated, and often drinking more than intended. With careful questioning and open discussion of the signs and symptoms, Mr. I. agreed to attend an outpatient treatment program. Interestingly, once sober, Mr. I.'s hypertension was able to be controlled with propranolol alone.

sideration, although the most important treatment of these medical complications is total abstinence. Physicians will also be asked to intervene in withdrawal syndromes; these syndromes generally require medical intervention, although recent practices have shown that many can be managed safely in the outpatient setting with proper supervision. Treatment of the dependence syndrome itself is a more complicated matter. Total abstinence must always be considered the goal even though relapses are usually encountered. The primary care physician must consider various levels of treatment from a simple referral to community support, such as AA, to referral to a full treatment program. It is important to be familiar with the local resources so that support for your patients is easily accessible. Referral phone numbers for AA are almost always in the telephone directory, and most communities have a variety of substance abuse programs. Medications can also be used to treat addictions. Disulfiram for alcoholism, and naltrexone or methadone for opiate addiction have been used for over 20 years. Most recently, naltrexone has been approved by the Food and Drug Administration (FDA) for the treatment of alcoholism; it has been demonstrated to be a useful adjunct to psychological treatment. Similarly, nicotine replacement therapy as an adjunct to behavior therapies for nicotine addiction has been shown to be helpful. Other medications, including buspirone, have shown promise in the treatment of alcoholism and major medication development programs are currently under way for all addictions. Finally, many substance abusing patients test limits, and primary care physicians need practice dealing directly with noncompliance with recommendations. Finding ways to motivate patients at various stages of addiction to change their behaviors is challenging but very rewarding. Understanding the long-term outcome and finding creative ways to intervene are the goals for treatment.

CONSIDER CONSULTATION WHEN . . .

- The patient is noncompliant with treatment regimen or relapses
- The patient's substance abuse has led to potentially life-threatening complications
- The patient has significant psychiatric symptoms in addition to the substance abuse
- The family is overwhelmed by the patient's condition
- The patient has complicated withdrawal symptoms, possibly including seizures and/or delirium

Annotated Bibliography

DuPont RL, McGovern JP: *A bridge to recovery—an introduction to 12-step programs,* Washington, D.C., 1994, American Psychiatric Press.

This interesting and brief review of AA and related 12-step programs may be useful to clinicians who are unaware of the ways these programs can help substance abusing patients turn their lives around.

Galanter M, Kleber HD: *Textbook of substance abuse treatment,* Washington, D.C., 1994, American Psychiatric Press.

This textbook provides a thorough review of all treatment modalities for alcoholics and other substance abusers. The writing is clear, and all major treatment modalities are reviewed.

Lowinson JH et al: *Substance abuse—A comprehensive textbook,* Baltimore, 1992, Williams and Wilkins.

A weighty tome, the *Comprehensive Textbook* is the standard review text for psychiatrists preparing for addiction subspecialty examinations. Topics are covered in great depth and this text is appropriate for the serious student of addiction.

Vaillant GE: *The natural history of alcoholism,* Cambridge, Mass, 1983, Harvard University Press.

Based on prospective evaluation of more than 600 men followed for upwards of 40 years, this landmark report is probably the most detailed evaluation to date of the pathways into and out of alcoholism.

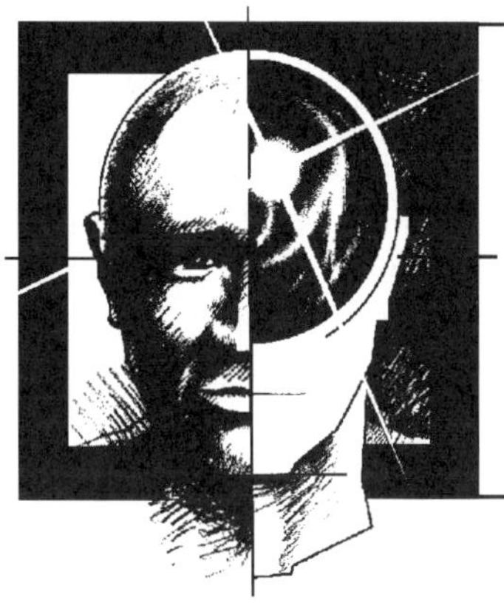

chapter 15

Eating Disorders

Richard W. Hudgens, MD

There are three disorders characterized by maladaptive eating behavior and the results of that behavior that commonly come to the attention of physicians. *Anorexia nervosa* is a well-defined syndrome of dieting and extreme weight loss. It usually occurs in women, begins in youth, and is driven by an exaggerated fear of fatness. *Bulimia nervosa* is marked by binges of eating large amounts of food in short periods of time. It is accompanied by a feeling that the process is out of control, and it is often followed by extreme psychological or physical discomfort. Purging of the food, usually through self-induced vomiting, follows the binge. Excessive exercise is also common. Although bulimia nervosa may appear as a syndrome in its own right, it is more often a symptom cluster that seen in other psychiatric disorders, especially major depression, obsessive-compulsive disorder (OCD), alcoholism, and anorexia nervosa. Anorexia nervosa and bulimia nervosa are considered psychiatric disorders that are usually susceptible to improvement or cure through nutritional correction, psychotherapy, and the somatic treatments such as psychoactive drugs or electroconvulsive therapy (ECT). *Obesity,* which is far more common than the first two conditions, is not considered a psychiatric disorder or the product of one. However, certain types of psychotherapy have a role to play in the management of this chronic affliction.

Primary care physicians are consulted by people with all three of these disorders. Obesity is obvious and readily acknowledged by patients. However, the symptoms of anorexia nervosa and bulimia nervosa may be hidden and lied about by patients, who may come to their doctors complaining of the physical consequences of their aberrant behavior. These patients may say nothing about the behavior itself or the emotions that accompany it.

Anorexia Nervosa

Historical Recognition of the Syndrome

From ancient times, involuntary starvation through poverty or torture has been a familiar phenomenon. The same is true of the cachexia caused by cancer and by chronic infections like tuberculosis. Such diseases have long been recognizable by accompanying signs, such as fever, tumors, and pervasive exhaustion. However, in centuries past there have also appeared occasional cases of young people who were neither febrile nor suffering from cancer and who voluntarily starved themselves to a skeletal condition while continuing physical activity and stubbornly resisting all persuasions to eat properly. Some of these people were ascetics who fasted for religious purposes. However, in seventeenth-century Britain there were published a few detailed and eloquent reports of men and women whose illnesses resembled anorexia nervosa in all essential respects.

The definition of anorexia nervosa as a distinct syndrome finally came about in the 1860s and 1870s, when Marcé and Lasègue in France and Gull in England independently developed thorough clinical descriptions. The ravages of starvation were described, as was the curious mental state that often accompanied it: "Whatever the duration of their abstinence, they experience a distaste for food which the most pressing want is unable to overcome. . . . Deeply impressed, whether by the absence of appetite or by the uneasiness caused by digestion, these patients arrive at a delirious conviction that they cannot or ought not to eat. In one word, the gastric nervous disorder becomes cerebro-nervous" (Marcé, 1860). The frustration encountered by caregivers was also recognized: "The delicacies of the table are multiplied in the hopes of stimulating the appetite, but the more the solicitude increases, the more the appetite diminishes. What dominates in the mental condition of the hysterical patient is, above all, the state of quietude . . . Not only does she not sigh for recovery, but she is not ill-pleased with her condition" (Lasègue, 1873). The oldest descriptions of anorexia nervosa have neither been exceeded in accuracy nor equaled in style and charm in all the succeeding years.

The cause or causes of the illness are as mysterious now as they were 120 years ago, although theories abound now as they did then. For a time after 1914, when Simmonds described a wasting disorder that followed infarction of the pituitary, many cases of anorexia nervosa were erroneously attributed to that cause. However, by 1949 the rarity of Simmonds' disease was acknowledged. Anorexia nervosa is now recognized as a complex disorder of unknown etiology affecting emotions, behavior, and physical state; as sometimes remitting but often chronic; and as having fatal outcome in a significant minority of cases.

Diagnosing Anorexia Nervosa

History

A new case of anorexia nervosa usually involves a teenage girl (90% to 95% of cases are female patients) who begins to diet in response to the belief that she is fat, whether or not she actually is. When she reaches her target weight she may continue to diet to emaciation, obsessed with a fear that if she stops dieting she will lose control and become obese. She typically underestimates the extent of her thinness; despite confrontation by others and despite looking at herself in the mirror, she has a distortion of body image. Menstruation stops, sometimes even before significant weight loss has occurred.

Consultation with a physician is usually at the insistence of family members, who have been increasingly worried about their relative's weight loss and frustrated by her air of bland unconcern and stubborn refusal to eat enough.

Patients with anorexia nervosa employ several methods of achieving and maintaining a low weight. They are usually not altogether forthcoming about how they do it and may conceal important aspects of their behavior, lying when questioned. Anorexia nervosa can be described in terms of two types—restrictive and binge eating/purging (Box 15-1, Table 15-1). In the restrictive subtype of the disorder, patients successfully control their weight by eating tiny amounts of food. They may take pride in the discipline this entails. In the binge-eating/purging subtype, patients purge, usually by inducing vomiting after eating. People with the latter subtype eat much more in response to normal hunger after hours or days of fasting than those with the restrictive subtype. Laxatives, enemas, and diuretics are also employed. These techniques are inefficient ways of losing weight, but even if the patient knows that, she may continue them in response to feelings of fullness and bloating. Appetite-suppressing drugs, especially those containing the readily available phenylpropanolamine, may be used in large amounts, resulting in increased restlessness and anxiety. If amphetamines are used, as is more rarely the case, toxic psychoses and persistent depression may result. Finally, patients often engage in excessive exercise to burn off calories. It is striking to see such frail-appearing young women walking, biking, running, or lifting weights for hours on end.

Despite their evident skinniness, patients deny fatigue, except when the illness has proceeded to extreme emaciation. Appetite is often described as good until the later stages of starvation; *anorexia* is usually an inaccurate term.

The patients' preoccupations with food may lead to other extremes of behavior. They may pore constantly over cookbooks, spending much time preparing special dishes for their families that they themselves do not eat. They may steal food or shoplift other items they do not need. They may hoard food and hide it until it rots and comes to the attention of a dismayed family. It is not unusual for a teenager with anorexia nervosa to aspire to a career as a chef or nutritionist.

The history of anorexia nervosa in men is similar to that in women. The average age of onset is in the midteens, and the same attitudes about food and weight are present. Like girls with anorexia nervosa, these

BOX 15-1 ANOREXIA NERVOSA

DSM-IV DIAGNOSTIC CRITERIA

A. Refusal to maintain body weight at or above a minimally normal weight for age and height (e.g., weight loss leading to maintenance of body weight less than 85% of that expected; or failure to make expected weight gain during period of growth, leading to body weight less than 85% of that expected).

B. Intense fear of gaining weight or becoming fat, even though underweight.

C. Disturbance in the way in which one's body weight or shape is experienced, undue influence of body weight or shape on self-evaluation, or denial of the seriousness of the current low body weight.

D. In postmenarcheal females, amenorrhea, i.e., the absence of at least three consecutive menstrual cycles. (A woman is considered to have amenorrhea if her periods occur only following hormone, e.g., estrogen, administration.)

Specify type:

Restricting Type: during the current episode of Anorexia Nervosa, the person has not regularly engaged in binge-eating or purging behavior (i.e., self-induced vomiting or the misuse of laxatives, diuretics, or enemas)

Binge-Eating/Purging Type: during the current episode of Anorexia Nervosa, the person has regularly engaged in binge-eating or purging behavior (i.e., self-induced vomiting or the misuse of laxatives, diuretics, or enemas)

From American Psychiatric Association: *Diagnostic and statistical manual of mental disorders,* ed 4 (DSM-IV), Washington, D.C., 1994, American Psychiatric Press.

TABLE 15-1 ANOREXIA NERVOSA

DIAGNOSIS

Discriminating features

1. Refusal to maintain minimal body weight
2. Absence of medical illness to explain weight loss
3. Denial of seriousness of low weight

Consistent features

1. Amenorrhea
2. Intense fear of weight gain
3. Disturbance in perception of own weight and shape
4. Preoccupation with food and weight

Variable features

1. Begins in women under age 20
2. Absence of fatigue despite weight loss
3. Rigid perfectionism and obsessionality
4. Food binging and purging
5. Electrolyte disturbances
6. Withholding or lying about clinical information
7. Hoarding of food

boys typically engage in excessive exercise. The pursuit of excessive thinness is at variance with society's ideal of a muscular male body type; some boys with anorexia nervosa develop into obsessive body builders, bypassing the risks of starvation.

A special challenge is presented by "older" women with anorexia nervosa—patients whose illnesses began when they were in their 20s or later and patients whose illnesses began in adolescence but have continued untreated into adulthood or even well into middle age. They are more guarded than teenage girls about revealing items in their history that would betray the diagnosis, and they are more able to resist coercion into treatment because they are adults. They often come to a physician with gastrointestinal or other physical complaints that may be a consequence of starvation, repeated vomiting, or laxative abuse. They may come reluctantly to the physician, yielding to the importunities of worried relatives, and they may deny with straight faces that obsessions with food and weight, morbid fear of fatness, excessive dieting, and purging have dominated their lives for many years. The history has gone underground because the patient knows that revealing it may threaten her control over the maintenance of her thinness. For adults with anorexia nervosa, just as for adolescents, a separate history should always be taken from a reliable informant.

Mental Status

By the time the patient reaches the physician's office, her family may be in turmoil, and the emotion displayed by the patient may be chiefly anger at her "interfering" relatives. During the severest stages of the illness, most people with anorexia nervosa, regardless of age, are stubbornly resistant to handing over any measure of control to others, much less to physicians who want them to gain weight.

As long as she is allowed to pursue her dieting behavior, the patient initially denies depression or anxiety but expresses a horror of fatness. Her conversation betrays a preoccupation with food, eating, and appearance, subjects to which she keeps returning no matter how a physician may try to divert her from them. If the physician is alone with the patient and gives her enough time to talk about her life, the patient may reveal a host of worries and a mood of depression beneath her facade of cheerful unconcern. There may be rigid perfectionism and a need to be in control in many areas besides body weight. This can cause the patient to despair of ever being adequate.

Psychotic symptoms are not part of the typical clinical picture of anorexia nervosa. However, some patients so stubbornly insist they are fat, despite overwhelming evidence to the contrary, that the belief has all the force of a somatic delusion.

Physical Examination

The appearance of young women with severe anorexia nervosa is striking. They are invariably compared with concentration camp survivors, but they have considerably more energy. The skin is characteristically dry and sometimes yellowish in color. Scalp hair is brittle, and there may be fine hair, *lanugo,* over the body. A patient's temperature is typically low, the pulse is slow, and blood pressure is low. If the patient has been vomiting often, there may be calluses on the dorsal surfaces of her fingers and on her knuckles, as well as enlargement of the salivary glands. Another complication of vomiting is the passage of acidic stomach contents through the mouth, which may result in redness of the gums and palate and in erosion of the teeth. The latter progresses from a dullness of the tooth surface in early stages to a yellowed appearance as the enamel erodes and exposes the dentin.

Routine Laboratory Findings

The routine battery of laboratory tests is not likely to be of diagnostic help in anorexia nervosa. There are electrolyte abnormalities, such as high serum bicarbonate and low potassium, in a minority of patients with anorexia nervosa. These are not diagnostic. If starvation proceeds to dangerous levels, there are many other findings, some of which are discussed in the section on medical complications.

Differential Diagnosis

Since there is nothing quite like anorexia nervosa, diagnostic confusion is unlikely if the doctor has taken an adequate history from reliable sources. Patients who are chronically wasted from the effects of a medical disorder like acquired immunodeficiency syndrome (AIDS), cancer, or Addison's disease may be depressed, but their medical illnesses can readily be diagnosed by the history; by physical findings and laboratory results; and by the absence of the telltale attitudes towards food, eating, and body image that characterize patients with anorexia nervosa.

There are two psychiatric disorders that in their chronic stages may exhibit wasting from malnutrition: schizophrenia and major depression. The delusions and hallucinations usually prominent in schizophrenia make it unlikely to be confused with anorexia nervosa. When wasting does occur in schizophrenia, it is often attended by delusions that food is poisoned or by an apathy and lack of activity that is different from the behavior of someone with anorexia nervosa.

People suffering from major depression in the absence of anorexia nervosa may eat little when they are in an apathetic state. They usually profess to have no appetite, and their energy is depleted. The peculiar attitudes about eating are absent, as is the level of physical activity associated with anorexia nervosa. Age of onset is also a diagnostic clue; it is unusual for anorexia nervosa to begin later than the mid-20s. When a patient has a wasting disease that began in middle age or later, it is almost certainly not anorexia nervosa. If the patient is a man, the qualifier *almost* can be dropped.

Medical Complications

Medical complications in patients with anorexia nervosa stem from the following three causes: purging behavior, starvation, and treatment of starvation. With rare exception these complications disappear as nutritional recovery and behavioral changes proceed. When that happens, the physician does not need to chase down and fine tune every derangement of hemodynamics, hormones, or electrolytes. The body takes care of itself, and physiological processes are restored.

Purging behavior—vomiting, enemas, and laxative abuse—can lead to low potassium, sodium, magnesium, phosphate and chloride levels, as well as a high level of bicarbonate. Hypokalemia, which occurs in as many as one in seven patients, may lead to cardiac arrhythmias and disorders of conduction. Severe hyponatremia, which is more unusual, can lead to coma and death. In some cases with severe dehydration from vomiting or abuse of laxatives and diuretics, secondary aldosteronism develops, with hypernatremia, hypokalemia, and metabolic alkalosis. On the other hand, metabolic acidosis develops if enemas or laxative abuse is dominant and leads to significant loss of alkaline fluid from the colon.

Other serious and even potentially fatal consequences of purging include esophageal rupture from repeated vomiting and emetine poisoning of the myocardium from the great amount of ipecac sometimes ingested to induce vomiting.

The medical consequences of starvation in patients with anorexia nervosa are identical to those found in other conditions associated with starvation. Most prominent are muscle wasting, weakness, lowered levels of the hormones involved in reproduction with consequent amenorrhea, delayed gastric emptying with the consequent feeling of fullness after small amounts of food, a low serum protein level and edema, a high plasma cortisol level, osteoporosis (which may not be corrected after nutritional recovery), hypotension, and bradycardia. Most deaths from anorexia nervosa occur because of starvation.

The restoration of nutrition, the necessary first step in the treatment of anorexia nervosa, carries some risks of its own. This is especially true when tube feeding, intravenous glucose, or intravenous total parenteral nutrition are employed and when nutritional restoration is too rapid. Whenever possible, refeeding should be accomplished by the patient feeding herself; although the process may be slow, rapidity of refeeding can be dangerous.

In a starved patient the sudden influx of a large glucose load can uncover a deficiency of phosphate, which was not required for the fat metabolism that predominated during starvation, but which is required for glucose metabolism. The consequent depletion of phosphate from the tissues may among other things lead to an encephalopathy that can be fatal. Rapid refeeding, especially by tube, can lead to aspiration, acute pancreatitis, and dilation or even rupture of the stomach. Occasionally a patient with severe anorexia nervosa, who is finally coming to treatment, dies because of complications arising during the refeeding process.

Clues to the Etiology

The cause of anorexia nervosa is not known. Investigators have sought answers in the following three main areas: studies of the psychopathology and interpersonal relations of individual cases; epidemiological, follow-up, and family studies; and biological studies.

Psychopathology and Individual Case Dynamics

Studies of individual cases, which often take place while a patient is undergoing psychotherapy, have led to psychological theories of causation. By the time a patient enters treatment she is already sick, and she is preoccupied with food, eating, and body image. By that time considerable family turmoil has also been generated by the patient's alarming condition, her relatives' importunities, and the patient's refusal to heed them. Based on these observations, some workers have proposed that family conflict and issues of perfectionism, control, and weight-consciousness preceded the illness and were causative factors. This has not been proven, but such issues must be addressed in treatment of the patient with anorexia nervosa and in the counseling of her family. Whether or not they are of etiological importance, they are important at the time of treatment.

Epidemiology

Epidemiological studies lend some support to the idea that attitudes toward eating and weight may play causative roles in anorexia nervosa. Although the disorder affects only a small fraction of the general population, ranging from one to four cases per 100,000, it has a much higher incidence among young white women of the middle and upper socioeconomic strata in America and Europe. It is also among that group that weight-consciousness and aborrhence of fatness abound and are virtually a cultural norm, leading some theorists to postulate that when severe anxiety, depression, or OCD arises in a member of that population, it may be manifested as anorexia nervosa. In contrast the pursuit of thinness more rarely afflicts black women, men, or poor people, and anorexia nervosa is also rare in those groups. The connection between anorexia nervosa and the obsession with thinness obviously needs much further study. For example, after reading old case reports, some researchers have questioned whether a morbid fear of fatness, now one of the criteria for making the diagnosis of anorexia nervosa, was an important feature of the disorder in earlier centuries. This question also arises because of cases of self-starvation in Asia, in which patients who fulfill the criteria for the disorder except for the fear of obesity. Current diagnostic criteria for the syndrome may be too culture-bound.

Follow-up and Family Studies

Anorexia nervosa and bulimia nervosa are much more common among relatives of people with anorexia nervosa than among the general population. Monzygotic co-twins of subjects with anorexia nervosa have the highest incidence of the disorder (one half to two thirds in some studies) and a high incidence of bulimia nervosa. A genetic susceptibility to the illness is suggested by this, but many more studies are needed in this area.

Association with some other psychiatric disorders is suggested by studies of patients and their relatives and by follow-up studies. Attempts to divide anorexia nervosa into subsyndromes (in addition to the restrictive and binge-eating/purging types) have been made. For example, some patients show a clear depressive picture, some show a dominant obsessive-compulsive picture, and some show a picture of conduct disturbance with features of antisocial personality. Others present a clinical picture with a mixture of those features. Affective disorders, alcoholism, and OCD have all been reported in patients' relatives at a greater rate than in relatives of control subjects. Even though anorexia nervosa becomes chronic in a significant minority of patients, some of the patients who recover from anorexia nervosa later develop other disorders, including depression, anxiety disorders, OCD, and bulimia nervosa without the picture of anorexia nervosa itself. This suggests that there is no simple association between anorexia nervosa and any other illness, as was at one time postulated for major depression. Anorexia nervosa may have causes quite different from those of disorders that occur together with it. So far, no one knows.

Biological Studies

There are numerous biological changes occurring in anorexia nervosa. Along with the medical complications mentioned in the related section, derangements in the major endocrine systems have been described, as have disturbances—confirmed or inferred—in some neurotransmitter systems. The trouble is that starvation from other causes produces similar changes. Definite biological precursors of anorexia nervosa have yet to be described.

The peculiarities of eating behavior in anorexia nervosa and bulimia nervosa, as well as the suppression of reproductive function (with amenorrhea sometimes preceding weight loss), have directed attention to the hypothalamus with its involvement in the pituitary-gonadal system and its role in hunger and satiety. However, dysfunctions predictive of eating disorders or trait markers for them have not yet been described. In anorexia nervosa, studies of hunger vs. satiety leave many questions unanswered; the whole matter is clearly more complicated than appetite or the absence thereof. Every physician who has taken care of patients with eating disorders knows that lack of appetite is not the main drive for fasting in anorexia nervosa and that binge eating often occurs in the absence of any sensation of hunger.

Course and Outcome

Anorexia nervosa usually begins in the teens, and its onset is rare after age 25. Although it can be a devastating and sometimes fatal illness, most people recover from it; follow-up studies of varying lengths document full or partial recovery in over one half of the subjects. Some patients who recover and who never have anorexia nervosa again develop (or continue to have) other psychiatric disorders, such as depression, alcoholism, anxiety, panic disorder, or OCD.

From one fourth to one half of patients with anorexia nervosa continue to have the illness with varying degrees of severity, even after treatment, and it may run a fluctuating course throughout their lives. Mortality rates in long-term studies lasting over 20 years, are between 10% and 20%. The majority of deaths are from complications of starvation, and most of the rest are from suicide. This high incidence of suicide serves as a warning that concurrent depression should be treated vigorously. The use of ECT in anorexia nervosa is seldom reported in the literature and may be underemployed.

Poorer long-term outcome is predicted by late onset of the illness (after age 20) and late entry into treatment, by persistence of the illness for more than 2 years, by extremely low weight at the beginning of treatment, by purging as a significant means of weight control, by poor premorbid psychological adjustment, and by drug or alcohol abuse. The results of outcome studies suggest that early vigorous treatment may protect against chronicity, although this is not certain.

Treatment

Restoration of normal or near-normal weight through proper eating is a primary goal of treatment. This cannot be achieved, at least not for long, unless there is considerable reduction in the patient's psychological discomfort. Fear of fatness and anxiety that she will lose control of weight-maintenance make the patient reluctant to enter treatment. These become even more intense as she gains weight, especially if she gains weight rapidly. Many people with anorexia nervosa never enter treatment at all or leave it early, especially if they are adults and can avoid coercion.

At the beginning of treatment, hospitalization may be necessary. This is certainly the case if the patient is cachectic or especially fearful of weight gain. Medical complications can be better addressed in a hospital; patients are more likely to begin eating properly in a controlled environment; and psychotherapy and administration of medication can begin more intensively.

Many patients do not gain weight at all unless they are in a hospital, and short hospital stays may not be sufficient. That presents a problem in these days of high hospital costs and pressures to shorten stays to a few days, especially considering that inpatient treatment of 2 months or longer was not unusual in the treatment of anorexia nervosa a couple of decades ago. The process of virtually coerced weight gain followed by consolidation of that weight gain and concomitant reduction of fear can be aborted by too-early discharge from hospital treatment. Fortunately, partial hospital programs for the treatment of eating disorders have been developed in many places. Treatment there is less expensive, and insurance carriers are becoming more disposed to favor it.

Whether or not the patient is treated in a hospital, the methods for achieving nutritional goals are the same. There should be three meals per day, vitamin and mineral supplements if necessary, avoidance of food binging, avoidance of purging, avoidance of alcohol, and avoidance of excessive exercise. It is advisable to prescribe ahead of time the amount and type of food to be eaten, in conformity with guidelines of nutrition specialists. This practice is often anxiety-reducing, because the patient is relieved of peculiarly burdensome decisions (for her) about what to eat and how much. Some hospital programs measure the amount of food that is actually eaten; some only measure a patient's weight at various intervals. Weight goals are set at the beginning of treatment, as is the expected rate of weight gain, which often ranges from 2 to 3 pounds per week.

It is common for patients to resist weight gain. As it begins, they may develop peripheral edema, which is occasioned by rehydration in the presence of a low serum protein level. They are easily made to feel full because gastric emptying is delayed in people who have been starving. Patients' abdomens may protrude. These various bloatings distress them greatly. They may vomit after meals, and it may be necessary to keep patients in sight for an hour or so after they eat to keep that from happening. When certain privileges, such as visitors, telephone, recreation, and ultimate discharge, are linked to achieving weight goals in hospitalized patients, patients may surreptitiously drink water before being weighed. Tube feeding is occasionally necessary if patients absolutely refuse to eat, but total parenteral nutrition is a last resort and used in such patients only when tube feeding is contraindicated.

From the previous discussion it is obvious why adults with anorexia nervosa are more difficult to treat than children and adolescents. The physician cannot make them stay in treatment programs involuntarily unless a court can be convinced that they are an immediate danger to themselves, which is not usually the case. Indeed, the physician cannot make a child stay in treatment either, unless her parents are in agreement with the physician. Parents' resolution may waver as their daughter pleads for her release from treatment, driven by her fear of fatness.

Treatment of emotional distress, for example the fear of fatness, depression, obsessions, and family turmoil, must be successful or the restoration of nutritional status is short-lived. Psychotherapy and medications are commonly used.

In individual psychotherapy, therapy in a group with other patients who have eating disorders, or family therapy with parents, patients deal with such issues as fear of eating, obsessionality, the need for control, relationships with other people, and the individual problems at their particular stages of life. Therapy that also addresses a reorganization of eating behavior has been shown helpful.

Since the beginning of the era of pharmacotherapy, medication has been used in anorexia nervosa. Because depression and obsessional preoccupations are often part of the illness, antidepressant medications are often prescribed first. Results with the early tricyclic antidepressants (TCAs) have been mixed. Recent reports indicate good results from fluoxetine (Prozac). This makes sense, because fluoxetine and other new serotonin-selective reuptake inhibitors (SSRIs) have better antiobsessional effects than the older drugs. Interestingly, these drugs also seldom increase appetite. Therefore they may be more acceptable to the patient with an eating disorder who often has a good appetite, which torments her and which she is preoccupied with resisting.

Not surprisingly, drugs that specifically aim at increasing appetite usually miss the mark. Cyproheptadine, the serotonin antagonist, has had limited success. TCAs such amitriptyline (Elavil) may drive the appetite up, particularly for sweets. They are no longer the first antidepressants to try in this illness.

Before the advent of SSRI antidepressants, antipsychotic (neuroleptic) drugs were used more often than they are now in the treatment of anorexia nervosa. Their use is associated with reductions in anxiety and in the intensity of obsessions. Moreover, they may be associated with weight gain without a concomitant increase in appetite. The low-potency drugs thioridazine (Mellaril) and chlorpromazine (Thorazine) have been favored over the high-potency drugs because of the more prominent extrapyramidal side effects of the latter group, including dystonias, extreme restlessness

PEARLS & PERILS

ANOREXIA NERVOSA

- The self-destructive behavior in anorexia nervosa is driven by an obsessive fear of becoming fat and not by poor appetite.
- Long-term mortality from anorexia nervosa is 10% to 20%; death is almost always from either starvation or suicide.
- Major depression occurring in anorexia nervosa should be treated vigorously with drugs or ECT as well as with psychotherapy.
- Rapid refeeding in starvation, especially intravenously or by tube, can be dangerous and even fatal. It is best and usually sufficient for the patient to feed herself.
- The older the patient with anorexia, the more successfully she hides her history and evades treatment. Young teenagers with cooperative parents are the least difficult.

(akathisia), stiffness, and tremors. Because people with anorexia nervosa are not psychotic, the long-term use of antipsychotic drugs, with their risk of later causing movement disorders, is controversial.

ECT has been used in patients with anorexia nervosa when severe psychological symptoms of the disorder have not responded to pharmacotherapy and psychotherapy. No controlled study of this treatment in this disorder has been done; the few published reports are anecdotal and generally favorable. ECT should certainly be considered when a patient with anorexia nervosa also meets the criteria for major depression and has not responded to treatment with antidepressant drugs (see the Pearls & Perils box on p. 263). This mode of treatment is not often used in adolescents because of prejudices, even legal barriers, against its use in minors. This is in spite of an ample literature documenting its safety and efficacy in teenagers with the affective disorders, mania, and major depression. All the evidence we have so far indicates that we should treat anorexia nervosa early and vigorously, that an episode of illness will be shortened in this way and a chronic course may thus be less likely.

Bulimia Nervosa

Recognition of the Syndrome

The fact that people sometimes engage in short episodes of massive overeating has been known since ancient times. Bouts of overeating followed by vomiting were not deemed pathological among sybarites of the Roman Empire, who just wanted to make room for more food. However, in the past couple of centuries a connection has been made between food binging and mental derangement. *Bulimia* is an old term that has long been linked to psychopathology. Its predecessor word, *bulimy,* was defined in the *Oxford English Dictionary* as, "a morbid hunger chiefly occurring in idiots and maniacs." It was not thought especially common. If it was in fact not common then, it certainly is today.

For years it has been recognized that patients with anorexia nervosa sometimes break out of their restrictive dieting, overeat (at least by their own criteria), and induce vomiting to keep from losing control of their weight. By the 1960s, episodes of uncontrolled binge eating were also described (often in the course of affective disorders) in people of normal weight and in people who were overweight. By the 1970s researchers were describing a syndrome in which people (with or without anorexia nervosa or depression) ate great amounts in short periods of time, felt that the process was out of their control, experienced emotional distress, and purged themselves or engaged in excessive exercise to avoid gaining weight. Since then the phenomenon now called *bulimia nervosa* has been studied as a syndrome in its own right.

Diagnosing Bulimia Nervosa

History

Physicians see many people with bulimia nervosa in their practices. It occurs much more often than anorexia nervosa, but it is also much less obvious since most such patients are of normal weight or somewhat overweight. Furthermore they may not readily volunteer the information that they binge eat and purge, since it is embarrassing to admit that. The physician must ask. Bulimia nervosa is so common, occurring in American women at an incidence of from 1 in 50 to 1 in 10 (depending on the sample surveyed), that questions about it should be part of routine medical-history taking.

The typical person with bulimia nervosa is a young woman. There are individual variations in the history, since bulimia nervosa may or may not begin in the context of another psychiatric disorder (Box 15-2, Table 15-2). Even when no other disorder is present, bulimia nervosa is nevertheless attended by significant emotional symptoms. When it occurs during major depression, it is often a depression accompanied by overeating rather than by loss of appetite. Purging behavior, typically vomiting or using excessive laxatives or enemas, is in response to that and driven by the same feelings of disgust and fear of fatness that afflict patients with anorexia nervosa.

The patient with bulimia nervosa, whether or not she suffers from major depression, reports episodes of eating large amounts of food in short periods of time as often as 1 or 2 times a week or several times a day. She may or may not report that hunger precedes a binge; it can be precipitated by the mere presence of something to eat. Psychologically stressful circumstances can also be triggers, because food becomes a temporary fix for emotional tension, just as alcohol does. High calorie sweet foods are favored. An episode of overeating is followed by the discomfort of abdominal distension and by emotional distress. The person feels helpless disgust with herself, a depressed mood, an anxious fear of fatness, and an overwhelming urge to get rid of the food she has just eaten.

Vomiting is the favored means of purging. Laxatives, enemas, and diuretics, much less efficient as methods of weight control, are also employed, as is compulsive overexercising. Sticking fingers down the throat is the most common means of inducing vomiting. Emetics, which may be taken in toxic amounts, are used less commonly. Vomiting gets easier to do as time passes. Simply leaning over the sink or toilet bowl may eventually work for the accomplished vomiter.

People with bulimia nervosa hate the fact that they

DSM-IV DIAGNOSTIC CRITERIA

BOX 15-2 BULIMIA NERVOSA

A. Recurrent episodes of binge eating. An episode of binge eating is characterized by both of the following:

(1) eating, in a discrete period of time (e.g., within any 2-hour period), an amount of food that is definitely larger than most people would eat during a similar period of time and under similar circumstances
(2) a sense of lack of control over eating during the episode (e.g., a feeling that one cannot stop eating or control what or how much one is eating)

B. Recurrent inappropriate compensatory behavior in order to prevent weight gain, such as self-induced vomiting; misuse of laxatives, diuretics, enemas, or other medications; fasting; or excessive exercise.

C. The binge eating and inappropriate compensatory behaviors both occur, on average, at least twice a week for 3 months.

D. Self-evaluation is unduly influenced by body shape and weight.

E. The disturbance does not occur exclusively during episodes of Anorexia Nervosa.

Specify type:
Purging Type: during the current episode of Bulimia Nervosa, the person has regularly engaged in self-induced vomiting or the misuse of laxatives, diuretics, or enemas
Nonpurging Type: during the current episode of Bulimia Nervosa, the person has used other inappropriate compensatory behaviors, such as fasting or excessive exercise, but has not regularly engaged in self-induced vomiting or the misuse of laxatives, diuretics, or enemas

From American Psychiatric Association: *Diagnostic and statistical manual of mental disorders,* ed 4 (DSM-IV), Washington, D.C., 1994, American Psychiatric Press.

DIAGNOSIS

TABLE 15-2 BULIMIA NERVOSA

Discriminating features

1. Persistent and recurrent binge eating in the absence of low weight
2. Inappropriate compensatory behavior (fasting, purging, or excessive exercise) in the absence of low weight

Consistent features

1. Feeling of loss of control over eating during the episode
2. Preoccupation with food and weight
3. Extreme psychological or physical discomfort after binging
4. Rebound binging after fasting

Variable features

1. Young female
2. Co-morbid with depression, obsessions, or substance abuse
3. Physical signs of self-induced vomiting
4. Concealing history of binging and purging
5. Amenorrhea
6. Electrolyte abnormalities

binge and purge, and they are ashamed of those behaviors. They overeat and vomit when they are alone. They take pains to conceal the behavior, hiding the vomitus if there is no conventional way to dispose of it. They search for ways to control their food binging. A common technique is to keep as little food around as possible. A strict routine helps them control the urge to overeat, and breaking that routine can open the door to bulimic behavior. A young woman may keep no food in her dormitory room at college. When she is home on vacation and faced with a well-stocked pantry, her family may discover that entire pies mysteriously disappear.

One popular but misguided method of controlling the urge to binge is fasting. This backfires because it causes bouts of increased hunger, which lead to even more overeating. A common story is of a high-school girl who skips breakfast, stays away from the school cafeteria at lunch, and then attacks the refrigerator when she gets home in the middle of the afternoon. Once such hunger-driven binges start, the patient finds them especially difficult to control. She continues eating well past the point when sensations of hunger should have been quelled.

Examination of the Patient

During the initial examination, many patients with bulimia nervosa exhibit anxiety, depressed mood, and preoccupation with fear of weight gain; the syndrome is often part of an episode of major depression. Telltale physical signs are few. Weight is usually normal or moderately above normal. There may be erosion of tooth enamel, redness of oral mucosa, enlargement of the parotid and submaxillary salivary glands, and calluses on the dorsal surfaces of the fingers; all of these are signs of the repeated induction of vomiting. The physician treating a patient with bulimia nervosa must be alert to possible hypokalemia from the loss of potassium through vomiting and the use of laxatives and diuretics. Other electrolyte derangements and serious complications of purging are discussed in the section on medical complications of anorexia nervosa.

Clues to the Etiology

Psychological and biological causes have been postulated for eating disorders. This is touched on in the section on the etiology of anorexia nervosa. Research stemming from such theories has not yet uncovered the causes of bulimia nervosa.

In bulimia nervosa, interpretation of biological studies is not confounded by the presence of starvation, as it is in anorexia nervosa. Moreover, since bulimia nervosa usually remits within a reasonable length of time, the same subjects can be studied in sick and healthy states. Some recent investigations stem from the knowledge that opioids in the central nervous system (CNS) and certain neurotransmitters (for example, serotonin and norepinephrine) influence appetite and mechanisms of satiety. Cerebrospinal fluid (CSF) and neuroimaging studies offer promise, but definite answers are not available so far. A satisfactory biological model for bulimia nervosa needs to account for the obsessions that drive bulimic behavior and the symptoms of major depression that are often present, as well as the apparent failure of satiety mechanisms.

Epidemiological studies demonstrate that bulimia nervosa is a common affliction. Estimates of its incidence vary widely, depending on the strictness of diagnostic criteria used and on the population studied. Prevalence may be as high as 2% to 10% of the population, with white adolescent girls and young women of middle or higher socioeconomic groups most at risk. Like anorexia nervosa, bulimia nervosa rarely occurs in men. As stated in the previous section, people with both anorexia nervosa and bulimia nervosa share demographic characteristics with those large elements of the American and European populace who most prize thinness and who worry about weight and diet often.

Family studies of bulimia nervosa report that relatives have increased prevalence of affective disorders, both major depression and bipolar disorder; of substance abuse disorders; and of obsessionality. These are the same syndromes that commonly appear in the patients themselves; more often than not, bulimia nervosa is co-morbid with something else, usually major depression. In bulimia nervosa, as in other psychiatric disorders, premorbid personality traits and subjects of habitual concern may be expressed in exaggerated form during the illness itself. If exceedingly weight-conscious women happen to develop depression, OCD, or alcoholism, they may also be at greater risk of becoming bulimic in the course of those disorders. Maladaptive eating patterns may increase, anxiety about weight may be intensified, and binge-purge behavior may then develop.

Course and Outcome

Full-fledged bulimia nervosa, meeting the diagnostic criteria of DSM-IV, is at one end of a continuum of behavior. A large minority of white American teenage girls and young women admit to bothersome preoccupation with weight, virtually chronic dieting, and occasional episodes of vomiting to get rid of particularly burdensome amounts of food. Although there has been an insufficient number of follow-up studies thus far, it is the general impression of physicians and investigators that this behavior and bulimia nervosa itself become less common as the subjects get older. The duration of bulimic behavior over several years and an extreme frequency of purging predict a poorer outcome.

For many patients in whom the rate of binging and purging diminishes over time, the physician's goal may shift from a major emphasis on controlling bulimia to an emphasis on treating the disorder with which it is co-morbid. When bulimia occurs during the course of another psychiatric illness (as is usually the case), the ultimate outcome depends on the outcome of the other disorder. When the latter subsides, bulimic behavior improves or goes away altogether. Follow-up studies demonstrate good outcomes for patients with bulimia nervosa whose depression, OCD, or other disorders are adequately treated and poorest outcomes for patients with poor premorbid psychological adjustment or with substance-abuse disorders.

Treatment

Treatment of people with bulimia nervosa is much easier than treatment of those with anorexia nervosa. In fact, it is not unusual to find patients who were successfully treated for major depression by their family doctors, having never confessed their secret binging and purging, and who were cured of bulimia nervosa without their physicians even knowing they had it.

The principles of treatment are restoration of conventional eating patterns and elimination of fasting as a means of weight control, avoidance of alcohol and recreational drugs, and treatment of co-morbid conditions.

PEARLS & PERILS

BULIMIA NERVOSA

- Food-binging and purging, usually by vomiting, occur in as many 2% to 10% of Americans, but patients may not volunteer that they engage in such behavior. The physician must ask about it.
- White teenage girls or young women of middle or higher social strata—those who prize thinness and fear fatness the most—are most at risk for anorexia nervosa and bulimia nervosa.
- Patients with bulimia nervosa feel out of control, frightened, and ashamed of their binge-purge behavior.
- Bulimia nervosa usually occurs with another psychiatric disorder, such as major depression, OCD, or alcoholism, which must then also be treated.
- All classes of antidepressant drugs are useful in treating bulimia nervosa, even when depression is not present. Those antidepressant drugs that decrease obsessional thinking and do not increase appetite are the first choice.
- Fasting is bad whether it occurs in patients who have bulimia nervosa or who are obese, and it is a common trigger for uncontrolled food binging.

Restoration of normal, three-meal-a-day eating behavior and elimination of mini-fasts may take place simply after a physician's advice, or it may occur during the course of cognitive behavior therapy (CBT). However, it may not take place until the other requirements of treatment are fulfilled.

Alcohol should be avoided, even if the patient is not alcoholic, because of its stimulating effect on appetite and its sometimes disruptive effect on mood. Recreational drugs are to be avoided for the same reason as alcohol. For example, marijuana and cocaine both render mood more unstable and disrupt eating behavior, with marijuana driving appetite up and cocaine driving it down. Appetite-suppressant medications lead to rebound hunger and weight gain, and in the long run they are worse than useless.

Treatment of a disorder that may accompany bulimia nervosa usually means treatment of major depression, substance abuse, or OCD, although some other disorder may be present instead. It is especially fortunate that all types of antidepressant drugs tested so far have a beneficial effect in patients with bulimia nervosa. This is often true even when the syndrome is not accompanied by symptoms of major depression (see the Pearls & Perils box above). Although the TCAs have been successful in treating bulimia nervosa, common sense dictates that physicians might now better choose an antidepressant medication that is not usually associated with weight gain or increased appetite. The SSRIs fulfill this requirement and also have a better record in the treatment of the obsessive-compulsive symptoms, which often afflict patients with bulimia nervosa.

Obesity: Psychiatric Issues

Obesity is not an eating disorder in any psychiatric diagnostic system, and no psychiatric disorder has been implicated in its cause. When obesity happens to coexist with a psychiatric disorder, such as depression or alcoholism, successful treatment of the psychiatric illness does not make the obesity go away. Rather, obesity is a common chronic medical disorder, presumed to be of multifactorial causes that are usually unknown, and the product of complex metabolic processes in which more calories have been taken in than expended. Obesity runs in families. Genetic predisposition is strongly suggested by twin studies and adoption studies; being closely related to people who are obese is a much more important determinant of obesity than being raised by people who are obese. Whereas revision of nutritional intake and behavior therapy have had some success in treating overweight children, adult obesity is rarely cured; people who are obese continue to be obese. After dieting, these people tend to return repeatedly to individual "set-points" of weight.

Although it is not a psychiatric illness, obesity should be considered in a chapter on eating disorders. Psychiatrists and other mental health professionals do get involved in the treatment of patients who are obese; people who are very overweight are often emotionally distressed by their obesity. Some obese people binge-eat, a behavior within the scope of psychiatry's concern. Psychotherapy has a role in the management of obesity in some circumstances.

There is scant evidence to support an old theory that obesity is the result of excessive eating caused by depressed mood and unhappiness. Rather the reverse is more likely; people who are obese suffer emotionally from the effects of obesity on their social relationships, employment, and medical condition. It is often this that leads them to psychiatrists or nonmedical therapists. As discussed below, psychotherapy of some type is part of the comprehensive treatment of obesity. Medication for the patient's frustration or depressed mood is not indicated unless the patient's symptoms fulfill criteria for an affective disorder; antidepressant drugs are not an effective treatment for unhappiness. Furthermore, many antidepressant drugs increase appetite and weight, and the appetite-suppressing effects of the newer SSRI drugs is almost always short-lived.

Binge eating in people who are obese is typically the result of fasting and is usually not accompanied by purging behavior or by the anorectic preoccupations that characterize bulimia nervosa. Patients who are overweight fast in an effort to lose weight rapidly, but their appetites catch up with them. Even a short fast, such as skipping breakfast and lunch, can produce that rebound effect. Some studies have found that people who are obese and have poor emotional adjustment or drug or alcohol abuse are the ones most likely to binge-eat. Treatment of this binging with antidepressant medications has not had the success enjoyed by the antidepressant treatment of bulimia nervosa. The binging will not stop unless the fasting stops.

Many programs for the treatment of obesity include individual or group psychotherapy, which addresses patients' specific eating behaviors as well as the emotional conflicts arising in their personal lives, schools, or jobs. The most comprehensive programs recognize the chronicity of the disorder and emphasize control and the establishment of a healthy life-style rather than cure. They include nutritionally-monitored very low calorie diets (VLCD) with low fat content, avoidance of fasting, a prescribed program of daily exercise, and psychotherapy to aid in the establishment of new eating behavior. Such programs result in significant weight loss, much of which is of course later regained. However, there is evidence that a significant minority of those completing a program of many months' duration do not return to their original weight and do live healthier lives, even though they may remain overweight. The biggest problems here, as in the case of so many treatments in the field of medicine, is with compliance. Many people quit rigorous programs before the time prescribed for them has elapsed. Even when they finish such programs, they often fail to maintain a routine of regular exercise and disciplined eating.

Many people have found that control of obesity and maintenance of a healthy life-style is enhanced by membership and regular attendance at meetings of lay organizations such as Overeaters Anonymous (OA) and Weight Watchers. As the name indicates, OA is patterned after Alcoholics Anonymous (AA), and views obesity as the result of food addiction that is analogous to alcohol or drug addiction. Members proceed through a 12-step program of recovery, just as members of AA do. Professionals are divided as to whether this approach makes sense; a person cannot abstain from food in the same way he can abstain from alcohol. The model is not a true fit, but many find it useful. Weight Watchers, which stresses the eating of prescribed foods and systematic attention to weight, also involves group support and the establishment of healthy eating behavior. People suffering from the chronic illness of obesity try these and other such programs and stick to the one that works best, if they are fortunate enough to find one.

Despite all these efforts, obesity endures, and the number and variety of proposed remedies are measures of an inability to control it. It has been estimated that the dieting industry consumes thirty billion dollars per year. If the war on obesity has not been a medical success, it has at least been a commercial success for entrepreneurs who capitalize on Americans' desire to be thin.

CONSIDER CONSULTATION WHEN . . .

(FOR ANOREXIA NERVOSA)

- Weight loss is accompanied by symptoms of major depressive disorder or obsessive-compulsive disorder
- Alcohol or drug dependence is suspected
- Weight loss is extreme
- Weight loss continues despite treatment
- Hospital care is required because of weight loss or severity of emotional distress

Annotated Bibliography

American psychiatric association practice guideline for eating disorders, *Am J Psychiatry* 150:207-228, 1993.

These guidelines include current standards of care and summaries of the clinical course and treatment of anorexia nervosa and bulimia nervosa. The bibliography includes literature through 1992.

Bliss EL, Branch CHH: *Anorexia nervosa: its history, psychology, and biology,* New York, 1960, Hoeber.

This is an old text with excellent case descriptions that will never be out of date.

Giannini AJ, Slaby AE, editors: *The eating disorders,* New York, 1993, Springer-Verlag.

This comprehensive multiauthored text deals with obesity as well as anorexia nervosa and bulimia nervosa.

Halmi KA, editor: *Psychobiology and treatment of anorexia nervosa and bulimia nervosa,* Washington, D.C., 1993, American Psychiatric Press.

Here is another good book that complements the Giannini text cited above.

Kaplan AS, Garfinkel PE, editors: *Medical issues and the eating disorders: the interface,* New York, 1993, Brunner/Mazel.

This source is indispensable for physicians treating eating disorders.

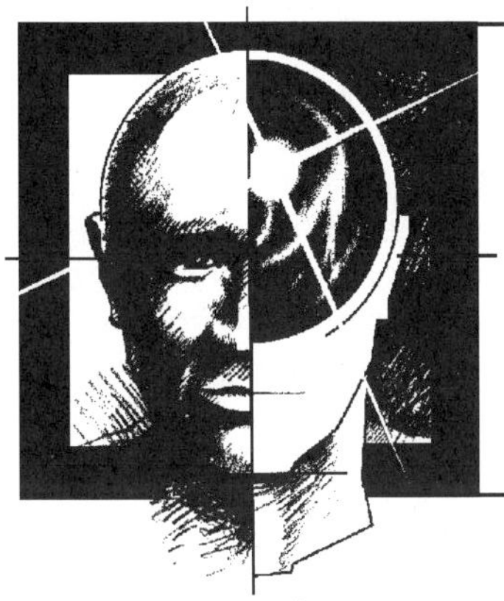

chapter 16

Somatoform Disorders

Carol S. North, MD and Samuel B. Guze, MD

Clinical Relevance: Importance and Scope of the Problem

Somatoform disorders present some of the most confusing and difficult problems in the practice of medicine. Somatoform disorders often go unrecognized in clinical practice, even by the most highly skilled physicians and psychiatrists. Nonrecognition of somatoform disorders results in unnecessary medical and surgical procedures, patient dissatisfaction with medical care, and frustration of physicians. With some basic background and vigilance, the physician can circumvent most of these problems. This chapter defines somatoform disorders, points out clinical indicators to alert the physician to the presence of these disorders, explains how to recognize and diagnose them, and finally describes their management. Because somatization disorder and conversion disorder are the most prevalent somatoform disorders and because they are the best understood of this set of disorders, this chapter focuses on these two disorders.

History of Somatization and Conversion Disorders

Hysteria, the precursor to somatization disorder, was well known by the ancient Egyptians long before the time of Hippocrates. Hysteria was thought to be caused by a wandering uterus, hence the name *hysteria,* derived from the Latin word for uterus. The association of the uterus with hysteria may have sprung from the observations that this is predominantly a disorder of women and that gynecological symptoms, such as menstrual and reproductive complaints, are central to the clinical presentation.

In the ninth century, hysteria was conceptualized as a purely physical disorder. However, by the Middle Ages hysteria was viewed not as a medical condition but as a spiritual disorder of evil and demonic possession. In the seventeenth century, an English physician named Sydenham reawakened medical interest in hysteria. Sydenham observed that hysteria could simulate almost any medical disease.

More than a century ago, Briquet provided the first systematic description of hysteria with a series of 430 cases that he studied for a decade. He observed that dramatic and medically unexplained complaints were characteristic features of the disorder and that patients with these complaints were extremely impressionable and emotionally labile. He described hysteria as a serious illness with devastating effects on patients and their families. Briquet and his contemporaries, Reynolds and Charcot, classified hysteria as a disorder of the central nervous system (CNS). Although Briquet recommended the term *hysteria* be dropped because of its pejorative connotations, the condition's name was not changed until almost a century later.

Kraepelin, another contemporary of Briquet, also studied patients with hysteria. His observations showed that the characteristic features of the disorder included tendency to exaggerate, emotional instability, and severe social disability. His patients complained of hallucinations. Around the turn of the century, patients with hysteria of Janet, Savill, and Breuer and Freud began to exhibit dual personalities, a popular new trend in psychiatric circles. As discussed in the Special Issues section, patients with somatization disorder are often captured by new psychiatric or medical "trendy" illnesses.

In the first half of the twentieth century, the concept of hysteria focused on the histrionic personality traits associated with the disorder, submerging the characteristic unexplained medical traits. However, in the 1960s and 1970s researchers at Washington University in St. Louis revived the model of hysteria as a "medical model" syndrome, defining it on the basis of multiple unexplained medical complaints in multiple organ systems; the histrionic personality components were considered secondary. Criteria for the diagnosis proposed in the classic work of Perley and Guze required the presence of at least 25 of 59 possible medically unexplained symptom complaints in at least 9 of 10 possible symptom groups. In honor of the first systematic observer of hysteria, Guze in 1970 suggested the name *Briquet's syndrome* for the disorder. This name has gained popularity in many sectors, but it has not been universally embraced.

Current official criteria for psychiatric disorders published by the American Psychiatric Association grew out of original criteria established by research efforts of the Washington University group in the 1970s. These official criteria use the term *somatization disorder* in place of the older term *hysteria*. This new name follows the tradition of defining the disorder based on its multiple unexplained somatic complaints. Although the criteria for Briquet's syndrome describe a more cohesive disorder that is more relevant to epidemiological research than the criteria for somatization disorder, in clinical practice the less cumbersome somatization disorder criteria are used in making the diagnosis.

The term *conversion* was originated by Freud, who applied it to symptoms he viewed as resulting from substitution of somatic symptoms for repressed emotions. According to Freudian theory of conversion, mental conflicts are converted into physical and mental symptoms through unconscious mechanisms of symbolism (the symptom serves as a symbol of the conflict) or of primary gain (that is, the desire to enact the patient role). Conversion symptoms were recognized as part of hysteria until 1980, when official DSM-III criteria separated conversion and somatization into distinct categories. At that juncture, somatization disorder followed the Washington University group's model of a polysomatoform disorder, and conversion disorder continued with Freudian concepts of psychological conflicts manifesting as somatic phenomena. Somatization disorder has been well validated as a diagnosis through studies that have defined core symptoms, delineated it from other disorders, documented family transmission, and demonstrated stability of diagnosis on follow-up examinations. Such studies have not yet been completed for conversion disorder.

Clinical Features

Somatization Disorder

Diagnosis

According to the DSM-IV definition, patients with somatization disorder have a history of significant symptoms in at least the following four categories: pain, gastrointestinal symptoms, sexual symptoms, and pseudoneurological symptoms (Box 16-1, Table 16-1). To qualify as significant, each symptom must be medically unexplained; this includes known effects of drugs or alcohol to which the individual was exposed. When a related medical condition is present, a symptom qualifies only if it or the social or occupational impairment it causes are in excess of that expected from the degree of the associated medical condition. By definition, somatization disorder must begin by age 30. Any patient with a new onset of multiple medically unexplained somatic complaints in the fourth decade of life or older should be considered undiagnosed until a medical evaluation indicates otherwise.

Patients with somatization disorder often display histrionic (dramatic) behaviors. The current definition of somatization disorder, departing from its historical roots in hysteria, does not require a hysterical presentation, nor is such a presentation pathognomonic of this disorder. Some patients may assume the apparent opposite emotional stance, expressing inappropriate

DSM-IV DIAGNOSTIC CRITERIA

BOX 16-1 SOMATIZATION DISORDER

A. A history of many physical complaints beginning before age 30 years that occur over a period of several years and result in treatment being sought or significant impairment in social, occupational, or other important areas of functioning.

B. Each of the following criteria must have been met, with individual symptoms occurring at any time during the course of the disturbance:

(1) *four pain symptoms:* a history of pain related to at least four different sites or functions (e.g., head, abdomen, back, joints, extremities, chest, rectum, during menstruation, during sexual intercourse, or during urination)
(2) *two gastrointestinal symptoms:* a history of at least two gastrointestinal symptoms other than pain (e.g., nausea, bloating, vomiting other than during pregnancy, diarrhea, or intolerance of several different foods)
(3) *one sexual symptom:* a history of at least one sexual or reproductive symptom other than pain (e.g., sexual indifference, erectile or ejaculatory dysfunction, irregular menses, excessive menstrual bleeding, vomiting throughout pregnancy)
(4) *one pseudoneurological symptom:* a history of at least one symptom or deficit suggesting a neurological condition not limited to pain (conversion symptoms such as impaired coordination or balance, paralysis or localized weakness, difficulty swallowing or lump in throat, aphonia, urinary retention, hallucinations, loss of touch or pain sensation, double vision, blindness, deafness, seizures; dissociative symptoms such as amnesia; or loss of consciousness other than fainting)

C. Either (1) or (2):

(1) after appropriate investigation, each of the symptoms in Criterion B cannot be fully explained by a known general medical condition or the direct effects of a substance (e.g., a drug of abuse, a medication)
(2) when there is a related general medical condition, the physical complaints or resulting social or occupational impairment are in excess of what would be expected from the history, physical examination, or laboratory findings

D. The symptoms are not intentionally produced or feigned (as in Factitious Disorder or Malingering).

From American Psychiatric Association: *Diagnostic and statistical manual of mental disorders,* ed 4 (DSM-IV), Washington, D.C., 1994, American Psychiatric Press.

indifference in the face of seemingly tragic and overwhelming medical events, a sign termed *la belle indifférence.* For example, a patient may describe vomiting buckets of blood until passing out with no trace of emotional concern.

The speech of patients with somatization disorder tends to be circumstantial and vague, which presents difficulties in eliciting a medical history. Descriptions of their symptoms are often dramatic, exaggerated, and extremely colorful, with sometimes bizarre and even outlandish examples. For example, one patient described her menstrual pain as rivers of fire in her belly and stated that it was so severe she had to double over to crawl to the toilet. Another patient reported that her headache was so severe that it felt like a bomb had blown off the top of her head. A patient diagnosed with mitral valve prolapse reported that when she felt upset she had "leaking" in her chest.

Certain red flags in the medical history should alert the physician to the possibility of somatization disorder. A complicated medical history with multiple diagnoses, multiple failed treatments, and an associated voluminous medical record is often the first clue. There are a number of other features, none of which are pathognomonic by themselves but when combined with other clues should also alert the physician. These include multiple allergies or medication intolerances. One patient reported that she was allergic to every antibiotic and pain killer ever made. She said that when she was given intravenous penicillin on two occasions, it caused a cardiac arrest; both times she was revived by the heroics of a cardiopulmonary resuscitation (CPR) team. Neither episode was documented in her medical record. Other features include complaints of many disorders (often disorders that have been popularized in the media) for which no well-integrated structural or pathophysiological models are known or for which the patient does not fit the definition of the syndrome. Examples of these disorders include chronic fatigue syndrome, fibromyalgia, hypoglycemia, chronic pain syndromes, temporomandibular joint syndrome, premenstrual syndrome, reflex sympathetic dystrophy, tension headache or migraine, irritable bowel syndrome, atypical chest pain, and multiple en-

DIAGNOSIS

TABLE 16-1
SOMATIZATION DISORDER

Discriminating feature

1. Medically unexplained somatic complaints in four or more organ systems:
   - Four or more pain symptoms (e.g., back, joint, extremity, rectal, or chest, or head pain, or dysmenorrhea)
   - Two or more gastrointestinal symptoms (e.g., nausea, vomiting, diarrhea, or abdominal bloating)
   - One or more sexual symptoms (e.g., dyspareunia, anorgasmia, menstrual complaints, or sexual indifference)
   - One or more pseudoneurological symptoms (e.g., paralysis, pseudoseizures, aphonia, blindness, deafness, diplopia, or amnesia)

Consistent features

1. More than 95% of cases are women
2. Onset is usually in adolescence to early adulthood but must begin before age 30
3. Tends to be chronic condition
4. Multiple psychosocial and interpersonal problems

Variable features

1. Patients often have psychological complaints, but they may refuse all consideration of psychological problems
2. Sometimes complicated by substance abuse (including iatrogenic)
3. Spouses often have drug or alcohol abuse, antisocial personalities, and physical abusiveness

vironmental allergies ("allergic to everything").

The family history often reveals further evidence, such as somatization disorder, antisocial personality disorder, criminality (for example, a prison history), and substance abuse in family members. Although it is not diagnostic, such information can alert the physician to search for further data supporting the diagnosis of somatization disorder.

The social history may also provide clues to the diagnosis. Childhood histories of abuse and dysfunctional or substance-abusing family backgrounds are commonly reported by these patients. They often live with or marry people who are alcoholic or sociopathic. The school or work history may be characterized by excessive disruptions because of medical problems and interpersonal difficulties. Despite this, if the employer is sympathetic and the patient does good work when she is healthy, she may have a long and apparently stable history with that employer.

Patients with somatization disorder rarely provide sufficient detail about their extensive medical history in the initial medical visit to allow the physician to make a diagnosis of somatization disorder. They are characteristically unreliable historians. When presenting to a medical specialist they may focus on their chief complaint and downplay or even entirely omit mention of their extensive symptoms in other multiple organ systems. Therefore it is important to persist in tracking down medical records and obtain more history from others who know the patient. Making the diagnosis may require the accumulation of symptoms over time, since the patient voices new symptom complaints to the physician as her symptom focus changes and evolves. Combining the patient's complaints elicited over time with those documented by other sources is often necessary to establish the diagnosis with confidence.

Natural History

Although by definition, somatization disorder must begin before age 30, it typically begins in the decade after puberty. The disorder is a chronic, lifelong condition with fluctuations in symptom severity, although prolonged, complete remissions rarely occur. On follow-up examination after several years, most women (90%) with the disorder still meet criteria for the diagnosis and few new diagnoses are found to explain the symptoms. However, men meeting criteria for somatization disorder have a greater likelihood of being found subsequently to have a medical disorder that explains the symptoms.

Social complications of somatization disorder include marital difficulties (which are often associated with sexual symptoms); occupational impairment; parenting problems; and multiple social problems such as stormy interpersonal relationships, legal problems related to divorce and other interpersonal problems, and family difficulties. Patients with somatization disorder report being confined to bed an average of seven days out of each month. An area of special concern for medical professionals is these patients' pattern of extensive use of medical services that results in unnecessary multiple medical and surgical procedures and treatments, which thereby increases the risk for complications and additional morbidity, as well as opportunities for claims of medical damages. Smith and colleagues at the University of Arkansas demonstrated that patients with somatization disorder seek health care excessively and at considerable expense, generating as much as 9 times the cost of other medical patients.

Suicide attempts are common in somatization disorder. In one sample, 51% of patients with somatization disorder had made suicide attempts. Completed suicide is fortunately not a common outcome of somatization disorder, but risk increases when co-morbid substance abuse is present. However, in any disorder in which suicidal gestures are encountered some gestures have the potential to result in unanticipated death. All suicide attempts, whether medically serious or trivial, are socially disruptive to families and other contacts of these patients.

Differential Diagnosis

Somatization disorder is most often confused with medical conditions. Certain indicators in the medical history indicate somatization disorder. These include distribution of complaints in multiple organ systems, and a lack of evidence of medically or structurally documented abnormalities or laboratory indicators over years of evaluation. Somatization disorder baffles physicians, as documented by a study by Tomasson and colleagues that showed that despite lack of medical documentation, 86% of patients received a medical diagnosis, with a mean of 2.8 medical diagnoses.

Somatization disorder not only generates medically undocumented somatoform symptoms of multiple medical disorders that patients do not really have, but it also produces "psychoform" symptoms of multiple psychiatric disorders that are not diagnosed. Two thirds of all patients with somatization disorder complain of current psychological symptoms. In fact, psychological symptoms are the most common main symptom complaint in somatization disorder, occurring in 25% of cases. More than one half of all patients with somatization disorder report prior treatment for psychiatric symptoms.

The most common psychological symptoms expressed by patients with somatization disorder are anxiety and depression. People who have somatization disorder report more depressive symptoms than do patients without somatization disorder who actually meet full criteria for major depression. Sometimes the distinction of somatization disorder from depressive and anxiety disorders can be quite problematic. Mood disturbance, hopelessness, suicidality, and vegetative symptoms such as fatigue and appetite disturbance that constitute criterion symptoms of major depression also serve as criterion symptoms of Briquet's syndrome and are highly prevalent in somatization disorder. Conversely, patients with depressive disorders often report hypochondriacal and somatic symptoms.

However, in patients without somatization disorder who are depressed, somatic complaints are not a lifelong pattern but are temporally associated with the depressive episode. Furthermore, depression in the absence of somatization disorder does not produce the multiple symptoms in multiple organ systems that help differentiate somatization disorder from depression. Patients with a major depressive episode describe it as a distinct change from how they usually feel, which is different from the worsening of the usual state described by patients with somatization disorder.

Anxiety disorders generate many somatic symptoms, especially cardiorespiratory symptoms (for example, palpitations, shortness of breath, and dizziness). Anxiety disorders are differentiated from somatization disorder symptoms, in which symptom complaints are lodged not just in the cardiorespiratory system but also in multiple organ systems. Symptoms of panic disorder occur by definition during panic attacks; in somatization disorder they must also occur at other times to be counted toward the diagnosis.

Patients with somatization disorder also complain of psychotic symptoms, including hallucinations, and for this reason somatization disorder is sometimes confused with psychotic disorders. However, their psychotic-like symptoms differ qualitatively from the stereotypical voices of schizophrenia that talk to each other or engage in a running commentary. Visual hallucinations of sexually symbolic objects, such as snakes, little naked (sometimes green) men running across the room, and cartoon figues, are more characteristic of the pseudopsychotic symptoms of somatization disorder, as are voices telling the person to harm someone she despises or would like to harm. Patients with somatization disorder also report episodes of physical hyperactivity and other manic-like symptoms, such as jitteriness, distractibility, sexual promiscuity, and excessive spending of money; however, on closer examination these symptoms do not fit the characteristic episodic nature of bipolar disorder and therefore this diagnosis is not warranted.

Patients with somatization disorder studied in academic centers almost always meet criteria for one or more other psychiatric syndromes. However, in primary care settings the rates of psychiatric comorbidity may be somewhat lower. The somatization disorder usually precedes the onset of the other psychiatric disorders, which by definition makes somatization disorder the primary diagnosis.

Other common co-morbid psychiatric disorders include drug and alcohol use disorders, to which these patients are subject. Most patients with somatization disorder are also found to meet criteria for a personality disorder, and some experts feel that somatization disorder arises from a personality pathology. Pennebaker and Watson argue that somatization disorder belongs not on Axis I where it is currently classified, but on Axis II with the personality disorders.

Genetics and Family History

Somatization disorder is a familial disorder, especially in women. It runs in affected families along with the male-dominant antisocial personality disorder. Patients with somatization disorder have first-degree male relatives with increased rates of antisocial personality disorder and, through the association with antisocial personality disorder, alcoholism. Female relatives of women with somatization disorder have increased rates of somatization disorder and also of antisocial personality disorder. A complication to understanding the relationship of these two disorders in families is the phenomenon of assortative mating. Women with somatization disorder tend to pair off with men who are antisocial and alcoholic, who further add these other conditions to the family illness patterns.

The familial associations of somatization disorder described in family studies have been confirmed by twin studies that have provided even more definite evidence of a genetic link. Torgerson showed that concordance rates of somatization are nearly 3 times higher in monozygotic twins (29%) than in dizygotic twins (10%). Adoption studies have provided the most compelling evidence of genetic contribution to the familial association of somatization disorder and antisocial personality disorder. Adopted offspring of biological parents with antisocial behavior studied by Cadoret and colleagues showed much higher rates of somatoform symptoms and diagnoses of somatization disorder than did adoptees without antisocial biological parentage.

Somatization and antisocial personality disorders are associated within individuals as well. Rates of antisocial personality disorder in women with somatization disorder may be as high as 25%. People with antisocial personality disorder also have more somatoform symptom complaints than do people without this disorder.

Epidemiology

Somatization disorder is not one of the most prevalent psychiatric disorders, occurring in 1 of 50 women in the general population. In certain populations it is much more prevalent; somatization disorder occurs in 9% of medical and surgical inpatients, 10% of psychiatric inpatients, 17% of patients with irritable bowel syndrome, 27% of women undergoing hysterectomies for noncancerous indications, 26% of first-degree female relatives of patients with somatization disorder, and 41% of female felons. Tertiary medical settings attract patients with somatization disorder, who gravitate toward centers of medical expertise as they search for answers for their multiple medically unexplained symptom complaints. Somatization disorder is also more prevalent among lesser educated populations.

Somatization disorder is almost exclusively a women's disorder, although it is well documented to occur in men, too. When somatization disorder occurs in men, it is considered to be a more severe condition than in women, as shown by its higher co-morbidity rates of alcoholism and depression.

BOX 16-2 CONVERSION DISORDER

DSM-IV DIAGNOSTIC CRITERIA

A. One or more symptoms or deficits affecting voluntary motor or sensory function that suggest a neurological or other general medical condition.

B. Psychological factors are judged to be associated with the symptom or deficit because the initiation or exacerbation of the symptom or deficit is preceded by conflicts or other stressors.

C. The symptom or deficit is not intentionally produced or feigned (as in Factitious Disorder or Malingering).

D. The symptom or deficit cannot, after appropriate investigation, be fully explained by a general medical condition, or by the direct effects of a substance, or as a culturally sanctioned behavior or experience.

E. The symptom or deficit causes clinically significant distress or impairment in social, occupational, or other important areas of functioning or warrants medical evaluation.

F. The symptom or deficit is not limited to pain or sexual dysfunction, does not occur exclusively during the course of Somatization Disorder, and is not better accounted for by another mental disorder.

Specify type of symptom or deficit:
With Motor Symptom or Deficit
With Sensory Symptom or Deficit
With Seizures or Convulsions
With Mixed Presentation

From American Psychiatric Association: *Diagnostic and statistical manual of mental disorders,* ed 4 (DSM-IV), Washington, D.C., 1994, American Psychiatric Press.

Conversion Disorder

Diagnosis

The hallmark of conversion disorder is the presence of one or more symptoms or deficits relating to voluntary motor or sensory function (Box 16-2; Table 16-2). The symptoms may suggest a general medical condition, but classically the symptoms are "pseudoneurological," suggesting illnesses such as multiple sclerosis or seizure disorder. Symptoms of conversion disorder are by definition medically unexplained, and they either cause significant social or occupational impairment or warrant medical evaluation. The following four types of conversion symptoms are recognized: (1) symptoms with motor deficit (for example, paralysis or weakness of a limb, difficulty walking because of weakness or balance problems, aphonia, and urinary retention); (2) symptoms with sensory deficit (such as numbness, blindness, tunnel vision, deafness, and hallucinations); (3) seizures or convulsions; and (4) mixed symptom types. The most common main complaints documented in patients with conversion disorder are numbness, aphonia, ataxia, fits, paralysis, and blindness.

According to the Washington University group, whose work was reviewed by Boffeli and Guze, the presence of pseudoneurological symptoms defines conversion disorder in atheoretical terms without the need to invoke the role of psychological mechanisms in the etiology or pathogenesis of the disorder. However, established criteria of the American Psychiatric Association require documentation of psychological factors associated with the onset or exacerbation of symptoms, such as emotional conflicts and stressors. An example of psychological factors associated with conversion symptoms is that of a woman who the morning after her husband told her he was going to leave her woke up to find herself completely paralyzed from the waist down. A problem with this requirement is that it is difficult to operationalize psychological factors into objective measures, and as a result no data are available to support this requirement in the criteria. Therefore a creative physician might always be able to hypothesize a connection between personal events and pseudoneurological symptoms.

DIAGNOSIS

TABLE 16-2
CONVERSION DISORDER

Discriminating features

1. One or more pseudoneurological symptoms relating to voluntary sensory or motor function
2. The four types of symptoms are motor deficit, sensory deficit, seizures or convulsions, and mixed types
3. Differentiated from somatization disorder by lack of many symptoms in many organ systems

Consistent features

1. Men more often have conversion disorder than somatization disorder (but women predominate in both disorders)
2. Onset usually age 10 to 35, but it may begin at any age
3. Isolated conversion symptoms are rare in the absence of another disorder (beware conversion diagnosis)

Variable features

1. 20% to 30% of patients are found to have a medical illness that explains the symptoms
2. Prognosis for individual symptoms is favorable, but long-term prognosis is for recurrence of same or new symptoms
3. Onset of symptoms in middle age or later greatly increases chance for medical explanation (beware conversion diagnosis)
4. Somatization disorder and antisocial personality are common co-morbid conditions

Natural History

Conversion disorder can begin at any age, although its onset is most often between the ages of 10 and 35. The onset of conversion symptoms in middle age or later should seriously raise the possibility of an occult neurological or general medical source for the symptoms. A sizable proportion, 20% to 30% of patients with conversion disorder, are later found to have a medical illness that in retrospect accounts for the symptoms. Approximately one third to one half of patients with symptoms diagnosed as conversion symptoms who do not have somatization disorder are later found to have a documented neurological disease. In contrast, only 10% of patients with somatization disorder who have conversion symptoms are found to have a medical illness that explains the symptoms.

The long-term prognosis of conversion disorder is poor, with two thirds or more of all patients remaining symptomatic at follow-up examinations an average of 6 years later. Other conversion symptoms, as well as additional psychiatric problems, commonly develop even though the original conversion symptom may have disappeared.

The extreme degree of social and occupational disability that is characteristic of somatization disorder is not necessarily associated with conversion disorder. The prognosis of conversion disorder tends to follow that of the co-morbid psychiatric disorder, with patients who have somatization disorder faring the worst. Often compensation and other psychosocial factors, including monetary or legal compensation factors and interpersonal conflict, are present in the individual's current situation. Compensation factors are more common in male patients with conversion symptoms, and they may be important in dealing with conversion symptoms in military and criminal justice settings.

The prognosis for specific conversion symptoms is relatively favorable, with recovery typically within 2 weeks. Two thirds of individual conversion symptoms are absent at follow-up examinations an average of 6 years later. However, symptom recurrence is common, occurring at a rate of 20% to 25% within 1 year. Favorable prognosis of conversion symptoms is associated with acute onset, an identifiable associated precipitating stressor, brief duration of symptoms before treatment, and high intelligence. Conversion symptoms with the poorest outcomes include pseudoseizures and conversion tremors.

Isolated conversion symptoms in the absence of another disorder, psychiatric or physical, are uncommon, and those unassociated with a psychiatric disorder are much more likely to be found later to have a specific medical illness that explains the symptom. Therefore the old term *conversion reaction* is a useless diagnosis and in fact potentially dangerous if it leads the physician to abandon further medical work-up. In cases of apparent isolated conversion symptoms without overt evidence of a major psychiatric disorder, physicians are encouraged to resist the temptation to attribute the symptom to psychological processes. Although it is frustrating for physicians to deal with unexplained phenomena such as this, nothing is gained by making unwarranted assumptions about etiology or diagnosis. To make premature and arbitrary conclusions about the etiology of isolated conversion symptoms only invites the passage of time to prove a conclusion wrong. Instead, the physician must learn to accept uncertainty.

Differential Diagnosis

In conversion disorder, as in somatization disorder, the main differentiation to be made is from medical (predominantly neurological) disorders. This process is similar to the differentiation of somatization symptoms from medically based symptoms. Conversion syndromes are commonly seen in patients with a variety of documented neurological conditions, including seizure disorders, head injuries, tumors of the CNS, frontal lobe lesions, cerebrovascular accidents, acute encephalitis, delirium, Klinefelter's syndrome, and multiple sclerosis.

Somatization disorder is differentiated from conversion disorder by the greater number of symptoms and their wide range of distribution in different organ systems. The most common psychiatric diagnosis in patients with conversion symptoms is somatization disorder. More than one half of the inpatients with conversion disorders on neurology wards have been found to qualify for a diagnosis of somatization disorder. Conversion disorder is also associated with the diagnosis of antisocial personality disorder. More than one third of general medical patients with conversion disorder meet criteria for somatization disorder or antisocial personality.

Depressive syndromes have also been found in association with conversion disorder. However, closer examination has revealed that this depression is usually secondary depression in individuals with preexisting somatization disorder or antisocial personality disorder. There is little evidence of association of conversion disorder and primary mood disorder. Therefore the physician is cautioned not to stop screening for psychiatric disorders when depression is recognized, because there is usually another important diagnosis (somatization disorder or antisocial personality disorder) lurking behind the scenes.

Genetics and Family History

Little is known about family transmission of conversion disorder. An isolated study of familial psychiatric illness found considerable diagnostic heterogeneity, a reflection of the fact that patients with conversion disorder are probably not a unified group. The known co-morbidity of somatization disorder and antisocial personality disorder with conversion disorder might suggest the presence of somatization disorder and antisocial personality disorder in relatives of patients with these co-morbid disorders, although not necessarily in relatives of patients without them.

Epidemiology

Conversion symptoms are relatively prevalent. It has been estimated that up to 25% of hospital inpatients have had conversion symptoms at some time, and around 10% of psychiatric consultations on general hospital medical and surgical inpatients are for conversion symptoms. Conversion disorder is more prevalent in women than men, with 75% and possibly 90% of cases occurring in women. Conversion disorder is more common in lesser educated, lower socioeconomic populations.

Other Somatoform Disorders

These disorders include hypochondriasis, pain disorder, body dysmorphic disorder, somatoform disorder not otherwise specified (NOS), and undifferentiated somatization disorder (a category of somatoform symptoms not meeting criteria for any of the other somatoform diagnoses). Minimal published data are available on these other somatoform disorders, and therefore little can be said about their natural history, genetic and familial patterns, epidemiology, and treatment.

Hypochondriasis is defined as a period of at least 6 months of preoccupation with having a serious disease, caused by the misinterpretation of bodily symptoms and despite appropriate medical evaluation and reassurance. The term *hypochondria* has carried multiple meanings in modern as well as historical cultures, and therefore it is an imprecise term that may encompass a wide variety of contexts. The focus of body dysmorphic disorder is an imagined defect in a person's physical appearance that is accompanied by marked and excessive concern about slight physical anomalies such as an excessively large nose, asymmetry of physical features, dissatisfaction with the alignment of one's teeth, or a woman's preoccupation with her breasts as being too small or too large. The category of somatoform disorder NOS includes somatoform disorders of sufficient severity that fail to meet criteria for other established somatoform disorders. Included in this category is pseudocyesis, a false belief of being pregnant without supporting objective physical signs such as enlarged abdomen, disappearance of menstruation, breast engorgement, and fetal movements.

It is not clear whether hypochondriacal disorders, body dysmorphic disorders, and other somatoform disorders are best classified with the somatization disorders or whether they are equally associated with delusional somatic complaints of chronic schizophrenia or somatic perseverations of obsessive-compulsive disorder (OCD).

PEARLS & PERILS

DIAGNOSIS OF SOMATOFORM DISORDERS

- Red flags for a diagnosis of somatization disorder are a complicated medical history with multiple diagnoses, multiple failed treatments, and a voluminous medical record.
- Any patient with new onset of multiple medically unexplained somatic complaints in the fourth decade or older should be assumed to have an organic condition until a medical evaluation documents otherwise.
- The depression described by patients with somatization disorder is a worsening of their usual state, as opposed the distinct change from usual feelings described by patients without somatization disorder who are experiencing a major depressive episode.
- Pseudoneurological symptoms are characteristic of patients with conversion disorder, who do not display the multiple somatoform symptoms in multiple organ systems characteristic of somatization disorder.

Pathophysiology

The pathophysiology of somatoform disorders is unknown. The lack of known pathology in these disorders may lead physicians to dismiss these patients as playing games, simulating, and pretending illness that they do not have. It is important for the physician to recognize that although these patients do not have the serious medical illnesses their symptoms suggest, somatoform disorders are often severely disabling illnesses with considerable personal suffering and emotional anguish. These are serious disorders requiring specific responses from the physician.

Treatment

Importance of Diagnosis

Brown and Smith (1988) have observed, "The first major obstacle in dealing with somatization disorder patients is making the diagnosis." Somatization disorder is especially vexing and perplexing to the physician if it is not recognized, and it may lead to considerable medical morbidity. Because of somatization disorder's proclivity to mimic medical conditions and the fact that it is often seen by nonpsychiatric physicians, all clinicians must be remain alert to the possibility of the condition (see the Pearls & Perils box above). Although making the diagnosis can be somewhat laborious, the amount of guidance the diagnosis can give physicians dealing with these often difficult cases makes the effort worthwhile.

Psychiatric Consultation

Busy physicians may become disheartened about their ability to help patients with somatization disorders, in part because of the magnitude of difficulties they have experienced with them and the tremendous amount of physicians' time that they can absorb. A common automatic response is to refer the patient to a mental health professional as quickly as possible to get the patient out of a medical practice. Patients with somatization disorder may resist seeing a psychiatrist because of the implication that "it's all in my head." Psychiatric consultation is useful only when it is acceptable to the patient, and consultation is preferable to a transfer out of the provider's practice, which patients may perceive as a personal rejection. Patients with somatization disorder who also have psychological symptoms may gravitate to psychiatric care on their own, but this is not often the case. Some patients may blame any emotional difficulties they experience on the medical problem they believe they have, contending that if the physician could just find and fix the medical problem there would be no basis for the emotional response. ("If the pain would just go away then I wouldn't be so depressed!") When the patient rejects psychiatric care, the total burden of care rests with nonpsychiatric physicians. If the primary physician is vigilant for this disorder and can make the diagnosis, the patient can often be managed effectively without psychiatric referral.

General Treatment Strategies

Little empirical data exists on the most effective treatment of somatoform disorders, and no prospective treatment trials have been reported in the literature. However, a general consensus on medical model treatment principles in the literature can guide the physician. In one of the few systematic studies to examine treatment practices, Smith and colleagues reported that psychiatric consultation to the primary physician of patients with somatization disorder to confirm the diagnosis and recommend conservative treatment reduced health-care expenditures without adversely affecting health status or patient satisfaction with health care.

Treatment recommendations are similar for all of the somatoform disorders, and they are modelled on established principles of treatment for somatization disorder. The most important role of the physician managing somatization disorder is orchestration of treatment. This includes initiation of all referrals to medical specialists, informing consulted medical specialists of the patient's somatoform disorder, and discouraging unnecessary procedures and treatments. Because patients with somatization disorder tend to consult large numbers of specialists for extensive complaints in multiple organ systems, careful central management of their overall treatment plan can protect them from unnecessary treatments and procedures, dangerous treatment interactions and other iatrogenic complications, and gradual removal of all expendable body organs over time. Therefore if at all possible, referrals for specialty care should be made by one primary physician, who might in some cases be the patient's psychiatrist. This practice also allows the physician to set limits on the doctor-shopping to which these patients are prone.

The goal of treatment of somatization disorder is not to cure it (because a cure is not known) but to manage the illness and prevent complications. The first principle in treating these patients invokes the portion of the Hippocratic oath that says, "do no harm." The physician's natural tendency is to want to do something for the patient, when in actuality it is often more beneficial for these patients to avoid "doing" for them.

The ultimate goal is not to remove all sources of the patient's discomfort whatsoever (which is impossible) but to aim for the patient to be able to live with her symptoms, rather than continuing to regard them as serious or requiring emergency or surgical intervention (see the Pearls & Perils box below). To achieve these ends it is necessary to develop a lasting, empathetic relationship with the patient. Genuine and compassionate interest by the physician helps bond patients with somatization disorder within the physician-patient relationship. The best strategy is to give the patient regular outpatient appointments so she does not have to generate symptom complaints to be seen, thus avoiding the reinforcement of somatoform symptoms

PEARLS & PERILS

MANAGEMENT OF SOMATOFORM DISORDERS

- The goal of treatment of somatoform disorders is not to cure but to manage the illness and prevent complications.
- Effective management requires orchestration of treatment by the patient's primary physician, whether that person be a psychiatrist, family physician, or other medical specialist. Orchestration of treatment includes initiation of all referrals to medical specialists, informing the patient's medical specialists of the somatoform disorder, and discouraging unnecessary procedures and treatments.
- The quality of the relationship of the primary physician with the patient is critical to the management of somatization disorder. Regularly scheduled office visits, physical examinations, and listening to the patient's complaints in a sympathetic but nonreactive manner are key elements.
- Physicians treating patients with somatoform disorders are advised to avoid proceeding to invasive treatments and procedures unless sufficient objective evidence warrants such action. These patients complain vociferously of many symptoms, underscoring the value of resisting the temptation to act on the magnitude of specific complaints unless objective indicators are present. (However, this is not to imply that these patients cannot develop serious illness; a physician must not dismiss their complaints without a reasonable effort to substantiate or rule out documentable medical illness.)
- Patients with somatoform disorders are at risk for substance abuse, both iatrogenic and illicit. Therefore caution is indicated when prescribing potentially abusable substances for these patients who tend to elicit prescriptions with their often vocal complaints of insomnia, anxiety, depression, or pain.
- Although suicide gestures are common in somatization disorder, completed suicide is rare.

in the physician-patient relationship. It is recommended that a physical examination be performed at the appointment, because this demonstrates the physician's caring concern and interest, as well as a desire to understand what the patient perceives as her real problem. This strategy naturally directs the physician to listen to the patient's complaints and examine her instead of proceeding directly to extensive medical evaluations and procedures.

When no medical explanation can be found for a given symptom with the treatment plan described in this chapter, the patient is reassured that the physician has paid serious attention to the symptom and found that there is no medically worrisome cause for it; furthermore she sees that the physician will continue to monitor her for signs of serious disease. Often this is enough to satisfy the patient. Despite this, some patients are more demanding and insist on further evaluation, sometimes threatening to find a "more expert" physician who by virtue of superior medical skill will find the cause of the symptoms. On one hand it is undesirable for the physician to be manipulated into performing further tests or procedures by pressure from the patient, but on the other hand there is value in making some effort to keep these patients from leaving a practice because then they shop for another physician who will perform unnecessary tests and procedures. If the physician who understands somatization disorder does not treat the patient, another physician who may not understand or even recognize the disorder will.

However, the physician is ultimately advised not to compromise the standard of care to satisfy these patients' demands. When the patient threatens to change physicians the clinician can acknowledge to her that she has the power to terminate the relationship, but he can also provide the opinion that this would be a regrettable error. Experience has shown that few patients change physicians as a result of the physician's consistency in following the principles of management outlined here, and many patients even feel more comfortable with a physician who sets clear limits.

Eventually unnecessary costs and risks of exhaustive medical evaluations of all symptoms should become apparent to the physician treating somatization disorder, and a decision made to limit more extensive evaluation to situations when objective physical findings are present or when the history is compellingly suggestive of a medical disorder. When this judgment becomes difficult, the problem may be resolved by discussing the case with a trusted colleague rather than defaulting by ordering more medical tests. These decisions must also be balanced with continuing awareness that patients with somatoform disorders are not immune to developing other medical conditions, and the physician must maintain vigilance for other treatable medical problems when presented with objective signs or otherwise convincing clinical pictures. Unfortunately, when these patients become medically ill the differentiation of a somatoform disorder from medical symptoms sometimes becomes even more difficult.

Physicians are discouraged from telling patients, "It's all in your head." It is more helpful to become comfortable with the uncertainty of medically unexplained somatic symptoms, offering to patients the honest conclusion of, "I don't know what is causing the symptoms." The physician and the patient may be comforted by the fact that additional time may clarify the origin of the symptoms. However, when time does not provide answers the physician is left without an explanation for the patient about her symptoms. Admitting to a lack of an explanation is preferable to telling the patient that she is imagining the symptom (which she may not be if an occult medical cause exists). This strategy allows the physician to offer potential options for treatment of psychiatric co-morbidity or for palliative relief of distress, including several classes of medications, such as antidepressants, antianxiety agents, and sedative agents, which are sometimes beneficial. Caveats in the use of these agents in patients with somatoform disorders are discussed on p. 281.

Behavioral Management

Somatoform behavior is encouraged by environmental reinforcement, such as attention for fainting spells by the family who gather at her side and rush her to the emergency room; similarly, symptoms can be attenuated or extinguished by removal of such rewards. The family can be advised to monitor the effects of their own behaviors on the patient's response. Excessive inquiry by the physician into symptoms at appointments encourages patients to focus on symptoms and is therefore best avoided.

Although attention to symptoms can encourage more symptoms, some attention to symptoms can be a useful tool. Because these patients often feel that physicians do not understand them or respond appropriately to their distress, allowing them to ventilate their difficulties helps to strengthen the rapport with the physician. Therefore physicians are advised to listen to complaints but to refrain from responding to them with further medical work-ups if there are no objective signs.

Over time, the physician may begin to inquire into the patient's social and interpersonal difficulties, which conveys to the patient that the most important and interesting aspect of her is not her symptoms. The additional concern and support for the patient demonstrated by inquiry into her psychosocial life also helps her begin to discuss her psychosocial problems, which are almost invariably part of the disorder and its sequelae. This in turn provides opportunities for supportive psychotherapy and guidance in practical problem-solving. As the physician-patient relationship grows more secure, the patient's dependence on the relationship enhances the physician's leverage in working with the patient to change her behavior. Leading the patient to work on real interpersonal difficulties and other psychosocial problems is more productive than allowing litanies of complaints of somatoform symptoms generated at repeated office visits. These excessive symptom complaints can often be managed positively with praise for the patient for enduring her symptoms.

It is important for the physician to realize that because these patients' lives revolve so heavily around their symptoms, their care can become excessively demanding if special attention is not paid to the physician-patient relationship from the start. Therefore getting the diagnosis right and then setting limits and boundaries in advance is a healthy medical practice that protects physicians from personal encroachment by patient demands. These limits build patient perceptions of professionalism and competence of the physician and a sense of security in a relationship with well-defined boundaries. Patients who have the habit of calling often between appointments might be informed that the general office policy limits phone calls to one per week unless it is a bona fide emergency. Patients may test limits early in the relationship, but once the limits are defined for them, they can often respect them.

In the inpatient setting, behavioral shaping of somatoform and conversion syndromes by reward contingency and redirection may hasten improvement. At the start, all the patient's hospital privileges are removed with the explanation that she must maintain total bed rest to avoid worsening her condition. She is told that as she shows signs of clinical improvement she will gain privileges that are appropriate for each level of function achieved. This positive framework helps redirect the patient from perceiving the program as punishment and reacting angrily toward the physician. It also allows patients with conversion symptoms to "save face" as symptoms are confronted not directly but allowed to resolve in the overt context of healing and improved functioning. Placebos such as saline injections intended to encourage these suggestible patients to believe they are recovering may have dramatic immediate effects, but their use is discouraged because of the dishonesty required to administer them and because in the long run they reinforce patients' concept of themselves as medically ill.

Patients with somatization disorder can behave seductively toward physicians, who need to be especially cognizant of professionalism and boundaries with these patients. Social physical contact other than a handshake is not recommended, especially early in the relationship. Use of the patient's title and last name (for example, Mrs. Smith) helps maintain appropriate distance. When patients cross boundaries (such as trying to hug, kiss, or sexually touch the physician), such incidents are best handled by prohibiting further boundary violations, discussing the incident with another professional, and documenting the consultation. Referral to another physician may be necessary if the issue cannot be resolved relatively quickly.

The practice of confronting patients directly about the reality of their symptoms is generally not recommended, nor is presenting them with the diagnosis of a somatoform disorder, a difficult concept for patients to understand. The suggestion that the symptoms are not real alienates the patient and results in an unnecessarily adversarial relationship, with the patient believing that the physician does not know what he is talking about. Patients interpret such confrontations as implying that the physician thinks they are either crazy or lying, with neither concept perceived by patients as respectful. It is not useful to argue whether the symptoms are real; it is more helpful to recognize that the patient's pain seems real to her.

Psychotherapy

Patients with somatoform disorders tend to develop little insight over time. Insight-oriented and expressive psychotherapies are usually ineffective for somatization disorder. There is no evidence to suggest that hypnosis, sodium amytal interviews, or other techniques aimed at helping the patient to remember, relive, abreact, or work through alleged traumas and awakened emotions are helpful. Patients with somatization disorder already rely too heavily on emotional responses and need no further encouragement of this behavior. Such techniques may in fact be harmful by allowing the patient to focus therapeutic attention away from the behaviors and problems at hand, blame others for her problems, and avoid working to find genuine solutions.

At best, patients with superior verbal abilities can achieve improved insight into the mind-body connection of stress and physical symptoms. Patients often accept the suggestion that responses to stress and pressure influence normal human physiology and can generate symptoms in many people. Physicians may help patients with somatization disorder learn that their headaches do not necessarily indicate that they have a brain tumor or anything else seriously wrong. Sometimes these normalizing explanations for symptoms spark a reaction of genuine relief.

A useful technique is to explain that such symptoms may continue to bother people for a while or from time to time, and to predict that this will probably be the case for the patient's current symptoms. Sometimes the patient "proves" the physician wrong, and the symptoms disappear altogether. Conversely, if the patient continues to be symptomatic, the physician can help the patient remember the earlier prediction that this might happen. Behavioral change in these patients is typically gradual, proceeding over months and possibly years. Over the long haul, the best strategy is empathetic engagement coupled with helping patients appreciate the natural association of increased physical symptoms with stressful times.

Psychiatric Symptoms and Psychotropic Medications

Symptoms of other psychiatric disorders routinely reported by patients with somatization disorder may complicate treatment if they are not recognized within the context of somatization disorder. The most difficult aspect of these commonly reported psychoform symptoms is that they provide a smokescreen for the treatment of the primary disorder (somatization disorder) if they become the focus of treatment. Complaints of anxiety and panic symptoms may invite physicians to prescribe benzodiazepines, and pain complaints invite the use of narcotics. Patients with somatization disorder are at greatly increased risk of abusing these medications, which therefore should be limited and closely monitored. Psychiatrists treating these patients may have to detoxify them from benzodiazepines and pain medications prescribed by other physicians who, not suspecting this disorder, may have inadvertently contributed to iatrogenic drug dependence. Buspirone, a relatively new nonaddictive antianxiety agent, can sometimes be useful for management of anxiety. Additionally, the sedating properties of antihistamines such as hydroxyzine can aid in management of insomnia and daytime anxiety.

Patients with somatization disorder who require abusable substances such as benzodiazepines or narcotics for documented medical conditions should be carefully monitored, and the pills in their prescriptions should be counted to prevent the escalation of dosage to which these patients are prone. Before the prescription of abusable drugs, a history of substance use disorder should be explored and documented in the chart. Ground rules need to be established at the outset, and the patient should be advised that the abusable medication is a short-term remedy only or that further increases in dose will not be forthcoming. When informed of the abuse potential of benzodiazepines, many patients exhibit cautious judgment in desiring to minimize their use or even avoid taking them at all. Although it may be tempting to prescribe antipsychotic agents for anxiety or insomnia when benzodiazepines are not a reasonable choice—especially when patients complain of psychotic-like symptoms—antipsychotic medications are not a good choice because of the potential for development of tardive dyskinesia, a potentially irreversible syndrome.

Unfortunately there is no medication available specifically for the treatment of somatization disorder. A useful philosophy is to encourage patients to deal with their emotional symptoms without resorting to pharmacological solutions whenever possible.

Because a goal in treating somatization disorder is simplification of the medication regimen, the physician should avoid the puritanical desire to remove all seemingly unnecessary or harmful medications immediately. In this effort, patients can be reassured that medications they need will not be withdrawn. Whereas the virtue of removing unnecessary and excessively complex medications is valued, the abrupt discontinuation of one or more medications can be problematic because of the well-known physical withdrawal effects of stopping benzodiazepines and antidepressants, as well as psychological withdrawal. It can be pointed out that symptoms experienced while withdrawing from one of these medications may be caused by too much medication rather than not enough.

Treatment of Co-Morbid Psychiatric Disorders

Admissions to psychiatric facilities for patients with somatization disorder are usually the result of complaints of depression or suicidality. Patients with somatization disorder commonly lose their depressive symptoms within a few hours or days of being on the ward and away from the interpersonal and other psychosocial precipitants of their symptoms, even if they have had no specific treatment for their depressive symptoms. This phenomenon supports the decision to wait 2 or 3 days before prescribing antidepressant medication to see if this will be the case. Otherwise, the clinical improvement may be incorrectly attributed to the medication.

Little is known about the epidemiology and management of major depression in relation to somatoform disorders. Somatization disorder patients meeting full criteria for major depression may benefit from the usual treatments for major depression. However, physicians are cautioned not to treat depressive symptoms without establishing a definite diagnosis of major depression. For patients with somatization disorder who develop major depressive features, treatment of the depression may improve the somatoform symptoms as the depressive episode resolves.

Good choices for antidepressants in these patients are the newer serotonin-selective reuptake inhibitors

(SSRIs), such as fluoxetine, paroxetine, and sertraline, because of their low risk profile compared with tricyclic antidepressants (TCAs) in this population prone to overdose in suicide gestures. The generally reduced side-effect profiles of these agents are also preferable, since patients with somatization disorder tend to be poorly tolerant of medication side effects. This latter problem advocates for the practice of starting psychotropic medications for these patients at low doses and increasing them slowly.

Antidepressant medications are also used in the treatment of chronic pain syndromes and for symptoms of irritable bowel syndrome, which are prevalent in these patients. Relief may be obtained at doses lower than those required to achieve antidepressant efficacy.

Suicide threats and attempts, even in patients with somatization disorder who rarely carry them to completion, must be taken seriously and dealt with carefully and vigorously, either by hospitalization or by close watch at home. If it can be determined that the suicidal crisis is related to an interpersonal problem that passed quickly, the patient is encouraged to state how things have changed and to demonstrate ways she can handle her difficulties without resorting to suicide. This critical piece of information must be documented in the chart. However, in the event that the patient cannot do this, she may require brief hospitalization while the interpersonal problem is being resolved. Restriction of privileges or seclusion administered nonpunitively ("for your own good," or "for your safety") after suicide gestures can dramatically reduce further suicidality.

Special Issues

Media attention and patient contact with disease-specific self-help groups such as those for chronic fatigue syndrome and for environmental allergies are on the rise and are thought to reinforce patients' medical appraisals of their symptoms. Patients with these syndromes may reorganize their identities around their alleged illness and pursue activities related to it with all-consuming vigor. These patients also visit alternative medical care providers such as homeopaths and natural healers whose professional sanctioning of these ideas may further entrench patients' conviction of serious medical disease.

Dissociative identity disorder, formerly known as multiple personality disorder (MPD), is a popular forum for such disease-related activities in patients with somatization disorder. A recent increase of reported cases of MPD to epidemic proportions has been attributed in part to spread through popular medical opinion and through the media. Most patients with MPD have been documented to meet criteria for somatization disorder, a diagnosis that can account for the symptoms of MPD. A more recent epidemic closely allied with MPD is the accusation of childhood sexual molestation by family members and more dramatically, of satanic ritual abuse, often arising in therapy designed to recover childhood memories of abuse. This entity tends to afflict the patients with somatization disorder who are also diagnosed with MPD, and it also tends to be uncovered by the same therapists who have an interest in MPD.

Conclusion

This chapter has reviewed the somatoform disorders with focus on the most prevalent and best understood diagnoses of somatization disorder and conversion disorder. Somatoform disorders have earned a reputation of being difficult to treat, but most of the difficulty lies with the lack of recognition of the disorder and failure to apply established principles of treatment. The goals of the physician treating patients with somatoform disorders are to orchestrate treatment, prevent complications of unnecessary medical procedures and tests, and assist the patient in navigating her way through interpersonal and other psychosocial problems that are inherent to these disorders.

CONSIDER CONSULTATION WHEN . . .

- Somatization disorder is suspected
- There are multiple unexplained medical complaints
- There are medically unexplained neurological complaints
- The patient demands additional evaluations or treatments when the medical situation does not warrant this
- The medical history does not add up

Annotated Bibliography

Andreasen NC, Black DW: *Somatoform and related disorders.* In *Introductory textbook of psychiatry,* ed 2, Washington, D.C., 1995, American Psychiatric Press.

This text, designed for medical students, is useful for all clinicians, physicians and nonphysicians, as well as mental-health and non-mental-health professionals, to achieve a basic and practical understanding of psychiatric disorders, their diagnosis, natural history, and treatment. The chapter on somatoform disorders provides complete information on the subject.

Goodwin DW, Guze SB: *Hysteria (somatization disorder).* In *Psychiatric diagnosis,* ed 4, New York, 1989, Oxford University Press.

This chapter provides physicians with an understanding of the diagnosis of somatoform disorders. This is achieved through atheoretical descriptions of these disorders without hypotheses about etiology, which have not been documented in these disorders. In particular, these disorders are described in terms of the core symptoms that define them, delineation from other disorders (exclusion criteria), family studies, and follow-up studies.

Othmer E, editor: Somatization disorder, *Psychiatr Ann* 18:330-362. 1988.

This special issue of this journal contains several seminal articles describing somatization disorder in general practice, guiding the physician on detection, diagnosis, and management of this disorder. It further updates the physician with recent data relating to co-morbid diagnoses and its presentation in the general medical setting.

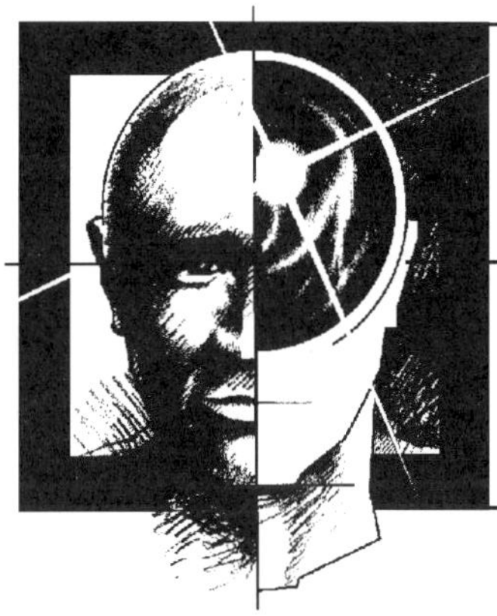

chapter 17

Dissociative and Factitious Disorders

Carol S. North, MD and Sean H. Yutzy, MD

This chapter covers two categories of psychiatric disorders: dissociative disorders and factitious disorders. These disorders are alike in that, in contrast to malingering, the alleged motivation for creation of the symptoms is not within conscious control. In other words, the motivation for both disorders is said to be unconscious. They are also alike in that little systematic information exists about either of them. These two categories of disorders differ in definition: dissociation is a *subjectively* reported perceptual disruption of an individual's experience of herself and/or her environment, whereas factitious disorders manifest actual *objective* medical findings that are fabricated by physical manipulation.

Dissociative Disorders

Perspective on Dissociative Disorders

Dissociation remains poorly understood despite a recent upsurge in the amount of published literature on dissociative disorders. The principal diagnosis in the category of dissociative disorders is dissociative identity disorder, formerly termed multiple personality disorder (MPD). Dissociative identity disorder is perhaps the most controversial disorder in psychiatry. It has divided the mental health field into polarized groups of enthusiastic believers and vocal skeptics. Reasonable professionals find their limits of credibility stretched by claims that multiple people can exist within one person, a situation not mitigated by the flamboyant symptom displays of patients with dissociative identity disorder. Chaos surrounds the occurrence of dissociative disorders in clinical settings and stems from staff division, the patient acting out, and a lack of unified and scientifically based clinical direction regarding the proper care for these patients.

Because of the lack of systematic study of dissociation, little empirical information is available. The field has advanced largely on anecdotal experience, poorly conceived studies, and polemical arguments that form the bulk of the published literature. Published investigations to date have suffered from a lack of adequate controls, selection bias, biased ascertainment, unwarranted conclusions from data, and a failure to address the most critical questions. Studies to validate dissociative identity disorders according to well-established traditions in medicine and psychiatry have not been performed, and therefore the diagnosis has not been scientifically validated. Therefore an academic review of this nonvalidated set of disorders encounters challenges posed by seriously limited literature.

A recent American epidemic of dissociative identity disorder has captivated the attention of both public and professional audiences and has resulted in record numbers of patients claiming to have the disorder and in accelerating numbers of professionals devoting interest to the disorder. As a result, mental health professionals are likely to see burgeoning numbers of patients with these complaints and to be exposed to an expanding professional literature regarding these disorders. The field's unprecedented rapid growth has outstripped available empirical evidence, leaving physicians to face clinical dilemmas with little informed direction. This chapter aims to help the physician sort through the morass of published literature and to point to some practical ways of understanding this confusing set of disorders and managing it in routine clinical practice.

The section on dissociative disorders addresses diagnostic and treatment issues and draws on available data and on the experience of medical model psychiatric professionals in dealing with these patients. Limitations of the published literature are identified.

History of Dissociative Disorders

The popularity and recognition of dissociative disorders has waxed and waned throughout medical history. Although the basic core manifestations of dissociation have remained constant, thoughts about the disorder have changed through different periods. Dissociation was first recognized in ancient Egypt in the form of spirit possession. In the Christian bible Jesus cast off evil spirits from a man named Legion whom modern authorities believe was afflicted with multiple personalities. Conceptualization of an association between dissociation and spirit possession persisted through the 1600s, 1700s, and 1800s; in these centuries several cases of multiple personalities were reported. These cases displayed prominent conversion features such as amnesia, paralysis, and aphonia. In the mid-1800s, the exorcism of evil spirits evolved into animal magnetism and then into mesmerism, which were forerunners of modern hypnosis.

The rapid rise in the popularity of hypnotism around the turn of this century was paralleled by the rise in popularity of multiple personality syndromes. This trend was met with a backlash of professional criticism and skepticism about therapists creating cases by suggestion and about patients beguiling their therapists by faking and acting out parts of separate personalities. Curiously, most of the reported cases of dissociative identity disorder have been concentrated in the United States and have been contributed by a small cluster of authors who have cross-referenced each other extensively.

In the first half of this century, attention to dissociative disorders diminished to the point of near extinction. Historically, dissociation was considered part of the syndrome of hysteria, which is now called *somatization disorder.* It was not until the late 1960s that dissociation was separated from hysteria and given its own category in official diagnostic nomenclatures. Since then it has developed a large following by those who believe dissociative disorders are common.

With the dramatization of famous cases such as *The Three Faces of Eve* and *Sybil,* the popularity of dissociative identity disorder has made exponential gains and in the 1980s and 1990s has erupted into an epidemic that has placed it prominently in national magazines and on television talk shows. A parallel rise in professional interest in the disorder has resulted in accelerating numbers of diagnosed cases and in a proliferation of reports in the literature. A professional society dedicated to the study and further recognition of dissociative disorders, the International Society for the Study of Dissociation, was formed in 1984 and acquired thousands of members in a short time.

The case of Sybil was the first to associate childhood abuse with dissociative identity disorder. Paralleling recent national attention to issues of child abuse, reports of child abuse histories in patients with dissociative disorders have proliferated. Some authors have characterized dissociative disorders as posttraumatic disorders that arise from childhood abuse. This interesting theory has had little empirical documentation but has nevertheless gained popular acceptance.

Clinical Features

The essential feature of dissociative disorders is a disrupted integration of the mental functions of consciousness, identity, perception of the environment, and memory. The most important diagnosis in this group of disorders is dissociative identity disorder. It is the best studied of these disorders and is by far the most represented in the literature on dissociation. Therefore this section focuses on the diagnosis of dissociative identity disorder. Other dissociative disorders, including dissociative amnesia, dissociative fugue, and depersonalization syndrome will also be briefly discussed.

Diagnosis

Dissociative Identity Disorder

Established diagnostic criteria for dissociative identity disorder are vague and allow considerable latitude

BOX 17-1 DISSOCIATIVE IDENTITY DISORDER

DSM-IV DIAGNOSTIC CRITERIA

A. The presence of two or more distinct identities or personality states (each with its own relatively enduring pattern of perceiving, relating to, and thinking about the environment and self).

B. At least two of these identities or personality states recurrently take control of the person's behavior.

C. Inability to recall important personal information that is too extensive to be explained by ordinary forgetfulness.

D. The disturbance is not due to the direct physiological effects of a substance (e.g., blackouts or chaotic behavior during Alcohol Intoxication) or a general medical condition (e.g., complex partial seizures).
Note: In children, the symptoms are not attributable to imaginary playmates or other fantasy play.

From American Psychiatric Association, *Diagnostic and statistical manual of mental disorders,* ed 4 (DSM-IV), Washington, D.C., 1994, American Psychiatric Press.

DIAGNOSIS

TABLE 17-1 DISSOCIATIVE IDENTITY DISORDER

Discriminating features

1. Two or more distinct personalities take control of the person
2. Amnesia between personalities
3. Not explained by substance abuse or medical condition

Consistent features

1. Vast majority are young women
2. Almost never occurs as a freestanding condition (2-4 other diagnoses)
3. Frequent co-morbid somatization and borderline personality (women), antisocial personality (men)
4. Multiple symptoms in multiple organ systems are classic features, as are multiple diagnoses and multiple failed treatments

Variable features

1. Effective treatment depends on co-morbid diagnosis
2. Prognosis is unknown but seems to follow co-morbid diagnosis
3. Substance use disorder is common; its detection and effects on therapy need attention

BOX 17-2

ADDITIONAL CORE SYMPTOMS OF DISSOCIATIVE IDENTITY DISORDER

1. Time distortion or time lapses
2. Report of behavioral episodes (of alternate personalities) by others that the individual does not recall
3. Notable changes in behavior associated with the use of a different name
4. Severe headaches associated with blackouts, seizures, dreams, visions, or voices (presumably switches between personalities)
5. Use of "we" to refer to self in conversation
6. Discovery of writings, drawings, or new articles of clothing in the patient's possession that are not recognized by the patient
7. Appearance of personalities with hypnosis
8. Hearing internal voices

and the opportunity for many different clinical presentations to qualify for a diagnosis. Essentially all that is required for the diagnosis is that the individual display two or more personalities (or personality states) that have amnesia for each other and take control of the body at different times. Additionally, the symptoms cannot be explained by a substance such as alcohol or a known medical condition such as temporal lobe epilepsy (Box 17-1, Table 17-1). In this context, *personality* is defined as an enduring pattern of behaviors that remains consistent across a wide range of situations and environments. Personality states are distinguished from complete personalities by their narrower range of occurrence, an even vaguer qualifier to an intrinsically vague concept.

Although the previously mentioned criteria are all that is technically needed to make a diagnosis of dissociative identity disorder, the vagueness of these criteria has led experts in dissociative disorders to determine the need to identify additional characteristic "core" features before concluding that the symptoms really fit the syndrome as intended by the definition (Box 17-2).

The diagnosis of dissociative identity disorder has not been validated by the five-phase process of Robins and Guze, which is patterned after the medical criteria of Sydenham and includes a clinical description of the syndrome, delineation from other psychiatric disorders, family studies, follow-up studies to ascertain stability of the diagnosis over time, and laboratory studies to define the unique characteristics of the syndrome. In particular, studies to delineate dissociative identity disorder from other psychiatric disorders, as well as family studies and follow-up studies, are lacking. However, such investigations are feasible. Therefore the remainder of the discussion of dissociative disorders proceeds with the recognition that these syndromes do not constitute validated diagnoses.

PEARLS & PERILS

DIAGNOSIS OF DISSOCIATIVE DISORDERS

- Multiple symptoms of multiple disorders are the most consistent feature of dissociative identity disorder. Patients with this disorder report many unexplained medical symptoms in many organ systems, as well as symptoms of all psychiatric diagnoses.
- Dissociative identity disorder almost never occurs alone. The average patient with this disorder meets the criteria for two to four other psychiatric diagnoses.
- Somatization disorder and borderline personality disorder are the most common coexisting disorders, and in men antisocial personality disorder is also common.

Other Dissociative Disorders

Dissociative amnesia, formerly termed psychogenic amnesia, is defined as a loss of memory for important personal information that is too extensive to be explained by ordinary forgetfulness and that occurs in the context of traumatic or stressful events or psychological conflicts. A *dissociative fugue* is characterized by an individual's sudden, unexpected travel from usual surroundings with no recollection of an autobiographical past. Typically the individual is confused about personal identity or may even adopt a totally new identity with complete amnesia for the former one. The new personality usually is more gregarious and uninhibited than the individual's usual character and shows no overt evidence of psychiatric illness aside from the identity switch. Lack of memory for the fugue state after recovering from it is characteristic. A *depersonalization disorder* is characterized by an individual who experiences one or more episodes of prominent feelings of detachment from oneself as if an outside observer of one's body or mind or as if in a dream. However, contact with reality is intact. These other dissociative conditions are not diagnosed if they are part of dissociative identity disorder.

By definition, dissociative disorders are not diagnosed if the symptoms occur only as part of another psychiatric disturbance such as posttraumatic stress disorder (PTSD), somatization disorder, or schizophrenia, or if the symptoms are caused by a neurological or other medical condition (such as head trauma or seizure disorder) or by the effects of a substance (such as alcohol or prescription or illicit drugs). Dissociative disorders are diagnosed only if the symptoms are significantly distressing or impair an individual's ability to function in social, occupational, or other important areas of life (see the Pearls & Perils box above).

Natural History

Ninety percent of the patients with dissociative identity disorder are women. Women with this disorder most often come to the attention of professionals in the mental health system; men with this disorder usually receive attention through the criminal system. The age of diagnosis is typically in the third and fourth decades, and the average time elapsed between symptom onset and the diagnosis of dissociative identity disorder is 6 to 7 years. The apparent onset of dissociative symptoms may be associated with stressful or traumatic situational difficulties.

Popular professional belief maintains that although dissociative identity disorder is seldom recognized until adulthood, its origins typically lie between the ages of 5 and 10 years. However, these claims are based on information retrospectively reported, often in the context of trying to connect the first onset of dissociative symptoms to alleged childhood molestation. As many as 96% to 98% of the cases of dissociative identity disorder have been reported to have been preceded by a history of childhood sexual abuse, but no methodologically adequate studies are available to document or refute such claims. Regardless, childhood sexual and physical abuse histories are commonly reported by these patients, often in graphic detail.

Dissociative symptoms often but not always appear to arise in the context of hypnosis, hypnotherapy, or guided imagery therapy. However, given the amount of media information and endorsement widely available, dissociation can now occur outside of any therapeutic context.

Although high-functioning patients occasionally have been described in the literature, patients with dissociative disorders are often psychiatrically and sometimes severely disabled. Little is known about the long-term prognosis, but the co-morbid disorders that usually accompany dissociative disorders (see the section on differential diagnosis) are chronic and disabling conditions with poor prognoses that indicate a guarded overall prognosis. The ultimate prognosis is thought to depend on the presence or absence of such co-morbid disorders. Overall improvement may be evident in middle age, which is also the documented course for the co-morbid diagnoses regardless of the presence or absence of a dissociative disorder. Recurrent episodes may occur during particularly stressful or traumatic periods of the individual's life.

Differential Diagnosis

Dissociative disorders must be differentiated from medical conditions, particularly neurological conditions such as head injuries, and from the effects of psychoactive substances that can lead to memory impairment (see Chapter 11). Unlike dissociative disorders, head injuries tend to result in circumscribed, retrograde memory loss that usually involves the period directly before the injury. Similarly, electroconvulsive therapy produces immediate retrograde temporary memory impairment with an occasional brief difficulty in generating new memories. In contrast, dissociative memory difficulties are typically anterograde (that is, the memory loss is restricted to a circumscribed period following a traumatic event), and are very specific to certain time periods surrounding personal traumas and to specified content such as an inability to recall certain personal information (such as name, address, current employment, or family). Characteristic dissociative complaints include an inability to recall memories before a certain age such as 7 or 8, and sometimes amnesia for an entire childhood. Similarly, patients may claim to lack any memory for a period such as between 6 and 12 years of age and throughout a period of alleged childhood incest experiences. Amnesia of a medical cause is not generally reversible, which is in contrast with the sometimes dramatic and sudden return of memories with dissociative amnesia—often in a flood of visualizations and flashbacks (especially when aided by hypnosis or guided imagery therapy).

A dissociative fugue must also be differentiated from complex partial seizures. With the latter, patients may wander, exhibit semipurposeful behavior, and display amnesia. Distinguishing features of seizure disorders are characteristic auras, motor abnormalities, stereotyped behaviors, perceptual alterations, postictal phenomena, and abnormal electroencephalographic (EEG) findings that evolve over time. True seizure episodes are brief and typically last less than 5 minutes and sometimes less than 1 minute, whereas dissociative episodes may last hours to days or sometimes periods of weeks or longer.

Dissociative identity disorder has been compared with syphilis in its proclivity to simulate a wide array of medical and psychiatric conditions. Patients with dissociation may report multiple unexplained medical symptoms in multiple organ systems that are indistinguishable from the pattern of patients with somatization disorder (see Chapter 16). Of the patients with dissociative identity disorder, 80% to 100% have been found to qualify for a diagnosis of somatization disorder. Conversion symptoms, including florid presentations such as limb paralysis and pseudoseizures, are commonly associated.

An elaborate diagnostic co-morbidity is the most consistent feature of dissociative identity disorder; therefore it has been characterized as a polysymptomatic, polysyndromic condition. The average patient with this disorder meets criteria for three or four additional psychiatric disorders. Severe depression is present in 70% to 100% of these patients, and approximately 75% of the patients report "high periods." Anxiety symptoms and panic attacks are prominent complaints and are present in the majority. Psychotic symptoms are reported by at least 90% of the patients, who report more psychotic symptoms than do patients with documented schizophrenia. Although these patients do not develop schizophrenia, one half of the patients with dissociative identity disorder erroneously receive this diagnosis during the course of their treatment.

Personality disorders have been diagnosed in 69% to 84% of those patients with dissociative identity disorder. The most prevalent Axis II disorder is borderline personality, with half of the patients meeting criteria; the next most prevalent personality disorder is antisocial personality, with one fourth to one half of the cases meeting criteria. Patients with dissociative disorders often have significant impulse control problems; eating disorders, particularly bulimia, are commonly associated. At least one half of the patients develop comorbid substance abuse.

Considerable disagreement surrounds the classification of the many co-morbid conditions for which patients with dissociative identity disorder technically meet criteria. Some experts maintain that dissociative identity disorder is the superordinate condition and subsumes all the (extensive) co-morbid psychopathology, whereas others argue that the other disorders are relevant, perhaps even more relevant than the dissociative identity disorder in terms of course, prognosis, and treatment. Our view is that dissociative identity disorder is most likely an epiphenomenon or a severity marker of its co-morbid diagnoses, most commonly somatization disorder and borderline personality disorder in women and antisocial personality disorder in men. The advantage of the multiaxial classification scheme of psychiatric disorders is that it allows diagnosis of all the relevant disorders, which facilitates the management of dissociative identity disorder within its larger and important multidiagnostic context.

Presumably, dissociative disorders must be differentiated from malingering, in which an individual may feign a loss of self-identity, amnesia for certain actions, and/or a lack of responsibility for actions of an alternate personality. For example, an individual might purposely enact a dissociative fugue with the clear intent to escape personal troubles such as legal action, financial consequences of bad debts, or military duty. In a famous case, the Hillside Strangler (Kenneth Bianchi) faked dissociative identity disorder skillfully enough to convince several experts. He used this disorder as a defense for his serial murders in court but ultimately failed.

The nature of the diagnostic criteria makes an accurate diagnosis of "real" dissociative syndromes a formidable challenge and hence renders the distinction between real and feigned dissociations virtually impossible. Hypnosis and amytal interview do not distinguish dissociative disorders from malingering, which may be successfully maintained even during these maneuvers. Although there is no simple technique to distinguish the two disorders, this task may be aided by identifying other signs of dissociative disorders (such as polysomatoform symptoms, suicide gestures, self-mutilation, childhood amnesia, and dissociative symptoms preexisting the current situation) that support the diagnosis through their known associations with it.

Genetics and Family History

Genetic transmission of dissociative identity disorder has not been established. No family studies (actual examination of family members) have been done, but family history studies (asking patients about their relatives) provide imperfect evidence through secondhand information from the patients. Family history studies have shown an increase in reported dissociative disorders among first-degree relatives of patients with dissociative identity disorder. One study found that the majority of parents of adolescents with the disorder have high rates of dissociative problems themselves. Children of patients with dissociative identity disorder have been reported to have frequent and severe psychiatric problems, including anxiety disorders, conduct disorders, learning disorders, and attention deficit disorders.

Many patients with a dissociative disorder have alcoholic family members, including at least one third of the fathers in one series. Because of the overwhelming co-morbidity of somatization disorder and borderline personality disorder in these patients, substance abuse and somatoform and antisocial and other personality disorders are not unexpected in family members. This array of psychiatric disorders in families would project an increased vulnerability for violent traumas and child abuse in the family environment. General experience with these families has identified dysfunctional families that commonly have authoritarian and excessively strict parenting patterns, extreme fundamental religiosity, and patterns of child abuse and neglect.

Epidemiology

Just half a century ago, dissociative identity disorder was thought to be so rare that it was considered nonexistent or extinct. However, the 1980s and 1990s have witnessed a precipitous and exponential increase in reported cases that has appropriately been labelled an epidemic. In part this increase may stem from increased public and professional awareness of the diagnosis and result in heightened identification of the disorder among previously undiagnosed cases, but the increase may also relate to an increase of the symptoms reported among a highly suggestible pool of individuals.

No adequate studies have been performed to estimate the prevalence of dissociative identity disorder in the general population. Depending on the definition used, the prevalence of dissociative identity disorder has been estimated to be between 1% and 5%, but "florid" cases are thought to be limited to 1 out of every 500 people. These estimates may be unreliable as a result of methodological problems, including an inadequate definition of the disorder and biased ascertainment of cases. Some reports suggest that dissociative identity disorder is more prevalent in selected populations such as prostitutes (5%), psychiatric inpatients (13%), forensic patients (39%), and exotic dancers (50%).

Proponents of the validity of dissociative identity disorder claim that the disorder continues to be grossly underdiagnosed because of lack of professional awareness and general closed-mindedness. Others, however, believe that the disorder is wildly overdiagnosed by a subset of physicians who tend to find high rates of the disorder in the populations with which they work; they also believe that highly suggestible individuals are vulnerable to developing it through iatrogenesis. Until more specific and reliable criteria for dissociative identity disorder are available and applied to systematically selected and representative population samples, meaningful population estimates of prevalence cannot be ascertained.

Pathophysiology

The pathophysiology of the dissociative disorders is unknown. Claims have been made regarding physiologic differences between personalities, including reports of distinct responses of different personality states to alcohol, food, and allergens; differences in visual acuity and dominant handedness; and changes in handwriting. These claims, however, are subjective reports for which objective findings have not been documented. Reports of more objectively defined differences in respiration, heart rate, blood pressure, skin conductance, visual evoked potentials, and brain wave activity have been documented and interpreted as physiological manifestations of switching personalities. These changes may represent ordinary fluctuations of normal physiological mechanisms in association with changes in emotional state. However, such changes are not unique to dissociation and have been measured in other psychiatric disorders, including those commonly associated with dissociative disorders.

Psychological testing for dissociative identity disorder reveals characteristic profiles. Extreme hypnotizability and suggestibility have been documented through standardized tests of patients with dissociative disorders. The Minnesota Multiphasic Personality Inventory (MMPI) has had more application in dissociative disorders than has any other psychological measure. The typical MMPI profile shows validity scales consistent with exaggerations of disease, faking of symptoms, complaints of extreme distress, or pleas for help. The MMPI clinical scales show an elevation of all complaint areas to highly pathological extremes, with the highest clinical subscale being the "schizophrenia" score. Only the masculinity-femininity scale is not elevated; it tends to be low in women, which reflects stereotypical feminine interests and dependency. The MMPI profiles of patients with a somatization disorder or histrionic personality and those of patients with borderline personality disorder show patterns that are indistinguishable from those of patients with dissociative identity disorder. All of these disorders are characterized by exaggerations of disease and by extremely high rates of symptom complaints across the clinical scales.

Treatment

Proponents of dissociative identity disorder argue that because the presentation of the disorder is often covert, concerted efforts to elicit it are needed so that it can be properly treated. A long list of symptoms that contains features of practically every psychiatric disorder has been enumerated to alert a consideration of this diagnosis. No studies have documented these techniques to identify cases that fit established diagnostic criteria, and this practice has been criticized for its potential to lead to an overdiagnosis of dissociation. Unfortunately, in the zeal to uncover cases of dissociation, other important diagnoses are often overlooked. Because dissociative identity disorder rarely occurs in the absence of co-morbid psychiatric disorders, especially somatization disorder and borderline personality disorder, an exclusive focus on dissociative disorders results in a failure to diagnose these other important disorders, which bears directly on treatment and outcome. Therefore the first consideration when embarking on the treatment of dissociative disorders is to complete the psychiatric evaluation so that the important co-morbid disorders—perhaps the only important disorders—are not left unaddressed.

Proponents of dissociative identity disorder reason that it seems to be caused by splitting the consciousness into individual personalities because appropriate treatment of the disorder rests on helping the patient fuse the personalities into one—the "host" personality, or the individual who existed before allegedly breaking into two or more personalities. Because no controlled outcome studies of dissociative identity disorder are available, these treatment methods have not been documented empirically.

The therapy recommended by proponents includes encouraging and assisting patients to recall traumatic memories, usually memories of sexual molestation during childhood. Because individuals with dissociative disorders have been shown to be highly suggestible, care is urged in efforts to help these individuals recover their "lost" memories so that false memories are not created. Reported memories of sexual or physical abuse in childhood that have been forgotten and then recovered are presently the subject of heated controversy and suspicion. Some clinicians feel that experiences of childhood abuse are grossly underreported because of a lack of professional recognition and undue skepticism, but others assert that such instances are overreported and are iatrogenically induced by therapy or media influences. No reliable methods are available to differentiate recovered memories of actual childhood events from implanted memories, and therefore caution is recommended in interpreting such claims. In fact, the entire concept of memory repression has been challenged as being a theoretical construct that cannot be tested for its existence.

Proponents of dissociative identity disorder recommend prolonged treatment with intensive psychotherapy, and some use hypnotic techniques to help patients learn about and fuse their personalities. Because of the extreme suggestibility of these patients, caution is urged to avoid further splitting into alternate personalities. Some physicians advocate the avoidance of hypnosis altogether in these patients. Hypnosis and/or intensive psychotherapy that focuses on the personalities typically yields increasing numbers of new personalities that evolve during the therapeutic process.

Even successful fusion of the personalities does not result in remission and elimination of psychiatric disability, because many problems remain. These remaining problems include serious co-morbid disorders (such as somatization disorder, borderline personality disorder, and antisocial personality disorder) that are themselves disabling and require a great deal of time and skill to manage. Kluft, a leading proponent of the disorder, concedes that "treatment of MPD leaves one with single personality disorder, the state at which most patients enter treatment." Therefore continued therapy is routinely recommended for at least 1 to 2 years, and perhaps as much as 5 or 6 years of intensive therapy is necessary after successful fusion of the personalities. Although favorable treatment outcomes have been documented in anecdotal cases and small series of patients, common experience holds that relapse is characteristic, even among those who are apparently fused.

We recommend a diametrically opposite approach to treatment to that proposed by the proponents of dissociative identity disorder. Instead of interpreting the multiple and often exotic psychiatric and somatoform symptoms exhibited by these patients as evidence of switching personalities, physicians are directed to recognize these symptoms as ordinary, typical symptoms of the documented comorbid psychiatric disorders (somatization disorder and borderline and antisocial personality disorders). This orientation helps the physician steer through the smokescreen of dissociative symptoms while maintaining the perspective of the overall clinical picture, which includes familiar and well-validated disorders. Therefore physicians are reminded to remain focused on treating the co-morbid psychiatric disorders and to deal with dissociative symptoms as they occur in this context. Principles delineated in other chapters of this volume regarding the treatment of somatization disorder and personality disorders are relevant for the treatment of dissociative disorders and should be followed in managing patients with these co-morbid disorders—regardless of the extreme presentation of the dissociative symptoms.

Contrary to the opinions of proponents of dissociative identity disorder, we believe that the diagnosis and treatment of dissociation does not require any special background in the recognition of dissociation or in performing the complicated procedures for fusing the personalities. We believe that psychiatric professionals adequately trained in medical model psychiatry and proficient in routine management of somatization disorder and personality disorders are best equipped to manage dissociative disorders through well-established procedures for the treatment of these associated conditions.

A protocol of "benign neglect" used successfully in the treatment of somatization disorder also has been invoked as a successful treatment for patients with a dissociative identity disorder. Successful treatment of dissociative identity disorder with these methods has been documented by Coryell, Fahy and colleagues, Cutler and Reed, and Kohlenberg. These reports have described clinical techniques of ignoring the dissociative symptoms and focusing attention and encouragement to engage the patients in learning to solve their interpersonal and other psychosocial difficulties without relying on dissociation for coping.

Once therapy for these other disorders is underway, the dissociative symptoms remain to be managed. Skeptics encourage confronting the patient and forbidding her to discuss dissociative symptoms in a behavioral program that directly discourages displays of dissociative symptoms and rewards efforts focused on resolving situational problems. This method has been used effectively in anecdotal cases. However, these confrontational techniques carry the risk of alienating the patient, as well as some of her supports who may be invested in her dissociation.

A less confrontational method encourages therapeutic engagement of the patient by first obtaining a history of her dissociative symptoms (such as the names and descriptions of all her alternate personalities) and then informing her gently that although she may experience herself as different personalities, these personalities are just different aspects of herself, such as different feelings, urges, and behavior patterns. She is then encouraged to begin accepting these aspects of herself as part of herself and to become involved in the process of starting to solve her many problems and learning better ways to cope. Over time, the complaints of multiple personalities and the associated constellation of symptoms should begin to fade as she obtains positive attention for responsible behaviors and begins to achieve mastery in problem areas of her life.

Patients with dissociative disorders often have had previous treatment in settings in which the recollection of previous traumas such as childhood molestation is recommended for the purpose of confronting and psychologically working through the trauma. Such work often occurs in "survivor group" settings and encourages the patient to further entrench herself in a victimization role. Although such issues cannot be ignored, therapy must balance overcoming the trauma with helping the individual emerge from the victim role and develop an increasing sense of self-reliance and control over her destiny.

No medications have been documented to be of specific value for the treatment of dissociation. When a diagnosis of major depressive disorder (MDD) can be made, which is often a difficult distinction in these polysymptomatic patients, antidepressant medication may be appropriate for treating the depression. Serotonin-selective reuptake inhibitors such as fluoxetine are safer than tricyclic antidepressants in these often impulsive, self-destructive individuals who are

> **TREATMENT OF DISSOCIATIVE DISORDERS**
>
> PEARLS & PERILS
>
> - The first consideration is to complete the psychiatric evaluation. The most important aspects of treatment to address are the coexisting disorders, which are likely to be more relevant than the dissociative disorder for designing treatment and establishing prognosis.
> - Physicians are cautioned not to get lost in the smokescreen of dissociative, psychiatric, and medical symptoms but to remain focused on the overall clinical picture, which includes treatment of the more relevant coexisting disorders.
> - Established treatments for the usual coexisting disorders (somatization disorder and borderline personality disorder) are relevant for the treatment of patients with these dissociative disorders and should be followed, regardless of the extreme presentation of dissociation.

prone to overdoses. Anxiety complaints may tempt the physician to prescribe benzodiazepines, but caution is recommended with these medications in dissociative patients because of their high risk for abuse and dependence. The complete evaluation of these patients must always include attention to possible substance abuse disorders because of the high rates of such disorders in dissociative identity disorders. Standard chemical dependency treatment may be indicated if substance abuse is present. Although patients with dissociative disorders often complain of psychoticlike symptoms, these patients are not considered to have true psychosis; therefore antipsychotic medications are not indicated for the treatment of dissociative disorders, especially considering the potential for irreversible involuntary movement disorders such as tardive dyskinesia (TD).

Patients with dissociative disorders often display suicidal and self-destructive behaviors, such as self-mutilation by cutting themselves with razor blades, burning themselves with cigarettes, or inserting sharp or caustic substances into their vaginas, as exhibited by patients with borderline personality disorder. In environments in which these behaviors receive attention and positive rewards, such behaviors can escalate to constant suicidal gestures and a preoccupation with self-mutilation. A treatment team that is united in response to such behaviors by setting limits to discourage their repetition can greatly assist progress in therapy toward helping the patient find more appropriate ways to deal with her conflicts and obtain her ends.

Therapy with these patients can be extremely demanding, frustrating, and even harrowing, partly because these patients with their often severe borderline personality behaviors can be extremely manipulative and are skillful at carving deep divisions between caregivers. Differences of opinion among mental health professionals about the existence of dissociative identity disorder and the interpretation of its symptoms provide fertile ground for these behaviors to create havoc in the treatment team. Establishing firm boundaries early in treatment with agreement of the entire treatment team is essential for satisfactory management of these patients (see Pearls & Perils box to the left).

Special Issues

A recent trend in popular mental health and self-help circles is the identification of a childhood history of satanic cult abuse. Many therapists who diagnose and treat large numbers of patients with dissociative identity disorder are also involved with helping patients recover memories of satanic cult abuse, and many of the patients at risk for dissociative identity disorder are also at risk for developing these recovered memories. A popular genre of self-help books on uncovering forgotten childhood memories of abuse and satanic ritual abuse has spread these ideas through culture and often provides recommended reading accompanying child abuse survivor therapy. Patients exposed to this material through reading, the media, other patients, or through therapist suggestion and encouragement may describe macabre stories of extreme abuse at the hands of a satanic cult, often with stereotypical content involving ritualistic sexual torture, impregnation of young girls and sacrifice of the fetus, the importation of babies from third-world countries for sacrificial rituals, and the consumption of blood, urine, and human flesh—stories that push the outer boundaries of believability for most professionals.

Therapeutic recommendations by some proponents of dissociative disorders include blaming family members, particularly parents, for the abuse. Formal accusations against family members and the termination of family contact by such patients in large and growing numbers has led affected families to band together into a national group, the False Memory Syndrome Foundation, to deny these accusations formally, recover from alleged damages to their families and community reputations, support one another in trying to regain contact with their loved ones, and advocate against therapy designed to recover such memories.

In managing patients with allegations of sexual abuse on the basis of recovered memories, it is recommended that the physician maintain a neutral stance, neither accepting the claim uncritically nor rejecting it outright in providing recommendations to the patient. It is not the physician's role to be a detective, nor does further exploration of her memory (such as via hypnosis, guided imagery, or amobarbital) without external validation further enhance the validity of the memory as a reflection of past events. The physician is reminded to maintain the perspective of the overall clinical picture, to diagnose and treat the relevant co-morbid disorders and to help the patient learn to cope with and solve the interpersonal difficulties and other psychosocial dilemmas that are almost invariably present.

Physicians are encouraged to maintain an atheoretical stance on the etiology of the psychopathology in dissociative disorders. Childhood abuse has no more been shown to be a cause of dissociative disorders than it has been shown to be the etiological basis of somatization disorder or antisocial personality disorder, which are conditions that also are associated with childhood abuse. Maintaining such an agnostic stance enables the physician to proceed with treatment unencumbered by preconceived notions of the need to resolve childhood abuse issues to cure the disorder.

Factitious Disorder

Perspective on Factitious Disorder

The intentional production or feigning of physical or psychological signs or symptoms without an external incentive (Box 17-3, Table 17-2) represents some of the most interesting illnesses in psychiatry with their bizarre, colorful, dramatic, dangerous, and frustrating presentations. It is easy to appreciate the physician's (and the public's) fascination in trying to understand the following behavior(s)/claim:

> Self-destructiveness in injecting oneself with parrot feces, the grandiosity of claiming to be an oceanographic physicist working with Jacques Cousteau, the passivity of submitting to 48 lumbar punctures, the skill to stop breathing to unconsciousness, and the wanderlust for 423 admissions (Pankratz, 1981)

Unfortunately, scientific understanding of these disorders is still in its infancy because of numerous issues: (1) evolving conceptualization of the disorder, (2) changing descriptions of "typical patient" profiles, (3) difficulties inherent in establishing the diagnosis, (4) infrequent case identification, (5) difficulties in delimitation from co-morbid illness, (6) lack of significant follow-up studies, (7) lack of significant family studies, and (8) problematic management issues (such as patients providing misleading information, refusing treatment, failing to follow up). All of these factors preclude scientific validation of the diagnoses. The entire literature on factitious disorders consists of approximately 1000 to 2000 case reports, several collected series, several retrospective record reviews, anecdotal reports of treatment (single-case), and a substantial amount of academic review papers considering theoretical aspects. Nonetheless, few if any authors doubt the existence of the phenomenon and that the patients suffer. Review of the current knowledge from the vantage point of medical model psychiatry will help the physician access the available information to work with these patients. Caveats and pitfalls of assessment and treatment will be addressed so the physician will be able to advocate for his patient's best interest.

History of Factitious Disorder

Although Munchausen's syndrome is the most commonly described manifestation of factitious disorder, it appears to represent only the most extreme (and noto-

BOX 17-3 FACTITIOUS DISORDER (DSM-IV DIAGNOSTIC CRITERIA)

A. Intentional production or feigning of physical or psychological signs or symptoms.

B. The motivation for the behavior is to assume the sick role.

C. External incentives for the behavior (such as economic gain, avoiding legal responsibility, or improving physical well-being, as in Malingering) are absent.

Code based on type:

With Predominantly Psychological Signs and Symptoms: if psychological signs and symptoms predominate in the clinical presentation

With Predominantly Physical Signs and Symptoms: if physical signs and symptoms predominate in the clinical presentation

With Combined Psychological and Physical Signs and Symptoms: if both psychological and physical signs and symptoms are present but neither predominates in the clinical presentation

From American Psychiatric Association: *Diagnostic and statistical manual of mental disorders,* ed 4 (DSM-IV), Washington, D.C., 1994, American Psychiatric Press.

rious) form of what is in all likelihood an uncommon phenomenon.

The first known medical description of factitious illness was by Chowne in 1843 as cited in Enoch and Trethowan. Chowne identified a man with "great bodily weakness and depression," which was attributed to "an irritable testicle." Unilateral orchiectomy provided the man with some relief, but the relief was only temporary, and it was decided that the other testicle had to be removed.

In 1951, Asher borrowed the name *Munchausen* and applied it to patients who demonstrated pathological lying (pseudologia fantastica) and wandering (peregrination). The name was taken from Rudolf Eric Raspe's book, *Baron Munchausen's Narrative of His Marvelous Travels and Campaigns in Russia,* because of the colorful accounts and peregrinations of Baron Karl Friedrich Hieronymous von Munchausen. The Baron, a former calvary officer in the Russian army, had a reputation for being a raconteur of outrageous stories and wandering to find audiences.

Asher's eponym was subsequently faulted by Spiro because the term *Munchausen's syndrome* was "too closely associated with lying, swindling, and the negative connotations of these behaviors." Additionally, the label was considered to be a misnomer according to Nadelson because Baron von Munchausen was not known for seeking medical attention or for engaging in self-destructive acts. In 1988 Patterson wrote that there was no evidence that Baron von Munchausen believed his stories or was trying to deceive his listeners. It appeared that Raspe alone benefitted financially from the publication, and Baron von Munchausen was embarrassed as well as resentful of the unwanted fame it brought him. Nevertheless, Munchausen's syndrome remained the selected term because, as Nadelson wrote, "The Baron's name is a more charming, evocative, antique, and noble reference and makes a more mouthfilling phrase".

Numerous other pseudoscientific appellations have been applied to patients who exhibit signs or symptoms of Munchausen's syndrome, including "hospital hobos," "hospital addicts," "metabolic malingerers," and "peregrinating problem patients." In 1968, Spiro proffered the term *chronic factitious symptomatology,* which was in part included in the DSM-III in 1980.

Asher was more successful with his original descriptions of these patients and captured the essence of their medical presentation, which warrants repeating:

> The patient showing the syndrome is admitted to the hospital with apparent acute illness supported by a plausible and dramatic history. Usually his story is largely made up of falsehoods; he is found to have attended, and deceived, an astounding number of hospitals; and he nearly always discharges himself against advice, after quarreling violently with both doctors and nurses. A large number of abdominal scars is particularly characteristic of this condition (Asher, 1951).

Asher went on to describe several well-known varieties that resemble organic emergencies:

1. The acute abdominal type (laparotomaphilia migrans), which is the most common. Some of the patients have had surgery so often that the development of genuine intestinal obstructions from adhesions may confuse the picture.
2. The hemorrhagic type, who specializes in bleeding from the lungs or stomach or from other blood loss. These types are colloquially known as "haemoptysis merchants," and "haematemesis merchants."
3. The neurologic type, who has a paroxysmal headache, loss of consciousness, or peculiar fits.

Subsequent to Asher's description of Munchausen's syndrome, a disproportionate amount of the aforementioned body of literature focused on the evolving profile of the typical patient with factitious disorder as mostly male with a history of antisocial behavior (with or without criminality), multisystem complaints, sub-

DIAGNOSIS

TABLE 17-2
FACTITIOUS DISORDER

Discriminating features

1. Intentional production or feigning of physical or psychological signs or symptoms
2. Motivation = assume the sick role
3. No secondary gain evident

Consistent features

1. Intentionality is apparent (e.g., injecting feces, ingesting phenolphthalein)
2. Factitious disorder by proxy involves inflicting factitious symptoms on another (typically the patient's own child)

Variable features

1. May include psychiatric as well as physical scenarios
2. Patients with Munchausen's syndrome demonstrate extreme peregrination and repetitive visits to multiple medical centers geographically
3. Patients produce simple to complicated and imaginative syndromes
4. Many patients work in the health care field

stance abuse, and drifting behavior with numerous hospitalizations. Interestingly, contemporaneous with the early descriptions were a small number of reports identifying a different type of patient. These authors described factitious disorder in young, geographically stable women. These early reports were supported by the case series (collected from interview and hospital records) by Carney and by Reich and Gottfried. Together, both series contained a total of 65 women (76 patients total) who were mostly young female nonwanderers. Reich and Gottfried opined that approximately 90% of the patients with factitious disorder would not fit the typical profile of (male) Munchausen's syndrome.

In 1976, Sneed and Bell applied the term *dauphin of Munchausen's* to a case in which a mother was suspected of conspiring with a 10-year-old boy to present factitious recurrent urinary calculi. In 1977, Meadow applied the term *Munchausen by proxy* to an individual who fabricates signs or symptoms of illness in another person with the intention of indirectly assuming the sick role (Box 17-4). The term was usually applied to a parent-child interaction in which the parent assumes the sick role indirectly through the child. The child was not diagnosed with factitious disorder unless he or she was part of the conspiracy.

Two other potential variants of factitious disorder have been described in the literature, but no distinct patient profile has emerged. These labels are factitious disorder with predominantly psychological symptoms and factitious disorder with combined psychological and physical symptoms.

In 1980 the DSM-III formally codified factitious disorders. Establishing the criteria facilitated the development of a conceptual framework for all the "simulating" disorders: malingering, factitious disorder, and somatoform disorders. This paradigm was based on ascertaining whether a symptom was voluntarily or involuntarily produced and whether it originated consciously or unconsciously. A simulating spectrum model could be established with malingering (voluntarily produced symptom consciously constructed) at one end and somatoform disorders (involuntarily produced symptom unconsciously constructed) at the other. Factitious disorder would be placed between the poles because the symptom was voluntarily produced but unconsciously constructed (a nebulous concept at best).

In 1985, Jonas and Pope advocated avoiding the conundrum of attempting to ascertain voluntary control and consciousness of the symptom in favor of focusing on the objective features. In particular, they suggested studies "using modern diagnostic criteria, might assess the demographics, associated phenomenology, biological findings (if any), family history, treatment response and long-term outcome of a cohort of patients presenting particularly clear-cut factitious signs or symptoms."

Clinical Features

Diagnosis

Although the diagnostic criteria for factitious disorder (see Boxes 17-3 and 17-4) remain controversial and unvalidated, sufficient overlapping descriptive case material on factitious disorder with predominantly physical signs and symptoms exists to provide guidance to the physician in recognizing these patients. In what appears to be the more severe form, the physician would expect to find some (or all) of the following features: pseudologia fantastica, peregrination (wandering), antisocial behavior, substance abuse, an extraordinarily complex medical history with an above-average level of medical knowledge, and chaotic hospital course. Pseudologia fantastica is probably the most commonly identified facet of this illness and refers to the generation of innumerable fabrications that involve both medical information and life history. The descriptions are dramatic, flamboyant, plausible, intriguing, and almost always untrue. According to Asher, patients with this disorder "lie for the sake of lying." Peregrination is often uncovered in pa-

BOX 17-4 RESEARCH CRITERIA FOR FACTITIOUS DISORDER BY PROXY — DSM-IV DIAGNOSTIC CRITERIA

A. Intentional production or feigning of physical or psychological signs or symptoms in another person who is under the individual's care.

B. The motivation for the perpetrator's behavior is to assume the sick role by proxy.

C. External incentives for the behavior (such as economic gain) are absent.

D. The behavior is not better accounted for by another mental disorder.

From American Psychiatric Association: *Diagnostic and statistical manual of mental disorders,* ed 4 (DSM-IV), Washington, D.C., 1994, American Psychiatric Press.

tients who choose to divulge information about their multiple medical hospitalizations and treatment in various regions or states. Some patients eagerly describe prior extensive medical and surgical procedures but refuse to identify or allow contact with the health care providers. These patients may demonstrate a particular symptom and deny prior evaluation and/or treatment, but a physical examination reveals numerous surgical scars and other evidence, such as bus tickets or suitcases, that suggests traveling.

Antisocial tendencies are commonly described in these individuals but usually take the form of minor antisocial acts such as vagrancy, peace disturbance, petty theft, and misdemeanor drug transgressions. Substance abuse is a common problem, but these individuals are not often described as dependent.

The medical knowledge of these individuals can be astounding. Some can provide at initial presentation their diagnosis, the founder of the disease, and the "classic" description of their illness. While discussing their evaluation, they may directly and without deviation provide the information necessary to drive the medical decision algorithm. Even with patients who do not intentionally attempt to demonstrate medical knowledge, the physician may be alerted to this issue when the patient asks for certain medications by generic name or seems to be familiar with the hospital routine after a brief stay. A noteworthy clinical point is the common incongruence between what the patient describes as extremely serious medical illness and the lack of appropriate concern demonstrated by the patient (for example, an inpatient calmly relates to a physician the presence of gross blood in the saliva and urine [from a surreptitious finger stick], but the patient vigorously complains about the smoking restrictions in the hospital).

Chaotic hospitalizations are the rule with these patients. Their hospital stays begin quietly as the initial work-up proceeds. However, as the final laboratory work is processed or as the wound heals, the patient may begin to evolve "new symptoms." Additionally, the patient may develop difficulties with the hospital staff regarding policies and procedures. At this juncture these patients often sign out of the hospital against medical advice.

In the apparently "less severely ill" female patients with factitious disorder, the absence of the more flamboyant features may prove particularly troublesome in establishing the diagnosis. In Reich and Gottfried's large outpatient series of patients with factitious disorder, they did not describe pseudologia fantastica or peregrinations but rather single body system complaint(s) with fewer hospitalizations. These authors collected and described a number of presentations (with etiologies) of factitious illness, including: (1) sepsis (introduction of contaminant), (2) failure of wound healing (introduction of a foreign body or manipulation), (3) fever (manipulation of thermometer), (4) metabolic disturbance (such as diuretics), (5) inappropriate use of indicated or surreptitious illicit substances (such as insulin), (6) frankly simulated history and signs of illness, and (7) surreptitious introduction of blood to body cavities, secretions, and excretions.

Wallach identified a number of common illnesses associated with factitious disorder, as well as a lengthy list of uncommonly produced illnesses. Although space does not permit lengthy review, the identification of several serves the purpose of educating the physician about the extraordinary interventions these patients undertake to remain in the sick role. These interventions include simulation of pheochromocytoma by self-injection of metaraminol, isoproterenol hydrochloride, or epinephrine (along with addition of epinephrine to the urine); pancytopenia by the ingestion of alkylating agents; and liver disease precipitated by hypervitaminosis A or by excessive ingestion of retinol.

Two final remarks about these patients are warranted. First, a significant number of patients with identified factitious disorder with physical symptoms worked in the health care field. Aduan and colleagues reported a series of 13 patients with self-induced infections; 10 of these patients were nurses. In the Reich and Gottfried series, 28 of 39 patients worked in the health care field. Finally, the physician should be aware that the only limitations to a factitious complaint are the patient's intelligence, motivation, and ingenuity.

Rosenberg reviewed 117 well-documented cases collected from the literature that were considered to represent the phenomenon of factitious disorder by proxy. Rosenberg found that 98% of the perpetrators were the biological mothers (producing symptoms in their children) and estimated the mortality rate at 9%. The factitious symptoms represented a wide variety of body system(s) dysfunctions, including bleeding (44%), seizures (42%), central nervous system (CNS) depression (19%), apnea (15%), hematuria (13%), diarrhea (11%), vomiting (10%), fever (10%), rash (9%), hemoptysis (3%), and upper respiratory tract abnormalities (1%). (The percentages add up to more than 100% because of multiple factitious symptoms.)

The clinical features of both factitious disorder with predominantly psychological symptoms and factitious disorder with combined psychological and physical symptoms have not been adequately described.

Natural History

The natural course of factitious disorders is unknown.

Differential Diagnosis

The possibility that a physical illness is causing the sign(s) and/or symptom(s) must be thoroughly considered first. There are a number of common medical illnesses that often manifest as vague motor or sensory symptoms (such as multiple sclerosis, acute intermittent porphyria, systemic lupus erythematosus), which must be considered. Occasionally, serious consideration is given to truncating the medical evaluation of "difficult patients," but a thorough assessment should be completed before the psychiatric intervention. Mood and psychotic disorders can occasionally appear as somatic symptomatology but are usually easily excluded by a complete review of the case history and consideration of the diagnostic criteria.

A confident diagnosis of factitious disorder requires excluding other simulating disorders. Although somatization (involuntary production) is almost always part of a general differential, the voluntary production of a symptom is rarely considered. In an attempt to determine the voluntary and conscious production of a symptom, the physician usually must change his role to a more investigative stance. This change may require a range of new behaviors, including multiple interviews with the patient, increased observation of the patient, additional laboratory evaluation, interview of collateral sources, and possibly a room search. All of these activities are undertaken in the best interest of the patient to answer the diagnostic issue. Finally, potential external incentives ("secondary gain") need to be reviewed to facilitate the exclusion of malingering.

A correct diagnosis of factitious disorder does not prevent the patient from developing physical illness as a result of previous actions (such as bowel obstruction from adhesions, endocarditis). It also does not prevent the occurrence of a "natural" medical illness.

Genetics and Family History

The genetics and family history of factitious disorder are unknown.

Epidemiology

The epidemiology of factitious disorder is unknown.

Pathophysiology

The pathophysiology of factitious disorder is unknown.

Treatment

Once the diagnosis of factitious disorder has been confidently established, most authors suggest consultation with psychiatry. Unfortunately, no controlled trials regarding the psychiatric/medical management of these patients have been conducted. The treatment recommendations identified in the literature are based on case reports involving treatment of one or two patients. In fact, the core issue of how the patient should be confronted has not been settled. Stone advocated vigorous confrontation at an early stage of treatment if the patient is to be helped. Hollander and Hersh suggested that both the primary physician and the psychiatrist be involved in the confrontation. According to Eisendrath, Ford suggested that confrontation be performed in a manner that is neither hostile nor punitive, with the primary care physician and the psychiatrist both continuing to treat the patient. Some authors have suggested that patients should not be confronted. Physicians should be prepared for the possibility that the patient may sign out of the hospital against medical advice. Should the patient be engaged for treatment, the literature does not endorse any particular form of psychiatric intervention by controlled trial.

Conclusion

Dissociative and factitious disorders are alike in that they are allegedly motivated by unconscious factors and in that relatively little empirical information is available about them. Neither has been empirically validated as a medical diagnosis, but both continue to play a role in clinical practice. Dissociative identity disorder is perhaps the most controversial of all psychiatric disorders and has divided the mental health field. Many professionals do not believe the disorder even exists. The identification and treatment of dissociation has been widely promulgated in mental health and popular arenas without adequate scientific investigation. The physician who is confronted with one of these patients is advised to consider diagnostic comorbidity and the other psychiatric conditions for which effective treatment protocols have been established. More work on factitious disorder is needed to help physicians manage them effectively, but previous experience indicates that direct confrontation with the patient, although seemingly desirable, may result in abrupt termination of treatment.

CONSIDER CONSULTATION WHEN . . .

- Dissociation or factitious disorder is suspected
- The medical history does not add up

Annotated Bibliography

Aldridge-Morris R: *Multiple personality: an exercise in deception,* London, 1989, Erlbaum.

This British monograph about MPD is written from the skeptical point of view. It reviews the existing literature on the disorder, with well-placed dry humor in pointing out the ridiculous nature of the disorder's flamboyant presentation.

Fahy TA: The diagnosis of multiple personality disorder: a critical review, *Br J Psychiatry* 153:597-606, 1988.

This article examines the phenomenology of the recent epidemic of MPD and reviews the relevant literature. The author is critical of the recent literature for its lack of methodological attention to the reliability of diagnosis, the prevalence, and the role of selection bias. He contends that MPD has not been shown to represent a distinct psychiatric disorder and instead classifies it as a hysterical symptom.

North CS et al: *Multiple personalities, multiple disorders: psychiatric classification and media influence,* New York, 1993, Oxford University Press.

This timely monograph examines MPD from an empirical viewpoint using the Washington University model of psychiatric nosology. It describes the research that has been done on the disorders and provides an in-depth analysis of how MPD has developed over the years in relation to the media. Existing data on MPD are critiqued, and the current state of knowledge on the disorder is reviewed in terms of clinical description of the disorder, delineation from other disorders, family history studies, follow-up studies, and laboratory documentation. This critical and balanced approach provides a valuable guide to physicians who are trying to make sense out of this confusing and controversial disorder.

Piper A: Multiple personality disorder, *Br J Psychiatry* 164:600-612, 1994.

This article critically examines five aspects of the diagnosis and treatment of MPD. It criticizes the current diagnostic criteria as being vague and overinclusive, identifies the epidemic as being artefactually produced, examines the question of personal responsibility of patients with this disorder, examines the evidence for childhood trauma as being the hypothesized cause of the disorder, and criticizes the techniques for diagnosing and treating the disorder as reinforcing its symptoms.

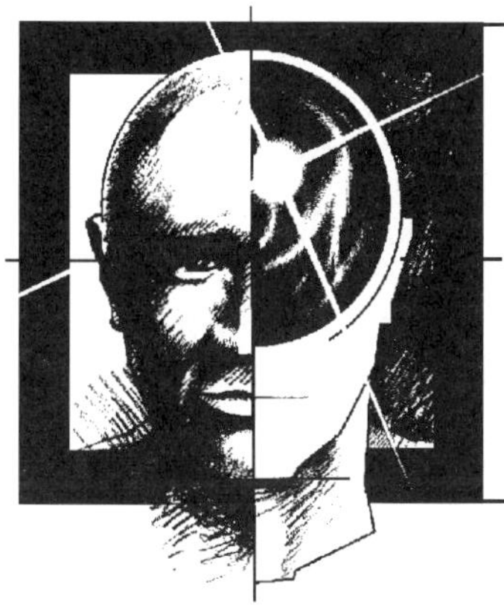

chapter 18

Personality Disorders

C. Robert Cloninger, MD, Dragan M. Svrakic, MD, PhD, Carmen Bayon, MD, and Thomas R. Przybeck, PhD

Clinical Features
Epidemiology and Presentation in Primary Medical Care
Natural History
Co-morbidity and Differential Diagnosis
Genetics and Family History
Pathophysiology
Treatment and Special Issues
Conclusion

The way that people learn from experience and adapt their feelings, thoughts, and actions is what characterizes their personality. More formally, personality can be broadly defined as the dynamic organization within an individual of the psychobiological systems that modulate adaptation to a changing environment. This includes systems regulating cognition, mood, personal impulse control, and social relations. Hence personality traits are enduring patterns of perceiving, relating to, and thinking about oneself, other people, and the world as a whole.

The diagnosis of a personality disorder requires that patients have chronic and pervasive impairments in their ability to work and to cooperate with others. These impairments include, for example, excessive dependency, perfectionism and rigidity, social detachment or inhibition, self-centeredness, or lack of empathy. Additionally, most patients with a personality disorder consistently have low self-esteem and handle stress poorly. The resulting subjective distress often leads them to complain to physicians and acquaintances about anxiety, depression, and worries about physical health. Finally, these patients have difficulty making healthy life-style choices related to their diets and personal activities (such as drinking, smoking, and exercising). Consequently, the personality and its disorders influence both objective and subjective aspects of physical health.

Nevertheless, these patients typically blame other people or unfavorable circumstances for their own personal, health, or social problems. This externalizing of responsibility is a result of two characteristics of personality disorders to which all physicians must be alert. First, people with personality disorders have a tendency to perceive their own deviant behaviors as perfectly adequate; in other words, personality disorders are ego-syntonic. Second, people with personality disorders try to change others instead of changing themselves; in other words, their attitude is alloplastic. Both of these symptoms of disease involve an effort to reduce patients' considerable subjective distress and to improve their perceived quality of life.

Systematic assessment of personality disorders is especially important because they are common and usually life-long disorders with extensive psychosocial disabilities. When antisocial personality disorder was the only disorder with reliable diagnostic criteria, the overall prevalence and importance of personality disorders was greatly underestimated. Now it is recognized that personality disorder is the primary psychiatric disorder in most patients with psychosocial impairment, particularly young adults. Approximately one sixth of the general population, one half of psychiatric outpatients, and two thirds of psychiatric inpatients and suicide attempters have personality disorders. Accordingly, diagnosis and treatment of any patient with psychosocial problems is incomplete without a systematic approach to assessing and classifying personality. For example, there is extensive heterogeneity in responses to antidepressant medications that cannot be predicted on the basis of depressive symptoms, co-morbid psychiatric syndromes, or subtypes defined by any other known characteristic. Nevertheless, two recent independent studies have confirmed that personality traits explain most of the variability in treatment response and can be used to help the physician select the most effective antidepressant for each individual patient.

Furthermore, the diagnosis of personality disorders can be made accurately with little time or expense once their essential features can be recognized and understood. Supportive treatment of subjective distress (such as compassionate listening, respect, and reassurance) is aimed at strengthening existing coping mechanisms. Simple cognitive-behavioral interventions that are not psychologically threatening (such as conceptualization of more adapted behaviors or education about life-style choices) may have many benefits beyond support. These additional benefits include reduced interpersonal conflict, increased compliance with treatment, and increased emotional satisfaction for the patient, the patient's family and friends, and the physician.

Clinical Features

Qualitative (Categorical) Diagnosis

The qualitative features that are diagnostic of a personality according to the American Psychiatric Association are summarized in Box 18-1 and Table 18-1.

First, the maladaptive response patterns must be stable and enduring; that is, these are generally life-long characteristics. Official criteria reported in DSM-IV require that the maladaptive pattern be "of long duration and its onset can be traced back at least to adolescence or early adulthood." In practice, however, a physician should be extremely careful distin-

BOX 18-1 A PERSONALITY DISORDER

DSM-IV DIAGNOSTIC CRITERIA

A. An enduring pattern of inner experience and behavior that deviates markedly from the expectations of the individual's culture. This pattern is manifested in two (or more) of the following areas:

(1) cognition (i.e., ways of perceiving and interpreting self, other people, and events)
(2) affectivity (i.e., the range, intensity, lability, and appropriateness of emotional response)
(3) interpersonal functioning
(4) impulse control

B. The enduring pattern is inflexible and pervasive across a broad range of personal and social situations.

C. The enduring pattern leads to clinically significant distress or impairment in social, occupational, or other important areas of functioning.

D. The pattern is stable and of long duration and its onset can be traced back at least to adolescence or early adulthood.

E. The enduring pattern is not better accounted for as a manifestation or consequence of another mental disorder.

F. The enduring pattern is not due to the direct physiological effects of a substance (e.g., a drug of abuse, a medication) or a general medical condition (e.g., head trauma).

From American Psychiatric Association: *Diagnostic and statistical manual for mental disorders,* ed 4 (DSM-IV), Washington, D.C., 1994, American Psychiatric Press.

guishing long-term maladaptation that is pathognomic of personality disorders from chronic personality changes that are caused by other mental disorders (such as chronic depression) or long-term situational factors. The maladaptive pattern must also be inflexible and pervasive; that is, it must be manifest in a wide range of personal and social contexts (for example, at home, at work, and with family and friends) and not in isolated aspects of a person's life. Finally, there must be substantial evidence of subjective distress, impaired social and occupational function, or both. Subjective distress refers to low self-esteem and limited problem-solving skills, which often lead to anxiety, depression, and hypochondriasis. Social and occupational impairment in people with a personality disorder results from their lack of mature goals and values.

Individuals with personality disorders have a peculiar capacity to elicit strong emotions from other people. They are often described with negative labels, such as aggravating, unlikable, difficult, or bad. Alternatively, they may be seductive or dependent and elicit inappropriate emotions or actions, such as sexual interest or the urge to rescue. Even professionals may have difficulty treating them with respectful objectivity because of a blurring of traditional personal boundaries. Such loss of objectivity occurs because the patient's deeply felt assumptions about other people may often elicit interpersonal responses that are appropriate to the patient's assumptions. A person's assumptions about himself and others often become self-fulfilling prophecies because of these automatic mechanisms of affect transfer. If someone smiles at another person, communicating appreciation, it is natural for the recipient to experience feelings of social attachment and to smile back automatically. Likewise, if someone frowns, communicating anger, it is natural to feel defensive in preparation for their angry attack. For example, many patients with personality disorders are suspicious and hostile about others' motives. This distrustful attitude is communicated in many verbal and nonverbal ways, and it often elicits disagreement or frank hostility from others. These uncooperative responses reinforce the original negative assumptions of the patient, which in turn lead to further alienation.

This vicious cycle of affect transfer can only be interrupted by professional objectivity combined with patience and compassionate respect for the person's disability. Such objectivity arises from recognizing the overall meaning and implications of a patient's pattern of interpersonal signals, so the patient's verbal and nonverbal communication take on diagnostic and therapeutic, rather than personal, significance. In optimal therapeutic relationships, patients should be patiently hopeful and physicians should be objectively caring. Whenever physicians become aware of strong positive or negative emotions toward a patient (counter-transference reactions), they should be alert to the possibility that the patient has a personality disorder (see the Pearls & Perils box on p. 304).

In addition to these consistent features of all personality disorders, there is much variation in specific styles of thinking, feeling, and relating. DSM-IV distinguishes three clusters of personality disorders (odd, dramatic, and anxious), but features of more than one cluster commonly occur in the same patient. Furthermore, each cluster is subdivided into discrete subtypes (Table 18-2), but most patients with a personality disorder have features of more than one subtype (for example, narcissistic, histrionic, and antisocial symptoms usually occur together).

Unfortunately, categorical classification systems, including DSM-IV, have failed to help physicians deal with personality disorders efficiently. The most prominent practical problem is that categorical systems do not establish a prescriptive relationship between diagnosis and treatment. In most other medical and psychiatric fields, clinical diagnosis directly indicates optimal treatment. However, in the field of personality disorders, this fundamental goal has not been achieved. The DSM-IV system usually yields multiple personality diagnoses for individual patients. In such cases, treatment priorities are easily confused. Typically, the most prominent symptoms clinically, which are not necessarily the most urgent ones to treat, are likely to be treated most vigorously. For example, people who are

DIAGNOSIS

TABLE 18-1

QUALITATIVE DESCRIPTION OF PERSONALITY DISORDERS

Discriminating feature

1. A maladaptive pattern of responses to personal and social stress that is stable and enduring since the teenage years, inflexible and pervasive, and causing subjective distress and impaired work or social relations

Consistent feature

1. Strong emotional reactions elicited from others (such as anger or the urge to rescue)

Variable features

1. Odd or eccentric behavior
2. Dramatic or impulsive behavior
3. Anxious or fearful attitude

PEARLS & PERILS

RECOGNIZING PERSONALITY DISORDER

- Personality disorder is the primary disorder in most patients with psychosocial impairment, especially young adults.
- No demographic group is protected from personality disorder.
- Individuals with a personality disorder impress others as irrational or excessively emotional because their behavior and interactions are dominated by unregulated, basic emotions (such as fear, anger, and disgust) without integration with mature goals and values.
- Strong emotional reactions to a patient, such as anger or an urge to rescue, suggest the possibility of personality disorder in the patient, inappropriate expectations by the physician, or both. (A patient may say, "I often get under the skin of other people," or "I don't know why people are always trying to protect me or tell me what to do when I don't want their help.")
- When there is a past history of a suicide attempt or psychiatric hospitalization, further review of school, work, and social behavior usually confirms presence of personality disorder. (A characteristic statement is, "I don't like or trust many people.")
- Transient immature behavior can occur under unusual stress and should be distinguished from the enduring and pervasive maladaptation typical of personality disorders or personality changes caused by other chronic mental and physical disorders.
- A pattern of consistently blaming other people and external circumstances for one's problems in a wide range of personal and social contexts is the essential diagnostic feature of personality disorder. (A common complaint is, "I often feel used, manipulated, or betrayed by others.")
- Patients with a personality disorder handle stress poorly and are often mildly depressed, anxious, or hypochondriacal. (The patient may state, "Many things upset, bother, or frustrate me," or "Nothing ever goes easy for me.")
- Severe pain and prolonged inability to work are seldom attributable to personality disorder alone. (The patient might say, "My health is just fair—not so bad that I cannot work, but not excellent.")
- When personality disorder is suspected, quantitative personality tests are unbiased, reliable, efficient, and inexpensive diagnostic tools that do not require referral.

TABLE 18-2

QUALITATIVE CLUSTERS AND SUBTYPES OF PERSONALITY DISORDERS ACCORDING TO DSM-IV

Cluster	Subtype	Discriminating features
Odd/Eccentric	Schizoid	Socially indifferent
	Paranoid	Suspicious
	Schizotypal	Eccentric
Dramatic/Impulsive	Antisocial	Disagreeable
	Borderline	Unstable
	Histrionic	Attention-seeking
	Narcissistic	Self-centered
Anxious/Fearful	Avoidant	Inhibited
	Dependent	Submissive
	Obsessive-compulsive	Perfectionistic
Not Otherwise Specified	Passive-aggressive	Negativistic
	Depressive	Pessimistic

narcissistic are likely to be treated for their excessive self-centered behaviors, even though it is their chronically fragile and low self-esteem that generates most of the typical narcissistic symptoms. Furthermore, DSM-IV classifies personality disorders into some syndromes that are symptomatically similar to some Axis I disorders (for example, paranoid personality and delusional disorder, schizotypal personality and schizophrenia). Consequently, the observed personality syndromes are commonly treated with nonspecific symptomatic treatments that are analogous to treatments already proven effective for the corresponding Axis I disorders (for example, neuroleptics for paranoid personality disorder). Such symptomatic treatments are generally inferior to those derived from the understanding of the underlying causative mechanisms. On the positive side, categorical models convey vivid, clinically useful information about rare prototypical cases, that is, cases that perfectly fit their corresponding "pigeon-hole" in the classification.

Detailed checklists of diagnostic features are available for each of the personality disorder subtypes listed in Table 18-2. Reliable structured interviews are available to make such diagnoses, but the interviews take 90 minutes or more to complete, and as noted, they usually produce multiple diagnoses. Consequently, other approaches are needed in practical clinical work.

Quantitative (Dimensional) Diagnosis

Qualitative terms such as *inflexible* and *enduring* require subjective judgments and produce little precision in the general diagnosis of a personality disorder. When an effort was made in the past to diagnose a personality disorder in such general qualitative terms, the reliability of diagnosis was low. In contrast, criteria for more specific subtypes increase reliability but produce many overlapping diagnoses. Fortunately, quantifiable components of personality have recently been identified that reliably distinguish all patients with a personality disorder from other people with other or no psychopathological disorder. These basic features of all personality disorders are referred to as character, which involves an individual's concepts and self-conscious emotions about his goals and values.

The following three dimensions of character have been distinguished: self-directedness, cooperativeness, and self-transcendence. Self-directedness quantifies the extent to which an individual accepts responsibility for control of his goals and habits rather than blaming other people and circumstances for his behavior; self-directed people are responsible, purposeful, resourceful, self-accepting, and dutiful. Cooperativeness quantifies the extent to which a person identifies with other people and feels like an integral part of society; cooperative people are tolerant, empathic, helpful, compassionate, and principled. Self-transcendence quantifies the extent to which a person feels like an integral part of the universe as a whole; self-transcendent people are imaginative, self-forgetful, faithful, spiritual, and idealistic. Highly creative individuals have achieved a high level in all three character dimensions, but many well-organized (that is, mature) people have a lower level of self-transcendence. For highly mature and creative people, life is full of challenging opportunities, people are generally trustworthy and nice, and most things ultimately work out right, even if they do not see how at the moment.

It has been repeatedly demonstrated that poorly developed character traits, especially self-directedness, increase the risk for personality disorders substantially (Table 18-3). Hence most individuals with a personality disorder have difficulty accepting responsibility, setting long-term goals, accepting their own limitations, or overcoming obstacles they encounter in life. Usually, but not always, they are also uncooperative. That is, they tend to be intolerant of others, insensitive to other people's feelings, and selfish; they often have difficulty trusting and confiding in other people; and they are often hostile and revengeful when others disappoint them; but they are quick to take advantage of others in an unprincipled manner when the opportunity arises.

In some exceptional cases, individuals with a high level of self-directedness can be maladapted as well. Specifically, people who are narcissistic or antisocial may be highly self-directed; in other words, they can be quite resourceful, purposeful, and thus quite successful in pursuing their narcissistic or antisocial goals. However, their low cooperativeness (for example, intolerance of others, revengefulness, and low empathy) may interfere with social relations to the extent that they have a personality disorder.

The degree of self-directedness is indicated in responses to questions about the person's goals in life, self-esteem, and ability to overcome obstacles. In a busy medical setting, this information may be most often elicited in discussions about life-style choices that are important for long-term health and prevention of disease (such as attitudes toward weight control, dietary balance, exercise, smoking, and drinking) and ways of relaxing and coping with stress. The more mature people are, the more clear their goals are and the more disciplined sequence of steps is that they are taking to accomplish their goals despite obstacles and initial failures. Immature people (that is, individuals with personality disorders) are unsure about their goals and unable to accept criticism or acknowledge their limitations. Consequently, when immature people are successful, they exhibit vanity; when they have problems, they blame other people and circumstances to avoid feelings of shame. They wish things were better but are not self-confident or determined enough to do whatever it takes to fulfill their wishes. As noted, patients with personality disorders usually also exhibit a low degree of cooperativeness. The components of cooperativeness (social tolerance, empathy, helpful-

DIAGNOSIS

TABLE 18-3

QUANTIFIABLE (DIMENSIONAL) FEATURES OF PERSONALITY DISORDER

Discriminating and consistent features

1. Low self-directedness, which includes an irresponsible, blaming attitude, no mature goals, resourcelessness, helplessness, poor self-esteem, and undisciplined behavior
2. Low cooperativeness, indicated by the patient being intolerant of others, lacking empathy, unhelpful, revengeful, and unprincipled

Variable features

1. Low persistence
2. Low reward dependence (odd cluster only)
3. High novelty seeking (dramatic cluster only)
4. High harm avoidance (anxious cluster only)

ness, compassion, and ethical principles) are self-explanatory and can be easily examined in the primary medical care as well.

Whereas undeveloped character traits represent the core features for determining the presence or absence of personality disorders, other quantifiable traits are used for differential diagnosis of the DSM-IV clusters (eccentric, dramatic, and anxious) and discrete subtypes of personality disorders. The different clusters are distinguished by aspects of personality that regulate automatic emotional responses such as anger, fear, and disgust. Such basic emotions are regulated by those components of personality that are called temperament, which develop in infancy and persist stably throughout life. Four dimensions of temperament have been identified and are labelled *novelty seeking, harm avoidance, reward dependence,* and *persistence.* Individuals who are highly novelty-seeking are impulsive, quick tempered, extravagant, and they dislike rules; such high novelty seeking is characteristic of individuals with antisocial, histrionic, and other erratic personality disorders. Individuals with a high degree of the harm-avoidance trait are anxious, fearful, shy, and fatigable; high harm avoidance is characteristic of avoidant and other anxious personality disorders. Individuals with low degrees of reward dependence are socially indifferent, aloof, cold, and independent; such low reward dependence is characteristic of schizoid and other odd personality disorders. Individuals who have high levels of persistence, such as some patients who are mature and some who are obsessional, are industrious and persevering, whereas those with little persistence are easily discouraged. Factor analyses have repeatedly supported the validity of the three DSM-IV clusters of personality disorders (eccentric/odd, anxious/fearful, erratic/dramatic) except that symptoms for obsessive-compulsive personality disorder tend to load separately from other personality disorders thus forming a fourth cluster. The fourth temperament dimension, persistence, has been repeatedly shown to correlate with symptoms for obsessive-compulsive personality disorder.

Temperament traits regulate the primary emotions of fear (harm avoidance), anger (novelty seeking), and attachment and disgust (reward dependence). People with personality disorders often impress others as irrational or excessively emotional because their behavior and interactions are dominated by extreme temperament traits that are only weakly modulated by character traits. Such individuals typically have rather primitive patterns of emotional responses in which behavior is dominated by the three elementary emotions. In contrast, mature people have a more complex emotional life that includes a broad spectrum of "secondary" emotions such as pride, humility, compassion, empathy, equanimity, and patience. The likelihood of a well-adapted temperament and mature character is high when these complex emotions are prominent.

Each of the character and temperament dimensions are normally distributed quantitative traits. They vary independently of each other, so all possible combinations of values on each dimension can occur. The presence or absence of any personality disorder can be defined as inadequate character development, which is indicated by low self-directedness or low cooperativeness. Furthermore, different personality subtypes can each be distinguished by a unique combination of values on the temperament dimensions. For example, histrionic personality disorder is characterized by high novelty seeking, low harm avoidance, high reward dependence, and sometimes low persistence. Antisocial personality disorder has the same temperament profile except that reward dependence is low.

The seven-factor model of temperament and character provides simple and practical guidelines for the integration of categorical and dimensional models of personality disorders. As described in Table 18-3, poorly developed character traits represent the consistent features typical of all personality disorders, whereas individual variation in the temperament dimensions (that is, the specific temperament profile) represents the distinguishing features of discrete personality disorders. Clearly this multidimensional model retains the benefits of categorical clinical diagnosis, because each temperament profile corresponds to one of the traditional personality disorders. It is easy to remember the discriminating features of most personality disorders as the extremes of a cube with three dimensions defined by novelty seeking, harm avoidance, and reward dependence (Figure 18-1).

In addition to providing vivid information about

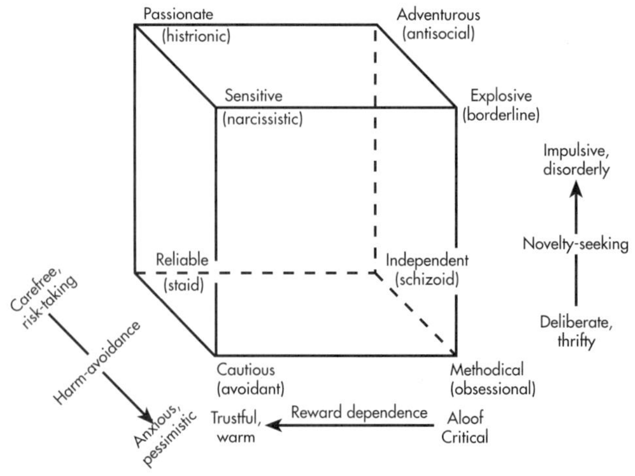

FIGURE 18-1 Temperament cube.

prototypical patients, categorical labels for the different multidimensional configurations also remain useful for purposes of description and prediction of course. On the other hand, quantified individual traits constituting the overall temperament profile are readily available for more precise diagnostic and treatment analyses. In general, for efficiency of assessment and for analysis of etiology and pathophysiology, it is helpful to be aware that the underlying clinical variation in personality disorders involves a small number of quantitative dimensions rather than a set of discrete diseases.

Several reliable self-report questionnaires are available to allow quantitative ratings of personality dimensions for differential diagnosis of personality disorders. Different models that distinguish normal and abnormal personality have been discussed in detail elsewhere by Stack and Lorr. The most commonly used are the Minnesota Multiphasic Personality Inventory-2 (MMPI-2), the Neuroticism-Extraversion-Openness (NEO) inventory, the Millon Clinical Multiaxial Inventory, and the Temperament and Character Inventory (TCI). The Millon Clinical Multiaxial Inventory is designed for use only with clinical psychiatric patients and is not appropriate for general medical patients. Comparisons of the TCI, NEO, and MMPI-2 show that the TCI is more comprehensive and better discriminating than the other two for the differential diagnosis of personality disorders. The seven-factor dimensional model of temperament and character described here is the most comprehensive model of personality currently available and has been validated in the general population and in psychiatric patients for the diagnosis of personality disorders. The personality dimensions are all assessed by the TCI, which consists of 240 true/false questions. The TCI can be self-administered in about 35 minutes at home or in the office. Copies of the test and services for scoring and interpretation are available from the authors.

Epidemiology and Presentation in Primary Medical Care

Between 11% and 23% of individuals in the general population are diagnosed as having a personality disorder according to the categorical criteria in Table 18-1. However, there is no natural subdivision between more mature and less mature people when quantitative ratings are made by people themselves or knowledgeable informants. Using the sum of self-directedness and cooperativeness scores as the measurement of maturity, one in every three individuals in the general population is noticeably less mature than others to those who know that person. Accordingly, for descriptive purposes here, the least mature sixth of the population (that is, the bottom 17%) is distinguished as having "severe" or "definite" cases and the next sixth is noted as having "mild" or "possible" cases.

Psychiatric patients with personality disorders are more often less educated, have more marital difficulties, and are unemployed more often. Data about the demographic features of personality disorder in the general population are summarized in Table 18-4. Patients with a personality disorder are more likely to be men, not white, never married, unemployed, and high-school dropouts, and they rarely attend religious services. Additionally, patients with personality disorders are usually young adults, because personality disorders are likely to remit with increasing age, as described in the Natural History section. However, except for age and church attendance these demographic differences are small, and no demographic group is immune to personality disorders.

Regarding general health, patients with a personality disorder are less likely to report that their health is excellent and more likely to say that it is only fair, presumably because somatic anxiety is weakly correlated ($r = .35, P < .01$) with low self-directedness. However,

TABLE 18-4

DEMOGRAPHIC FEATURES OF PERSONALITY DISORDER IN A SAMPLE OF 800 INDIVIDUALS REPRESENTATIVE OF THE GENERAL ADULT POPULATION OF METROPOLITAN ST. LOUIS

	Personality disorder		No personality disorder	
Feature	Severe (n = 141) %	Mild (n = 131) %	Average (n = 276) %	Mature (n = 252) %
Male	59	47	40	36
Not white	19	24	17	15
Never married	23	13	8	9
Unemployed	6	8	4	3
Did not graduate high school	17	15	13	7
Rarely attend religious services	56	38	27	19

many report their health as good to very good. Likewise, 27% of patients with a personality disorder report that their health impairs their ability to work, compared with 19% of those without a personality disorder. Most patients with personality disorders do complain of significant bodily pain during the month before they are questioned, but this is only slightly more common than it is in other people (51% vs. 40%) and seldom severe (6%). Overall, the excess of physical health complaints in patients with a personality disorder is consistent but small. This suggests that the physical health of a patient with a personality disorder is usually not impaired much more than is attributable to hypochondriasis and other aspects of mental health.

In contrast, patients with personality disorders differ substantially from others in their histories of past psychiatric problems (Table 18-5). Use of psychotropic medications and mental health counseling are only weakly associated with personality disorders. However, psychiatric hospitalization occurs in 8% to 14% of patients with personality disorders and only 4% of others. Among the 6% of the general population with a history of psychiatric hospitalization, 39% have severe personality disorders and another 22% have mild personality disorders. Likewise, about 7% of the general population report a past suicide attempt; of these, 46% have a severe personality disorder and another 21% have a mild personality disorder. Accordingly, the possibility of a personality disorder should be carefully evaluated in any patient with a past history of psychiatric hospitalization or a suicide attempt.

The detection of a personality disorder is helpful in treatment because it alerts the physician to the common subjective distress and psychosocial disability of the patient. Many patients with personality disorders are nervous or sad much of the time, whereas others are rarely so (Table 18-6). For example, patients with severe personality disorders are 13 times more likely than mature people to report that they were unable to cheer up much of the week before they are questioned. (13% vs. 1%). Accordingly, reports of anxiety and depression have different diagnostic and treatment implications depending on the presence or absence of a personality disorder, as is discussed later.

Natural History

The requirement of early onset and enduring impairment assures extensive chronicity for personality disorders. However, in a general population sample of varying age, people with personality disorder are often younger than people without personality disorder; for example, in the St. Louis Health Survey, the average age varied from 40 years in people with severe personality disorders to 46 years in mature individuals. The proportions of individuals with severe and mild personality disorders are shown by age in Table 18-7. This association of personality disorders with younger age indi-

TABLE 18-5

LIFETIME HISTORY OF PAST PSYCHIATRIC TREATMENT IN THE GENERAL POPULATION

	Personality disorder		No personality disorder	
Psychiatric history	**Severe (n = 141) %**	**Mild (n = 131) %**	**Average (n = 276) %**	**Mature (n = 252) %**
Medication	32	35	27	23
Counselling	32	23	19	18
Hospitalized	14	8	4	4
Suicide attempt	17	8	4	2

TABLE 18-6

NERVOUSNESS AND MOOD IN THE PAST MONTH IN THE GENERAL ADULT POPULATION

	Personality disorder		No personality disorder	
Psychiatric history	**Severe (n = 141) %**	**Mild (n = 131) %**	**Average (n = 276) %**	**Mature (n = 252) %**
In the past month, much of the time are you. . . ?				
Nervous	25	13	7	2
Downcast	27	24	8	1
Unable to cheer up?	13	8	4	1

TABLE 18-7

PREVALENCE OF PERSONALITY DISORDER BY AGE

Personality status	Age group 18-24 (n = 85) %	25-39 (n = 286) %	40-59 (n = 241) %	60+ (n = 191) %
Personality Disorder				
Severe	34	17	17	11
Mild	22	16	14	17
No Personality Disorder				
Average	32	33	33	39
Mature	12	34	36	33
Total %	100	100	100	100

cates maturation (that is, remission of the personality disorder) with increasing age in some cases. In particular, three dimensions of personality change substantially with age according to both longitudinal comparisons of the same people at different ages and correlations of age and personality in cross-sectional studies of the general population. Novelty seeking decreases with age by approximately 18%, and older individuals become less impulsive (more reflective), less rule-breaking (more orderly), and less quick-tempered (more stoical). Cooperativeness increases markedly in most children during school age and then increases by 12% on average after age 18. Self-directedness increases markedly in most people during adolescence and young adulthood, increasing on average by 9% after age 18.

The decreasing prevalence of personality disorders with age is attributable to the increased development of both self-directedness and cooperativeness with age. The additional tendency for novelty seeking to decrease with age explains the finding that patients with impulsive personality disorders, such as antisocial and borderline personality disorders, show even more improvement than patients with anxious or eccentric personality disorders. The best documented finding about change in personality disorders is the remission of criminal behavior in individuals with antisocial personality disorders. In a prospective 30-year follow-up study of children, Robins found that 39% of 82 patients with antisocial personality disorder settled down and matured; that is, they became more responsible and conscientious and they reduced their criminal activities and substance abuse. In Robins' study, 12% of patients were judged to be in remission and 27% were much improved. Maturation usually occurred in the fourth decade (ages 31 to 40), but there was no age at which improvement was not possible. Of those improving, 20% did so by age 30, 50% improved between ages 31 and 40, and 30% improved after age 40. Regardless of age, they nearly always remained impulsive (high novelty seeking), risk-taking (low harm avoidance), and aloof (low reward dependence), but they also became mature enough to maintain work and family life in a stable manner.

When asked to explain how the transition to maturity was achieved, patients with personality disorder usually point to meaningful emotional experiences and valued life opportunities. These include events like marriage to a caring and responsible spouse; obtaining a job that permits the development of skills and self-respect, as well as hope about opportunities for advancement; and religious conversion. The emergent changes often are sudden and associated with a new perspective on life, which cannot be achieved by logic, medication, or advice alone. Such emotional experiences and emergent insights lead to new goals and values. The basic temperament traits stay nearly the same, but they can be satisfied by mature goals and values.

Co-Morbidity and Differential Diagnosis

Transient mood states, like depressive episodes, may alter personality function temporarily. Increases in anxiety or depression lead to moderate increases in harm avoidance, but they do not alter other aspects of temperament. Self-directedness and cooperativeness may also be transiently reduced during depressive episodes. Consequently a person with no enduring personality disorder may act immature when depressed or under stress. The diagnosis of a personality disorder should be based on enduring patterns of behavior and not on limited episodes of anxiety or depression.

Adolescent use of alcohol or drugs usually leads to an arrest in character development. Mature problem-solving skills, goals, and values do not develop maturely when a person relies on drug abuse for pleasant thrills or relief of worries. Once abstinence is achieved, character development may proceed. Meanwhile, the diagnosis of personality disorder is justified on the basis of a person's inner experience (way of thinking and feeling) and behavior (impulse control and social relations) regardless of explanations such as drug abuse or social deprivation.

Most patients with psychoses have co-morbid personality disorders. In fact, it has been suggested that personality disorder increases vulnerability to psychosis, particularly when self-transcendence is high, because such individuals are prone to magical ideation and perceptual abberations. Alternatively, a personality disorder may represent an early manifestation of the psychotic illness. Further prospective studies are needed to evaluate whether clinical features of patients or external influences (such as drug use or stress) can distinguish patients whose personality disorders will deteriorate into psychosis from other patients with personality disorders. In most cases, psychoses in patients with personality disorders are brief reactive psychoses, but they may also be chronic psychoses, such as schizophrenia. A personality disorder should be diagnosed in addition to other diagnoses, because it may add useful information about the patient's behavior and treatment.

Patients with personality disorders also commonly have co-morbid psychiatric syndromes related to anxiety, depression, and substance abuse. The risk and severity of these co-morbid syndromes vary quantitatively with the degree of immaturity. For example, the severity of depression in the week preceding a survey was measured in the general population using a scale developed by the NIMH Center for Epidemiological Studies (CES) (Table 18-8). The CES depression scale indicates a high probability of major depression when there are many depressive symptoms (scores of 21 or more) and a high probability of minor depression or dysthymia with moderate depressive complaints (scores of 16 to 20). Using these reports, the risk of major depression varies from 2% in mature individuals to 42% in people with severe personality disorders, and minor depression varies from 2% to 16%. Alcoholism, indicated by lifetime reports of three or more problems on the Michigan Alcoholism Screening Test,

TABLE 18-8

PSYCHIATRIC SYNDROMES CO-MORBID WITH PERSONALITY DISORDER IN THE GENERAL ADULT POPULATION

	Personality disorder		No personality disorder	
Co-morbid psychiatric syndromes (n = 252)	**Severe (n = 141) %**	**Mild (n = 131) %**	**Average (n = 276) %**	**Mature (n = 252) %**
Depression*				
Major	42	30	11	2
Minor	16	13	13	2
Alcoholism†				
Definite	28	17	12	8
Possible	12	18	16	10
Cigarette smoking				
Ever	77	72	68	56
Pack/day	54	48	41	31
Current	45	40	34	23
Eating disorder				
Binging	31	25	15	9
Purging	6	6	4	4
Panic Attacks	20	17	11	6
Phobias				
Specific	37	36	25	22
Social	42	37	20	14

*Depression based on Center for Epidemiological Studies-Depressed Scale (CES-D) (16 to 20, minor; 21+, major).
†Alcoholism based on the Short Michigan Alcoholism Screening Test (SMAST).

varies from 16% in mature individuals to 37% in severe personality disorder. The extent of cigarette smoking and symptoms of eating or anxiety disorders are inversely correlated with the degree of maturity. Accordingly, subjective distress and difficulty handling stress are prominent features of all personality disorders (see the Pearls & Perils box below).

Genetics and Family History

Genetic and environmental factors interact in complex ways to influence the risk of developing a personality disorder. Robust findings from many family studies show that relatives of individuals with personality disorders often have incomplete forms of the same disorder with mild or partial features. Likewise, parents with no personality disorder may produce one or several children with a severe personality disorder. Furthermore, in family studies, including studies of adopted-away children whose biological parents have personality disorders, the risk of personality disorder in children is increased by the number of disorders and their severity in their biological parents. Additionally, studies of adoptive parents and family environments show that the risk of a personality disorder depends on the severity of psychosocial disorganization of the family in which a child is reared. All these observations about twins, adoptees, and families are explained by the hypothesis that there is quantitative inheritance of the individual personality dimensions that influence the risk of a personality disorder, rather than the separate inheritance of individual personality disorders.

More specifically, the four dimensions of temperament are each moderately heritable. The genetic heritabilities of each temperament dimension is about 50%, according to twin and adoption studies. Each temperament dimension is also inherited independently of the others. Surprisingly, social learning in the family environment does not influence temperament traits at all. In other words, parents do not influence the basic emotions or temperaments of their children during rearing. Consequently, the biological parents with particular temperament traits increase the risk of those same traits in their adopted-away children.

However, parents can influence character. The three dimensions of character are only weakly heritable, but they are substantially influenced by social learning in the family environment shared by siblings. Family environment explains about 35% of variability of character traits such as self-directedness and cooperativeness. Consequently, psychosocial disorganization in the rear-

PEARLS & PERILS

TREATING PERSONALITY DISORDER

- Patients with personality disorders usually require a multifaceted treatment plan that combines psychotherapy and pharmacotherapy.
- Effective treatment requires much work, patience, and empathy.
- There is no age at which improvement is impossible.
- Compassionate support and reassurance can be safely provided without giving direct advice.
- Creativity in inventing new techniques, strategies, or methods is encouraged to help patients deal efficiently with the common and frustrating "no-way-out" situations.
- Direct advice on personal and social problems is generally counterproductive in patients with personality disorder because they become dependent, noncompliant, or resentful.
- Personality change is based on emotional experiences that alter basic assumptions and views about oneself, others, and the world.
- Prognosis is especially poor in patients who have never had a meaningful relationship with at least one person.
- The patient should be asked to define her treatment goals with subsequent realistic evaluation of the likelihood of success, which is central to patient selection. Initially, these goals should be as simple and concrete as possible (for example, to develop certain social skills, or to reduce alcohol use). In many cases, successful completion of this initial phase motivates the patient to define other, more complex treatment goals and to continue treatment.
- Focus on healthy life-style choices, (such as those concerning diet, exercise, and stress management) is a beneficial approach to personality disorders in primary medical care settings.
- Personality disorder can complicate medical treatment and herald the onset of severe mental disorders.
- Psychotropic medications may be beneficial to facilitate personality change, but they are inadequate without guidance and interpretation about experience, as can be provided in expert psychotherapy.
- Noncompliance with medical treatment or emergence of marked emotional instability warrants further evaluation by psychological testing, or if acceptable to the patient, referral to specialists for an expert opinion about diagnosis and treatment.
- Relapses and recovery are expected features of treatment with chronic disorders such as personality disorders. Consultation with colleagues helps to avoid giving up or developing inappropriate attitudes.

ing environment of a child has a substantial influence on character development and the risk of immature personality disorder. Parents should be educated and supported in their efforts to provide a character-building milieu tailored to the temperaments of their individual children. Mature character development is most likely in homes that provide security and definite limits on behavior in a warm, compassionate manner, as well as encouraging self-directed choice and the value of respect for other people.

Pathophysiology

Personality disorders can be understood in terms of the dynamic interactions among the components of a complex adaptive system. Temperament dimensions are inherited biases in adaptive responses to environmental stimuli. The biased adaptive-response patterns, in turn, constrain the way character matures; that is; they modify the way people view themselves, others, and the world at large. Theoretical discussion of the quantitative biodynamics of personality development is considered in detail elsewhere by Svrakic and colleagues (1996). Here only key empirical findings are summarized about temperament, which accounts for most of the neurobiological risk for developing a personality disorder.

The four temperaments influence differences between individuals in their responses to associative conditioning. For example, harm avoidance levels predict the formation of conditioned signals of punishment but not reward. In other words, individuals with a high tendency toward harm avoidance are more prone to worry because they acquire warning signals about danger more readily than others. Individual differences in harm avoidance are correlated with the number of serotonin$_2$ receptors in platelets. Noradrenergic mechanisms also appear to be involved in harm avoidance, and Joyce and colleagues showed that high levels of harm avoidance in women predict response to the noradrenergic antidepressant desipramine in major depression.

Likewise, reward dependence levels predict the formation of conditioned signals of reward but not punishment. In other words, individuals who are highly reward dependent are more sensitive to the exchange of signs of appreciation and approval. High reward dependence levels predict high morning cortisol levels in major depression and also antidepressant responses to serotoninergic drugs such as clomipramine and nefazodone.

Novelty-seeking levels predict quick reaction times and sensitivity to incentive activation of behavior by novelty and conditioned signals of reward. Novelty seeking is at least partly modulated by dopaminergic mechanisms; high novelty seeking appears to depend on low release and rapid reuptake of dopamine. Striatal uptake of dopa in patients with Parkinson's disease is strongly correlated with novelty seeking but not with other temperament dimensions. The gene locus encoding the dopamine D_4 receptor contributes to individual differences in novelty-seeking levels in two independent reports. Dopamine inhibits the release of prolactin, and high novelty seeking is strongly correlated with high plasma prolactin levels in the general population.

Given these individual differences in temperament, it is possible to predict the course of character development. For example, a personality disorder (that is, low self-directedness and cooperativeness) is most likely when the temperament profile combines high harm avoidance, low reward dependence, and high novelty seeking. Family environment and chance events may also influence the emergence and remission of a personality disorder. In contrast, mature character is most likely when the temperament profile combines low novelty seeking, low harm avoidance, and high reward dependence.

Treatment and Special Issues

Individuals with personality disorders perceive their aberrant life-styles as adequate and justified, and they seldom seek or accept psychiatric treatment. Occasionally they may seek help in the following situations: (1) when they are requested by others to do so (usually a spouse or parents); (2) when maladaptive behaviors culminate in unbearable marital, family, and career circumstances; and (3) when other mental problems (such as subjective distress, anxiety, depression, or substance abuse), or somatic problems (for example, obesity) complicate their clinical picture. In general, patients who have personality disorders require a multifaceted treatment plan that often combines psychotherapy and pharmacotherapy.

There are two major barriers to effective management of personality disorders that are entirely within the control of the physician. The first obstacle is the common loss of professional objectivity and personal involvement. Inappropriate personal involvement is signaled by the development of strong emotions (positive or negative) and is usually called positive or negative counter-transference. Such involvement can be corrected by using the incipient development of such feelings as a signal to reassess diagnosis and treatment. Discussions and counseling with colleagues are useful because even strong counter-transference feelings sometimes persist unrecognized.

The second preventable error in management is to give direct advice. Direct advice about personal and social problems is counterproductive in patients with personality disorders because they usually become dependent, noncompliant, or resentful. Occasionally, some patients who have antisocial, narcissistic, or schizoid personality disorder represent an exception to this general rule. These patients are at low risk of developing excessive dependency, and at least initially, they need precise structure and direction. However, it is most beneficial to provide guidance and support without giving direct advice. All that is usually required in supportive therapy is compassionate attention, respect for the dignity of other human beings despite their flaws, and reinforcement of available coping mechanisms.

When tempted to make an exception to the rule of not giving direct advice, the physician should remember that change in personality does not come from advice or logic. People change only when they are not satisfied with themselves and their relationships. In other words, personal growth only arises from emotional experiences that stimulate new insights and feelings about oneself and the environment. This fact reminds physicians that guidance and consultation involve joint evaluation of options and encouragement to practice skills in solving problems. In contrast, direct advice robs patients of the opportunity to become more self-reliant or to learn from their failure to do so.

If a patient is noncompliant with important medical treatments despite supportive therapy and simple cognitive-behavioral approaches to life-style management, additional evaluation may be needed. This can involve reevaluation of the diagnostic assessment by psychometric testing, as described in the section related to the recognition of personality disorders. Either before or after this testing, referral to a psychiatrist may be indicated for an expert opinion about diagnosis and treatment.

However, the physician should always keep in mind that substantial personality change, which is often needed by people with personality disorders, involves an extensive reorganization of internalized concepts and coping mechanisms and thus requires precise diagnostic analyses, specific treatment strategies, and, above all, expert training. Likewise, the use of psychotropic medications for the treatment of personality disorders requires at least an initial consultation with a psychiatrist knowledgeable about personality disorders. The expert diagnosis and treatment may include any of several available psychotherapy approaches alone or more often, combined with pharmacotherapy. The major points relevant to psychotherapy and pharmacotherapy of personality disorders are summarized in the following sections.

Psychotherapy

As already noted, many patients with personality disorders do not recognize or admit their psychopathological conditions. Often they resist and resent psychiatric diagnoses and any form of mental health treatment. Accordingly, it is prudent to let the patient define her treatment goals and then realistically evaluate the likelihood of successful outcome. Initially, these goals should be as simple and concrete as possible (for example, to develop certain social skills or to reduce alcohol use). In many cases, successful completion of this initial phase motivates the patient to define other, more complex treatment goals and to continue treatment. An alternative approach in a busy medical practice is to focus primarily on issues that are related to physical health but offer an adequate basis for the diagnosis and treatment of the personality disorder. For example, a systematic focus on healthy life-style choices provides a nonthreatening basis for evaluation of a patient's goals, values, habits, and skills (that is, their personality). Choices about diet, weight control, exercise, smoking, drinking, and ways of relaxing and managing stress are appropriate for discussion with a physician and do not threaten or stigmatize the patient. Discussion of these choices with a patient can provide a guiding stimulus for her developing more self-direction and constructive planning about her life. Patients' discipline in working toward their chosen goals is an indicator of their maturity. If they do not succeed at first, they can learn more about setting goals and personal growth by learning to take smaller steps at a time. In this process, patients usually learn to accept their strengths and limitations and to forgive themselves for mistakes and failures. Self-acceptance and acceptance of others usually progress hand in hand. Such patient guidance is a simplified and nonthreatening form of cognitive-behavior therapy (CBT) and can be safely practiced in a busy primary care office.

As a rule of thumb in the psychotherapy of personality disorders, it is optimal to use combinations of theoretical orientations (psychodynamic, cognitive, and behavioral) and formats (individual, group, family, and marital), whether these are carried out by an individual or a multidisciplinary team. An increasing number of professionals ignore ideological barriers dividing schools of psychotherapy, and attempt both technical synthesis (eclecticism) and theoretical synthesis (integration) of various orientations. Different approaches to psychotherapy are complementary, and each can contribute to the overall efficacy of the treatment of personality disorders. Dynamic schools have been traditionally regarded as helping patients understand conflicting internal motivations, behavioral schools assist patients in changing the most disruptive behaviors, and humanistic approaches assist patients in achieving what might be called *cooperative self-assertiveness* or *altruistic individualism.* No one approach is invariably superior to the others. Most therapists, regardless of their orientation, pursue all three of them. Dynamic (insight-oriented) therapies may be usefully complemented by humanistic and behavioral (action-oriented) ones, because personality change only occurs when concepts and insights are integrated into everyday behavior and social interactions. Individual sessions are usually combined with group sessions, and they elaborate on relevant group experiences, that is, those reflecting the most disruptive maladaptive behaviors. Group interactions are considered useful for helping patients with personality disorders acquire social skills. However, some patients with schizoid, borderline, or avoidant personality disorder may resist this format because it is difficult for them to share their intimate experiences with a large group of people, to be exposed, and to tolerate the confrontations that are likely to occur in group therapy.

Pharmacotherapy

Psychotropic medications may be beneficial to facilitate personality change, but they are inadequate without the guidance and interpretation about experience that can be provided in psychotherapy. In general, there are two approaches to the pharmacotherapy of personality disorders: (1) specific or causal therapy, which is aimed at correcting neurochemical disturbances underlying deviant behavior traits, and (2) symptomatic therapy, which is aimed at correcting target symptoms of personality disorders.

The central idea behind causal pharmacotherapy of personality disorders is that enduring personality changes may result from drug-induced changes in neurobiological dispositions to specific personality traits. The seven-factor psychobiological model of personality, in contrast to categorical and factor-analytically derived models, provides testable hypotheses about treatable underlying mechanisms of extreme behavior variants. The basic rationale is that temperament traits are stable neurobiological dispositions that are difficult to change either by voluntary effort or by psychotherapy alone. As discussed in the pathophysiology section, several lines of evidence support the hypothesis that distinct brain neural circuits and neurotransmitter networks constitute the neurobiological substrate of observable temperament traits. Personality disorders are postulated to reflect extreme variations in these complex adaptive networks with consequent liability to deviant moods and idiosyncratic learning styles, which ultimately lead to maladaptive behaviors. This concept has important ramifications for both research and clinical practice, since it provides testable guidelines for the neurochemical manipulation of the underlying trait vulnerability. For example, preliminary evidence suggests that the responses to antidepressants of different patients with major depressive disorder (MDD) can be predicted to a substantial degree by their temperament and not by the number, type, severity, or course of their depressive symptoms. Clinically, patients who are highly sensitive to social approval (that is, those who are highly reward dependent) are most likely to improve when taking serotonin-selective reuptake inhibitors (SSRIs) such as fluoxetine or nefazodone. In contrast, those who are highly fearful but not socially dependent are most likely to improve when they take noradrenergic uptake inhibitors such as desipramine. If further work confirms and refines the nature of the relationship between temperament and therapeutic response, improved treatment outcomes can be expected.

Phenotypic similarity between some personality disorders and some Axis I disorders have also served as a rationale for treating patients who have personality disorders with drugs used for schizophrenic and mood disorders. However, symptomatic pharmacotherapy should not be based on the categorical diagnoses of personality disorders for two basic reasons. First, the efficiency of drug treatments is best evaluated on a behavioral (symptom) level. Secondly, the target symptoms likely to respond to particular drugs are not unique to patients with any specific diagnosis but are shared by various personality disorders. In general, symptomatic pharmacotherapy of people with personality disorders focuses on aggression and behavioral dyscontrol, mood and anxiety dysregulation, and psychotic symptoms (including cognitive distortions).

Aggression

It is useful, although sometimes difficult, to distinguish different types of aggression. The most common form of aggression occurs when a quick-tempered person is provoked by frustration or threats. This is often called *affective aggression* and is common in people who are impulsive-aggressive (that is, those who are highly novelty seeking and have a low tendency toward harm avoidance). Aggression that appears to be unprovoked sometimes occurs in patients with cerebral instability documented by an abnormal electroencephalogram (EEG) and is often called *ictal aggression,* regardless of any associated personality traits. Predatory aggression, or cruelty, involves hostile revengefulness and taking pleasure in victimizing others, often with intact impulse control; such predatory aggression is most common in individuals who have low levels of cooperativeness, which is most likely in antisocial and borderline personality disorders. Lastly, organic-like impulsivity is often accompanied by poor social judgment and aggression; it is best distinguished from other impulsive-aggressive syndromes by prominent distractibility, inattention, and emotional lability (as is characteristic of patients with frontal lobe lesions). Additionally, such patients often manifest high somatic anxiety with panic and cardiorespiratory symptoms, muscular tension, and motor restlessness.

Multiple double-blind trials have shown that lithium carbonate is often beneficial in the treatment of affective aggression. It helps individuals who are impulsive-aggressive be more reflective, or think about consequences before acting on impulse. To a lesser extent, it may help reduce cruelty and lack of cooperativeness, but this may be an indirect result of reducing impulsivity, which often is a predisposing influence in the development of hostility and revengefulness. Likewise, low-dose neuroleptics may be useful for modifying old habits and assist in reducing affective or predatory aggression. Certainly, physicians deciding to use neuroleptics on a long-term basis need to consider the potential side-effects, such as tardive dyskinesia, and decisions should be made with carefully informed consent of the patient. Anticonvulsants, such as carbamazepine, reduce both the intensity and the rate of unprovoked angry outbursts in some patients regardless of normality of their EEGs. Double-blind trials have also shown that psychostimulants and catecholamine agonists, such as methylphenidate or pemoline, are often beneficial in the treatment of inattentive and hyperactive adults who are impulsive and aggressive, especially when the symptoms have begun in early childhood. Antidepressants (particularly SSRIs) are considered by some to be beneficial for certain impulsive personality disorders (for example, schizotypal and borderline personality disorders). Finally, monoamine oxidase inhibitors (MAOIs) such as tranylcypromine, are effective in some dysphoric states with somatic anxiety and hostility, and they are also recommended for adults who are hyperkinetic.

On the other hand, there are some relative contraindications for other drugs. For example, lithium should not be given to people who are antisocial but without aggression and impulsivity; it does not diminish nonaggressive antisocial behaviors (such as lying, cheating, and stealing), and it is poorly tolerated by people who are anxious and schizoid. Likewise, benzodiazepines and alcohol have disinhibiting effects on violence, reduce conditioned avoidance behavior (loosen inhibitions), and further impair passive avoidance learning in people who are impulsive and antisocial. The use of benzodiazepines seems appropriate only in nonaggressive behaviors, as are typical of patients with schizoid personality disorder.

Mood Dysregulation

Mood dysregulation includes chronic anxiety, emotional lability, emotional detachment, and depression or dysphoria. Patients with personality disorders often have both cognitive anxiety (that is, anticipatory worrying) and somatic anxiety (that is, concern about bodily pains and psychophysiological reactions). Cognitive anxiety is most responsive to benzodiazepines, whereas somatic anxiety is more responsive to MAOIs and SSRIs. Avoidant traits can be also effectively treated with either SSRIs or MAOIs. Some components of somatic anxiety, such as sweating, palpitations, diarrhea, and tremor, can be treated with beta blockers. Severe, psychotic-like anxiety responds to low-dose neuroleptics, but caution about prolonged use is necessary, as noted in the previous section. Emotional instability (manifested as severe mood swings) is usually responsive to lithium. Tricyclic antidepressants (TCAs), such as imipramine, tend to increase impulsivity and anger in emotionally unstable patients who have borderline and other personality disorders and should be used with extreme caution.

Emotional detachment, cold and aloof emotions, and disinterest in social relations (chronic asociality) is typical of people who are schizoid and schizotypal, to a lesser extent, people who are antisocial or paranoid, and to some who are narcissistic. In cases where these symptoms reflect an underlying depression, antidepressants (TCAs, SSRIs, or MAOIs) may help. Physicians should be cautious using TCAs with schizotypal personality disorder, because they may worsen or trigger psychosis. In many cases, emotional detachment responds to atypical neuroleptics such as risperidone, which may reduce social withdrawal and other features of eccentric personality disorders with less risk of extrapyramidal symptoms than typical neuroleptics. However, dose adjustment is crucial to maintain compliance because patients with personality disorders often have little tolerance for side effects.

Atypical depression and dysphoria, common in personality disorders, are rarely responsive to TCAs, but rather they respond to to SSRIs, MAOIs, or possibly neuroleptics (the latter are not drugs of first choice because of their potentially irreversible side effects and should only be used after careful consideration of the risk-benefit ratio). In fact, at least half of the patients with personality disorder who have atypical depression worsen when they take TCAs. In contrast, classic depressive episodes, which often complicate personality disorders, are treated with antidepressants, (including heterocyclics) in doses suggested for primary major depression.

Psychotic Symptoms

Acute, brief reactive psychoses may complicate most personality disorders. These are treated symptomatically, according to accepted pharmacological practices. In general, patients with personality disorder who are psychotic are likely to respond to and comply with low doses of powerful neuroleptics. Acute psychotic symptoms requiring medication may subside when environmental stressors are brought under control; thus physicians should be ready to lower the dose or discontinue the medication.

Some patients with personality disorders manifest chronic low-level psychotic-like symptoms, such as thought disorders (ideas of reference, magical thinking, odd fantasies, or suspiciousness), unusual perceptual experiences (illusions), and eccentric behaviors. These symptoms respond to low-dose powerful neuroleptics such as haloperidol. Some chronic cognitive disturbances, such as mild ideas of reference or suspiciousness, tend to subside when the background emotional tension is reduced. For example, alprazolam has been found to be beneficial in patients with borderline personality, particularly those with a history of drug abuse and suspiciousness. Again, long-term use of

TABLE 18-9

CHOICE OF DRUGS ACCORDING TO TARGET SYMPTOMS OF PERSONALITY DISORDER

Target symptom	Drug of choice	Contraindication
Behavioral dyscontrol		
Aggression/impulsivity		
Affective aggression ("hot temper" with normal EEG)	Lithium* Serotoninergic drugs* Anticonvulsants* Low-dose neuroleptics	?Benzodiazepines
Predatory aggression (hostility/cruelty)	Neuroleptics* Lithium	Benzodiazepines†
Organic-like aggression	Imipramine* Catecholamine agonists	
Ictal aggression (abnormal EEG)	Carbamazepine* Diphenylhydantoin* Benzodiazepines	Neuroleptics†
Mood dysregulation		
Emotional lability	Lithium* Neuroleptics	?TCAs
Emotional detachment	Atypical neuroleptics (risperidone)* MAOIs	?TCAs†
Depression		
Atypical depression/dysphoria	MAOIs* Serotoninergic drugs* Neuroleptics	?TCAs
Classical depression	Antidepressants*	
Anxiety		
Chronic cognitive anxiety	Serotoninergic drugs* MAOIs* Benzodiazepines	
Chronic somatic anxiety	MAOIs* Beta blockers	?Benzodiazepines
Acute and severe anxiety	Low-dose neuroleptics	
Psychotic symptoms		
Acute and brief psychotic episodes	Drug choice depends on the clinical picture; doses are usual or lower than usual	
Chronic and low-level psychotic-like symptoms	Low-dose neuroleptics*	

*Drug of choice.
†Major contraindication.

benzodiazepines is associated with high risk of drug dependence, particularly in patients with personality disorders, so these drugs should be prescribed only after careful consideration of the risk-benefit ratio. Additionally, their use should be carefully monitored for evidence of abuse or dependence.

Table 18-9 summarizes possible drug choices to be considered for various target symptoms of personality disorders. It should be emphasized again that advanced psychotherapy or the use of psychotropic medications for treatment of a personality disorder requires expert training or the close supervision by a psychiatrist. This is a rapidly advancing area of psychiatry, and decisions about the use of drugs with potential for serious side effects or dependence should be made carefully.

Conclusion

Personality disorders are the primary psychiatric illness observed in most patients with psychosocial complaints, particularly young adults. Personality disorders are present in one sixth of people in the general population, one half of all psychiatric outpatients, and two thirds of patients with a history of psychiatric hospitalization or suicide attempt. Reliable diagnosis of personality disorders can be made in routine clinical practice by brief assessment of the following two essential features: low self-directedness and low cooperativeness. These features indicate reduced ability to work and to get along with other people. Personality disorders are usually life-long disorders, but they can mature (remit) spontaneously or with treatment. Temperament components of personality disorder are moderately heritable, whereas character components are more influenced by family environment. Neurobiological findings about personality explain the benefit of differential pharmacotherapy for different subtypes of personality disorders. Supportive and cognitive-behavioral treatment of personality disorders within primary medical care is feasible and often benefits a patient's level of compliance with other aspects of medical treatment.

Acknowledgment

Supported in part by grants from the National Institute of Health MH-31302, AA-07982, and AA-08028

CONSIDER CONSULTATION WHEN . . .

- Strong emotional reactions to a patient occur, such as anger or the urge to rescue
- There is a history of suicide attempts or psychiatric hospitalization within the previous 5 years
- The patient expresses hopelessness or suicidal ideas
- The patient expresses revengefulness or destructive intentions
- The patient unexpectedly deteriorates in emotional, personal, or social adjustment

Annotated Bibliography

Beck AT et al: *Cognitive therapy of personality disorders,* New York, 1990, Guilford Press.

This book describes the application of CBT to each of the individual subtypes of personality disorders classified according to criteria of the American Psychiatric Association.

Cloninger CR: Temperament and personality, *Curr Opin Neurobiol* 4:266, 1994.

This article is a brief review of available data about the hierarchical structure and neurobiological basis of individual differences in personality. It includes an extensive annotated bibliography of recent research.

Cloninger CR et al: *The Temperament and Character Inventory (TCI): a guide to its development and use,* St. Louis, 1994, Washington University Center for Psychobiology of Personality.

This book provides a comprehensive description and bibliography of the seven-factor model of personality, including its psychobiological and genetic basis, psychometrics, normative data from the general and diverse clinical populations, and use and interpretation. It describes the practical clinical use of the TCI and available scoring and interpretation services for clinicians in practice. It can be ordered by fax at 314-362-5594.

Strack S, Lorr M, editors: *Differentiating normal and abnormal personality,* New York, 1994, Springer Publishing Co.

This book provides a comprehensive review of theories and measurement techniques for distinguishing normal and abnormal personality variants. Articles on alternative dimensional and categorical models are presented by their originators and compared critically.

Vaillant GE: *Adaptation to life,* Boston, 1977, Little, Brown and Co.

This book describes and clearly illustrates mature and immature psychodynamic mechanisms used to cope with life stress across the lifespan.

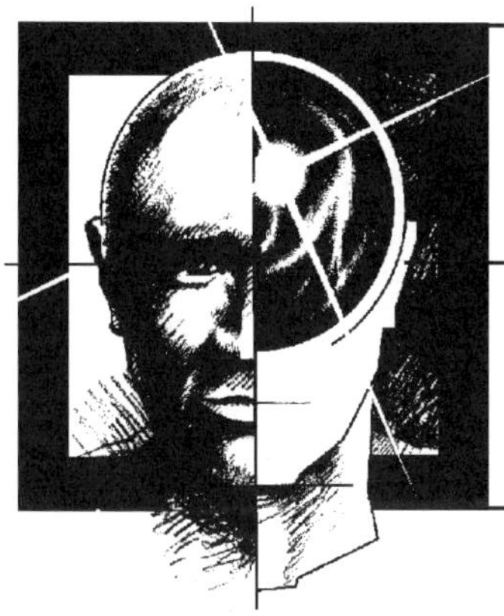

chapter 19

Trauma-Related Syndromes

Carol S. North, MD

Clinical Relevance: Importance and Scope of the Problem

People today face increasing threats to life and limb brought about by accelerating technological sophistication. Potential technological accidents include transportation accidents such as airplane, subway, train, and highway vehicle collisions; structural collapses of buildings and transportation structures such as stadiums and bridges because of architectural design flaws; and industrial accidents, including explosions and toxic chemical spills. Furthermore, modern technology has aided the intrusion of human terror into public life through the development of increasingly devastating means of wreaking death and destruction. Such technology in the hands of terrorist perpetrators across the globe has provided the means for bombs in crowded public structures, noxious gas leaks in congested subways, and shooting masses of innocent people in busy public settings such as post offices and courthouses. Finally, technology has crafted tools to heighten the massive human destruction of war, as witnessed by concentration camps, mass genocide, and nuclear bombs decimating entire metropolitan areas.

In addition to these new dangers, modern society continues to face age-old threats from natural disasters such as tornadoes, hurricanes, earthquakes, volcanoes, wildfires, and floods. Modern disasters may contain elements of both technological and natural catastrophes, such as the Mexico City earthquake, during which devastation was magnified by inadequate antiearthquake construction of buildings, and the Great Midwest Floods of 1993, in which water-containment procedures of the Army Corps of Engineers came under critical fire.

On a smaller but more endemic scale, rising problems with drugs and crime in American cities and the associated epidemic of gang-related violence that is concentrated in indigent areas make violent trauma a part of daily life. Even the most affluent neighborhoods are not immune to random violence and other traumas, such as motor vehicle accidents, assaults, rapes, robberies, carjackings, and murders, that are sporadic and shocking. In unsafe neighborhoods in which violence affects the lives of citizens on a routine basis, the population must cope with ongoing, repeated traumatization of such an extent and intensity that it may even mimic military combat settings.

Society's accelerating vulnerability to technological disasters, terrorism, and increasing violence in communities poses a heightened risk of trauma-related syndromes within the population. Therefore physicians can increasingly expect to encounter traumatized individuals in clinical practice and to find themselves in positions of leadership through helping community members cope with overwhelming violence in their midst. Such encounters can be expected both on a community-wide scale after major disasters and with ongoing endemic violence within communities. Physicians, with some review of posttraumatic syndromes and management techniques, can deal with these syndromes effectively in the community.

History of Posttraumatic Stress Disorder

Although the diagnosis of posttraumatic stress disorder (PTSD) is relatively new in official psychiatric nomenclature, posttraumatic syndromes are well known throughout history and have been described in soldiers of the American Civil War, the Crimean War, and World War I as syndromes of physical and nervous exhaustion and under names such as *soldier's heart* and *shell shock*. PTSD has been best studied among combat veterans, especially in Vietnam veterans throughout the 1980s and 1990s. The current term PTSD first appeared in DSM-III in 1980, and the criteria have been refined in subsequent editions of the diagnostic manual.

An extensive, relatively new body of literature addresses the development of adult psychiatric syndromes in relationship to reports of childhood trauma, especially childhood sexual abuse. In particular, the literature on dissociative disorders indicates that the vast majority of patients with these disorders report childhood abuse (often severe and in some cases allegedly at the hands of satanic cults). These reports have provided a stimulus for theories of dissociative disorders as posttraumatic syndromes that arise from childhood abuse.

Clinical Features

Diagnosis

PTSD is officially classified with the anxiety disorders in the current psychiatric diagnostic classification scheme. DSM-IV criteria for PTSD are summarized in Box 19-1. PTSD is the only psychiatric disorder that is defined in relation to a stressor, and it is the only psychiatric disorder for which a psychosocial cause is implicated in the diagnostic criteria. The single most important aspect of the diagnosis of PTSD is that a trauma causing physical injury or threat to life or limb to the individual must be identified, or the individual must have witnessed or confronted such an event (Table 19-1). For example a person may be an eyewitness to a violent act or learn that a close family member faced an acute life-threatening trauma. Additionally, the traumatic event must evoke a response of intense fear, helplessness, or horror.

Qualifying types of traumatic events include violent personal assault (such as kidnapping, mugging, physical assault, rape, or torture); violent accidents (for example, motor vehicle accidents, falling from a building or a cliff, or being crushed by heavy machinery); natural and manmade disasters; military combat; being taken hostage; detainment in a concentration camp or as a prisoner of war; and being diagnosed with an acute life-threatening illness. Witnessing a violent injury or death, or unexpectedly seeing a dead body or dismembered body parts qualifies as a traumatic event, as does learning of a sudden, unanticipated death or violent injury of a family member or close friend. Nonviolent events such as watching a scary movie, being fired from a job, or being served with divorce papers are not considered qualifying events.

Posttraumatic symptoms evoked by the traumatic event are divided into the following three categories: persistent reexperiencing of the event, persistent avoidance of reminders and numbing responses, and persistent arousal responses. Symptoms of persistent reexperience include distressing intrusive memories, vivid visual images of the event, dissociative "flashback" episodes in which the person relives the event, and recurring or distressing dreams of the event. For example, a survivor of a mass-murder episode complained of being tormented by unrelenting visual images that she described as "snapshots" of the victims' heads being blown apart as they were shot at point-blank range by a large-bore gun. Persistent avoidance and numbing responses include active avoidance of reminders of the event (for example, going out of the way not to travel near the location of the event), "psychic numbing" or "emotional anesthesia," restricted range of emotional expression, loss of interest in previ-

DSM-IV DIAGNOSTIC CRITERIA

BOX 19-1 POSTTRAUMATIC STRESS DISORDER

A. The person has been exposed to a traumatic event in which both of the following were present:

(1) the person experienced, witnessed, or was confronted with an event or events that involved actual or threatened death or serious injury, or a threat to the physical integrity of self or others
(2) the person's response involved intense fear, helplessness, or horror.

B. The traumatic event is persistently reexperienced in one (or more) of the following ways:

(1) recurrent and intrusive distressing recollections of the event, including images, thoughts, or perceptions.
(2) recurrent distressing dreams of the event.
(3) acting or feeling as if the traumatic event were recurring (includes a sense of reliving the experience, illusions, hallucinations, and dissociative flashback episodes, including those that occur on awakening or when intoxicated).
(4) intense psychological distress at exposure to internal or external cues that symbolize or resemble an aspect of the traumatic event
(5) physiological reactivity on exposure to internal or external cues that symbolize or resemble an aspect of the traumatic event

C. Persistent avoidance of stimuli associated with the trauma and numbing of general responsiveness (not present before the trauma), as indicated by three (or more) of the following:

(1) efforts to avoid thoughts, feelings, or conversations associated with the trauma
(2) efforts to avoid activities, places, or people that arouse recollections of the trauma
(3) inability to recall an important aspect of the trauma
(4) markedly diminished interest or participation in significant activities
(5) feeling of detachment or estrangement from others
(6) restricted range of affect (e.g., unable to have loving feelings)
(7) sense of a foreshortened future (e.g., does not expect to have a career, marriage, children, or a normal life span)

D. Persistent symptoms of increased arousal (not present before the trauma), as indicated by two (or more) of the following:

(1) difficulty falling or staying asleep
(2) irritability or outbursts of anger
(3) difficulty concentrating
(4) hypervigilance
(5) exaggerated startle response

E. Duration of the disturbance (symptoms in Criteria B, C, and D) is more than 1 month.

F. The disturbance causes clinically significant distress or impairment in social, occupational, or other important areas of functioning.

Specify if:
Acute: if duration of symptoms is less than 3 months
Chronic: if duration of symptoms is 3 months or more

Specify if:
With Delayed Onset: if onset of symptoms is at least 6 months after the stressor

From American Psychiatric Association: *Diagnostic and statistical manual of mental disorders,* ed 4 (DSM-IV), Washington, D.C., 1994, American Psychiatric Press.

DIAGNOSIS

TABLE 19-1
POSTTRAUMATIC STRESS DISORDER

Discriminating features

1. Requires a traumatic event that causes physical injury or threat to life/limb
2. Categories of symptoms are reexperiencing, avoidance and numbing, and hyperarousal
3. Lasts at least 1 month

Consistent features

1. Symptoms are a conglomerate of anxiety, depression, and dissociation
2. Higher rates in women
3. PTSD is more likely after more severe events (e.g., with terror, horror, large numbers of fatalities, or gruesome images)
4. PTSD is more likely with greater exposure to event (e.g., people trapped inside burning building have more severe exposure than onlookers)

Variable features

1. Psychiatric co-morbidity, especially anxiety and depressive disorders
2. Associated with prior psychiatric illness, especially cases with less serious trauma or with less exposure
3. Acute PTSD begins within 3 months of event; delayed onset PTSD begins at least 3 months after event; chronic PTSD persists at least 3 months

ously enjoyed activities, and feelings of detachment from others. Persistent arousal responses include difficulty falling or staying asleep, exaggerated startle responses such as jumpiness in response to loud noises, and hypervigilance. For example, a woman who survived a shooting massacre described no longer being able to sit in a room with her back to the door, and another woman complained that she now involuntarily scanned for a gun in the hands of every new person entering the room. Posttraumatic symptoms qualify for a diagnosis only if they were new after the trauma or if preexisting symptoms were greatly magnified after the trauma.

In PTSD, the symptoms must result in significant distress or social impairment. Symptoms of the disorder must be present for at least 1 month for the diagnosis to be made. Subclassification according to length of illness defines acute PTSD as lasting for fewer than 3 months and chronic PTSD as lasting 3 months or more. Delayed onset PTSD is defined by the passage of at least 6 months from the traumatic event to onset of the symptoms.

Researchers studying posttraumatic syndromes are interested in traumatic responses that may be present during the first month before a diagnosis of PTSD technically can be made. Therefore the diagnosis of acute stress disorder was first introduced in DSM-IV to describe a set of symptoms that occur after the same type of traumatic event as described for PTSD but do not meet full criteria for PTSD. Criterion symptoms of acute stress disorder include dissociative symptoms, persistent reexperiencing of the event, avoidance responses, and hyperarousal. As for the diagnosis of PTSD, the symptoms must interfere with a person's usual functioning. The symptoms must last for at least 2 days, and they must occur within the first month after the event.

The character of PTSD symptoms manifests differently in different populations. The post-Vietnam syndrome involves severe and vivid flashbacks, causing its sufferers to relive the war experience with immediate intensity. Compared to survivors of civilian traumas, combat veterans more commonly report emotional numbing, amnesia, social isolation, and survivor guilt. Survivor guilt has been dropped from the PTSD criteria because of its uncommon appearance in other traumatized populations. Combat veterans in general are a special population that is characterized by male predominance, preparation with combat-readiness training, expectation of military combat experience, and exposure to trauma (combat) that was often long-lasting and repetitive. Vietnam veterans also faced the special stress of the politically charged anti-war atmosphere on their return to American society, which undoubtedly placed an added psychosocial burden on them. War veterans would be expected to show different responses to combat traumas than other populations subjected to different traumas, such as community-wide catastrophes or random and singular acts of violence in the community. Therefore not only do members of these other populations face a different type of trauma agent, but they may also have different vulnerabilities to traumatic experiences and varied coping abilities. Finally, dissociative disorders of adults who report severe childhood traumas display a different set of symptoms than do survivors of violent adult trauma (see Chapter 17).

An important clinical aspect of posttraumatic experience is the recognition that although most people briefly develop at least some psychological symptoms after catastrophic traumas, most individuals do not become psychiatrically ill. The ability for most individuals to emerge from severely catastrophic events psychologically intact bears witness to human resilience and the capacity of the mind to process and cope with extremes of traumatic experience.

Natural History

Symptoms of PTSD may begin within hours, and they usually begin within a few days of the event. Delayed onset (by definition, longer than 6 months after the trauma) of PTSD is uncommon, but cases beginning later, as much as several years, after the event have been described. A study by Helzer and colleagues of Vietnam veterans sampled from the general population found that 16% of cases had delayed onset. However, World War II veterans studied by Archibald and Tuddenham showed no evidence of delayed PTSD. A 14-year follow-up study of survivors of the Buffalo Creek dam break and flood found that 20% of all PTSD cases identified were delayed cases (that is, they met PTSD criteria at the time of the follow-up study but not at the time of the index).

PTSD symptoms typically begin to fade within weeks of the event, but their character and intensity can vary over time. Helzer and colleagues found that approximately half of the cases in the general population resolve within 6 months. A resurgence of symptoms at the 1-year anniversary of the event is characteristic and may become an annual phenomenon with diminishing intensity in subsequent years. Such anniversary reactions are thought to be further stimulated by media attention reminding people of the event.

Chronic PTSD with symptoms persisting for many years has also been described. More than one half of PTSD cases in a community study were found to persist for more than 1 year. In a study by Helzer and colleagues, one third of PTSD cases persisted for at least 3 years. Chronicity is predicted by the presence of preexisting psychiatric disorders, neuroticism, a history of early separation from parents in childhood, and a family history of anxiety or antisocial behavior. Among disaster survivors, litigation is thought to keep symptoms alive, slowing the recovery process, which apparently rebounds relatively quickly once the litigation is completed. Prisoners of war appear to have the greatest chronicity. Engdahl and colleagues found that after 40 years, more than one half (58%) of World War II prisoners of war with PTSD met the criteria for active PTSD; Sutker's group found this number to be 90%.

Differential Diagnosis (Co-Morbidity)

PTSD is differentiated from acute stress disorder in that PTSD requires the persistence of symptoms for at least 1 month, as well as a greater number of symptoms in discrete groups. The diagnosis of acute stress disorder, unlike PTSD, requires an onset of symptoms within 1 month of the traumatic event. If an individual with acute stress disorder subsequently fulfills criteria for PTSD, the diagnosis is changed from acute stress disorder to PTSD.

PTSD is differentiated from adjustment disorder by the extreme nature of the stressor (physically injurious or life-threatening) required for PTSD, compared with the stressor in adjustment disorder, which can be of any type or severity. After an extreme trauma, symptoms that do not meet criteria for PTSD, acute stress disorder, or another psychiatric disorder might be diagnosed as adjustment disorder. This diagnosis might also be made for posttraumatic symptoms occurring in response to a nonqualifying type of stressor.

Other psychiatric disorders with symptoms that can be confused with PTSD include obsessive-compulsive disorder (OCD), which has obsessions and compulsions that are recognized by the individual as inappropriate and which do not occur in response to a traumatic event, and psychotic disorders, which have hallucinations and other perceptual disturbances that must be differentiated from the characteristic flashbacks of PTSD. PTSD should be differentiated from malingering in situations in which an individual stands to gain financially or personally (for example, eligibility for disability benefits or forensic determination of criminal responsibility).

According to DSM-IV, co-morbid psychiatric disorders associated with PTSD may include panic disorder, agoraphobia, social or other phobias, OCD, major depressive disorder (MDD), somatization disorder, and substance use disorders. The manual further states that no information is available on the extent to which these co-morbid disorders may precede or follow the onset of PTSD—meaning that they may occur as additional psychopathological conditions along with PTSD after a traumatic event or that they may be predisposing conditions. Further research is needed to determine these relationships.

The disaster literature has examined psychiatric co-morbidity with PTSD in some detail. Rates of psychiatric co-morbidity with PTSD found after disasters range from approximately 20% in studies of survivors of a volcano eruption and of a plane crash into a hotel to 89% in survivors of a multiple-agent disaster setting. MDD appears to be the most common co-morbid disorder.

General population studies find that other psychiatric disorders are twice as prevalent in people who suffer from PTSD than in the rest of the population. Approximately 80% of people with PTSD are found to meet criteria for an additional diagnosis. Disorders most closely associated with PTSD in the general population are OCD, mood disorders, and substance abuse. Three fourths of people with PTSD have a preexisting personal or family history of anxiety disorder.

Further work on psychiatric co-morbidity with

PTSD has been carried out in military combat populations. Veterans with PTSD have been found to have co-morbidity rates of up to 80%. The most commonly associated psychiatric disorders in veterans with PTSD are MDD, anxiety disorders, substance abuse, and antisocial personality disorder. Prisoners of war appear to have the highest rates of co-morbidity with PTSD, with more than 90% meeting criteria for a second diagnosis.

Co-morbidity of personality disorders with PTSD has been best studied in military populations. More than two thirds of Vietnam veterans with PTSD have been found to meet criteria for a personality disorder diagnosis. It is not clear to what degree associated personality findings may represent enduring changes in personality function as a result of the trauma, as well as to what degree they may reflect preexisting psychopathological conditions in people susceptible to traumatic events and posttraumatic difficulties.

PTSD symptoms overlap considerably with symptoms of other psychiatric disorders. Sleep disturbance, one of the most common PTSD symptoms, is also one of the criterion symptoms of MDD. Loss of interest in usual activities and difficulties concentrating, which are criteria for PTSD, are also criterion symptoms of MDD. The hypervigilance of PTSD is also seen in other anxiety disorders. Amnesia and feelings of numbness and detachment described in PTSD are hallmark symptoms of dissociative disorders.

Because of the great degree of symptom overlap, the validity of the separateness of PTSD as a clinical entity has been questioned. In essence, the diagnostic criteria for PTSD are an assimilation of symptoms of the following three recognized psychiatric categories: MDD, generalized anxiety disorder (GAD), and dissociative disorders. The documented overlap of PTSD with other disorders in traumatized populations may be at least in part a function of this overlap in symptom criteria. Controversy persists as to whether PTSD belongs with the anxiety disorders or whether it is more appropriately grouped with the dissociative disorders. Even more fundamentally, however, standard procedures for validation of PTSD as a distinct diagnosis have yet to be completed.

Genetics and Family History

The genetics of PTSD are unknown. A family history study by Davidson and colleagues of 36 patients who were military veterans with chronic PTSD found evidence of psychiatric illness in two thirds (66%) of the families. Substance abuse (60%), anxiety disorders (22%), and MDD (20%) were the most prevalent disorders in families. Only 6% of families had one or more members with PTSD. The familial association of PTSD with a variety of other disorders and not with PTSD argues against the assumption that PTSD as currently defined describes a unified syndrome.

Epidemiology

Between 1% and 14% of the general population have been found to meet lifetime criteria for an episode of PTSD. The experience of violent trauma is far more prevalent than the PTSD that may follow it. Most people who have such an experience do not develop PTSD.

The population study by Breslau's group found that 39% of the population had experienced a violent traumatic event and that the most common violent trauma was a violent accident or injury (9%); physical assault was next most common (8%). A study by Norris of a community sample of 1000 adults found that a higher proportion (69%) had experienced a traumatic event, including 21% who had experienced a traumatic event in the previous year alone. Robberies (25%) and motor vehicle accidents (23%) were the most common traumas. Men were significantly more likely than women to report a traumatic event, with 74% indicating such a history.

In the Breslau study, nearly one fourth (24%) of people who had experienced a traumatic event developed PTSD in relation to it. Overall, 9% of the population was found to have experienced an episode of PTSD. The type of event most likely to be followed by PTSD was rape among women, which resulted in PTSD in 80% of the cases. A general population study by Helzer's group found lower rates of PTSD—0.5% in men and 1.3% in women. In the Norris study, the lifetime rate of PTSD was 5%.

Studies conducted in psychiatric treatment settings yield high rates of PTSD and traumatization. The majority of psychiatric outpatients (68%) and inpatients (81%) report a history of physical or sexual victimization. Drug-abusing women in treatment almost universally (99%) report a history of violent trauma, and 59% of those with trauma qualify for a diagnosis of PTSD.

Rates of PTSD after disasters vary widely according to the type of disaster agent and the population affected. Studies of tornadoes, volcanos, mudslides, floods, and dioxin contamination have yielded rates of PTSD from 2% to 8%. Higher rates of PTSD were found among survivors of a plane crash into a hotel (22%) and among victims of a shooting massacre in a Texas cafeteria (29%). Even higher rates of PTSD (44% to 54%) have been recorded in studies of survivors of a dam break and flood, bushfires, and an airplane crash-landing.

Studies of Vietnam combat veterans have identified rates of PTSD in the range of 15% to 31%. Much higher rates of PTSD have been documented in prisoners of war (50% to 78%).

Risk Factors

Specific characteristics of evocative trauma agents predict human response to them. The highest rates of psychiatric difficulties are associated with disaster agents with the most severe elements of terror (that is, threat to life or limb), horror (witness to grotesque scenes), suddenness and unexpectedness of occurrence (tornadoes and plane crashes), long duration of impact (floods continuing for months), repetitive impact (repeated crests of floods in a single season), intensity of impact (sheer numbers of lives lost and catastrophic financial damages to communities), degree of personal damages (physical injury, total destruction of a home), and grief over loss of loved ones. Disasters with the additional element of causation by human factors, particularly willful acts of terrorism (for example, bombings and shooting massacres) even more than accidents by human error, are thought to evoke more pathological human responses.

The personal attributes of those individuals exposed to traumatic events predict both exposure to traumatic events and psychiatric response. Individual vulnerability to exposure to traumatic events varies among populations and individuals. Whereas certain freak accidents, such as plane crashes into buildings, and unprecedented terrorism, such as bombings of public buildings, are virtually equal-opportunity events, many traumatic stressors target special groups with attributes that increase the likelihood of exposure. For example, people who live on flood plains because they cannot afford land on higher ground are at a greatly increased risk of experiencing a catastrophic flood. People who cannot afford to live anywhere but in poor neighborhoods are at a greater risk of victimization by criminal violence than are those who live in more affluent areas. Demographic and personal characteristics found to predict exposure to violent trauma in the community include low education, male gender, early conduct problems, and an extroverted personality style. People with psychiatric disorders—especially illicit drug use disorders, alcoholism, and antisocial personality disorder—report a history of violent trauma in excess of that in the rest of the population.

Among military populations, preservice variables have been found to predict likelihood of combat exposure. These predictors include youthfulness, less education, a history of juvenile conduct problems, and preexisting psychiatric problems. Therefore those least likely to tolerate the horrors of combat are those most likely to be placed in combat.

Persons of any age, either gender, and any race may develop PTSD. Somewhat different factors are found to predict psychiatric illness after a traumatic event than those that predict the likelihood of exposure to the event. Among populations exposed to traumatic events, the demographic characteristics of survivors can further predispose them to a psychiatric disorder after the event. After disasters, women tend to have higher rates of PTSD than men. A low socioeconomic level and lack of education may predict a greater degree of postdisaster psychopathology. Although one study found that older people are at increased risk for psychiatric problems after disasters, a number of other studies have determined that age does not predict postdisaster adjustment. Personal support networks, or at least a perception of them, are associated with improved outcome after disasters; however, one study found that women may find spousal and social support burdensome after extreme stress. After a violent trauma in the community, female gender, youth, less education, and black race have been found to predict vulnerability to developing PTSD. Among combat veterans, combat-related PTSD has been found to be associated with lower educational achievement.

In all trauma-exposed populations, preexisting psychopathological conditions have repeatedly been found to be the greatest predictor of trauma-associated psychopathology. In populations surviving major disasters, predisaster psychiatric illness strongly predicts a person's psychopathological state after the disaster, especially in low-impact disasters and among less-exposed individuals. However, with increasing disaster intensity and greater individual exposure to the disaster agent, personal vulnerability becomes less predictive; more individuals with no history of psychiatric problems succumb to the psychological impact of traumas of a catastrophic magnitude that would theoretically overwhelm even the most resilient person.

Among combat veterans, the preservice psychopathological state is similarly predictive of postwar psychiatric adjustment. Even when controlling for the degree of combat exposure, combat-related PTSD and PTSD symptoms are predicted by preservice MMPI ratings of hypochondriasis, paranoia, depression, hypomania, psychopathic deviation, social introversion, and diminished masculinity. A history of juvenile conduct symptoms was found to predict PTSD symptoms in combat veterans in a general population sample. Antisocial personality disorder in combat veterans predicts drug and alcohol abuse but not PTSD. Postwar factors have also been found to predict the psychiatric outcome of combat veterans. Greater psychiatric difficulties have been reported among soldiers who experience other negative life events and who lack social supports or networks on returning home. In community survivors of violent trauma, preexisting psychiatric disorders also predict PTSD. PTSD is associated with a history of childhood behavior problems and with preexisting neuroticism, drug abuse (particularly cocaine and opiate abuse), anxiety, and depression.

Pathophysiology

The hypothalamic-pituitary-adrenal axis is one of the main hormonal systems mediating the physiological stress response, and it is considered pivotal in the generation of PTSD symptoms. Relative to healthy controls, patients with PTSD have been found to have an elevated urinary excretion of epinephrine and norepinephrine. Additionally, urinary excretion of cortisol is decreased and the plasma adrenocorticotropic hormone level is elevated. Central nervous system (CNS) lymphocyte glucocorticoid receptors have been shown to be up-regulated in PTSD, suggesting that PTSD symptoms may be generated through a mechanism of hypersensitivity of feedback inhibition of corticosteroids in the hypothalamic-pituitary-adrenal axis system.

Combat veterans with PTSD show heightened autonomic responses, including elevated heart rate, blood pressure, and electrodermal responses. Those suffering from PTSD are hypothesized to experience continuous and repeated autonomic arousal through conditioning of a persistent startle reaction as well as through their own internally generated imagery in the form of flashbacks and intrusive recollections of the traumatic event. Persistence or nonhabituation of the autonomic response to repetitive tone stimuli has been observed in Israeli combat veterans relative to controls and is thought to support a chronic autonomic arousal model of PTSD. However, it is not clear whether this nonhabituation phenomenon might relate to antecedent constitutional risk or to an acquired abnormality from the experience of trauma. Chronic autonomic arousal in PTSD may overstimulate the hypothalamic-pituitary-adrenal–axis and lead to exhaustion of adrenal cortical function. The suppression of affective arousal described in PTSD (emotional numbing) theoretically reflects this adrenal exhaustion.

Military veterans with combat-related PTSD have been found to show increased latency and decreased amount of rapid eye movement (REM) sleep, reduced Stage IV sleep, and lowered sleep efficiency. Nightmares related to PTSD occur in various stages of non-REM sleep, further supporting the theory that PTSD is a disorder of general hyperarousal.

Van der Kolk and colleagues postulate that endogenous opioids, especially enkephalins and endorphins, play a central role in neuroendocrine mechanisms of PTSD. Disturbances in reciprocal pathways between the CNS, the noradrenergic system, and the opioid peptide system are identified as a likely source of the extremely vivid character of posttraumatic flashbacks and nightmares. A study of Vietnam veterans with PTSD documented that after viewing a disturbing videotape dramatizing combat, pain ratings to a heat stimulus were significantly lower than they were among healthy controls who also viewed the film. Experimental administration of the opioid blocker naloxone in otherwise identical conditions resulted in normalization of the pain response equivalent to that of the controls. This restoration of veterans' pain response by naloxone suggests that the PTSD-associated attenuation of the pain response after the disturbing reminder of the trauma (akin to numbing in PTSD) is mediated by opioid systems.

Magnetic resonance imaging (MRI) studies provide evidence of reduced hippocampal volumes in PTSD patients compared with matched controls, and the hippocampal volume correlates with 24-hour urinary cortisol measurement. Ongoing stress with its resultant chronic corticosteroid stimulation in PTSD is hypothesized to exert a neurotoxic effect on hippocampal structures, which is potentially a source of memory impairment found to be in association with PTSD in some studies.

The *N*-methyl-D-aspartate (NMDA) receptor is postulated to play a role in the dissociative-like aspects of PTSD. Evidence for this role is that dissociative anesthetic drugs, such as ketamine and phencyclidine (PCP), that block the excitatory amino-acid neurotransmitters glutamate and aspartate at NMDA receptors have been shown to generate dissociative symptoms such as depersonalization, distortions of body image and time perception, analgesia, and amnesia. Further evidence for the connection of dissociation with fear and arousal states of PTSD is the finding that the administration of lactate, yohimbine, or m-chlorophenylpiperazine (m-CPP) can induce flashbacks and panic-like episodes in patients with PTSD (but not healthy controls).

Treatment

Because there are no empirical studies of treatment protocols for PTSD, the physician is best guided by the collective experience and recommendations provided by anecdotal report and the general observations of physicians who have treated large numbers of cases. The first task in management of posttraumatic syndromes is to complete a full diagnostic evaluation, which often reveals the presence of one or more important co-morbid conditions. The greatest potential error is abandonment of the diagnostic investigation once the presence of PTSD has been identified. The co-morbid conditions, most often mood and anxiety disorders, substance abuse, and personality disorders, can confuse and confound treatment if they are not recognized and managed. Treatment of these disorders in the usual manner is recommended along with specific attention to the PTSD; in fact these other disorders may overshadow PTSD in clinical importance, implications for management, and determination of outcome.

The mainstay of treatment for PTSD is psychotherapy. The treatment of PTSD begins with taking the history and giving the person an opportunity to share his or her experience. Studies of disaster survivors have repeatedly found that the most common means of coping is by talking about the event. Even though recalling the event to describe it to a listener might seem intrusive and traumatic for patients with PTSD, the act of recounting the trauma may serve to reduce it to words, which are then manageable. More importantly, recounting the experience sometimes helps to wear out the shocking aspects of the experience through mental accommodation by repeated exposure to the memories. Sharing the story with an interested listener also serves to dilute the concentration of the shocking material because it expands into a larger space that includes the listener. Recounting the trauma also begins to bond the storyteller to the listener, who is enlisted as a support person in this context. However, available data are not sufficient to determine when and under what circumstances a person should be encouraged or discouraged to talk about the experience or to avoid thinking or talking about it. Traumatized individuals relying on denial and avoidance as their only coping method may find abrupt confrontation with the full impact of the memory of the event overwhelming. Therefore proceeding cautiously and not pushing against resistance when pursuing discussion of the event are recommended, especially in the early stages after a traumatic event.

Group sharing of experiences after community-wide disasters can be especially helpful. A model for crisis intervention group work designed by Mitchell involves leading a 1- to 3-hour group session for as few as four to five people or as many as 45 to 50 individuals after a traumatic event. The method involves facilitating the sharing of group members' experiences of the event, their feelings and thoughts about it as it was originally unfolding and again in later phases, and the signs and symptoms of distress that members have experienced. It also includes the education of the group about common human experiences after such events, what to expect in terms of the evolution of emotions and symptoms, instruction on how to manage trauma-related stress, and recognizing signals of distress that indicate a need for professional help. Functions of this group work include providing a vocabulary for members to describe their responses, encouragement of open sharing and cognitive processing of the experience, legitimizing and normalizing their experience, developing support for one another, providing coping and problem-solving strategies, and identifying individuals at risk for serious psychiatric problems.

One of the most important aspects of therapy for posttraumatic syndromes is reassurance and normalization of the survivors' experiences of traumas. Most survivors of traumatic events do not develop psychiatric disorders. People recovering from severe traumas can benefit from understanding that their responses to the situation, which may seem abnormal or extreme to them, are simply normal responses to an abnormal situation and that the experience they went through might be expected to make virtually anyone experience psychological discomfort. Reassurance that most people in similar situations experience at least some PTSD symptoms and that these usually fade with time is extremely helpful to individuals seeking to make sense out of their unusual experience and their reactions to it. This "road map" for survivors of extreme traumas helps guide them through this uncharted territory of life experience that is foreign to most.

Survivors of extreme events begin to heal through cognitive processing of the experience. Grotesque and horrifying aspects of a disaster experience and military combat that are not supposed to be a part of life must be assimilated into the unique personal context of each individual's private system of meaning and organization of life and existence. This process may include philosophical and spiritual dimensions that lie within the individual's particular personal and cultural framework. Resources for this process may include an individual's place of worship and educational background, which indicates potential intellectual resources and utility of available reading materials.

Psychobehavioral techniques may be useful, depending on the individual's situation and abilities. These techniques include coupling progressive muscle-relaxation with specific desensitization techniques, in which the patient begins with vivid imagination of the traumatic scene and proceeds to graded physical reintroduction to the location or situation in which the trauma occurred. Special techniques to facilitate this process may include thought-stopping procedures, use of peaceful imagery, progressive muscle-relaxation techniques, and the identification and replacement of maladaptive cognitions with rational ideas (see the Pearls & Perils box on p. 328).

Medication by itself does not by itself induce the remission of PTSD, but partial symptomatic relief can sometimes be realized through pharmaceutical agents, as reviewed by both Friedman and Epstein. Avoidance of medication altogether is often preferable in the management of posttraumatic symptoms without comorbid disorders that dictate pharmacological intervention. Oversedation by psychotropic agents may inhibit or slow the necessary cognitive processing of the experience that is necessary for healing. No particular pharmacological treatment for PTSD has been determined to be effective. However, a number of theoretical considerations have suggested the potential value of various psychopharmacological agents. For ex-

POSTTRAUMATIC STRESS DISORDER

PEARLS & PERILS

- The most critical aspect of the diagnosis of PTSD is identification of an appropriate trauma, that is, experiencing an event that caused physical injury or threat to life or limb to the individual (or witnessing a violent event or learning that a close family member experienced an acute life-threatening trauma). Nonviolent stressors such as being fired from a job and being divorced do not qualify.
- Symptoms of PTSD derive from the following three psychiatric categories: anxiety, depression, and dissociation.
- The best predictor of psychiatric illness after disasters is the preexisting psychopathological state, especially in low-impact events or among those with mild exposure to the trauma. With increasing intensity of the event and exposure to it, more individuals with no past psychiatric history are prone to postdisaster difficulties.
- When PTSD is present, co-morbid psychiatric diagnoses are common and should not be overlooked.
- An important clinical aspect of posttraumatic experience is the recognition that although most people briefly develop at least some psychological symptoms after catastrophic traumas, most individuals do not become psychiatrically ill. This information is helpful to reassure people after traumatic events and to normalize their experience as a normal response to an abnormal event.
- The most commonly used coping method after a traumatic event for people with, as well as those without, PTSD is talking about the traumatic experience with a supportive listener. No particular medication has been found to be of specific value in the treatment of PTSD, but the use of medication for symptomatic relief may occasionally be of benefit.

ample, benzodiazepines and anticonvulsants have been hypothesized as reasonable agents to control the possible kindling role in the genesis of PTSD; tricyclic antidepressant agents (TCAs) have been hypothesized to dampen hyperarousal of PTSD through antipanic mechanisms as well as through enhancement of endogenous opioids and synergism of serotoninergic mechanisms. Clonidine, an $alpha_2$ agonist, may downregulate activation of sympathetic outflow from the locus caeruleus.

Various psychotropic agents, including TCAs (such as desipramine and nortriptyline), serotonin-selective reuptake inhibitors (SSRIs) (for example, fluoxetine and paroxetine), monoamine oxidase inhibitors (MAOIs) (for example, phenelzine), benzodiazepines, propranolol, lithium, clonidine, and anticonvulsants have all been tried with limited and anecdotal success. The overlap of PTSD with depressive and anxiety disorders complicates the assessment of the specific efficacy of these agents for PTSD. Knowledge of the efficacy of pharmacotherapeutic agents for PTSD awaits methodologically adequate drug trials.

Antipsychotic agents (major tranquilizers) have been found to have no place in routine treatment of PTSD because psychosis plays no known role in posttraumatic disorders. The risk of inducing the permanent effects of an involuntary movement disorder such as tardive dyskinesia (TD) with these agents makes them unattractive alternatives. Benzodiazepines (minor tranquilizers), seemingly useful for treating anxiety while reducing the hypothesized potential for brain kindling of seizure-like psychiatric phenomena in these patients, are limited as potential choices because of their habit-forming and abuse potential, especially in this population with documented liability for substance abuse and personality problems.

Special Issues

Social and political forces in the mental health field in the 1980s increased public attention to matters of child abuse and its potential long-term effects. These forces have helped mold popular conceptualizations of posttraumatic syndromes. In this climate, popular books such as Bass and Davis' *The Courage to Heal* have identified a host of psychopathological syndromes as adult sequelae of child abuse. These materials urge therapists and patients to work together to uncover memories of childhood abuse and resolve the traumatic experience as necessary to achieving mental health. A parallel, rapidly expanding professional literature identifies chronic adult posttraumatic syndromes as a consequence of childhood abuse. Multiple personality disorder (MPD) (currently termed *dissociative identity disorder*), which has rapidly grown to epidemic proportions in the last two decades, is the leading contender of adult syndromes postulated to arise from childhood abuse. A reported history of childhood abuse in 96% to 98% of cases of MPD has led proponents of the disorder to conceptualize it as a posttraumatic disorder caused by childhood abuse. Although this is an interesting hypothesis, no empirical documentation for it exists; however, it has gained popular acceptance as the explanation for the disorder.

Terr hypothesizes that extreme childhood traumas such as victimization by terrorism and witnessing violent acts promote posttraumatic depressive and dissociative syndromes in adult life. Other writers have noted an association of childhood victimization by abuse and violence with later aggression, criminality, and arrests for violent acts. From observations such as these, theories on intergenerational perpetuation of childhood abuse and violence (the "cycle of violence") have been generated. Whereas such trauma-related theories suggest potentially attractive explanations for these phenomena, direct empirical data pertaining to the subject are sparse.

A relevant study by Mullen and colleagues has examined the relationship of childhood sexual abuse and adult mental health in women in a community sample. Although reports of childhood abuse were most prevalent among women from disrupted and dysfunctional homes and predicted several types of adult psychopathological conditions, the authors made several cautionary statements. They indicated that rather than abuse being the direct causal factor, other explanations for the association might be found. These explanations could include the possibility that sexual abuse could represent a marker for other variables that might be the operative causal factors in adult psychopathological conditions, or at least part of a broader etiological scenario.

Further analysis of the Mullin and colleagues data showed that although a report of sexual abuse predicted adult psychopathological disorders beyond what other predictive factors contributed, other problems in the childhood home life were important predictors of the sexual abuse as well as of the psychopathological state independent of the sexual abuse. This study illustrates the importance of examining all the factors together rather than restricting the focus to childhood sexual abuse as a predictor of adult psychopathological conditions in a social and environmental vacuum. Lack of attention to these principles has led to unwarranted and unsupported conclusions about dissociation and other disorders as posttraumatic syndromes with etiological roots in childhood trauma and abuse. To reiterate earlier statements, the only psychiatric disorder whose definition is etiologically based on traumatic experience is PTSD.

Conclusion

Although PTSD is a relatively new entity in official psychiatric criteria, trauma-related syndromes have been recognized for ages. Considerable work has yet to be completed to further define it, delineate it from other psychiatric syndromes, and categorize it. PTSD comprises symptoms of the following three classes of psychopathology: dissociation, anxiety, and depression.

Little systematic, data-based information on treatment is available in the published literature. No particular medication has been found to be of specific value in the treatment of PTSD. The physician is advised to search for co-morbid psychiatric disorders that are often present and to treat them in the usual manner, using medications such as antianxiety and sedative agents when necessary for symptomatic relief. A general rule is to avoid medication if possible. The general mainstay of treatment is the provision of a supportive psychotherapeutic environment for emotionally traumatized individuals to ventilate feelings; reassurance of the normalcy of their feelings and experiences after extreme events; and help working to find ways to process, cope with, and heal from the trauma. In this setting, time heals, and the physician functions to facilitate that healing.

CONSIDER CONSULTATION WHEN . . .

- A patient has experienced an extreme traumatic event with threat to life or limb (e.g., being run over by a train, kidnapped at gunpoint and multiply raped, or assaulted with intent to kill), especially with: a history of previous psychiatric problems; co-morbid psychiatric disorder such as substance abuse, depression, or anxiety disorder; inadequate social support or significant other life problems; inability to function or severe subjective emotional distress.

Annotated Bibliography

Wilson JP, Raphael B, editors: *International handbook of traumatic stress syndromes,* New York, 1993, Plenum.

This tome of more than 1000 pages is the ultimate information source on trauma-related syndromes, as well as an extremely useful handbook for clinicians and researchers. Written by the top authorities on the subject in the world, this book covers a wide range of topics, including theoretical and research methodology strategies; war trauma and civil violence; trauma from torture, detention, and internment; disaster-related syndromes; trauma syndromes in children and adolescents, including violence, incest, and transgenerational syndromes; dissociative disorders; intervention strategies; and social policy.

Ursano RJ, McCaughey BG, Fullerton CS, editors: *Individual and community responses to trauma and disaster: the structure of human chaos,* Cambridge, 1994, Cambridge University Press.

This comprehensive and scholarly volume, written by an international collection of leading researchers in the field, covers the entire range of extreme traumas and disasters: technological, natural, and manmade. Empirical studies and observational reports, as well as practical clinical methods of debriefing victims and helpers and providing psychological relief, are presented.

Lystad M, editor: *Mental health response to mass emergencies: theory and practice,* New York, 1988, Brunner/Mazel.

This text is a volume of a "refereed" book series, ensuring the highest academic quality of its content. An internationally respected field of researchers has provided contributions to this readable text that covers individual and community responses to disaster, social and clinical intervention programs, and public/education/planning programs with practical material that can be directly implemented in communities.

Allen RD, editor: *Handbook of post-disaster interventions,* Corte Madera, Calif., 1993, Select Press. (A Special Issue of the *Journal of Social Behavior and Personality* 8(5):1993.)

This practical handbook was written for three audiences: clinicians responding to disaster survivors, organizers of a mental health response following a disaster, and researchers interested in the field of trauma and disasters. It contains useful information on the treatment of psychological trauma for clinicians, strategies and issues for designing a community disaster response, and a review of the academic literature on the subject of disasters.

Journal of Traumatic Stress, New York, Plenum Press.

This journal of the International Society for Traumatic Stress Studies, and edited by BL Green, is an interdisciplinary forum for the publication of peer-reviewed original academic papers on the biopsychosocial aspects of trauma. Issues included are theory, research, treatment, prevention, education/training, and legal and policy concerns. Its topics include war, disaster, accident, violence or abuse, hostage-taking, and life-threatening illness. Published monthly, this journal is aimed as a primary reference for professionals who study and treat people exposed to extreme human traumas.

section three

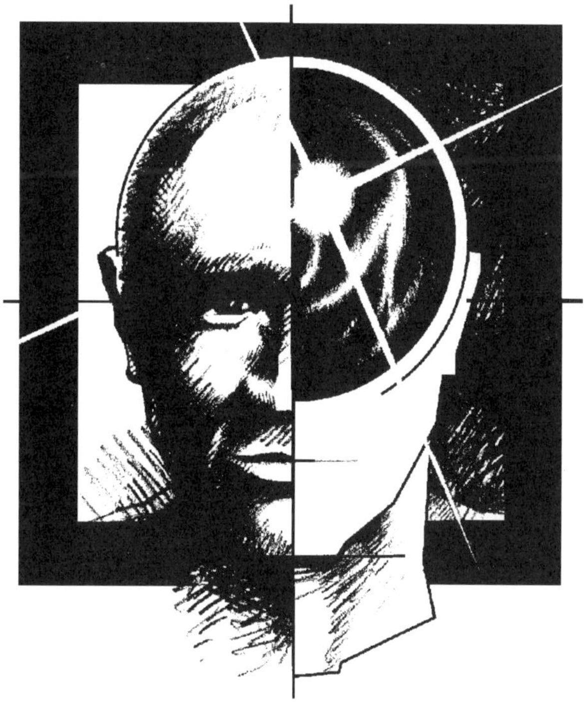

Important Topics in Clinical Medicine

Charles F. Zorumski, MD

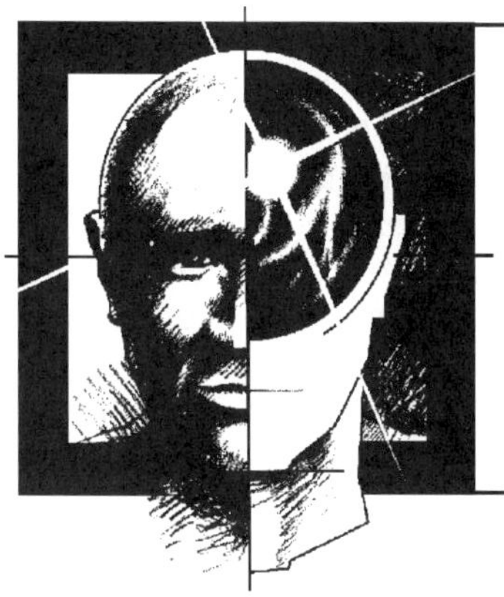

chapter 20

Psychotherapy

Samuel B. Guze, MD and Richard D. Wetzel, PhD

What is psychotherapy? What are its possible forms? What are the theoretical foundations of the different forms? How beneficial is it, and what are its risks and side effects?

As is often the case when considering vague but complex concepts, definitions offered in dictionaries leave the reader with general notions at best. The twenty-eighth edition of *Dorland's Illustrated Medical Dictionary* provides the following definition: "treatment of mental disorders and behavioral disturbances using such psychological techniques as support, suggestion, persuasion, reeducation, reassurance, and insight in order to alter maladaptive patterns of coping and to encourage personality growth."

The third edition of the *American Heritage Dictionary of the English Language* offers, "treatment of mental and emotional disorders through the use of psychological techniques designed to encourage communication of conflicts and insight into problems, with the goal being personality growth and behavior modification."

The second edition of the *Oxford English Dictionary* (OED) proposes, "treatment of disease by 'psychic' methods. In mod. use, the treatment of disorders of the mind or personality by psychological or psychophysiological methods." The OED cites 1853 as the date of the first recorded use of the term.

Relating to the Patient

A brief review of standard textbooks of psychiatry reveals equally general definitions coupled with discussions of the various types of psychotherapy and some suggestions as to how to proceed in carrying out such treatments. Even though psychotherapy is difficult to define, almost all schools of psychotherapy recognize that the physician-patient relationship is central both to the practice of medicine and to the practice of psychotherapy. The first task in psychotherapy is to understand, develop, and maintain the relationship with the patient. This relationship is an important tool in any physician's armamentarium.

The physician, especially the physician with ongoing responsibility for the patient, can and ought to play an important role in providing a psychotherapeutic relationship, whether the patient's illness is cancer, stroke, arthritis, depression, panic attacks, acquired immunodeficiency syndrome (AIDS), diabetes, tuberculosis, or epilepsy. In fact, any patient confronting an illness associated with chronic or recurrent pain, disability, or early death must be considered a candidate for psychotherapy.

Psychotherapy nearly always implies important and personal communication with the patient. The patient must come to believe that the physician is genuinely sympathetic and interested in helping the patient understand his medical condition (when there is one) and overall situation. The patient must develop confidence that the physician respects the patient's personhood and sympathizes with his symptoms, suffering, and relevant experiences. Patients are likely to come to such conclusions by the therapist's action and communication.

Psychotherapeutic interaction with patients depends on showing sympathy, respect, patience, and interest. The patient's concerns, worries, fears, and other difficulties must guide the interaction. Psychotherapeutic communication requires much careful and attentive listening. In general, the patient should be doing most (but not all) of the talking if the exchange is to be maximally useful and therapeutic. The patient must be encouraged to talk more, steadily providing more information. "Tell me more," "And then what happened?," "How did you feel?," and "What did you do or say?" are a few examples of therapist responses designed to show that the interviewer really is interested in what the patient has to report or say. These responses elicit more information and indicate to the patient that the process involves serious participation from the patient.

In addition to encouraging questions, the physician may offer comments such as, "You were upset," "You sound angry even now," "You sound hurt," "I wonder if you showed that you were upset (angry, hurt)", and "I wonder how much it still troubles you." Such comments make it clear to patients that it is proper to consider their feelings and to try to describe them as well as possible. Patient responses can then be moved along by returning to the basic requests of, "Tell me more about that," and "I'd like to understand that better."

Some patients may have difficulty responding. When this is the case, the patient may be told, "You seem to find it hard to talk about such things," or "Are you aware that it is not easy for you to talk about these feelings?" The specific words or phrases are not what is important. Asking simple straightforward questions, pointing out fairly obvious observations, or making relatively obvious inferences help the patient continue talking and thinking about his experiences. If the patient can be encouraged to talk about feelings, troubles, worries, or fears, progress is being made.

As the patient talks more openly and freely, the physician can try to tie together what the patient says with the presenting problem. For example, the physician may say, "I wonder if you see any connection between what we have just talked about and what brought you to see me." If the patient offers some relevant observations, the physician can suggest, "This is worth more discussion and thinking." Again, the goal is to encourage the patient to talk about feelings, experiences, and circumstances that are relevant to the clinical problem and to the patient's ways of coping with the disorder and its associated difficulties.

At an appropriate time and in the hope that the patient will be helped to cope more optimally, the physician can suggest that the patient's illness is causing problems that might benefit from some discussions. Once more, the exact language is not important. The aim is to make clear that the physician is interested in the patient's concerns and circumstances and wants to be helpful. All patients appreciate such interest. Patients interpret the physician's interest as evidence that the physician cares and recognizes the human being involved in the illness. Even patients who are not certain that such discussions make sense usually respond favorably to the physician's interest if an adequate relationship has been established. In any case, increased trust, confidence, and hope are often the result of such strategies. Expression of interest in and concern for the patient can never be delegated successfully to another person or associate of the physician.

Dealing with the Patient's Illness

When the therapeutic relationship is adequately developed and working well, the focus usually turns naturally to educating the patient and clarifying the patient's understanding of the illness or related problems. The patient's temperament and personality and their impact on the patient's reaction to the illness and treatment are also a central focus of the psychotherapeutic program. The discussion generally deals with the patient's attitudes, coping style, important relationships, and life circumstances, since these factors interact with the patient's illness and course.

Again, this requires the patient to have confidence and trust the physician. Such confidence and trust are strengthened by the way the physician interacts with the patient in all spheres. The psychotherapeutic relationship requires from the physician a supportive, encouraging, and sympathetic approach that communicates a desire and willingness to respect the patient's concerns and needs.

The psychotherapeutic relationship permits the physician to make observations and suggestions that may be uncomfortable or even unwanted by the patient at times. Usually, patients can tolerate and accept such communications when the relationship is properly established. Furthermore, the proper psychotherapeutic relationship permits the patient to disagree with the physician in a way that fosters further exploration and greater mutual understanding. The goal is always to help the patient understand as much as possible about the illness or other problems and about the patient's ways of interpreting and dealing with these.

It should now be clear that psychotherapy can and should be part of an appropriate treatment plan in patients whose clinical problems warrant the time and effort. In this light, psychotherapy is a process rather than a thing. It is a process designed to establish and cultivate the right kind of therapeutic relationship. It includes important educational and learning goals. As already indicated, these should be seen as means to help the patient understand his medical or psychiatric problem in a context of individual and social circumstances, family and other personal relationships, and individual temperament and personality. Because the physician is uniquely qualified to understand the disease processes in his area of specialization, the treatments involved, and the usual reactions of patients to the illness and its treatment, it is unlikely that the physician can find someone else better qualified to help the patients understand and deal with these problems.

Within this context of care, concern, patient support, and education, any empirically validated approach to curing, improving, or ameliorating the patient's illness, concerns, or life fits easily, whether the approach is psychotherapeutic or pharmacological. It can also be readily seen that the process of psychotherapy, as described so far, should never be reserved solely for the psychiatric physician.

Dealing with the Patient's Life

Since patients, like physicians, are complex human beings, they come with problems other than their relationship with their physician and the burdens of their illness. A patient's job, economic situation, marriage, family, school, and other problems can absorb the time and energy the patient needs to deal with her illness. It is well accepted that stress can exacerbate (but not usually cause) an existing medical or psychiatric problem. The caring physician, sensitive to the additional life burden imposed by such problems, can offer simple counsel or referral to appropriate sources of help for these nonmedical problems. When patients do better, their illnesses often do better as well. This is the situation in which referral to psychologists or other nonmedical professionals is most likely to help the patient and the physician.

Psychotherapy as Rehabilitation

This concept of psychotherapy and the way it is carried out has been termed *rehabilitative psychotherapy* because it is based on certain fundamental principles in rehabilitation medicine. As in much of rehabilitation medicine, the focus is less on etiology and more on disability. In most treatment programs in rehabilitation medicine, the emphasis is not on how the injury or disability was caused but on the nature and severity of the disability and on the individual's personality and temperament, since these factors affect the patient's energy, motivation, flexibility, and cooperation. Clearly, the approach to psychotherapy advocated here is similar; it is not primarily focused on etiology, which is still largely unknown in psychiatry and psychology, but on helping the patient cope with disability and on increasing self-confidence and skill in achieving optimal solutions to clinical and life problems.

Other Views of Psychotherapy

Psychotherapy as an Investigative Tool in Psychiatry

Even though the term itself and the general concepts associated with psychotherapy were in use before Freud and were often associated with discussions about the use of hypnosis, it is to psychoanalytic practice and theory that physicians must turn to understand the development of certain kinds of thinking and practice concerning psychotherapy. Freud believed and taught that the analytic method was a procedure capable of advancing the scientific understanding of personality and psychiatric disorder. With some modifications, many psychiatrists and psychologists believe this. Obviously psychotherapy is used by only a few therapists to the extent that it is considered an investigative tool in psychiatry.

The Psychodynamic Model in Psychiatry and Psychology

Since Freud and the advent of psychoanalysis, practitioners in the psychodynamic tradition have been guided by the conviction that dynamic psychotherapy deals with unconscious psychological forces crystallized during early development. These are centrally responsible for many or all psychopathological conditions. Psychopathology, according to this model, represents an adjustment or compromise between instinctive drives, personality needs, defenses, and the environment. Many would add the family genetic background to this mix. In other words, psychodynamic psychotherapy has been understood to be directed at identifying and correcting the mechanisms that were thought to be formed by the original etiological factors that lead to or maintain the current psychiatric or psychological problems.

Thus psychodynamic psychotherapy in its varied permutations reflects a set of related beliefs concerning the central causes of psychopathology. Crucial to these beliefs is the concept of defenses, particularly repression, emphasized by Freud. Repression in this context refers to the hypothesis of motivated unconscious forgetting. The presumption is that a fundamental psychological process for forgetting painful and frightening memories exists in at least some humans. It is argued that this unconscious process is called into action to protect the individual from the associated fear, guilt, other unacceptable emotion, or unwanted social consequences of fully experienced emotion. Whereas the repression may leave the individual without any memory of the repressed experience, it is often not entirely complete and the individual experiences a variety of psychopathological disturbances.

However, it must be understood that little evidence exists from systematic controlled studies to support the concept of repression except from the clinical reports of psychotherapists who accept the idea to begin with. The absence of credible scientific evidence for the existence of repression is not hard to understand. Studies designed to eliminate or minimize the effects of therapists' suggestions to patients are almost impossible to implement. To start with, it would be considered unethical to expose patients or other subjects to experiments involving the serious inculcation of different and perhaps contrasting beliefs about their early experiences and relating the beliefs to current symptoms or illnesses. Additionally, it would be hard to accept the idea that a skeptical therapist in a controlled study would perform the same way as a therapist convinced about the role of repression and unconscious dynamics. It would also be difficult, if not impossible, to match and select experimental and control subjects in terms of their previous knowledge about and acceptance of dynamic psychology and psychiatry, since these ideas are widespread and believed by many people to be scientifically established.

According to some experts, laboratory experiments carried out under controlled laboratory situations by psychologists interested in the retention and loss of memories, which have generally failed to uncover evidence in favor of repression, may suffer from the difficulty of generating the level of sustained emotional involvement in their experimental subjects that is seen regularly in clinical situations where patients are suffering from a range of distressing and disabling emotional disturbances. Others find this concern of little import.

The absence of satisfactory evidence supporting the existence of dynamic repression does not prove that the hypothesis is invalid, but it does mean that a reasonable level of skepticism is called for in approaching the subject. The widespread epidemic in the United States of the often-correlated phenomena of recovered memories of childhood sexual abuse, reports of satanic ritual abuse, multiple personality disorder, and other "dissociative" phenomena (all of which depend on dynamic repression as the central explanation) may attest to the consequences of uncritical acceptance of what remains an unproven and probably unprovable concept. However, popular fads may not depend on the belief systems of mental health professionals alone.

Psychotherapy based on the belief that the causes of psychiatric disorders are known and can be found in the unconscious psychological residues of early development and experience can be characterized as etiology-directed. Such psychotherapy assumes that these psychological processes are to be recognized and confirmed by exploring free associations, dreams, symptoms, projective tests, and transference phenomena (the belief that the patient's reactions to the physician reflect unconscious tendencies to transfer repressed feelings and attitudes from childhood to a substitute for the patient's parents or other close relatives). Some modifications of traditional psychodynamic psychotherapy are still based on the same beliefs concerning etiology, but they also reflect efforts to shorten the process or to compensate for the inability to apply the full process because of limited time and money or because the illness is too severe to hope that psychotherapy will be successful. These modifications (ego psychology) focus on the assets or strengths the patient brings to the situation and try to increase coping ability, frustration tolerance, and similar aspects. To this extent, such modifications are less driven by assumptions about etiology and more by the rehabilitation model a physician espouses.

As noted, considerable widespread disagreement exists about the evidence for these psychodynamic theories and practices. Many experienced and thoughtful individuals are skeptical about the validity of the formulations and interpretations derived from efforts to plumb the "dynamic unconscious" with the associated causal ideas that are closely linked to the basic concept.

Assumptions that the causes of a psychiatric disorder are well known and adequately understood are not confined to psychoanalytically oriented psychotherapists. Such overconfidence can also easily be found in some cognitive therapists, rational-emotive therapists, and in biomedically oriented psychiatrists.

In other words, nonetiologically based rehabilitation psychotherapy is predicated on the belief that patients can often benefit from frank discussions with the physician about anything of importance to the patient. Most of the doubters prefer the belief that the etiology of most psychiatric disorders is unknown or imperfectly understood, although they believe or hope that extensive genetic, epidemiological, and neurobiological research is beginning to point to potential causal factors.

However, many of these skeptics recognize that some psychotherapeutic strategies are often helpful in treating a wide range of clinical problems. A number of psychotherapeutic approaches have been suggested and implemented that do not depend on any unproven theories of etiology. These approaches are based on the goals of helping patients understand their disorders better and improving their abilities to cope more effectively with the consequences of their conditions and associated disability.

Psychotherapy need not be based on any specific causal hypothesis to recognize and work with certain widely accepted assumptions about people in pain, in distress, fearful about their futures, or contemplating serious disability or early death. Nearly all such people can benefit from the opportunity to review, consider, and discuss what is happening to them with an individual whom they trust and in whom they place confidence. Such discussions should be meant to clarify patients' understanding of their conditions and situations, help them acknowledge and express their emotions and feelings, and explore various ways of coping better. When such discussions are properly carried out, they often provide important emotional support, stimulate greater confidence in a patient's ability to manage optimally, and convey a sense that a patient is not entirely alone in dealing with the particular problems she is confronting.

Ideally, nonetiologically directed psychotherapy should be an integral part of the strategy for treating all patients. In fact, all interaction with the patient should be carried out within a psychotherapeutic framework. Eliciting the initial history and continued elaboration of the history, conducting repeated and ongoing evaluations of the patient's mental status, explaining the illness and the elements of the treatment, and discussing possible complications and prognosis all offer rich opportunities for helpful psychotherapeutic intervention.

Problematic Practices Related to Psychotherapy

The widespread practice in most managed care systems of assigning responsibility for psychotherapy to another mental health professional, most often a social worker or counsellor, appears to be derived from a number of assumptions, possibly erroneous, about psychotherapy.

Instead of understanding psychotherapy as an integral part in the treatment of many patients that is to be interwoven with the other elements of care, it is conceptualized as a separate and distinct therapeutic effort designed to cure the patient ultimately or to do whatever can be done to achieve the goal within a defined number of visits.

Since there is so little evidence to support such a concept, the practice appears to be irrational. It separates the care of the patient into two different realms—one for the consideration of physical phenomena and the other for psychological phenomena. In fact, since in many managed care programs the mental health component is "carved out" (meaning that professionals in different organizations and systems are involved in the care of the individual patient), the worst of the Cartesian distinction between mind and body is revealed; professionals in the separate systems often do not know one another, do not professionally interact except for a rare telephone call, and often have widely divergent views about the patient. Hardly anyone knowledgeable considers such an arrangement desirable or truly defensible.

There is nothing quite comparable to this approach to patient care elsewhere in medicine. No other clinical field has been subjected to such carve-outs in which the responsible physician, in this case the psychiatrist, has as little overall responsibility for what is being done with the patient. The point being made here is not that other mental health professionals have no important role to play in the care of many patients. Quite the contrary: such professionals can be helpful but not by practicing independently of the responsible physician.

In an optimally organized arrangement, many patients require only a brief consultation with a psychiatrist and can then be referred to a psychologist, social worker, nurse, or other professional. Such patients might include those with marital problems, dissatisfaction at work, problems coping with parents, interpersonal conflicts, or other similar problems. In each case, the psychiatrist's initial responsibility includes ascertaining whether such problems are associated with recognizable psychiatric disorders. If such an association exists, the psychiatrist considers the appropriateness of treating the patient personally rather than referring the patient to a nonpsychiatric colleague. If the problem does appear to be linked to a psychiatric disorder but affects a medical disorder, such a referral might be in order. Of course, the psychiatrist should remain in touch with the colleague to be sure that the patient in fact did not have an associated psychiatric condition that had not been recognized earlier.

Sometimes, even in the presence of a diagnosable psychiatric disorder, referral to a nonpsychiatric colleague might be appropriate, especially if the psychiatrist concludes that medication is not indicated for a patient. However, in all cases the psychiatrist should continue to monitor the patient's course and response to treatment. This could often be handled by brief discussions with the other colleague, but it might sometimes warrant another face-to-face encounter with the patient and even the patient's family.

Because of the impact of psychoanalysis, many people (including a large percentage of psychotherapists) think of psychotherapy as a specific form of treatment, akin to surgery or medication, to be administered by experts trained to carry out the arcane procedures. Psychotherapy is not recognized as appropriate and helpful primarily as part of a comprehensive and integrated approach to the care of certain patients. It is not entirely surprising, then, to see managed care arrangements in which providing psychotherapy is approached in the same way that other specific interventions are approached. Thus physicians have the current situation in which specialists in psychotherapy are provided along with other specialists. These psychotherapy specialists (predominantly social workers and counselors) are defined as parallel to other medical specialists, with responsibility for providing a specific intervention independent from other interventions and typically without any real coordination or oversight by any knowledgeable physician.

The thinking behind these arrangements, in addition to basic cost considerations, is that if psychotherapy is considered important, it should be provided just as laboratory, x-ray, or other technical services are provided. However, unlike the situation with these other services, psychotherapy is provided without recognizing or appreciating the need for an integrated approach to care at the level of the individual patient with a particular set of clinical problems. In medicine this vital coordination is generally provided by the responsible physician (most often a primary care physician). When it comes to patients with psychiatric problems, especially disabling problems, such responsibility and oversight should be coordinated by a psychiatrist, but it seems generally totally absent or minimal in most managed care systems.

It is likely that this failure reflects an antecedent failure to understand and appreciate the validity of psychiatric illness. Even in the face of strong financial pressures, it seems unlikely that the present dominant arrangement for the care of psychiatrically ill patients would have spread as it has unless those in charge disparage the suffering and disability associated with significant psychiatric illness. If a physician does not take psychiatric disorders seriously, she is unlikely to devise a system for providing care that is appropriate.

At the same time, the present dominant arrangement is predicated to a considerable degree on the scientifically unsubstantiated view that psychotherapy offers the hope of identifying etiological factors responsible for the presenting psychopathological problem.

It is a curious combination of ideas; psychiatric disorders are not too serious, so too much money should not be spent treating them (specifically, the best-trained and most experienced professional, the psychiatrist, should not be used except in the most limited circumstances). At the same time, efforts to discover the causes of the psychiatric condition should be emphasized through psychotherapy that is largely provided by people whose scientific training and clinical experience has been quite limited.

In other words, psychotherapy for patients with significant psychiatric illness should be part of an integrated clinical approach with a psychiatrist responsible for overseeing the entire intervention. When a primary care physician has had appropriate training, the oversight might be that of the primary physician. Psychotherapy independent of diagnostic evaluation and reevaluation or of other therapeutic interventions such as drugs, electroconvulsive therapy (ECT), diet, and physical rehabilitation represents a sad retreat from the comprehensive strategy called for in the care of patients with chronic, recurrent, painful, or disabling disorders.

As discussed, psychotherapy provided under a psychiatric or mental health carve-out arrangement in which there is little useful and effective communication between the psychotherapist and the rest of the medical team is usually suboptimal and often more costly than necessary. Independent psychotherapists typically see patients as much and as often as the plan permits. A physician using such psychotherapy guided by the psychodynamic tradition can always find much to talk about in any patient. Therefore the natural tendency is to provide as much psychotherapy as the plan permits. Thus there is a serious question as to whether such carve-out arrangements are really cheaper, in addition to the question about their theoretical justification.

Another issue relevant to psychotherapy is the meaning of illness. For some patients and some psychotherapists, this is an important aspect of psychotherapy. These individuals are predisposed to search for and often find meaning in all important life experiences, including illnesses. Typically, efforts to give meaning to illness or other suffering involve plausible stories that may be independent of scientific validity. These stories or interpretations during psychotherapy occasionally may seem to be helpful to the patient, even when they clearly have no scientific basis. However, it must be clearly recognized that such meaning is quite different from what physicians have always understood by etiology (see the Pearls & Perils box to the right).

PEARLS & PERILS

PSYCHOTHERAPY

- The first task in psychotherapy is to understand, develop, and maintain the relationship with the patient.
- Psychotherapeutic communication requires a lot of careful and attentive listening.
- The goal is to help the patient understand as much as possible about the illness or other problems and about his ways of interpreting and dealing with these.
- Rehabilitative psychotherapy focuses less on etiology, which is still largely unknown, and more on disability. The emphasis is on helping the patient cope with the disability and increase self-confidence and skill in achieving optimal solutions to clinical and life problems.
- Many skeptics recognize that some psychotherapeutic strategies are often helpful. However, assumptions that the causes of psychiatric disorders are known and understood are not confined to psychodynamically oriented psychotherapists.

Conclusion

Psychotherapy can provide much needed emotional support, the chance to discuss and understand one's self better, an opportunity to consider the meaning of one's illness and related experiences, a safe and protected situation in which to explore various options and possibilities that take into consideration one's personal attributes and circumstances, and a special environment in which frustrations and anger may be freely expressed. The psychotherapeutic process can also lead to hypotheses about etiology, but it does not allow for the critical testing of such hypotheses. Psychotherapy offers no way to control for the preexisting assumptions of the therapist or the patient, nor for the effect on the patient's communications of the therapist's interpretations and suggestions. And, significantly, the psychotherapeutic process does not allow one to determine the causal relationships between phenomena of interest considered during psychotherapy and the patient's clinical problems. Nevertheless, psychotherapy, especially when based upon a rehabilitation strategy, is fully compatible with the medical model. Only those who believe that psychotherapy is the best path to identifying etiology are likely to object seriously to the basic arguments presented here (Guze 1992).

Annotated Bibliography

Guze SB: Psychotherapy and the etiology of psychiatric disorders, *Psychiatr Dev* 3:183-193, 1988.

Guze SB: *Why psychiatry is a branch of medicine,* New York, 1992, Oxford University Press.

Guze SB, Murphy GE: An empirical approach to psychotherapy: the agnostic position, *Am J Psychiatry* 120:53-57, 1963.

The above three references provide a fuller consideration of the concepts underlying the medical model for psychiatry and the basis for rehabilitative psychotherapy.

Spence DP: *Narrative truth and historical truth,* New York, 1982, W.W. Norton and Company.

This is a clear discussion of the problems inherent in all psychotherapeutic interpretation.

Sulloway FJ: *Freud, biologist of the mind,* New York, 1979, Basic Books.

This is an excellent history and critique of psychoanalytic thought and practice.

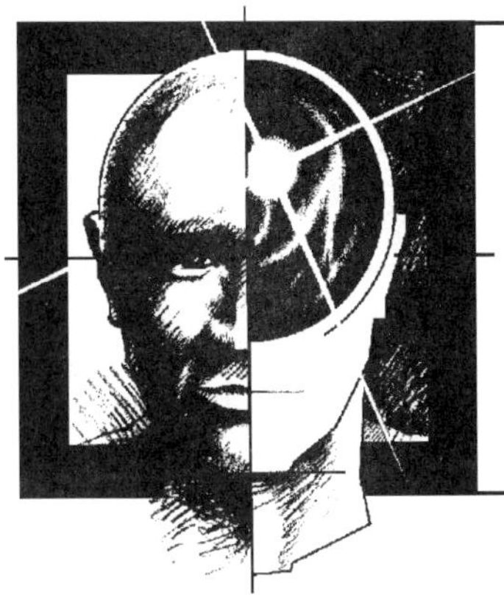

chapter 21

Pharmacotherapy

John G. Csernansky, MD

Most of the major classes of psychotropic drugs used today were discovered through serendipity in the 1950s and 1960s. For example, the monoamine oxidase inhibitor antidepressants (MAOIs) were discovered when the "activating" effects of iproniazid, a prototype MAOI, were noticed in patients being treated for tuberculosis. Until recently, new members of each major psychotropic drug class were highly similar (that is, "me-too drugs"), developed by making slight modifications to the chemical structures of the original drugs. Too little was known about the underlying causes or physiology of severe mental disorders to permit more innovative approaches to drug development.

Psychotropic drug development is now surging forward because of two new innovations. First, new drugs are being designed by targeting particular neurotransmitter receptors or other proteins (for example, monoamine transporters) that are hypothesized to be related to the pathophysiology of severe mental disorders. Second, an increasing number of neurotransmitter receptors and other proteins have been discovered by molecular biologists using cloning techniques, thereby providing new targets for drug action. In addition to these new approaches, psychotropic drugs continue to be discovered by empirical observation—for example, the anticonvulsants for the treatment of patients with bipolar disorder. Thus a variety of new drugs have become available for the treatment of patients with psychotic, affective, and anxiety disorders that are substantially different from the classic drugs developed in the 1950s and 1960s. These drugs include clozapine and risperidone for the treatment of schizophrenia; carbamazepine and valproate for the treatment of bipolar disorder; fluoxetine, sertraline, and paroxetine for the treatment of depression; and clomipramine and fluvoxamine for the treatment of obsessive-compulsive disorder (OCD). For the first time since the discovery of the original psychotropic drugs, physicians must choose from among drugs with substantive differences in efficacy and side effects to treat their patients.

In this chapter, the clinical characteristics of the major classes of psychotherapeutic drugs are reviewed, and guidelines for drug use and for evaluating the scientific literature in this area are provided. Detailed discussions of the pharmacokinetics and pharmacodynamics of psychotherapeutic drugs can be found in other texts.

Major Classes of Psychotherapeutic Drugs

Antidepressants

Contrary to some popular beliefs, antidepressant drugs are not stimulants. They only relieve symptoms of depression in patients whose moods are disordered. In other individuals, they have no perceptable effects other than their side effects (such as sedation). The efficacy of antidepressant drugs has been best demonstrated for individuals with major depressive disorder (MDD). The symptoms of MDD have been summarized in Chapter 8 and include low mood, hopelessness, guilt, suicidal thoughts, insomnia, loss of appetite and weight, and loss of sex drive. These symptoms gradually remit during treatment, usually after a delay of 1 to 2 weeks. Among patients with MDD, approximately two thirds respond to antidepressant drugs. MDD can be successfully treated with antidepressant drugs whether it occurs in patients with unipolar or bipolar mood disorder. Attempts have been made to treat other mood disorders with antidepressant drugs, but in these cases the efficacy of treatment is much less certain. These other disorders include minor depressive disorder, dysphoria associated with some personality disorders, and cyclothymia.

There are three major classes of antidepressant drugs (Table 21-1). Tricyclic antidepressants (TCAs) (including imipramine, amitriptyline, desipramine, and nortriptyline), MAOIs (for example, phenelzine and tranylcypromine) and serotonin-selective reuptake inhibitors (SSRIs) (such as fluoxetine, sertraline, paroxetine, and fluvoxamine). Additionally some individual drugs are difficult to classify (for example, trazodone and bupropion) and have been labelled heterocyclics. These groups of drugs have equivalent efficacy but are distinguishable by their side effects. The side effects of TCAs derive from the following three major mechanisms: (1) muscarinic cholinergic receptor blockade, (2) α_1-adrenergic receptor blockade, and (3) quinidine-like effects on cardiac conduction. In the case of the anticholinergic effects of the TCAs, dry mouth, blurry vision, constipation, urinary hesitancy, and sedation are common and occur in a dose-dependent fashion. Blockage of α_1-adrenergic receptors can cause problematic hypotension, which can then lead to faintings

TABLE 21-1

ANTIDEPRESSANT DRUGS

Drug (generic name)	Recommended doses (mg/day)	Recommended blood level (as noted)	Half-life (hours)
Tricyclic antidepressants			
Amitriptyline (AMI)	75-200	AMI + NTP > 200 ng/ml	30-46
Clomipramine	150-300		22-80
Desipramine (DMI)	75-200	>150 ng/ml	14-40
Doxepin	75-300		8-24
Imipramine (IMI)	75-200	IMI + DMI > 180 ng/ml	8-24
Nortriptyline (NTP)	75-150	75-150 ng/ml	18-80
Protriptyline	20-40	70-170 ng/ml	50-140
Serotonin-selective reuptake inhibitors			
Fluoxetine	10-60		24-100
Fluvoxamine	100-300		12-18
Nefazodone	300-600		2-4
Paroxetine	20-40		18-24
Sertraline	50-150		20-26
Trazodone	150-600		4-8
Monoamine oxidase inhibitors			
Pargyline	75-150		
Phenelzine	45-75 (calculate dose by body weight: 1 mg/kg)		
Selegiline	5-10		
Tranylcypromine	10-30		
Other			
Bupropion	15-300		10-16

and falls. MAOIs can also commonly cause hypotension. However, when foods or other drugs containing tyramine or adrenergic agonists are consumed along with an MAOI, sudden and severe hypertension can occur (that is, hypertensive crisis). The classic MAOIs are irreversible and nonselective with respect to the isoenzyme of monoamine oxidase inhibited. More recently developed drugs are selective (for the monoamine-oxidase A isozyme) and reversible inhibitors of monoamine oxidase (for example, meclobamide). These selective MAOIs appear to have fewer and less severe side effects. The SSRIs are the best tolerated of all antidepressants, and they are surprisingly safe even in overdose. Their side effects are nausea, headache, insomnia, agitation, and sexual dysfunction (for example, delayed orgasm), attributable in all likelihood to their serotonin-enhancing actions.

There is no simple explanation for the approximate one third of patients who do not respond to antidepressant drugs. In some cases, the dose of drug and duration of treatment have been inadequate. However, when this is not the explanation, there is usually no other that can be found. The efficacy of antidepressant drugs has been variously enhanced by adding lithium, thyroid hormone, and more recently, the anxiolytic, buspirone. However, when drug therapy fails, electroconvulsive therapy (ECT) should be tried (see Chapter 22).

The approach to drug treatment of depression has thus far been focused on presynaptic mechanisms. That is, TCAs and SSRIs block the reuptake of biogenic amines (such as serotonin and norepinephrine) into the presynaptic terminals where they are ordinarily destroyed. In the case of the MAOIs, monoamine reuptake is not blocked, but metabolism of the amine by monoamine oxidase after reuptake into the presynaptic terminal is prevented, thus spilling the monoamine back out into the synaptic cleft. Additionally, chronic treatment with many of these drugs decreases the functioning of inhibitory presynaptic autoreceptors, which variously slow monoamine synthesis and release, as well as the firing rate of the cell. In all cases, the net effect of treatment appears to be an increase in the rate of monoamine transmission, and among the monoamines, changes in serotonin transmission appear to be most essential.

Development of new antidepressants drugs is turning to postsynaptic mechanisms. For example, some antagonists (such as trazadone and nefazodone) at postsynaptic serotonin receptors ($5\text{-}HT_{2a}$ and $5\text{-}HT_{2c}$) appear to have antidepressant efficacy. Perhaps mixtures of drugs acting on both presynaptic and postsynaptic mechanisms will soon be used to increase efficacy and expand the type and number of patients successfully treated.

Anxiolytics

Benzodiazepines are the most commonly prescribed anxiolytic drugs in the United States (Table 21-2). They are far safer and less likely to cause physical tolerance than the barbiturates and meprobamate, which they have replaced. Benzodiazepines act by binding to specific sites on the γ-aminobutyric acid (GABA) receptor-chloride channel macromolecular complex and thereby enhance the actions of that inhibitory transmitter. These drugs have a variety of effects in addition to anxiolysis, including sedation, muscle relaxation, and seizure inhibition. From the point of view of this chapter, these other actions may be considered side effects; however, benzodiazepines are used as hypnotics, muscle relaxants, and anticonvulsants in other settings. Recently, drugs such as zolpidem and buspirone, which are distinct from the benzodiazepines, have been developed. Zolpidem binds to specific subtypes of benzodiazepine sites on the GABA receptor-chloride channel macromolecular complex, and buspirone acts as a partial serotonin-autoreceptor ($5\text{-}HT_{1a}$) agonist.

Anxiety has been experienced by all people. In some individuals, anxiety is only transient, but it is of such severe intensity that treatment with a drug is indicated. In others, anxiety along with other symptoms becomes a chronic problem and necessitates treatment. DSM-IV lists a variety of such anxiety disorders, including generalized anxiety disorder (GAD) and panic disorder. However, anxiolytics are prescribed much more often for anxiety as a single symptom than for one of these DSM-IV anxiety disorders.

As mentioned, sedation is a common side effect of the benzodiazepines. The fact that the degree of sedation caused by different anxiolytics varies has been exploited to promote the use of some drugs in this category as anxiolytics (drugs with little sedation) and some as hypnotics (drugs with more sedation). A serious drawback to the use of benzodiazepines is that physical tolerance and dependence develops. Withdrawal syndromes have been described, although they are usually mild and difficult to distinguish from the reemergence of the original symptoms of anxiety for which treatment was given. Tolerance and withdrawal phenomena have been more commonly described for drugs with relatively short half-lives (such as alprazolam and lorazepam). In rare cases, seizures and even delirium tremens have been described after stopping chronic benzodiazepine use. Given the propensity of these drugs to cause tolerance, chronic use should be avoided. In cases where the symptoms of a chronic anxiety disorder warrant long-term drug treatment, the use of buspirone (for GAD) or an antidepressant (for panic disorder or OCD) is preferred.

Simple anxiety that is unresponsive to an anxiolytic drug has not been described. The capacity to experience the effects of an anxiolytic drug, unlike that for the antidepressant or antipsychotic effects of drugs, appears to be consistently present in all people, whether they have anxiety disorders or not. However, the response of patients with GAD panic disorder, or OCD to drug therapy is less predictable. The reasons for lack of response in such patients are unknown.

There are two major avenues for the development of new anxiolytic drugs. The first involves elucidating the role of serotonin in the pathophysiology of anxiety and anxiety disorders, thereby identifying new drugs that act through serotoninergic mechanisms to relieve anxiety. Buspirone is a prototype drug in this class. Other azapirone drugs, such as gepirone and ipsapirone, have also been shown to have similar anxiolytic effects. Their lack of ability to cause tolerance and sedation recommend them for use in the long-term treatment of GAD. The TCAs and the SSRIs, particularly fluoxetine and fluvoxamine, are also being used for the treatment of panic disorder and OCD. The second avenue of anxiolytic-drug development involves the discovery of drugs that act specifically on particular benzodiazepine-type binding sites on a subunit of the GABA receptor-chloride channel macromolecular complex. Zolpidem, although not a benzodiazepine in chemical structure, may be considered one of the first examples of this new drug category.

TABLE 21-2

ANXIOLYTIC DRUGS

Drug (generic name)	Recommended dose (mg/day)	Half-life (hours)
Benzodiazepines		
Alprazolam	0.5-2.0	6-20
Chlordiazepoxide	10-75	10-30
Clonazepam	1-10	20-40
Clorazepate	15-60	50-80
Diazepam	2-20	15-60
Lorazepam	2-6	8-20
Oxazepam	20-60	6-20
Beta-blockers		
Atenolol	50-100	6-8
Metoprolol	100-200	2-4
Nadolol	40-80	15-20
Propranolol	40-80	2-6
Other		
Buspirone	20-60	2-4

Antipsychotics

Until the discovery of antipsychotic drugs in the early 1950s, there were few effective treatments for psychotic illnesses. The one exception to this rule was ECT (see Chapter 22). During the 1960s and 1970s a multitude of antipsychotic drugs were developed and marketed, all of which shared a common pharmacological action in that they blocked dopamine (D_2) receptors. In the last several years, attempts have been made to develop antipsychotic drugs that act through atypical mechanisms (for example, mixed serotonin-dopamine antagonists). These attempts, although only partially successful, have so far resulted in the marketing of two new drugs, clozapine and risperidone. Others are likely to follow soon.

Antipsychotic drugs, also called *neuroleptics,* are used for the treatment of psychotic symptoms when they occur in a variety of psychiatric disorders (Table 21-3). The most common illness in this category is schizophrenia, and antipsychotic drugs are the mainstay of treatment for this potentially disabling condition (see Chapter 13). Some individuals develop com-

TABLE 21-3

ANTIPSYCHOTIC DRUGS

Drug (generic name)	Recommended dose (mg/day)	Recommended blood level (as noted)	Half-life (hours)
Chlorpromazine	100-1000	30-100 ng/ml	20-40
Clozapine	300-900	>350 ng/ml	6-30
Fluphenazine	2-20	0.2-2.8 ng/ml	20-40
Haloperidol	2-20	5-16 ng/ml	12-30
Loxapine	15-160		20-40
Mesoridazine	25-400		20-40
Molindone	10-100		15-30
Perphenazine	8-64	0.8-2.4 ng/ml	20-40
Pimozide	2-6		50-80
Risperidone	2-8		2-8
Thioridazine	50-600		20-40
Thiothixene	6-60	2-15 ng/ml	20-40
Trifluoperazine	4-20		20-40

plex delusions in the absence of other symptoms of schizophrenia; these individual are classified as having delusional disorder. Patients with bipolar disorder also commonly receive neuroleptics when psychotic symptoms complicate either manic or depressive states (see Chapter 8). Additionally, patients with unipolar depression may also develop hallucinations and delusions that require such treatment. Finally, psychotic symptoms can occur after the use of hallucinogens or stimulants, and neuroleptics are also useful in mitigating these temporary conditions.

The side effects of antipsychotic drugs can be divided into two categories. First, neurological side effects can occur as the result of dopamine-receptor blockade in the nigrostriatal pathway and can include pseudoparkinsonism and dystonia. Akathisia, neuroleptic malignant syndrome, and tardive dyskinesia have also been linked to such unwanted dopamine-receptor blockade but with less certainty. Second, a variety of other side effects can occur as the result of the drug-induced blockade of receptors for other neurotransmitters, such as acetylcholine (blurry vision, urinary hesitancy, constipation, and confusion), norepinephrine (orthostatic hypotension and sedation) and histamine (sedation). A variety of antipsychotic drugs with high potency and relative selectivity in relation to other neurotransmitters (such as haloperidol, fluphenazine, and thiothixene) are available that have few of the second category of side effects. Only older, low-potency drugs (for example, chlorpromazine and thioridazine) are seriously troubled by these side effects, calling into question the continuing use of such drugs in the 1990s.

Unfortunately, the neurological side effects of antipsychotic drugs are not so easily avoided. Whereas the antipsychotic effects of neuroleptics are thought to occur through the blockade of dopamine D_2 receptors in mesolimbic brain regions, the neurological side effects are thought to occur through the blockade of the same receptors in the caudate nucleus and putamen. Separating these actions has been difficult; however, the recent advent of so-called *atypical antipsychotics* holds promise. These drugs, which include clozapine, risperidone, remoxipride, olanzapine, seroquel, and sertindole, appear to have similar (or in the case of clozapine, superior) efficacy and yet fewer concomitant neurological side effects. The presumed mechanisms for these differences are at least twofold—the blockade of only a select population of mesolimbic dopamine receptors and the concomitant blockade of other neurotransmitter receptors (such as serotonin) that selectively mitigate the interruption of dopamine transmission in the nigrostriatal pathway.

Today, approximately 50% of patients with chronic schizophrenia do not respond adequately to conventional neuroleptics. Among schizophrenic patients in their first episode, this rate of nonresponse may be lower (approximately 20%). There is no clear explanation as to why patients with apparently similar clinical presentations respond differently; differences in neurobiological parameters are presumed but unproven. Of patients with schizophrenia who are refractory to conventional neuroleptics, 30% to 50% respond to the atypical drug clozapine. Although the more widespread use of clozapine is limited by its propensity to cause agranulocytosis, the availability of this drug is critical for a substantial minority of patients.

Current attempts at further antipsychotic drug development are being focused on developing additional atypical drugs that are more easily administered. It is hoped that such drugs will be effective with minimal neurological side effects (through specificity of their sites of action) and that they will treat a much higher proportion of patients than current atypical drugs. The latter goal will only be fully realized when physicians have developed a thorough understanding of the pathophysiology of schizophrenia and know the particular circuits involved, as well as their component neurotransmitter receptor targets.

Mood Stabilizers

The first mood stabilizer is hardly a drug at all but an ion. Lithium was discovered in 1949 by John Cade, an Australian psychiatrist. Cade, looking for toxic substances in the urine of patients with bipolar disorder, administered combinations of urea and uric acid (the latter substance was thought to be protective) to rodents and noticed a calming action of the uric acid. This was in all likelihood because he had given the uric acid as its most soluble salt, lithium urate. From this observation, he discovered the calming effects of lithium carbonate, which he then administered to patients with bipolar illness. His choice of dose (600 mg 3 times per day) was highly fortunate even if it was an accident, and all 10 of his first patients improved dramatically.

Today, there are two classes of mood-stabilizing drugs: lithium salts and anticonvulsants (Table 21-4). In the first category, lithium carbonate is still the most common compound administered, given in a slow-release preparation administered twice daily (Lithobid), or in several regular preparations. Lithium citrate is available as a liquid, and it can be used when compliance with lithium carbonate capsules is in question. At least three anticonvulsants are now known to have mood-stabilizing properties. The first discovered mood stabilizer was carbamazepine, and clinical trials have now demonstrated the efficacy of this compound in acute mania and depression, as well as its use as a prophylaxis against episodes of bipolar disorder. Evidence

TABLE 21-4

MOOD-STABILIZING DRUGS

Drug (generic name)	Recommended doses (mg/day)	Recommended blood level (as noted)	Half-life (hours)
Lithium preparations			
Lithium carbonate	900-1800	0.6-1.5 mEq/L	20-24
Lithium citrate	900-1800	0.6-1.5 mEq/L	20-24
Anticonvulsants			
Carbamazepine	600-1200	6-12 μg/ml	30-36
Clonazepam	2-5		20-40
Sodium valproate	1000-2000	30-100 μg/ml	10-20

is also accumulating to show that sodium valproate is similarly effective. Although there is less evidence for clonazepam, this drug appears to be promising according to anecdotal reports.

The dosing of lithium carbonate and lithium citrate should be carefully guided using blood level monitoring. Serum concentrations of 0.5 to 1.2 mEq/L are usually optimal. For both carbamazepine and sodium valproate, blood levels are obtainable and can be used to guide dosing. However, there is no evidence that optimal efficacy is obtained for the treatment of bipolar disorder using blood level ranges developed for the treatment of seizures.

As alluded to, mood-stabilizing drugs are useful for the treatment of manic episodes and for reducing the risks of future episodes of mania. Mood-stabilizing drugs are also effective, although somewhat less so than antidepressants such as TCAs, in treating episodes of bipolar depression. However, when used as antidepressants in this way, they are not likely to precipitate a "switch" of the patient from depression to mania. Characteristics that may identify those patients with bipolar disorder who are most effectively treated with anticonvulsants rather than lithium have been suggested to be rapid cycling and a negative family history for bipolar disorder. Mood-stabilizing drugs have also been proposed as treatments for other psychiatric disorders that have a cyclical or oscillating character, such as cyclothymic disorder and intermittent explosive disorder. However, firm evidence from controlled clinical trials demonstrating efficacy in these situations is lacking. Mood-stabilizing drugs have also been suggested as adjunctive treatments to be added to neuroleptics for the treatment of refractory cases of psychoses, such as schizophrenia or schizoaffective disorder. However, the evidence from controlled trials remains inconclusive in this situation.

The common side effects of lithium include nausea, diarrhea, tremor, lethargy, polyuria, and weight gain. Reversing initial concerns, the drug is now known to be relatively free of cardiovascular side effects. T-wave flattening and inversion is common but benign. However, lithium should not be given to patients with sick sinus syndrome, since it can aggravate the bradycardia associated with this syndrome and occasionally precipitate cardiac arrest. Since lithium inhibits the release of thyroid hormone (T_4) from the thyroid gland, the drug may cause hypothyroidism and goiter. None of these side effects, including the effects on the thyroid gland, demand that the lithium be stopped. In the case of lithium-induced hypothyroidism, thyroid hormone can be given to overcome it. There remains concern regarding the chronic effects of lithium on renal function, in particular the development of interstitial nephritis, which might then lead to irreversible decreases in creatinine clearance. Although this side effect appears to be much rarer than originally thought, renal function should be routinely monitored to detect it. Lithium is also known to cause cardiovascular abnormalities in the fetus, particularly when given during the first trimester of pregnancy.

In overdose, lithium can be lethal. Delirium, followed by coma, cardiovascular collapse, and death is the usual progression. Monitoring of lithium serum concentrations as the sole guide to treatment during overdose can be dangerous, since the serum concentrations may change rapidly and unpredictably, and may not always faithfully reflect tissue levels of the drug. Clinical judgment and repeated examinations are an essential accompaniment to blood level monitoring. Lithium overdose is surprisingly treatable with renal dialysis.

The common side effects of anticonvulsants include sedation, nausea, weakness, ataxia, diplopia, and nystagmus. They are dose-dependent and can be mitigated by dose reduction. Oddly, carbamazepine can also exacerbate psychotic symptoms in some patients. Carbamazepine is also well known for its capacity to cause leukopenia. Although this rarely leads to agranulocytosis, blood counts should be monitored during carbamazepine treatment, particularly during the first 6 weeks. Sodium valproate lacks many of the side effects of carbamazepine. However, sedation and increases in liver enzymes are common. Many anticonvulsants, including carbamazepine and sodium valproate, can cause cranial-facial birth defects and therefore should be avoided in pregnant patients.

Lithium is effective in treating approximately 70% of manic episodes but only 50% to 60% of depressive episodes in patients with bipolar disorder. Lithium's efficacy as a prophylactic treatment in patients with bipolar disorder lies approximately midway between these two estimates. The rates of success for treating the various aspects of bipolar disorder with anticonvulsants are less well defined, but they appear to be approximately the same as for lithium. When one mood-stabilizing drug has failed in treating a patient with bipolar disorder, others should be tried. Additionally, lithium and an anticonvulsant can be used together, and in some cases this combination has resulted in increased efficacy. For patients with bipolar disorder who are refractory to these mood-stabilizing drugs, ECT is indicated (see Chapter 22).

A larger arsenal of mood-stabilizing drugs would be desirable. When lithium was first discovered to be effective as a mood-stabilizing drug, other ions were explored as treatments also. However, this early effort was not successful. Current efforts in drug development are focused on testing the efficacy of other anticonvulsants, such as clonazepam. Moreover, considerable effort is being expended to understand the mechanisms of action responsible for the mood-stabilizing effects of carbamazepine and valproate.

Phases of Treatment

Most psychiatric illnesses are lifelong; none of the drugs available to treat them are curative. Whereas past efforts to treat psychiatric disorders have emphasized the treatment of acute episodes, current efforts are more directed toward maintenance treatment; that is, preventing episodes of illness. There are two important rationales for this change in emphasis. First, if the acute episodes of illness can be prevented, the costs of inpatient hospitalization needed to treat those episodes can be avoided. Second, evidence is accumulating that episodes of certain illnesses, such as schizophrenia, may unleash "toxic" processes that may worsen the prognosis and undermine the capacity for subsequent drug responses.

Treatment of Acute Episodes of Illness

Most patients begin treatment for psychiatric illness in the midst of an acute episode. In this situation, there is almost always agitation and a sense of urgency among the patient's family and friends. Treatment for an acute episode of psychosis, mania, or depression is often undertaken in the hospital. Speed of treatment is necessary because of the patient's agitation, the family's concern, and institutional pressures to reduce the duration of hospitalization. Unfortunately, most drug treatments for psychiatric illness have no immediate effects.

Antipsychotics are effective in some patients in a few days, but in the majority of patients, clinical response develops gradually over 2 to 4 weeks. Increasing the dose of antipsychotic drug has been shown not to speed the process, suggesting that the clinical response to antipsychotic drugs depends on intrinsic brain mechanisms with fixed latencies. The clinical response to antidepressant drugs also develops gradually. In most patients, the clinical response develops within 2 to 3 weeks. In some patients, longer periods are required. Therefore a physician should not come to the conclusion that a depressed patient cannot respond to an antidepressant until treatment has been underway for at least 6 weeks at therapeutic doses. In the case of mood stabilizers, such as lithium and carbamazepine, there are also latencies in response, usually on the order of 1 to 2 weeks. The only drug group for which there is no latency before a clinical response is the group of benzodiazepine anxiolytics. In this case the response is immediate.

The fact that most patients respond to psychotropic drugs after a latency period is at odds with the need to speed the treatment of acute episodes of psychiatric illness. However, as mentioned in the previous paragraph, increasing the dose of drug does not shorten the latency. The usual dose ranges for most psychotropic drugs are listed in Tables 21-1 through 21-4. Additionally, obtaining serum or plasma levels of psychotropic drugs can assist in achieving an optimal dose (see Tables 21-1 through 21-4). Among all psychotropic drugs, lithium offers the best example for this practice, because the therapeutic serum level range has been clearly established (see Table 21-4). Among neuroleptics, haloperidol blood levels are most interpretable because of the several studies done in this area and the fact that haloperidol has few active metabolites, which can render blood level monitoring of the parent drug meaningless. Among antidepressants, monitoring blood levels of nortriptyline has been best validated. Clinically useful blood level ranges are given in Tables 21-1, 21-3, and 21-4. Research to determine valid blood level ranges for other psychotropic drugs continues.

Using higher-than-optimal drug doses during the treatment of acute episodes of psychiatric illness is inadvisable for several reasons. First, unnecessary side effects that can complicate and slow treatment occur. Second, the patient is less likely to comply with long-term treatment with any drug given in excess. Third, the costs of newer drugs (for example, SSRIs) can be substantial, and excess dosing can be a financial burden to the patient. In some cases of depression, mania, and particular types of schizophrenic psychosis (that is, catatonic schizophrenia), ECT may work more quickly than treatment with a psychotropic drug. However, the use of ECT as a first therapy in such cases is still considered unusual and not the general rule.

Continuation Treatment

Continuation treatment is defined as drug treatment after the acute response to treatment has occurred but before the underlying episode has concluded. The period of continuation treatment may vary, but it almost always consists of weeks or months. Despite the fact the changes in symptoms may be few during continuation treatment, it is almost always necessary to sustain the initial efficacy of drug treatment. However, continuation treatment should not be confused with maintenance treatment (see the following section). An indicator of interrupting continuation treatment (that is, before the underlying episode of illness is over) is immediate relapse. In contrast, relapse during the maintenance phase of treatment often occurs weeks to months after drug treatment has been stopped. As drug treatments for psychiatric illness have become less troubled by side effects, there is little reason for interrupting treatment during the continuation phase. Such interruptions are most often done by patients themselves and lead rapidly to relapse and rehospitalization.

Maintenance Treatment

Increasing emphasis is being placed on the maintenance treatment of psychiatric illness. Although it is simple to undertake, patients and their families often do not understand the need for it. It is essential that patients with unipolar and bipolar mood disorders, schizophrenia, and other serious mental disorders understand that the illness does not conclude with its first acute episode. In most cases, these illnesses are lifelong, with episodes of illness interspersed with periods of wellness. As noted, many patients do not regain their original "baseline" after an acute episode of psychiatric illness. Therefore the prevention of such episodes should be a major goal for the management of psychiatric disorders.

In almost all cases, the same drug is used for acute and maintenance treatment. As described, acute treatment and maintenance treatment are bridged by the continuation phase. Clinical experts, at one time, often recommended that lower drug doses be used during the maintenance phases of treatment of depression and psychosis. However, this advice has become obsolete for two principal reasons. First, it is possible to achieve optimal doses of psychotropic drugs through the use of blood-level monitoring (see Tables 21-1, 21-3, and 21-4) and structured treatment protocols. Second, recently developed psychotropic drugs tend to have fewer side effects and are better tolerated without the need for dose adjustment. Today, maintenance treatment of depression, mania, and psychosis should be performed with the same drug used successfully for acute treatment and at the same dose.

Often, maintenance treatment is continued for an indefinite time. In patients with schizophrenia or bipolar disorder, this is usually the rule. In patients with unipolar depression, indefinite treatment with antidepressant drugs is becoming more common.

General Guidelines for Use of Psychotropic Drugs

The ideal psychotropic drug has the following characteristics: (1) it acts directly and specifically on pathogenetic mechanisms; (2) it benefits all patients with the indicated disorder; (3) it acts immediately; (4) it does not cause tolerance or dependence; (5) it is not toxic at therapeutic doses or after overdose; and (6) it has no side effects. Of course, no current drug meets these criteria, and for that reason, choosing among a number of imperfect drug options using clinical judgment remains an essential ingredient of practice. To optimally use the psychotropic drugs available today, the following guidelines are suggested (see the Pearls & Perils box below).

First, the patient's diagnosis should be established with as much certainty as possible. In this way, the physician can relate choices among the options to lit-

PEARLS & PERILS

GUIDELINES FOR DRUG THERAPY

- Before prescribing a psychotropic drug, the physician should establish the patient's diagnosis with certainty.
- The physician should develop a sequence of treatment options in decreasing order of predicted value.
- One psychotropic drug variable should be changed at a time.
- The physician should allow for time-dependent clinical effects.
- The minimum effective dose of the psychotropic drug should be used.
- The physician should rely on the results of controlled clinical trials to guide practice.

BOX 21-1

EXAMPLE OF A DRUG TREATMENT ALGORITHM

(1) Diagnosis of an outpatient with major depression. No prior history of treatment.
(2) Treatment with an SSRI for 4 weeks (paroxetine, 20 mg/day).
(3) If the patient has no response and no intolerable side effects, increased dose for 4 additional weeks (paroxetine, 40 mg/day)
(4) If no response, consideration of alternate drug (such as an MAOI), augmentation of the initial drug (for example, with lithium), or ECT. Continued treatment for an additional 4 weeks.
(5) If no response cessation of drug treatment and start of ECT.

(***Special Note:*** Options for drug treatment should be discussed in an open interchange with the patient. When choosing among some options (see step 4), there may not be clearly superior alternatives. In such cases, it is often wise to follow the patient's wishes. In this way, compliance later in treatment can be enhanced. Also, ECT may become the best treatment option at any point in treatment if symptoms become acutely severe or if suicidal ideation becomes intense and a rapid response is wanted.)

erature findings, and the patient's chances of responding to the first drug chosen are optimized. Second, the physician should develop a sequence of treatment options in decreasing order of predicted value (Box 21-1). None of the drug treatments available work in all patients. Therefore a physician usually prescribes one drug after another in a trial-and-error fashion. When the physician has faced this possibility from the outset of treatment, the trials can proceed more smoothly and without hesitation. Third, only one variable at a time should be changed. When searching for an optimal treatment, the physician can vary one or another drug and the dose of each drug. Although the desire to speed treatment may tempt a physician to change more than one of these parameters at a time, confusion usually follows from this practice. Additionally, if the physician does find a regimen that works, she may not know which of the drugs produced the desired therapeutic effect and the patient may become committed to continuation and maintenance treatment with unnecessary drugs. Fourth, it is important to allow for time-dependent clinical effects. Keeping in mind that almost all psychotropic drugs act gradually over time, the patient and the physician must have patience and resist the pressures of managed care. Fifth, the minimum effective dose should be used. Higher-than-optimal doses are likely to be associated with avoidable side effects, and opportunities for downward dose titration during continuation and maintenance treatment are rarely realized. Blood-level monitoring can assist in this endeavor in some cases (see Tables 21-1 through 21-4). Sixth, the physician should rely on the results of controlled clinical trials whenever they are available. The expert physician certainly should rely on his own unique clinical experiences, but he should not ignore data from controlled clinical trials. Compelling anecdotes can be misleading and should seldom be the basis for routine practice. Rather, clinical anecdotes should point the way for designing future controlled trials.

Development of New Psychotherapeutic Drugs

Clinical Anecdotes and Ideas

The development of new psychotropic drugs often comes about because of astute clinical observation. Such observation may occur when a drug is used in groups of patients not originally intended or when symptoms other than those originally targeted in the intended group appear to respond. Whatever the situation, the idea for a new drug treatment for one of the psychiatric disorders develops. However, single anecdotes are rarely a sufficient reason to launch a clinical trial. The physician or researcher usually collects reports of similar cases to show that the new treatment is plausible. The value of collecting and reporting such case series should not be underestimated. In the absence of a fundamental understanding of the pathophysiology of most psychiatric disorders, such reports can be the source of entirely new approaches to treatment.

Toxicity and Pharmacokinetic Trials

The first hurdle in the clinical development of a new drug is that it must be tested for its toxicity. Although toxicity will have been tested in a variety of animal species before the new drug is given to humans, only humans can report on the subjective mental effects of a drug. This phase of drug development, called *phase I,* is almost always carried out with volunteers who do not have psychiatric illness. Such trials are small, involving a few dozen subjects, and usually are designed to study the pharmacokinetics of the drug as well.

Preliminary Clinical Trials

The goals of the first clinical trials in patients, called *phase II,* are to evaluate efficacy and to detect unintended side effects. Patients with psychiatric disorders often are more or less sensitive to the sedation, dysphoria, or agitation caused by a psychotropic drug. Therefore these side effects are often difficult to evaluate in volunteers with psychiatric illness. Early clinical trials are often uncontrolled or only placebo controlled. In this way, only a preliminary estimation of the degree and type of efficacy can be made. Information about doses and latencies required for efficacy is also collected at this time, and it may be used in the design of subsequent larger trials. These trials usually involve relatively small numbers of subjects, perhaps 100 or so. Few definite conclusions about the potential for a new drug are drawn at this stage.

Controlled Clinical Trials

Controlled clinical trials, called *phase III trials,* are the mainstay of drug development. Usually the Food and Drug Administration (FDA) requires two phase III controlled clinical trials called *pivotal studies;* in each one the new drug is compared with a different existing drug for the indication. Whether an additional comparison with placebo is necessary varies for each new psychotropic drug. Since an existing drug may show only minimal efficacy in a controlled trial, the degree of efficacy of the new drug may not be properly evaluated when a placebo control is omitted. However, treatment of serious psychiatric disorders with placebo, particularly for an extended time, runs counter to many current treatment recommendations and may be unethical. Nonetheless, the theoretically ideal controlled trial compares the new drug with an existing drug and placebo simultaneously. In this way, both the absolute and relative efficacy of the new drug can be definitely tested. The results of such a trial are the firmest foundation for routine clinical practice.

Conclusion

It is difficult to overstate the importance of psychotropic drugs for patients with psychiatric disorders. The treatment of disorders such as schizophrenia and bipolar disorder was largely a disappointment before the discovery of such drugs. Today we have effective drugs for depression, anxiety, mania, and schizophrenic psychosis. There is hope that many patients with even the most severe disorders, such as schizophrenia and bipolar disorder, can lead relatively normal lives. The discovery of such drugs has also had a profound effect on our thinking about psychiatric illness. Before their discovery there were few clues to help physicians understand the pathophysiology of psychiatric disorders. Today, most theories about the neurobiology of psychiatric disorders were developed at least in part by reasoning backward from the discovered pharmacological effects of psychotropic drugs. Perhaps in the future, advances in our understanding of the etiology and pathogenesis of psychiatric disorders will drive new drug development.

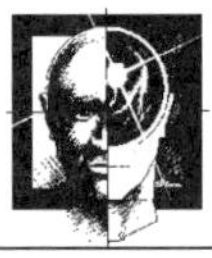

Annotated Bibliography

Bloom FE, Kupfer DJ, editors: *Psychopharmacology: the fourth generation of progress,* New York, 1995, Raven Press.

This large reference text provides an exhaustive compilation of reviews on the neurobiology of psychiatric disorders and the molecular mechanisms of psychotropic drug actions. Additionally, the use of each of the major classes of psychotropic drugs in the acute, continuation, and maintenance settings is reviewed. There are also selected chapters on new drug design and development and methodology of controlled clinical trials.

Gilman AG editors: *Goodman and Gilman's the pharmacological basis of therpeutics,* New York, 1990, Pergamon Press.

This book contains comprehensive information about the pharmacokinetics and pharmacodynamics of psychotropic drugs. Up-to-date guidelines regarding indications, dosing, and side effects can also be found.

Hollister LE, Csernansky JG: *Clinical pharmacology of psychotherapeutic drugs,* ed 3, New York, 1990, Churchill Livingstone, Inc.

This book is a concise, readable text that reviews the pharmacology and clinical uses of all major classes of psychotropic drugs. The chapter on each drug category can be read in a single sitting. Common side effects and clinically relevant drug interactions are also reviewed.

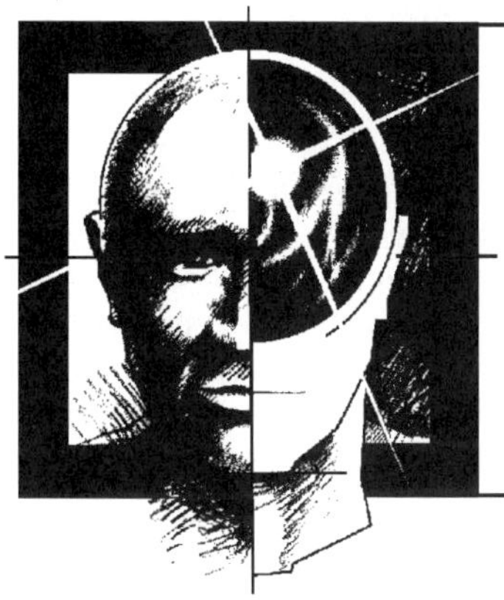

chapter 22

Electroconvulsive Therapy

Charles F. Zorumski, MD and Keith Eugene Isenberg, MD

Psychotropic medications are mainstays in the treatment of affective and psychotic disorders. However, a substantial minority of patients with these disorders either are medication resistant or cannot tolerate side effects of medication. Other patients have severe, life-threatening symptoms that preclude waiting for the delayed response associated with some medications. These severe symptoms include marked suicidal intent, starvation, and exhaustion. For these groups of patients, electroconvulsive therapy (ECT) can be an effective and safe alternative treatment. This chapter discusses the use of ECT in the management of psychiatric disorders, with particular emphasis on patients who have coexisting medical illnesses and on facilitating the involvement of nonpsychiatrists in the selection and implementation of this form of therapy.

Historical Background

The use of convulsive therapy for treatment of psychiatric disorders dates to Ladislaus von Meduna in the 1930s. Based on what was perceived as a "biological antagonism" between epilepsy and schizophrenia, Meduna hypothesized that induced seizures would have clinical benefit. Meduna examined the effects of camphor injections in patients with schizophrenia and observed improvement in about one half of the patients he treated. Problems with patient discomfort and the unreliability of camphor injections in producing seizures led to a search for other ways to induce therapeutic convulsions in humans. In 1938, Ugo Cerletti, Luigi Bini, and colleagues, after a series of observations in animals, administered the first electrically-induced therapeutic seizures in a human. The first patient treated was a 39-year-old man who was acutely psychotic with delusions, hallucinations, incomprehensible speech, and periodic mutism. A previous psychotic episode in this patient had responded well to pentylenetetrazol-induced seizures. Cerletti and Bini administered a series of 11 electrical treatments, and the patient demonstrated dramatic improvement in psychotic symptoms. The importance of Cerletti and Bini's observation is that it introduced a simple and effective way to induce seizures in people. In the early days of ECT, treatments were administered to unanesthetized patients. This caused a great deal of fear and was associated with a number of complications, including fractures, soft-tissue injuries, and hypoxia. ECT technique has undergone numerous changes since its inception, including the routine use of general anesthetics, muscle relaxants, and brief-pulse electrical stimulators. These innovations have maintained the therapeutic benefits of electrically-induced seizures but have greatly diminished a number of untoward effects previously associated with the treatment. ECT has been used to treat a variety of neuropsychiatric disorders, and has found its greatest utility in the management of acute psychotic disorders and major affective disorders, including both mania and depression.

Indications for ECT

Major Depression

Major depression is the psychiatric disorder most commonly treated with ECT. Because there are several classes of antidepressant medications with good clinical efficacy, ECT is typically reserved for use in selected groups of patients with depression (Figure 22-1). Foremost are patients who are unresponsive to

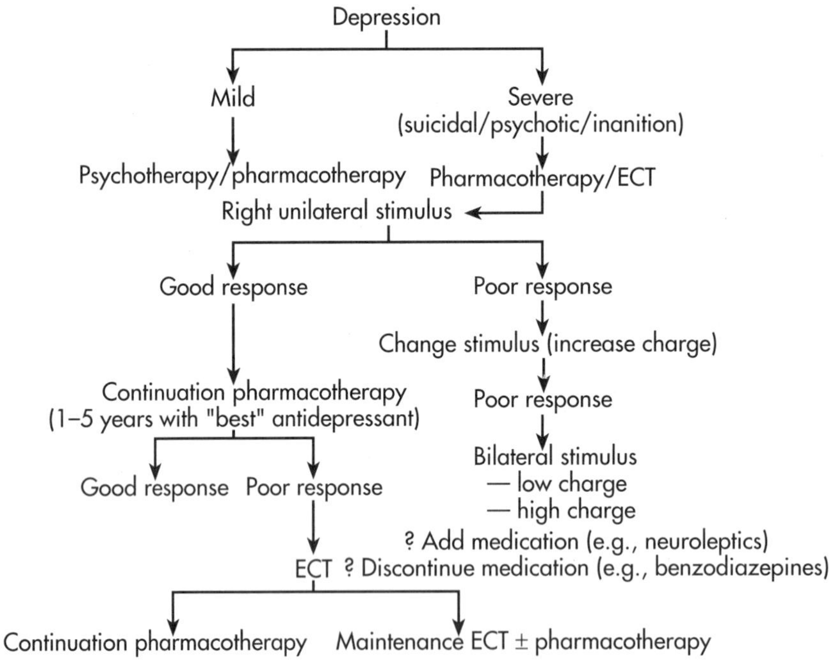

FIGURE 22-1 Use of ECT in the treatment of depression. ECT is usually administered to severely depressed patients as indicated by suicidality, psychosis, or severe disability; most patients will have failed multiple trials of pharmacotherapy and psychotherapy. A nondominant (right hemisphere) unilateral stimulus using an electrical charge that is at least 2.5 times the seizure threshold is usually the treatment of first choice. For patients with a poor response to nondominant hemisphere ECT, options include increasing the electrical charge or switching to low charge (minimally suprathreshold) bilateral ECT. Failure to respond to low-charge bilateral ECT should be followed by high-charge bilateral treatments. After a successful course of ECT, continuation therapy with an antidepressant medication diminishes the risk of relapse. Patients who subsequently relapse are candidates for maintenance ECT.

pharmacological treatments. These patients have often failed to respond to adequate trials of two or more antidepressants before referral for ECT. Several studies have demonstrated a favorable response to ECT in people who do not respond to medication, with significant to complete improvement of depressive symptoms in more than 50% of patients, depending on the criteria used to judge improvement. Failure to respond to pharmacotherapy is an important indication for the primary care physician to make a referral to a psychiatrist.

There are several groups of patients with depression for whom ECT might be considered a first-line treatment. These include patients with a history of medication nonresponse who have previously responded to ECT. If these patients relapse, a repeat trial of medications is usually not helpful, and ECT should be considered early. Patients who develop psychotic symptoms (delusions and hallucinations) in the context of major depression can be difficult to treat with psychotropic medications and typically require the combined use of an antipsychotic drug with an antidepressant. Patients with psychotic depression have a good response to ECT, and this form of treatment should be considered first-line for these patients.

The response of patients with major depression to psychotropic medications is often delayed for days to weeks. Because of this, patients with severe symptoms are sometimes referred for ECT early in their course. These include patients with severe suicidal ideation (particularly after a recent suicide attempt) or refusal to eat, in whom delays in treatment response could be life threatening. Assessment by the nonpsychiatric physician can help establish the presence of disabling depression as well as assist the psychiatrist with the management of concurrent medical complications that are all too common in these severely ill individuals.

In general, the more "endogenous" symptoms a depressed patient has, the more likely the patient is to respond to ECT. These endogenous features include marked psychomotor retardation or agitation, sleep disturbances with early morning awakening, a clear decrease in appetite with weight loss, and diurnal variation of symptoms with worsening in the morning and improvement as the day progresses. Such patients, particularly if they have no prior history of nonresponse to medication, have response rates of 80% or greater to ECT, making ECT one of the most effective forms of antidepressant treatment available. Some patients (approximately 10%) show a partial response to ECT. Individuals who fail to respond to ECT may benefit from subsequent pharmacotherapy with antidepressants.

There are patients with depression for whom ECT may be less useful. These include patients who develop depression in the context of somatization disorder and possibly obsessive-compulsive disorder (OCD). Additionally, patients with dysthymia, a chronic form (at least 2 years) of depression in which symptoms do not meet criteria for a major depressive episode, may have a less favorable outcome with ECT. However, periodic episodes of major depression arising in the context of dysthymia may respond well to ECT. In patients with dysthymia, a major difficulty is in judging ECT response relative to the patient's baseline level of symptoms. Regardless of depression subtype, some patients opt to receive ECT when presented with ECT as a highly effective treatment capable of achieving rapid results.

Mania

Most patients with acute mania respond well to mood-stabilizing medications (lithium, valproic acid, and carbamazepine) with or without antipsychotic medications. However, ECT can be an effective treatment for mania in patients who respond poorly to mood stabilizers or who cannot tolerate side effects of medication. As in depression, patients with severe manic symptoms (including marked agitation, assaultiveness, and exhaustion) may be appropriate candidates for early intervention with ECT, although there is little systematic evidence that there is a better response to ECT than to psychotropic medications. Some data suggest that 80% to 90% of patients with acute mania respond favorably to ECT. Patients who suffer multiple episodes of mania and depression in a single year, a type of bipolar affective disorder identified as *rapid cycling,* may note a reduction in the number of episodes after a course of ECT.

Catatonia

Catatonia is a syndrome of multiple causes characterized by motor and behavioral symptoms that include psychomotor retardation, mutism, posturing, and catalepsy (holding a posture for a long time). The most common disorder associated with catatonia is mania, although patients with schizophrenia, major depression, and several neurological and medical illnesses can also exhibit this symptom constellation. Catatonia, regardless of cause, has an excellent response to ECT, with marked improvement occurring over a few (three or four) treatments. However, it is not clear that catatonia responds better to ECT than to pharmacological treatment with antipsychotic medications or benzodiazepines.

Schizophrenia

Chronic symptoms of schizophrenia, including blunted affect, thought disorder, and long-standing delusions and hallucinations are refractory to most treatments, including ECT. However, patients with schizophrenia often experience acute exacerbations marked by agitation and worsening of hallucinations, delusions, and thought disorder. These acute exacerbations are usually responsive to adjustments in antipsychotic medications. ECT can also be effective in treating these acute decompensations, although ECT should be considered a second-line treatment. It is estimated that 70% to 80% of patients with schizophrenia in an acute relapse respond favorably to ECT. In contrast, only 5% to 10% of patients with chronic, residual symptoms of the disorder exhibit any clinical benefit from ECT. In the past, prolonged courses of ECT (20 to 30 treatments or more over several weeks, referred to as *regressive ECT*) were used to treat people with chronic schizophrenia. The benefits of this form of treatment are minimal at best, and they do not outweigh the marked memory impairment and confusion associated with protracted ECT courses.

Other Disorders

ECT has been used to treat a variety of other psychiatric disorders, including somatization disorder (hysteria), personality disorders, OCD, and alcohol and drug dependence. Although there are reports of benefits in some patients, it appears that ECT is not a useful treatment for these disorders. In these disorders, ECT should be reserved for patients who develop major depressive episodes that are unresponsive to pharmacological management or that are associated with severe symptomatology.

Patients with several neurological disorders may benefit temporarily from ECT. As described, marked psychomotor slowing and catatonia predict a good ECT response. Consistent with this, there is evidence that patients with Parkinson's disease, who exhibit marked motor slowing and are subject to depressive episodes, have both a good affective and motor response to ECT. The beneficial effects of ECT on the motor symptoms of Parkinson's disease appear to be independent of the beneficial effects on mood, because some patients without a mood disorder show motor improvement with ECT. The effects of ECT on motor symptoms are typically short-lived unless maintenance treatments at regular intervals are given. Long-term follow-up data on patients with Parkinson's disease treated with ECT are needed.

Repeated ECT treatments have anticonvulsant effects. Over a course of ECT, seizure threshold increases and seizure durations decrease. Historically, these anticonvulsant effects of ECT were used to treat refractory epileptic patients. However, there is no systematic evidence that ECT is as effective as presently available anticonvulsant medications, and the anticonvulsant effects of ECT are relatively short-lived, subsiding over days to weeks.

Contraindications to ECT

There are no absolute contraindications to ECT, but some groups of patients may be particularly vulnerable to complications from the treatments. ECT produces acute increases in cerebral blood flow (CBF) and intracranial pressure. In patients with space occupying lesions of the central nervous system (CNS), the change in intracranial pressure increases the risk of brain herniation and neurological decompensation. For these reasons, the presence of a space-occupying CNS lesion was previously considered an absolute contraindication to ECT. However, there have been several reports of patients with intracranial tumors who have been successfully treated with ECT for psychiatric disorders. All patients with space-occupying lesions must be considered at high risk for complications from ECT. Patients at greatest risk are those with focal neurological signs (particularly recent changes in the neurological examination), headaches, papilledema, or evidence of a shift in intracranial contents on brain imaging studies. Patients with small CNS lesions that are unassociated with any of these findings are at somewhat lower risk. Since changes in CBF and intracranial pressure are related to changes in systemic blood pressure, it is important to manage blood pressure changes associated with ECT carefully in patients who have CNS tumors. Patients with CNS tumors may also benefit from treatment with dexamethasone to limit swelling in the region of the tumor during ECT.

For weeks to months after a myocardial infarction or cerebrovascular accident, there is an increased risk of complications from general anesthesia. Additionally, the blood pressure and heart rate changes that accompany ECT add to this risk. Although ECT can be used in these patients, the relative risks vs. benefits must be considered carefully. It appears that the period of greatest risk is in the first 6 weeks after a myocardial infarction or stroke.

Cardiovascular Responses to ECT

During each ECT treatment, patients experience marked changes in cardiovascular function (Figure 22-2). Immediately after the electrical stimulus, parasympathetic tone is increased and there is a pronounced bradycardia or asystole lasting several seconds. This initial heart-rate slowing is prevented by pretreatment with anticholinergic medications (atropine or glycopyrrolate). During the generalized seizure, there are

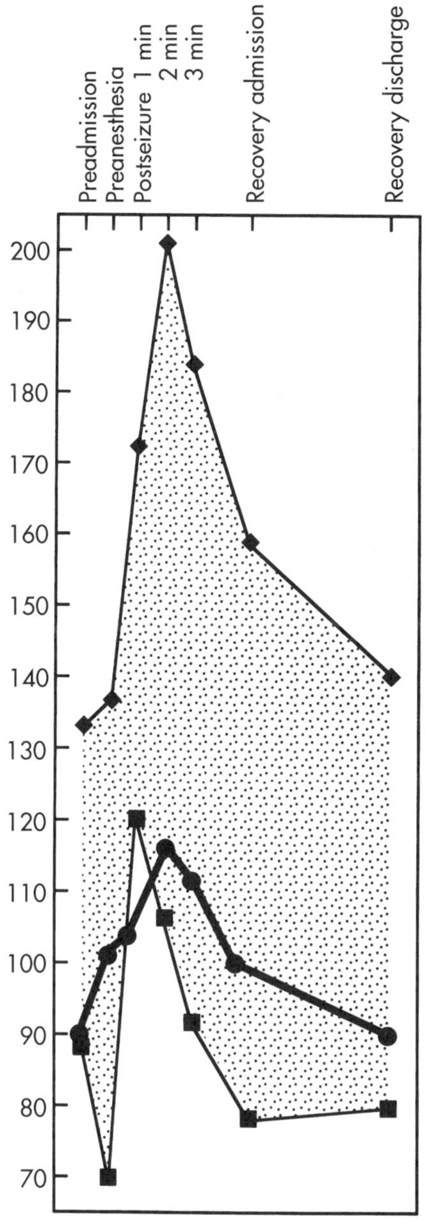

FIGURE 22-2 ECT-associated cardiovascular changes. ECT seizures are associated with sympathetic (central and adrenal) discharges that result in transient elevations of heart rate *(circles)* and blood pressure (*diamonds* and *squares* represent systolic and diastolic blood pressures, respectively). The graph shows typical changes encountered during a single ECT treatment. The timing of the measurements is indicated at the top of the graph. Note that the ECT-induced changes reverse rapidly after the treatment; by the time the patient has recovered sufficiently from the treatment to be discharged from the ECT area (about 45 minutes after preadmission), blood pressure and heart rate have returned to baseline.

marked increases in heart rate (typically 120 to 160 beats per minute) and blood pressure (systolic blood pressures as high as 220 to 250 mm Hg and diastolic pressures up to 120 to 150 mm Hg). The cardiovascular responses are believed to reflect the release of catecholamines during the seizure. The hemodynamic changes persist throughout the seizure and can last for 5 to 15 minutes or longer after the seizure. After the seizure, some patients develop a period of bradycardia that can last several minutes.

Patients with cardiovascular illnesses are at risk for myocardial ischemia and arrhythmias during ECT. Most ECT-induced arrhythmias and electrocardiographic (ECG) changes are time limited and do not require specific treatment. However, serious arrhythmias that compromise hemodynamic function require appropriate management. It is therefore mandatory that medications and equipment for cardiac emergencies be available in the ECT treatment room. Ventricular arrhythmias (tachycardia and fibrillation), myocardial infarction, and myocardial rupture are the most common causes of death during ECT. Despite the marked increases in blood pressure, the occurrence of a cerebrovascular bleed or a ruptured aneurysm in the context of ECT is extremely uncommon.

Several measures can be effective in improving the safety of ECT and in dampening the cardiovascular responses to the treatment. Careful pre-ECT evaluation of cardiac function is important, and appropriate treatment of underlying disorders should be initiated. One to two hours before an ECT treatment, routine oral cardiac medications should be administered. As described in the next section, the judicious use of beta blockers and nifedipine can also be helpful in selected patients. Patients at high risk for myocardial ischemia can be premedicated with nitrates.

ECT Technique

General Management

ECT treatments are usually administered with informed patient consent. This requires a thorough discussion with the patient, and if possible with the patient's family, of the ECT indications, procedure, risks, and benefits. This also should include a discussion of the risks of not treating the underlying disorder. Some patients who suffer from severe psychiatric disorders may be unable or unwilling to give informed consent. Administration of ECT is subject to various legal regulations, although many jurisdictions permit involuntary treatment in severe cases after proper legal review. In all cases of involuntary ECT, it is important to consider carefully the severity of the symptoms, the response to pharmacotherapy, and the consequences of treatment.

The evaluation of patients before ECT includes detailed psychiatric and medical histories and a thorough physical examination. The psychiatric history should include information about psychiatric diagnosis, indications for ECT, and prior responses to psychotropic medications and ECT. The medical examination should emphasize cardiovascular, respiratory, and neurological systems. Any prior history of surgical or anesthetic complications in the patient or patient's family should be documented, with particular emphasis on conditions that interfere with anesthesia (such as medication intolerance, pseudocholinesterase deficiency, or gastroesophageal reflux).

The pre-ECT laboratory evaluation need not be extensive, but it should emphasize potential problems identified in the history and physical examination. Minimal recommended tests include a complete blood count, serum electrolytes, and an ECG. Patients over age 50 and those with a history of cardiorespiratory illnesses should have a chest x-ray before treatment. Spine x-rays are not required for ECT, but they should be considered for patients with clear histories of major back problems. Routine neuroimaging studies are not necessary for most patients before ECT, but they should be obtained in patients with suspicious neurological histories and examinations.

Anesthesia

Before ECT, patients are not allowed to eat or drink for several hours (typically 6 to 8 hours). However, cardiovascular medications or medications to diminish gastric-acid secretion can be administered orally under supervision 1 to 2 hours before treatment.

In general, anesthetic standards for outpatient surgery are appropriate for ECT. These include standards for anesthetic administration and postoperative care. In some centers, ECT is administered in an operating room, whereas in others, ECT is given in a specialized suite. Before treatment, all patients are evaluated by the person administering the ECT anesthetic to minimize anesthetic risk and, in consultation with the treating psychiatrist, to maximize the therapeutic benefit. At the time of treatment, the patient's blood pressure, pulse, three-lead ECG, and level of oxygen saturation are monitored. A catheter is inserted in a peripheral vein, and two or three medications are routinely administered for each ECT session. For most patients an anticholinergic medication, usually atropine (0.4 to 0.6 mg, intravenous) or glycopyrrolate (0.2 to 0.4 mg, intravenous), is administered to inhibit the bradycardia that follows electrical stimulation. If oral secretions are a problem during ECT, the anticholinergic drug can be administered 30 to 60 minutes before treatment, intramuscularly. In many ECT centers, anticholinergics are administered to all patients. However, anticholinergics cause an increased heart rate that could compound the tachycardia that occurs during a seizure. This has led some ECT practitioners to use these medications on a case-by-case basis, with the anticholinergics being reserved for patients who have histories of bradyarrhythmias or who are on medications that compound the bradycardia that occurs during ECT. These medications include beta blockers (for example, propranolol and metoprolol), digoxin, and verapamil. Atropine has the added disadvantage that it is a centrally acting anticholinergic that could increase the memory impairment that occurs during a course of ECT. However, at doses of 0.4 to 0.6 mg, atropine tends to be well tolerated and is relatively inexpensive.

Before administering the anesthetic, patients are preoxygenated with 100% oxygen by mask. Oxygen is administered throughout the procedure until the patient resumes normal respiration. This usually takes about 10 minutes or less. The use of oxygen diminishes the risk of cardiac ischemia during ECT and may diminish cognitive side effects of the treatments.

Methohexital (1 mg/kg, intravenous), a short-acting barbiturate, is the most commonly used anesthetic for ECT. Methohexital has a rapid onset and short duration of action (5 to 10 minutes), and it is inexpensive. Potential problems with methohexital include respiratory depression at high doses and laryngospasm at low doses. Other anesthetics include thiopental, etomidate, ketamine, and propofol. Although most intravenous anesthetics, including the barbiturates, have anticonvulsant effects that could diminish the effectiveness of ECT, this seems to be most problematic with propofol and least problematic with ketamine. In adults, ketamine can produce significant side effects, including increased blood pressure responses during ECT and psychotomimetic effects.

In the early days of ECT, fractures of vertebrae and long bones, resulting from muscle contractions during the electrical stimulus, were major complications of treatment. Routine pretreatment with muscle relaxants has eliminated this problem. Succinylcholine (1 mg/kg, intravenous), a depolarizing muscle relaxant, is the agent of choice for use in ECT. The advantages of succinylcholine include rapid onset, brief duration of action (5 to 10 minutes), and low cost. Patients with neuromuscular disorders are at risk for developing severe hyperkalemia after the use of succinylcholine. This is because succinylcholine works by depolarizing muscle cells and causes an acute increase in extracellular potassium. Similar problems could occur in patients with recent trauma or burns. Patients with neuromuscular disorders are also at increased risk for developing malignant hyperthermia after succinylcholine use. Other patients have genetic or drug-induced alterations in the activity of pseudocholinesterase, the enzyme that degrades succinylcholine. Deficiencies in pseudocholinesterase can cause prolonged paralysis, requiring intubation and assisted ventilation. For patients with neuromuscular disorders or pseudocholinesterase deficiencies, nondepolarizing muscle relaxants such as atracurium may be used.

Despite the routine use of muscle relaxants, direct electrical stimulation of the jaw muscles during the ECT stimulus causes clenching of the teeth. To protect the teeth and tongue, patients treated with ECT have a bite block inserted in the mouth before electrical stimulation. The bite block can be removed after the electrical stimulus.

During an ECT-induced seizure there are marked increases in heart rate and blood pressure that typically last several minutes. In young, medically healthy patients, these cardiovascular changes are well-tolerated, but they could predispose patients with heart disease to serious arrhythmias or myocardial ischemia. Preoperative evaluation of patients taking cardiovascular medications may show the need to adjust their medication regimen before instituting ECT. In selected patients, blood pressure and heart rate can be controlled during ECT by premedication with esmolol (0.2 mg/kg, intravenous), a short-acting beta blocker, or labetalol (5 to 20 mg, intravenous), a combined β- and α-adrenergic antagonist. Esmolol may be the preferred drug because of its shorter duration of action. Since beta blockers enhance the initial bradycardic response to ECT, patients taking these medications are usually pretreated with an anticholinergic medication. Alternatively, the beta blocker can be administered intravenously after the electrical stimulation and the onset of generalized seizure activity. More serious sustained blood pressure changes can be blunted by premedication with calcium channel blockers such as nifedipine (10 to 20 mg, sublingually) 30 minutes before ECT.

The decision to use agents to control heart rate and blood pressure is best made on a case-by-case basis, involving anesthesiologists in the process. It is important to emphasize that ECT has been used as a treatment for more than 50 years and has had low morbidity and mortality from cardiovascular complications. Potential problems with agents used to treat the cardiovascular changes associated with ECT include hypotension and bradyarrhythmias. These side effects can pose serious risks to elderly patients treated with ECT, in whom falls are a major problem. In general, conservative management is recommended for the cardiovascular changes accompanying ECT. The most appropriate pharmacological treatments for hemodynamic changes are those that have a short duration of action.

Electrical Stimulation

Repeated generalized CNS seizures are necessary to produce the clinical benefits of ECT. Thus the goal of an ECT session is to induce a generalized seizure in the CNS under controlled conditions. Seizures are induced by passing a brief electrical current across the head from two electrodes that are positioned either bitemporally (bilateral ECT) or over the nondominant cerebral hemisphere (unilateral ECT). Presently, a temporoparietal electrode placement is most often used for unilateral ECT (Figure 22-3). For right-handed patients, electrodes are placed over the right cerebral hemisphere. Since most left-handed patients (approximately 70%) are left-hemisphere dominant for language, and since there is no evidence that the cerebral systems underlying mood are lateralized differently in left-handed people, a right-sided electrode placement is also appropriate for most of these patients as well. Both unilateral and bilateral forms of treatment are effective, but bilateral ECT is associated with significantly greater memory impairment and confusion. For this reason, nondominant unilateral ECT is the preferred initial mode of treatment for most patients. However, unilateral stimulation results more often in missed or partial seizures than bilateral stimulation unless the electrical dose is carefully adjusted. Additionally, for reasons that are unclear, some patients do not respond well to unilateral ECT, and the response to unilateral ECT is slower to develop.

ECT-induced seizures are typically monitored by a two-lead electroencephalogram (EEG) and by observing convulsive motor movements during the seizure. Because treatments are done with muscle relaxation, peripheral movements are usually monitored by occluding the flow of the muscle relaxant into a limb using an inflated blood-pressure cuff or tourniquet. To ensure the production of a generalized seizure, the isolated limb is usually ipsilateral to the side of the head that is electrically stimulated in unilateral ECT treatments. Electrical stimuli that are subconvulsive or that induce only focal seizure activity produce no clinical benefit. Similarly, treatments that abort seizure activity immediately after electrical stimulation diminish the effectiveness of the treatments. The typical duration of a seizure during ECT is 30 to 90 seconds as monitored by EEG. It is believed that seizures lasting less than 25 seconds are less therapeutic, but this is not well documented. In patients who develop very short seizures during ECT (less than 25 seconds), intravenous caffeine (250 to 500 mg) can be used to lengthen the seizures. Alternatively, reductions in the dose of anes-

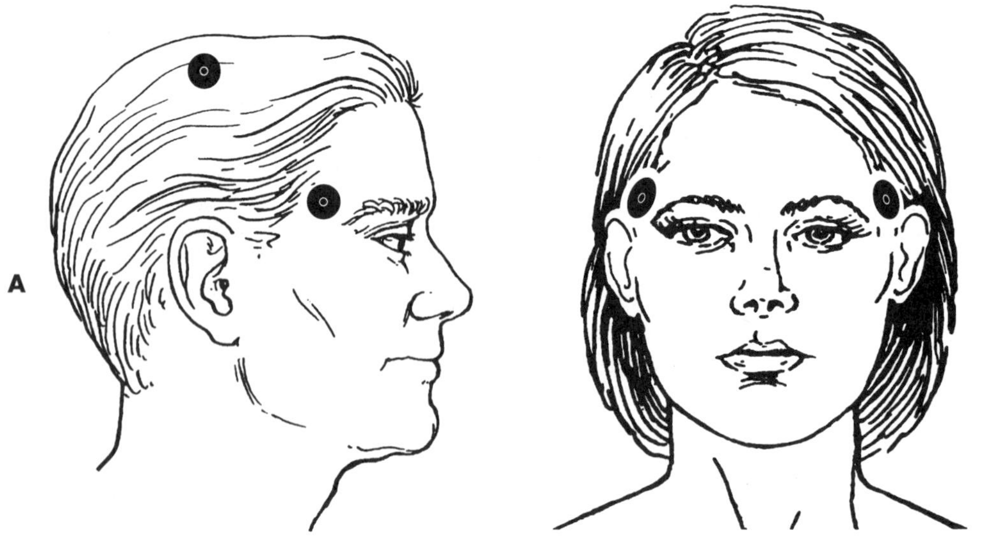

FIGURE 22-3 Electrode placement for ECT. Stimulation can be administered either unilaterally *(A)* or bilaterally *(B)*. Nondominant unilateral stimuli are administered using the d'Elia placement *(A)*, which is relatively memory-sparing compared with bilateral electrode placements. Before electrode application, the placement sites are cleaned with a saline-soaked pad and an electrical conducting gel is applied to the ECT electrodes. With constant current stimulators, a low amplitude, subconvulsive electrical stimulus is used to estimate the interelectrode impedance. Excessive impedance usually results from poor preparation of the electrode sites. To prevent electrical tissue burns, most constant current ECT stimulators have a failsafe that prohibits administering the convulsive stimulus if the interelectrode impedance exceeds certain values.

thetic agent lengthens seizures in some patients. Prolonged seizures, defined as seizures longer than 180 seconds on EEG, are terminated by an intravenous anticonvulsant, usually methohexital or diazepam. *Status epilepticus* is rare during ECT, and it is managed—in consultation with a neurologist—with agents typically employed for this problem when it arises in other settings.

Based on a series of elegant studies by Harold Sackeim and colleagues, it appears that the electrical dose used to produce seizures is an important variable in determining clinical response. With bilateral ECT, stimuli that are just above the seizure threshold (defined as the minimal amount of electrical charge needed to induce a seizure) produce good clinical effects. These low-charge bilateral treatments also appear to diminish the cognitive side effects of bilateral ECT. In contrast, unilateral ECT administered at minimally suprathreshold doses produces only limited clinical improvement despite inducing generalized CNS seizures of adequate duration. In contrast, administering unilateral treatments at electrical doses that are more than 2.5 times the seizure threshold greatly improves the efficacy of unilateral ECT and maintains the cognitive benefits of the treatment relative to bilateral ECT. Patients who fail to respond to high-charge unilateral ECT should be switched to bilateral ECT. A patient should not be considered an ECT failure unless a trial of high-charge bilateral ECT has been administered.

During the ECT stimulus, most of the current flow is shunted between the stimulating electrodes. This is because the resistivity of the scalp is much less than that of the skull (about 200 Ω/cm vs. 17,000 Ω/cm). It is estimated that less than 20% of the electrical stimulus enters the cranial cavity. Caution must be exercised in treating patients who have skull defects in the area where the electrodes are placed, since skull defects allow significantly greater current flow into the cranium and could result in electrolytic tissue damage.

ECT stimulators use either a constant current or a constant voltage output. Constant-current stimulators are used most commonly, and they have greater ease in quantifying the electrical dose since the amplitude of the output waveform is not dependent on the impedance between the electrodes. A major consideration in selecting an ECT stimulator is the electrical waveform generated by the stimulator. Most ECT devices use either brief electrical pulses (that is, a series of square wave pulses of specified amplitude and duration that rise and fall almost instantaneously) or sine-wave outputs. Compared with sine-wave generators, seizures can be induced at significantly lower charges using brief (0.5 to 2.0 msec) electrical pulses delivered at frequencies of 30 to 90 Hz for 0.5 to 8.0 seconds. The difference in seizure threshold arises from the fact that sine waves are inefficient stimuli that provide much of their current flow during neuronal refractory periods when action potentials cannot be generated. Brief-pulse stimulation is also associated with fewer cognitive side effects than sine-wave stimulation. For these reasons, it is recommended that only brief-pulse stimulators be used for ECT. Typical seizure thresholds using brief-pulse stimulation range from 25 mC to several hundred millicoulombs. Most ECT stimulators used clinically in the United States have maximal outputs of 500 to 600 mC. For comparison with stimulators used for cardioversion, this is equivalent to less than 100 watt-seconds (joules), assuming an interelectrode impedance of about 200 Ω.

Side Effects and Risks of ECT

ECT requires the use of general anesthetics and electrical stimulation, and ECT-induced seizures are associated with marked changes in cardiovascular function. Additionally, ECT is often used in the treatment of psychiatric disorders in patients with serious medical illnesses. As a result, ECT is associated with a small but definite risk of death. It is estimated that an ECT-related death, defined as a death occurring within 24 hours of a treatment, occurs in about 2 to 4 of every 100,000 treatments. This risk is not significantly greater than the risk for general anesthesia alone. Since most centers administering ECT give fewer than 1000 treatments per year, most physicians rarely encounter an ECT death. The cause of death is most often an adverse cardiovascular event (myocardial infarction, myocardial rupture, or ventricular arrhythmia). In weighing the risk of death, it is important to consider that untreated major psychiatric disorders are also associated with significant risks of morbidity and mortality from suicide and deterioration in general health. About one in six individuals with severe depression commits suicide—an enormously greater risk than that associated with ECT.

Confusion and memory impairment are major side effects of ECT. It is important to emphasize that cognitive impairments are adverse effects of the treatment and play no role in the therapeutic effects of ECT. After an ECT treatment there is a period of postictal and postanesthetic confusion lasting several minutes to several hours. During this period some patients become agitated and require treatment with benzodiazepines or antipsychotic medications. This immediate post-ECT confusion may worsen with increasing number and frequency of ECT treatments. The memory impairment associated with ECT consists of both retrograde and anterograde components. In general, memory is worst for events occurring during the ECT course, although some patients have deficits in the recall of past information as well. ECT-induced memory loss tends to improve with time after the cessation of an ECT course, returning to baseline levels within about 6 to 8 weeks in most patients. Since certain psychiatric disorders, particularly depression, are associated with deficits in concentration and information recall, many patients report that their memory function is actually improved after a successful course of ECT, compared with a baseline defined when they were ill. Some patients report longer-lived deficits in autobiographical memories after ECT, but these have been difficult to document systematically. Memory impairments, like postictal confusion, worsen with increased number and frequency of treatments. Furthermore, bilateral ECT produces significantly greater memory impairment than nondominant-hemisphere unilateral stimulation. It also appears that the cognitive side effects of ECT are increased by the use of high electrical charges to induce seizures and perhaps by high doses of anesthetic medications and CNS-active anticholinergic drugs. The influence of electrical dose on memory and the role of electrical dose in ECT efficacy provide persuasive arguments for titrating seizure threshold and adjusting the administered electrical dose carefully in individual patients. Similarly, unilateral ECT should be the treatment of first choice for most patients. Despite advances in ECT technique, it is clear that memory effects of ECT are a serious limitation of this treatment.

Other time-limited side effects of ECT include muscle soreness, nausea, vomiting, and headaches. The muscle soreness results primarily from fasciculations produced by succinylcholine, but direct muscle depolarization during the electrical stimulus and movement during the seizure contribute in some patients. Before the use of muscle relaxants, fractures of long bones and vertebrae were complications of ECT, but these are extremely rare in patients adequately treated with muscle relaxants. In patients with a prior history of back, joint, or bone problems, careful monitoring of muscle relaxation is important. The nausea, vomiting, and headaches that some patients experience after an ECT treatment usually respond to simple interventions (antiemetics or analgesics).

Patient acceptance of ECT can be difficult to achieve. In part, difficulties with acceptance reflect anxieties typically associated with any medical procedure. Clear communication of indications, benefits, and risks to patients and their families verbally, in written form, and when available in video form diminishes anxiety as well as being part of the informed consent process. Unfortunately, routine premedication for anxiety (for example, with benzodiazepines) is undesirable because of possible inhibition of seizure induction and perhaps because of an adverse impact on ECT efficacy. Unfavorable perception by the general public, to the extent that this influences use of ECT, may reflect bowdlerized media portrayals. More recent accurate accounts, such as that provided by Manning, will hopefully facilitate acceptance of ECT by patients, families, and the general public.

ECT in Patients with Concurrent Medical Illnesses

Treatment of psychiatric disorders in patients with severe medical illnesses can be difficult, because many psychotropic medications have side effects that limit their use in this population. Of particular note are the cardiovascular side effects of tricyclic antidepressants (TCAs) and low potency antipsychotics (such as chlorpromazine and thioridazine). The newer generation psychotropic medications, particularly the serotonin-selective reuptake inhibitors (SSRIs), have more favorable side-effect profiles that may make these drugs better choices in medically ill patients. However, the effectiveness of SSRIs in medically ill patients has not been thoroughly studied. Because of its rapid effectiveness and relative safety, ECT is an important consideration in treating medically ill patients who have major affective or psychotic disorders. Although there are no absolute contraindications to ECT, patients with severe cardiovascular illnesses are exposed to marked hemodynamic changes during ECT. In effect, ECT is a form of myocardial stress with significant changes in heart rate and blood pressure. To diminish the cardiovascular risks of ECT, nonpsychiatric physicians are often involved in the evaluation of medically ill patients before ECT, and at times they may be asked to participate in the administration of treatments.

ECT has been successfully used to treat patients who have a variety of cardiovascular illnesses. Consultation with a physician knowledgeable about the management of cardiovascular disorders may suggest management that minimizes ECT-related cardiovascular stress (for example, antihypertensives). Most medications used to treat cardiovascular illnesses, including hypertension, present no specific problems during concurrent use with ECT. A possible exception is reserpine, which has been associated with ECT-related deaths. Certain antiarrhythmic drugs (such as phenytoin, procainamide, and lidocaine) increase seizure threshold and make it more difficult to induce therapeutic seizures. The presence of uncompensated congestive heart failure presents significant anesthetic and ECT risks. After appropriate medical management, patients with congestive heart failure can be treated successfully with ECT, although they remain at risk for decompensation. Patients with cardiac pacemakers can be treated with ECT provided that there is adequate grounding of the electrical equipment used to administer treatments. A pacemaker magnet should be available at the time of treatment to help control heart rate if necessary. Patients with vascular aneurysms can be treated with ECT, but careful attention should be paid to limiting the hemodynamic changes. Similarly, patients who have had cardiac surgery—including valve replacements, coronary artery bypass grafts, or cardiac transplants—have been treated successfully with ECT. The valve-replacement patients are typically on anticoagulant medications. These medications can be used concurrently with ECT without inordinate risk.

There are risks associated with the use of ECT in patients with respiratory illnesses (emphysema, bronchitis, and asthma), since the treatments require general anesthesia. However, respiratory illnesses do not preclude the use of ECT. Endotracheal intubation is not routinely used for ECT, and in general it is to be avoided because of the need for multiple treatments and hence multiple intubations over several weeks. Intubation is usually reserved for patients with severe gastroesophageal reflux, although conservative management with medications that diminish gastric acid secretion (such as cimetidine, ranitidine, and omeprazole) and cricoid pressure during ECT are the preferred modes of management. Theophylline is used in the treatment of some patients with respiratory disorders, and it has been associated with prolonged seizures and *status epilepticus* during ECT. For this reason, it is recommended that theophylline levels be kept as low as possible (less than 20 μg/ml) or that the medication be discontinued during a course of ECT.

Numerous patients with diabetes mellitus have been treated successfully with ECT. Before treatment, blood sugar is monitored by finger stick and should be between 80 and 250 mg/dl. In patients receiving insulin, the morning dose is usually withheld until after ECT, when patients can resume oral intake. ECT is reported to have variable effects on blood sugar levels in diabetic patients, but these effects do not appear to be a significant clinical problem provided that patients are monitored closely throughout their ECT courses.

Patients with coexisting neurological and psychiatric disorders have been treated successfully with ECT. Blood pressure and heart-rate changes in patients with CNS tumors or cerebrovascular disorders should be monitored carefully and limited to the extent possible. Although spontaneous seizures after ECT have been described, patients with epilepsy are not at marked risk during ECT. In fact, there may be a diminished incidence of seizures during ECT, since the treatment has anticonvulsant effects. Patients taking anticonvulsant medications for the treatment of a seizure disorder should continue taking these medications throughout their ECT course, since there are substantial risks associated with discontinuing or diminishing the dose of these agents in patients who are epileptic.

Intraocular pressure increases during ECT. However, these changes are short-lived and usually do not present a clinical problem. Patients with glaucoma should continue their routine medications during ECT. One potential problem concerns the use of ECT in patients treated with ecothiophate eye drops. Ecothiophate inhibits pseudocholinesterase and has been associated with prolonged paralysis after use of succinylcholine.

ECT has been used successfully to treat major psychiatric disorders during pregnancy and has not been associated with significant complications in the mother or the fetus. The decision to use ECT during pregnancy requires involvement of the patient's obstetrician. Routine intubation of the mother or intensive fetal monitoring during ECT do not seem warranted based on the published literature. A delivery suite should be available for patients in the later stages of pregnancy in the unlikely event that an emergent delivery is required.

ECT Course

A typical course of ECT consists of 6 to 12 treatments administered once daily, 2 or 3 times per week. There have been attempts to speed the ECT course by giving multiple treatments at a session (two to four seizures per session). However, there is little evidence that administering multiple treatments per session enhances the clinical response, and multiple treatments increase the risk of memory impairment. The number of treatments in an ECT course depends primarily on the clinical response and the side effects of treatment, most notably memory loss and confusion. Fixed courses of treatments for all patients are inappropriate because the response to ECT can vary greatly from patient to patient. Once a stable degree of improvement is achieved, ECT treatments are usually discontinued and the patient is started on continuation pharmacotherapy. All patients who respond to ECT need some form of maintenance treatment, since there is a significant risk of relapse (approximately 80%) without treatment during the 3 to 6 months after a successful ECT course. The maintenance treatment is usually an antidepressant medication that the patient has not failed in the past. In some patients, ECT is used as a maintenance treatment; when used for this purpose, it is administered on a schedule of decreasing frequency starting with once-weekly treatment and gradual tapering to once-monthly treatment. Maintenance ECT is usually administered on an outpatient basis, and difficulties with this form of treatment include memory impairment and inconvenience for patients and their families. Despite these limitations, maintenance ECT is appropriate for patients who have previously failed multiple medications but who have a good response to an acute course of ECT.

ECT and Psychotropic Medications

There is little evidence that concurrent use of psychotropic medications enhances the beneficial effects of ECT, but certain side effects of medication could increase the adverse effects of ECT. For example, medications with significant anticholinergic effects (such as TCAs, antiparkinsonian drugs, or low-potency antipsychotics) could compound the memory impairment associated with ECT. Some evidence suggests that benzodiazepines may diminish the beneficial effects of unilateral ECT, presumably by increasing seizure threshold. Similar concerns exist with anticonvulsants used for mood stabilization (such as valproic acid or carbamazepine). Certain medications (such as bupropion, clozapine, amoxapine, and maprotiline) may predispose a patient to prolonged seizures during ECT, but the evidence supporting this is limited. Lithium appears to increase the cognitive impairments of ECT and may be associated with spontaneous seizures and other neurological complications during ECT. Phenelzine, a monamine oxidase inhibitor (MAOI), has been reported to inhibit pseudocholinesterase and could prolong the apnea produced by succinylcholine.

For most patients, psychotropic drug use should be limited during an ECT course. Patients who are severely agitated and psychotic can be treated with high-potency antipsychotic drugs (for example, haloperidol or thiothixene) during a course of ECT. Severely anxious patients can be treated with low doses of a shorter-acting benzodiazepine (such as lorazepam or alprazolam). For temporary sleep disturbances, zolpidem or chloral hydrate are reasonable choices. To the extent possible, the use of anxiolytic and hypnotic medications should be limited during an ECT course.

ECT Mechanisms

Since the mechanisms underlying major psychiatric disorders are poorly understood, it is not surprising that the mechanisms responsible for the beneficial and adverse effects of ECT are poorly understood. As noted years ago by Seymour Kety, a renowned neurochemist, the problem lies not in detecting changes in cerebral function after ECT, but rather in determining which of the changes are important and which are irrelevant. In considering the mechanisms of ECT, it is important to recall that the one constant across numerous studies is that the therapeutic benefits of ECT require the repeated induction of generalized CNS seizures. Thus considerable effort has been directed toward understanding how generalized seizures alter CNS function. Unfortunately, most major neurochemical systems that have been studied have shown some form of alteration after ECT (or electroshock in animals), making it difficult to be confident of the role played by any one system.

Based on available data, certain mechanisms seem unlikely to be involved in the effects of ECT. For example, anesthetic medications have little to do with the therapeutic benefits. Similarly, there is no convincing evidence that ECT produces structural brain damage, and thus ECT does not produce its effects by damaging the CNS. The memory-impairing effects of ECT are also unrelated to the therapeutic benefits. Most of the innovations in ECT technique have been aimed at maintaining the therapeutic benefits while eliminating, to the extent possible, the cognitive-impairing effects of the treatment. The routine use of unilateral electrode placements, brief-pulse stimulators, and titrated electrical doses are three notable examples.

It is presently believed that the therapeutic and adverse cognitive effects of ECT result from changes in neurotransmitter biochemistry and receptors. Leading candidates include the biogenic amine and muscarinic cholinergic transmitter systems. Since many psychotropic medications alter the function of biogenic amine transmitter systems (norepinephrine, dopamine, and serotonin), there has been intense interest in examining the effects of ECT on these systems. Unequivocal effects of ECT on biogenic amine systems have been observed, some of which are consistent with current hypothesis (β-adrenergic receptor down regulation) and others that are inconsistent (increases in serotonin$_2$ receptor binding). Other plausible hypotheses suggest that changes in neuroendocrine systems, biochemical second-messenger systems, or CNS gene expression ultimately underlie the effects of ECT.

Another line of thought postulates that the anticonvulsant effects of ECT are important in the clinical benefits. Again, the mechanisms of these effects are not certain but could involve changes in the γ-aminobutyric acid (GABA), opioid, or adenosine transmitter systems. Indeed, it is interesting that caffeine (an adenosine receptor antagonist) is used in ECT to prolong seizures that have become extremely short over a series of treatments, suggesting the importance of the adenosine system in seizure termination. The anticonvulsant hypothesis of ECT is attractive given the usefulness of certain anticonvulsants as mood stabilizers, and it could account for beneficial effects in both mania and depression. Unfortunately, at present there is no direct evidence demonstrating that any specific neurochemical or neurophysiological effect of ECT, exclusive of a generalized CNS seizure, is critical for the clinical effects observed.

Conclusion

ECT is an extremely powerful and dramatic treatment for certain psychiatric disorders (see the Pearls & Perils box below). ECT is most useful in the management of severe affective disorders, psychotic states, and catatonia. In some cases ECT can be life-saving. The beneficial effects of ECT depend on producing a generalized seizure in the CNS, but certain characteristics of the electrical stimulus, particularly in nondominant hemisphere ECT, are also important. The major risks of ECT include a small chance of death from cardiovascular complications and time-limited problems with memory loss and confusion. ECT is appropriate for treating psychiatric disorders in patients with concurrent medical and neurological disorders, and it may be preferred over certain psychotropic medications. In high-risk medical patients, particularly those with severe cardiac illnesses, a thorough understanding of the hemodynamic effects of ECT coupled with a careful analysis of the risk-to-benefit ratio is mandatory. The nonpsychiatric physician can enhance the effectiveness of ECT by recognizing its efficacy, assisting with patient selection, and actively participating in efforts to minimize risk.

PEARLS & PERILS

ECT OVERVIEW

- ECT is a safe and effective treatment for major depression, mania, catatonia, and acute schizophrenic episodes.
- ECT is administered under general anesthesia with muscle relaxation.
- The therapeutic effects of ECT require the repeated induction of generalized CNS seizures.
- There are no absolute contraindications to ECT. Patients with CNS tumors, particularly those with focal neurological signs or evidence of increased intracranial pressure, are at risk for decompensation.
- Each ECT treatment is associated with significant increases in blood pressure and heart rate. These effects need to be considered carefully when treating patients with cardiovascular illnesses.
- Confusion and memory impairment are time-limited side effects of ECT. The risk of memory impairment can be diminished by use of nondominant hemisphere electrical stimulation.

Annotated Bibliography

Abrams R: *Electroconvulsive therapy,* ed 2, New York, 1992, Oxford University Press.

This book provides an excellent, well-referenced overview of ECT, and it is a must for any serious ECT practitioner. For primary care physicians, the book presents a good discussion of cardiovascular changes associated with ECT and the use of ECT in medically ill patients.

American Psychiatric Association Task Force: *The practice of electroconvulsive therapy: recommendations for treatment, training and privileging,* Washington D.C., 1990, American Psychiatric Press.

This book contains the recommendations of the American Psychiatric Association concerning the use of ECT. The rationales for specific recommendations are clearly outlined. This book is also a must for ECT practitioners.

Coffey CE, editor: *The clinical science of electroconvulsive therapy,* Washington, D.C., 1993, American Psychiatric Press.

This book contains excellent overviews of a number of important topics in ECT and is written by leaders in the field. Both clinical and research issues are considered in this work.

Devanand DP et al: Does ECT alter brain structure? *Am J Psychiatry* 151:957, 1994.

This paper presents an excellent overview of whether ECT causes damage to the CNS. Based on a careful review of the existing clinical and preclinical literature, the authors conclude that there is no systematic evidence supporting the hypothesis that ECT alters brain structure.

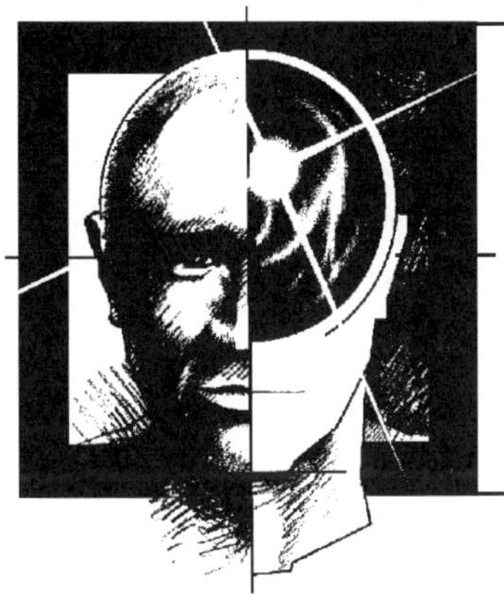

chapter 23

Psychiatric Genetic Counseling

Steven O. Moldin, PhD

Analyses of family, twin, and adoption data have generally been quite consistent in supporting the influence of genetic factors in the etiology of major mental disorders (Box 23-1), and a firm knowledge base about their familial transmission now exists (Box 23-2). Within the last 10 years, numerous claims of gene localization have been made for several mental disorders, and in every case so far efforts to replicate the original finding have failed. Either genetic analysis of new families failed to yield similar evidence, or evidence for gene localization disappeared in the original sample of families when more members were analyzed or when more informative genetic markers were typed. Consequently, the precise mode of familial transmission of any mental disorder remains unclear and no specific gene has been conclusively identified.

Although traditional methods of genetic analysis have led to the mapping of Mendelian disorders such as adult polycystic kidney disease and Huntington's disease to the human genome, they are less likely to be successful in the investigation of genetically complex mental disorders, where environmental factors and multiple genes of small relative effect likely influence disease expression. Recent advances in high-throughput genotyping and high-resolution genetic mapping that have led to localization of multiple genes involved in another genetically complex disease (diabetes) have raised hopes considerably that disease-susceptibility genes may be found for mental disorders. These discoveries may be enhanced as the U.S. Human Genome Project (USHGP) nears its ambitious goal of mapping and sequencing the entire genome. The USHGP, with an estimated cost of $3 billion that makes it the largest scientific project funded by the federal government since the Apollo Moon Project, will provide a better understanding of genetically complex diseases like mental disorders. Perhaps its great benefit will be the development of more exact ways of screening and diagnosing; this ultimately may lead to specific genetic cures.

The ultimate detection of disease susceptibility genes will lead to an increased probability that genetic testing will become available and accessible to many individuals at increased risk. The emergence of the biotechnology industry greatly increases the likelihood that these findings will be rapidly translated into widely available test kits and diagnostic products. Entrepreneurial pressure may also lead to the development of commercial and academic "genetic testing services" that would not be regulated under current Food and Drug Administration (FDA) procedures. Furthermore, the potential of generating all of this genetic information about individuals raises serious questions of potential discrimination and strongly demonstrates that all consumers must be informed about the meaning of genetic risk and genetic testing. The Institute of Medicine Committee on Assessing Genetic Risks noted in its 1994 report, "Interpretation and communication of predictive test results in psychiatry will be particularly difficult. To prepare for the issues associated with genetic testing for psychiatric diseases in the future, psychiatrists and other mental health professionals will need more training in genetics and genetic counseling." This report goes on to say, "Since genetics education and counseling are likely to be provided increasingly by primary care practitioners, these practitioners will need training to help them perform these functions appropriately and to know when to refer patients to specialized genetics personnel."

This chapter provides an overview to the basic principles of psychiatric genetic counseling and serves as a useful framework to primary care physicians to

BOX 23-1

MENTAL DISORDERS WITH A GENETIC COMPONENT TO ETIOLOGY

Psychotic disorders

Schizophrenia
Schizoaffective disorder

Mood disorders

Bipolar disorder (manic-depressive illness)
Severe depression

Substance-related disorders

Alcohol dependence

Childhood disorders

Attention-deficit hyperactivity disorder
Autism
Chronic tics and Tourette's disorder

Anxiety, somatoform, and eating disorders

Generalized anxiety disorder
Obsessive-compulsive disorder
Panic disorder
Phobia
Somatization disorder
Anorexia nervosa
Bulimia nervosa

Personality disorders

Antisocial personality disorder
Schizotypal personality disorder

BOX 23-2

FACTS ABOUT THE FAMILIAL TRANSMISSION OF MENTAL DISORDERS

- Analyses of family data consistently support the hypothesis of familial aggregation.
- Analyses of available twin and adoption data support the influence of genetic factors.
- Familial transmission does not follow a clear Mendelian pattern in most families.
- Risk to illness in relatives increases markedly with the degree of genetic relatedness.
- Environmental factors are necessary for illness expression.

address questions about recurrence risks, familial inheritance, and the future availability of genetic testing for mental disorders.

Epidemiology of Heritable Mental Disorders

Interpretation of the familial risk to a mental disorder requires knowledge of the rate of disease in the general population. Without such knowledge, one cannot determine whether illness occurring in the relatives of an affected individual is occurring at a rate higher than what would be expected by chance. Table 23-1 shows the lifetime rates of several mental disorders. Interpretation is straightforward; for example, 1 out of 100 individuals in the U.S. population will develop schizophrenia during their lifetime. This table also shows risks to first-degree relatives (parents, offspring, and siblings) of an affected individual. These are approximate figures determined from a comprehensive literature review and are simplified; for example, the risk to parents of an individual with schizophrenia is nearly one half the risk to children. The risk figure shown is pooled across siblings, children, and parents. The heritable form of depression appears to include those cases of "severe" depression where the individual was hospitalized, incapacitated, or psychotic during a depressed period.

Models of Familial Transmission

The presence or absence of a mental disorder is an observable characteristic *(phenotype)* of a person that is produced by his genetic constitution *(genotype)* in conjunction with the environment. Mathematical models exist in genetic epidemiology to represent the ways in which genes and environment produce the pattern of disease transmission in families and populations.

Single Major Locus Models

The single major locus model assumes that a disease is due to the presence of a mutation in one of the different forms *(alleles)* of a single gene, which lies at one position on a chromosome *(locus)*. Such diseases are called *Mendelian,* because their pattern of familial transmission follows rules developed in 1865 by Gregor Mendel from his breeding experiments with pea plants. Environmental factors that affect disease expression are not transmitted from generation to generation; that is, they are not shared among family members. More complex single-locus transmission is possible, in which there is absence of disease in individuals known to carry the mutant allele. The single gene in such cases is *incompletely penetrant,* and patterns of disease transmission deviate from Mendelian expectations.

Medical genetics courses taught in U.S. medical schools typically focus exclusively on the variety of known Mendelian disorders with autosomal dominant, autosomal recessive, or X-linked modes of inheritance. Over 4000 rare human diseases are inherited as simple Mendelian traits and are meticulously catalogued in successive editions of McKusick's classic text, *Mendelian Inheritance in Man.* However, there is no substantive evidence for the primary involvement of a single major locus in the transmission of any mental disorder. Disease patterns in most families are incompatible with single major-locus transmission, even after allowing for incomplete penetrance. This in no way weakens the evidence that there is a genetic contribution to the etiology of mental disorders; rather, alternative models are needed to better explain familial transmission.

TABLE 23-1

EPIDEMIOLOGY OF MENTAL DISORDERS

Population	Approximate lifetime morbid risks: Schizophrenia	Bipolar disorder	Severe depression	Obsessive-compulsive disorder	Panic disorder	Generalized anxiety disorder	Alcohol dependence	Phobia	Anorexia nervosa
General population	1%	.8%	4%* 8%†	1.5%	3.5%	3.5%	14%* 3%†	4%-11%	.1%
First-degree relatives of an affected individual	9%	8%	9%* 18%†	17%	15%	19.5%	27%* 5%†	12%-31%	5%-10%

*Risk to males; †Risk to females.

Multilocus Models

Disease transmission can be the result of the combined effect of two or more genes. These multilocus models can be divided into the following three categories: multifactorial-polygenic, mixed, and oligogenic models (Box 23-3).

The multifactorial-polygenic model assumes that disease is caused by the additive action of multiple genes that are each of small and approximately equal relative effect *(polygenes)* or by environmental risk factors transmitted (shared) within families. Shared environmental risk factors and polygenic effects increase an individual's *liability* to disease. Liability is assumed to follow a normal distribution in the population; that is, some individuals have high values, some have low values, but most cluster around the middle of the distribution. Everyone in the population has a liability score, but only those with liability scores above a threshold have the disease. It is not the disease *per se,* but rather liability to the disease, that is transmitted in families. Neither genetic nor environmental factors that augment liability are sufficient for disease expression; both are necessary. The greater the genetic contribution to liability (a predisposition or *diathesis*), the lesser of an environmental effect is required to precipitate disease. The polygenic model is a submodel, in which transmissible risk factors are polygenes only. In such cases, environment is still important, but it is idiosyncratic environmental events not shared among family members (for example, a blow to the head or obstetric complications) that contribute to liability.

Mixed models are multilocus models in which disease transmission is due to the effect of a single major gene and the effect of transmissible environmental factors or polygenes. Essentially, the mixed model is a marriage between the single locus and multifactorial-polygenic models.

An oligogenic disease phenotype is one influenced by a limited number of loci called *quantitative trait loci* (QTLs), which are each of small and approximately equal effect. The only difference between QTLs and polygenes is simply one of degree. Oligogenic models (from the Greek *oligos* meaning *few*) posit a small number of QTLs that confer disease susceptibility. The probability of identifying and mapping a given QTL to the genome increases as the total number of QTLs influencing a disease decreases. Risch analyzed risk ratios for classes of relatives and found statistical evidence for the interaction of a small number of such multiple-disease susceptibility loci with a polygenic background in the inheritance of schizophrenia. Similar results have been obtained in analyses of recurrence risk patterns from family studies of cleft lip with or without cleft palate. Several QTLs involved in the transmission of diabetes may have been identified recently. However, recent computer simulations have shown that whereas it may not be difficult to detect one of several QTLs, a much greater number of new families is required to replicate the original finding.

BOX 23-3

MULTILOCUS MODELS THAT EXPLAIN THE GENETIC TRANSMISSION OF MENTAL DISORDERS IN MOST FAMILIES

Multifactorial-polygenic models
Mixed models
Oligogenic models

Multilocus models explain why patterns of familial aggregation are irregular and how disorders skip generations. For example, in schizophrenia, nearly 90% of offspring of affected individuals do not develop schizophrenia; nearly 90% of ill individuals have two parents who are not schizophrenic; and over 60% of affected individuals do not have an affected first- or second-degree relative. However, genetically predisposed unaffected individuals can still transmit an augmented genetic predisposition. Gottesman and Bertelsen conducted a clever study of monozygotic twins discordant for schizophrenia and found that the rate of schizophrenia in the offspring of the affected twins was approximately the same as in the offspring of their nonaffected co-twins. Individuals known to have a schizophrenia genotype (by virtue of having an identical twin with schizophrenia), but who did not develop schizophrenia, transmitted augmented genetic liability to their offspring.

Multilocus models explain the familial aggregation of physical diseases like hypertension, atheroma and coronary artery disease, ulcers, many cancers, diabetes, and cleft lip with or without cleft palate. Discussion on the genetics of these and other common adult diseases are presented in the outstanding book, *The Genetic Basis of Common Diseases,* edited by King, Rotter, and Motulsky.

What To Avoid in Genetic Counseling: Lessons from the Eugenics Movement

Breathtaking advances in the science and technology of human genetics bring the danger that genetic knowledge and information will be misused. The USHGP has established an Ethical, Legal, and Social Implications (ELSI) program to answer and address such anxieties as scientific research is being processed and applied by the public. Future misuse of scientific information hopefully can be avoided through an acknowledgment and understanding of past abuses in human genetics.

Whereas clinical genetic counseling efforts historically have always focused on helping individual families, a movement developed in the early part of the 1900s to apply the principles of genetics to change the genetic make-up of the population. Termed *eugenics,* this movement closely intertwined a rudimentary interpretation of Mendelian principles of inheritance as understood at that time with a desire to define individuals who displayed deep-seated problems such as criminal behavior, prostitution, unemployment, chronic alcoholism, and mental handicaps as "genetically inferior" and therefore socially undesirable.

Studies lacking scientific merit conducted at the time provided a justification for the proliferation of eugenic policies throughout Europe and the United States. A series of coercive measures were broadly instituted to implement the segregation, institutionalization, and sterilization of mentally impaired individuals. The first involuntary sterilization law in the United States was passed by the state of Indiana in 1907; the thirty-second and last state (Georgia) to enact eugenics legislation did so in 1937. It is estimated that at least 100,000 individuals (at least 60,000 involuntarily) were sterilized in the United States during the time of the active implementation of these laws. Most states included mental retardation, insanity, and criminality as reasons for involuntary sterilization; many also included chronic alcoholism, epilepsy, and prostitution. The low point of eugenics was reached in Nazi Germany, where a national eugenics law was introduced in 1933 and where compulsory sterilization was followed by the active killing of individuals with congenital malformations, mental disorders, and other inherited conditions such as Huntington's disease.

In addition to being ethically and morally untenable, eugenics practices were scientifically flawed and bound to fail in their attempts to decrease the incidence of severe mental disorders. As discussed, environmental factors are required to precipitate such genetically complex conditions, and multiple genes required to predispose an individual to them. Many psychiatrically normal individuals in the population may transmit at least one of the genes predisposing a person to a given mental disorder.

Although eugenics has become a discredited field, the medical community must always remain vigilant. A recently published controversial book dealing with the heritability of intelligence has raised the threat of finding different polymorphic markers in the genomes of individuals from different racial or ethnic groups and then using genetic technology in a biased manner to implement discriminatory social policies. The ongoing work of the ELSI research team in collaboration with the National Institutes of Health (NIH) is of tremendous importance in establishing guidelines to protect the privacy, autonomy, and ethical values of affected individuals and family members. Eugenics and other practices to avoid in genetic counseling are presented in the Pearls & Perils box below.

Origins and Definition of Genetic Counseling

When Sheldon Reed first coined the term *genetic counseling* in 1949, he formalized a set of activities that had gone on since the beginning of the century. These early activities were guided by the broad appli-

PEARLS & PERILS

PSYCHIATRIC GENETIC COUNSELING

- The genetic counselor should be sensitive to the counselee's cultural and racial values.
- The physician should reinforce the counselee's autonomy to make decisions and provide empathic therapeutic responsiveness to the counselee's needs.
- It is important to strictly maintain confidentiality.
- It is necessary to obtain informed consent for genetic testing (when available).
- The physician should avoid directiveness and paternalism.
- Any given reproductive option should not be presented as the "correct" one for the individual or society.
- Genetic counseling should not be conceptualized as a means to reduce the incidence of a genetic disorder.
- The physician should not bombard patients with information they are unable to integrate into their own personal life experiences.
- Counseling should not be limited to the provision of risk figures only, nor should the discussion of risk be limited to only a statistical interpretation.
- Genetic counseling should never be provided over the telephone.
- The physician should not provide predictive genetic testing (when available) to asymptomatic individuals without adequate pretest and posttest genetic counseling.
- The physician should not be hurried, uninterested, or unwilling to listen and answer questions.

cation of Mendelian principles of inheritance and took the form of guidance and advice on problems such as mental retardation, neural tube defects, schizophrenia, and cleft lip or palate. The efforts of early pioneers like Reed and Edward Dight led to the opening of the first genetic counseling clinics at the University of Michigan in 1940 and the University of Minnesota in 1941.

A useful definition of genetic counseling is given by Harper in his book *Practical Genetic Counseling:* "Genetic counseling is the process by which patients or relatives at risk of a disorder that may be hereditary are advised of the consequences of the disorder, the probability of developing or transmitting it and of the ways in which this may be prevented, avoided, or ameliorated." Above all else, genetic counseling is a process of communication, with the general goals of providing patients and at-risk family members with information about a disorder and with information that allows them to make informed reproductive and other decisions. Genetic counseling guidelines are given in the Pearls & Perils box on p. 369 and are discussed in the following paragraphs. The goal of counseling is never reduction of disease incidence by presenting a reproductive decision as the correct one for the patient or for society; such a goal is explicitly eugenic.

Cultural and Racial Sensitivity

Adequate provision of genetic counseling services increasingly requires the adoption of a multicultural perspective; this is crucial when the socioeconomic status, race, or culture of the primary care physician or genetic counselor differs markedly from that of the counselee. Relevant didactic materials incorporated into medical school curricula, as well as into medical practice in public hospital settings, can provide the primary care physician with a broad multicultural perspective on the psychosocial needs of a range of patients. However, genetic counseling with individuals from diverse cultures will likely raise complex psychological issues, and a physician's acute self-awareness of personal biases and prejudices is essential.

Maintaining the Counselee's Autonomy to Make Decisions

The traditional principles guiding the genetics profession require respect of the autonomy and decision-making capacity of the patient in a nondirective manner. This concept includes respect for the patient's experience, knowledge, and values as valid bases for decision-making. In nondirective counseling, the counselor persuades the patient that she has the capacity and ability to make and carry out her own decisions. Directive interventions focus on the ideal choice or decision; there is an attempt on the part of the counselor to persuade the patient to pursue a specific course of action. Directiveness may be inadvertently applied in subtle or covert ways if the counselor's attitudes, value judgments, and preferences toward risk and illness communicate more than objective information.

A nondirective approach is required in the genetic counseling of mental disorders. In many ways, the goals of nondirective genetic counseling resemble what the cognitive behavioral psychotherapist tries to accomplish—that is, the correction or restructuring of inaccurate cognitive perceptions to allow the patient to develop more decision-making autonomy.

Empathic Responsiveness to the Counselee

Genetic counseling requires a supportive environment for counselees to both emotionally and intellectually integrate the information provided to them. Provision of a supportive environment is especially important in psychiatric genetic counseling, given the devastating emotional effect that severe mental disorders have on affected individuals and their family members. An experience-oriented approach to genetic counseling is highly recommended, in which the experiences, attitudes, and perceptions of the patient becomes central. This necessitates active involvement of the patient in the counseling process and clear identification by the counselor of the objective of the counseling visit for the patient. Although the counselor shows some directiveness by introducing the necessary elements of the counseling sessions (for example, history taking, risk calculation and interpretation, and information delivery), the content of the genetic counseling sessions must be oriented toward the experience and expectations of the patient as determined through constant feedback. Information that is scientifically pertinent but considered unrelated by the patient to her decision-making process must be avoided. Such an experience-oriented approach to genetic counseling permits empathic responsiveness to the counselee and provides support to make informed decisions. In this sense, the experience-oriented approach resembles that taken in the modern psychoanalytic therapeutic approach of the highly influential theorist Heinz Kohut. The counselor provides a highly empathic, nondirective, and nonjudgmental environment and serves the function of organizing and processing genetic information that the counselee will later have to do for herself.

Maintaining Confidentiality: Avoiding Genetic Discrimination

The future development of genetic testing to identify one or more disease-susceptibility loci may set the stage for dramatic improvements in diagnosis and perhaps treatment. However, such advances may bring serious social problems. *Genetic discrimination* is discrimination against an individual or his relatives because of real or perceived differences from the typical genome. This definition specifically excludes those individuals who at the time of the discriminatory act are affected. Although the Americans with Disabilities Act of 1990 may play a potential role in proscribing genetic discrimination and regulating the use of genetic information by insurers, many have argued that discrimination on the basis of genotype should be considered a separate category. A number of states (including California, Wisconsin, and Ohio) have enacted or considered legislation specifically addressing the issue of genetic discrimination.

Distinguishing and classifying individuals at different risks is the central activity of the commercial insurance industry. Whereas life-insurance companies presently do not require genetic tests in underwriting, this is probably a reflection of high testing costs and the rarity of most genetic disorders for which testing is available. However, development of presymptomatic tests for common mental disorders, together with marked reductions in cost that accompany multiple testing conducted on the same sample, may lead to a genetic testing requirement for medical or life insurance. Given that serious mental disorders are associated with high medical costs and increased mortality, it is likely that information generated from genetic testing for mental disorders will be used by insurance companies to deny coverage to or limit coverage of at-risk individuals.

The central role of confidentiality in health-care delivery has been recognized since the time of Hippocrates. A crucial aspect of the doctor-patient relationship is the latter's perception that he can disclose potentially embarrassing or stigmatizing information without fear of adverse consequences. Several ethical questions raised by the Ad Hoc Committee on Genetic Testing/Insurance Issues appointed by the American Society of Human Genetics must also be raised in the genetic counseling of mental disorders. How much should a patient be told about the potential future implications of genetic testing or counseling for insurance reimbursement or coverage? Should patients be advised to obtain life insurance before being counseled? Should genetic information be excluded from medical records before release to insurance companies? What are the legal and ethical responsibilities of the primary care physician who has knowledge and access to genetic information? When is a patient competent to waive his right of confidentiality? The answers to these and other complex questions must evolve as the ethical, professional, and legal responsibilities of the primary care physician evolve in the managed care era.

Tentative suggestions can be made in accordance with the practices adopted at Washington University's Center for Psychiatric Genetic Counseling (WUCPGC), which was established by the Department of Psychiatry in 1993. Before counseling occurs, patients are encouraged to review life- and disability-insurance policies and to be aware of the possible implications that test results may have for future health care and employment. Patients are informed that the information to be provided may hurt their potential future access to health, life, or disability insurance if they attempt to obtain third-party reimbursement. Likewise, patients are informed of the potential for future limited access if they discuss their visit to a psychiatric genetic counseling center with their primary care or other physician or if they discuss the information provided to them during the course of counseling. Such a discussion could become part of a medical record to which insurance companies would have access. Patients are assured that all forms of genetic information are considered confidential and will not be disclosed without the individual's consent. Information will not be revealed to a spouse without written permission.

Informed Consent

It is often difficult for patients, especially those with mental disorders, to imagine how fully genetic counseling results may affect their lives. This will certainly be the case with establishment of future presymptomatic screening and predictive testing programs. Obtaining informed consent in those circumstances is therefore essential to help guarantee the legal and ethical responsibilities of the practitioner. Box 23-4 shows guidelines for obtaining informed consent to the future presymptomatic screening and testing for mental disorders. Such informed consent must be consistent with requirements of the local Institutional Review Board (IRB) and in accord with state and federal guidelines. Some subjects with mental illness may lack the ability to give informed consent; in those cases, consent of a legally authorized representative is required. A related question concerns whether relatives can be asked to give substitute permission for subjects unable to give consent themselves. In several

BOX 23-4

GUIDELINES FOR OBTAINING INFORMED CONSENT TO THE FUTURE PRESYMPTOMATIC SCREENING AND TESTING FOR MENTAL DISORDERS

- Inform the patient of the current state of knowledge about the genetics of the disease.
- The decision to take the test should be informed and carefully considered. An individual should never be coerced under any circumstances.
- If available, recommend that the genetic test be performed on an affected family member in conjunction with a full psychiatric examination to confirm the presence of the disease in the family.
- Inform the patient that all information is strictly confidential unless the patient waives his right (for example, to request third-party reimbursement).
- Obtain the patient's commitment to be psychiatrically evaluated and interviewed regarding his attitudes toward predictive testing.
- Obtain the patient's commitment to participate in both pretest and posttest genetic counseling.
- Inform the patient of all possible testing outcomes (such as the presence of a specific genetic mutation or the size of a mutation)
- The patient should be accompanied to testing and counseling sessions by a companion (parents, spouse, or close friend but not a sibling).
- Always give the results face-to-face and never over the telephone or by mail.
- Carefully explain the meaning of test outcomes as related to that individual's risk to disease, given the roles of predisposing multiple disease susceptibility loci and precipitating environmental factors.

states there are laws designating a series of relatives who may give substituted judgment for treatment decisions. The situation is more ambiguous when consent is for participation in a voluntary predictive-testing program. A carefully designed consent process with the involvement of the local IRB may overcome such problems.

Development of Psychiatric Genetic Counseling

Research is needed to investigate the demand for psychiatric genetic counseling and the training or knowledge base of genetic counselors currently servicing individuals with a personal or family history of mental disorder. In the only empirical study of psychiatric genetic counseling needs, Turlington and Moldin mailed a survey to members of the National Society of Genetic Counselors. Results obtained from 282 respondents show that 14% of patients seen by counselors nationwide (over 12,000 individuals) had a personal or family history of a mental disorder. This figure likely represents a lower limit of the actual need for psychiatric genetic counseling, given that centers do not explicitly market such services. The results showed that whereas psychiatric genetic counseling knowledge and skills are in demand, less than 13% of counselors surveyed had received formal training in psychiatric genetic counseling; between 61% and 92% of counselors rated different aspects of their knowledge base and ability to provide services in the area of psychiatric genetic counseling as fair or poor.

The fundamental problem in increasing access of patients to psychiatric genetic counseling is that genetic service providers at academic medical centers typically have developed considerable expertise in rare Mendelian conditions but not in genetically complex diseases. Psychiatric outpatient service providers have little formal background in genetics. This vacuum in service delivery led to the creation of the WUCPGC. Other similar specialty services may open in the psychiatry departments at Indiana University and the University of Pittsburgh.

Representative Psychiatric Genetic Counseling Scenarios

Patients requesting psychiatric genetic counseling services typically can be seen in one visit that lasts from 2 to 3 hours. Representative counseling scenarios include the following situations: (1) couples planning a pregnancy, where one of the expectant parents or a relative has a mental disorder. They desire to know the risk to their unborn child; (2) couples with one or more children, where one of the parents or a relative has a mental disorder. The visit is often precipitated by the child's exhibition of behavioral problems. The couple desires to know their child's risk and possible prodromal signs and symptoms; (3) couples who have adopted or will adopt a child who has one or both biological parents suffering from a mental disorder; and (4) individuals with a family history of mental disorder who desire to know their own risk. Commonly, counselees provide family histories in which two disorders (such as bipolar disorder and alcoholism) are present in the family. Although most patients have some knowledge of genetic components to major mental disorders like schizophrenia and bipolar disorder, they often lack knowledge of the role of genetic factors in the transmission of alcohol dependence.

Stages in Psychiatric Genetic Counseling

The stages of psychiatric genetic counseling are presented in Box 23-5 and are discussed in the following paragraphs. It is essential during each stage to follow genetic counseling "pearls" of advice and to avoid the "perils."

Identify the Goal

The first step in psychiatric genetic counseling is to identify the goal of the patient's visit and the questions that she wants answered. This determines the emphasize that should be placed on a specific content area. For example, greater emphasis should be placed on discussion of prodromal signs and symptoms for a couple who are concerned about an 18-year-old child who is acting unusual than for the counseling of an expectant couple who are more interested in knowing and understanding the magnitude of risk to an unborn child. Identifying and answering specific counseling questions is the key to maintaining patient satisfaction.

The stated reason for the visit may not be the primary reason. Occasionally, psychiatric genetic counseling is requested by affected individuals who have been frustrated in their dealings with the traditional mental health system. A request for psychiatric genetic counseling is a way to obtain access to an alternate service where emotional support can be obtained.

Accurate Diagnosis

Accurate diagnosis is essential in genetic counseling. Psychiatric diagnostic procedures have undergone a renaissance in the last 20 years, in that structured and explicit criteria now exist for mental disorders and such criteria result in high interrater agreement. Assessments made through the use of a structured diagnostic interview yield diagnoses of much greater reliability.

Accurate diagnostic assessment can be facilitated through administration of the Minnesota Multiphasic Personality Inventory (MMPI), an objective self-report psychological test of psychopathological state that takes about 1 hour to complete, and through the Diagnostic Interview for Genetic Studies (DIGS), a new state-of-the-art clinical interview developed for the Genetics Initiative sponsored by the National Institute of Mental Health (NIMH).

Attempts must always be made to see affected individuals face-to-face. However, in many cases affected individuals in the family requesting psychiatric genetic counseling are unwilling or unable to come in for a full diagnostic assessment. Although counselees often have knowledge of the diagnosis and treatment of affected relatives, unstructured questioning is usually not fruitful. In these cases the Family Instrument for Genetic Studies (FIGS) is administered to available family members. The FIGS was developed for the NIMH-sponsored Genetics Initiative and is a structured guide for gathering information about relatives to make diagnoses of mood disorders, schizophrenia, substance abuse or dependence, and schizophrenia-related personality disorders. Individuals are asked to provide information about another person (such as an affected relative) and not about themselves. The FIGS provides a comprehensive approach by which family history data on psychiatric hospitalizations, death by suicide, and other clinical information can be collected. Use of the FIGS provides increased specificity in the differential diagnosis of psychotic and mood disorders, as well as in the detection of substance abuse. The sensitivity of the FIGS is increased when information is collected from multiple informants, and the instrument can be administered to knowledgeable relatives over the telephone. The administration time varies depending on the particular family history. Copies of the DIGS and FIGS can be obtained by writing the author.

Diagnostic issues that arise during psychiatric genetic counseling are presented in Box 23-6 and discussed in the following section. Strategies to resolve the first three issues in Box 23-6 involve careful ad-

BOX 23-5

STAGES IN PSYCHIATRIC GENETIC COUNSELING

- Define the goal.
- Obtain a complete family history.
- Establish an accurate diagnosis.
- Evaluate the counselee.
- Provide education.
- Emphasize that liability to illness (not illness *per se*) is transmitted.
- Emphasize that environmental factors are required to precipitate disease.
- Estimate recurrence risks.
- Discuss the magnitude of recurrence risks.
- Discuss the burden of illness on the patient and the family.
- Discuss the possibility of modification of the burden of illness or the risk.
- Discuss prodromal symptoms.
- Provide support in the decision-making process.
- Discuss anticipated future developments.
- Follow up the patient's visit.

ministration of the DIGS or FIGS and supplementation with information from medical records. An assumption derived from the empirical literature is that the genetic predispositions *(diatheses)* for major mental disorders are independent; that is, having a diathesis for schizophrenia does not increase risk for alcoholism. In cases of co-morbidity, different risk calculations and counseling are independently provided for each co-morbid diagnosis. In cases where it is not possible to clearly rule out a diagnosis, diagnostic ambiguity is acknowledged to the patient, and genetic counseling (including recurrence risk estimation) is provided for both disorders. For example, a patient may be told, "We cannot be certain if your mother had schizophrenia or bipolar disorder. If we assume she had schizophrenia, your son's risk to schizophrenia is 14% and his risk for bipolar disorder is not elevated above the general population risk. If we assume that your mother had bipolar disorder, your son's risk for bipolar disorder is 13% and his risk for schizophrenia is not elevated above the general population risk." In cases where available FIGS, DIGS, or medical records information support a diagnosis of schizoaffective disorder, risks for both bipolar disorder and schizophrenia are discussed.

Depressive symptoms are nonspecific and can occur secondarily to a variety of physical and mental disorders. Consequently there are many individuals who meet the DSM-IV criteria for major depression but who do not have a heritable form of depression. Consideration of empirical research findings suggests that heterogeneity within the depressive spectrum, and the fourth issue from Box 23-6, may be resolved by identifying severe depression as the more heritable condition. *Severe* refers to cases of depression where the individual has been hospitalized, incapacitated, or psychotic during a depressed period or when a patient has experienced multiple episodes.

Blacker and Tsuang estimate that 65% to 74% of unipolar relatives of bipolar patients have a bipolar diathesis, and that 5% to 12% of people with unipolar depression in the population may have a bipolar diathesis. However, no validated predictors exist to distinguish "bipolar diathesis" patients with unipolar depression from "nonbipolar diathesis" patients with unipolar depression. The fifth issue from Box 23-6 may be resolved in the following way: risk for severe depression is determined when the affected relative has severe unipolar depression and there is no bipolar disorder in the family. When an affected relative has bipolar disorder and there are cases of severe unipolar depression in the family, counseling is provided under two conditions. First, the physician assumes that all cases of depression are genetically separate from cases of bipolar disorder. Counseling is independently provided for both. Only relatives with a diagnosis of bipolar disorder are counted as affected when counseling is provided for bipolar disorder, and only those affected with severe depression are counted as affected when counseling is provided for depression. In the second condition, the physician assumes that depressive and bipolar relatives have the same diathesis. All relatives with either severe depression or bipolar disorder are counted as affected, and counseling is provided for bipolar disorder. In this way, a range of risk for bipolar disorder and an independent estimate of risk for unipolar depression are provided, with the explanation that it is unclear whether relatives with unipolar depression have a bipolar or a unipolar depressive diathesis.

BOX 23-6

TYPICAL DIAGNOSTIC ISSUES IN PSYCHIATRIC GENETIC COUNSELING

1. Is the diagnosis schizophrenia or a psychotic mood disorder?
2. Is substance dependence present in the family?
3. Is there co-morbidity (e.g., substance dependence and bipolar disorder)?
4. Is a reported case of unipolar depression diagnosable as genetic or nongenetic?
5. When does a relative's diagnosis of unipolar depression augment one's risk for bipolar disorder?

The Family History

Collecting medical and psychiatric family information is a crucial step in genetic counseling and is facilitated by constructing a pedigree. Accurate pedigree construction is fundamental to the provision of services and provides an unambiguous and permanent record of genetic information in the family. Reliable information is generally available only on first-degree and second-degree relatives (uncles and aunts, nephews and nieces, grandparents, grandchildren, half-siblings) of the at-risk individual.

A standardized nomenclature for human pedigrees has recently been proposed by Bennett and colleagues. Circles are used to identify women, and squares are used for men. Affected individuals are shaded; with two or more co-morbid conditions, the symbol is partitioned accordingly. Slashes are drawn through the symbols for individuals who are dead, and the at-risk individual is indicated by a diagonal arrow. A horizontal line connects two parents and is also used to connect members of a sibship; a vertical line connects different generations.

Counselee Evaluation

Discussion of risk and other information during the genetic counseling session is often stressful. Therefore it is always necessary to evaluate the counselee's mental status, coping skills, and abilities to understand and process genetic counseling information. Affected counselees must always be evaluated regarding their treatment status, clinical stability, and understanding of the illness. Individuals requesting counseling who are actively psychotic, clinically depressed, or demonstrate impaired competency or judgment in any way must be given a referral to an appropriate mental health professional or a more intensive assessment session. At this point, possible postponement of genetic counseling may be discussed.

Education

Patients should be presented with a balanced and objective clinical description of the disease under consideration, available treatment options, and potential future developments. Basic clinical information is especially helpful to unaffected spouses and can have a powerful effect on their decision making. For example, a study conducted by Targum and colleagues found that about one half of unaffected spouses of patients with bipolar disorder would not have married or had children if they had known more about bipolar disorder before making these decisions. A patient's understanding of the illness can be facilitated by the provision of brochures published by the National Alliance for the Mentally Ill (NAMI; telephone numbers: 800-950-6264 or 703-524-7600) or the NIMH (telephone number: 301-443-4513). The pamphlet by Gottesman and Moldin entitled *Schizophrenia and Genetic Risks: A Guide to Genetic Counseling* available from NAMI is currently the only educational material that is specifically dedicated to a discussion of genetic counseling issues for a mental disorder.

Explaining Complex Genetic Transmission

A central role of psychiatric genetic counseling is to dispel myths and clarify the complex role that both genes and environment play in etiology. A common misconception is that genetic involvement means that at-risk individuals are destined to have the disorder. Often individuals think in terms of 100% risk; patients who have received genetic counseling for Mendelian disorders commonly think in terms of 25% or 50% risks. Patients must be counseled that neither genetic nor environmental factors are sufficient and that both are necessary for illness expression. An analogy may be made to the overburdened camel whose back was broken by the addition of a single straw. Genetic and environmental risk factors each contribute to an individual's liability for the disorder; when liability increases beyond a certain threshold, illness results. Counselees must be reminded that environmental assets can decrease liability; thus positive environmental experiences can compensate for high genetic liability. Another analogy that patients find helpful is the case of cigarette smoking and lung cancer. Some individuals (presumably with low genetic liability) smoke multiple packs of cigarettes for years and do not develop lung cancer. Other individuals (presumably with moderate to high genetic liability) smoke for brief periods and develop lung cancer. Still others (presumably with a very high genetic liability) who never smoke develop lung cancer after brief exposure to milder risk factors.

Environmental Risk Factors

Patients commonly ask about environmental risk factors that contribute to the liability to develop mental disorders. An example of a clear relationship between a disorder and a risk factor is alcohol dependence and prolonged heavy alcohol ingestion. Given the high co-morbidity between alcohol dependence and depression, individuals with augmented risks for either depression or alcohol dependence are counseled specifically regarding the risk of prolonged heavy alcohol ingestion. Individuals with enhanced liability to schizophrenia or bipolar disorder are also sensitive to psychotic symptom development after abusing alcohol, amphetamines, phencyclidine, cocaine, or other illicit substances. Parental death during childhood and other stressors that reflect loss or separation (actual or symbolic) can trigger depression. Several prescription medicines and physical illnesses also can trigger illness in genetically predisposed individuals.

Nonspecific stressful life events are the environmental factors that typically play the greatest role in triggering the onset of serious mental disorders. Such stressors are quite often idiosyncratic; that is, they are situations or events unique to an individual that are not shared within families and thus are difficult for the physician to detect. This explains the frustration and inability of many parents of affected individuals to find significant triggering life events in their child's history. The idiosyncratic nature of such events often leads to confusion on the part of counselees as to the role of environmental factors; illness onset is viewed as "predetermined" or "genetically hard-wired" because clear precipitants cannot be identified. It is essential to carefully explain that an event that may not be stressful for them or most people may have been sufficiently stressful to a genetically predisposed individual to trigger illness onset.

Recurrence Risks and Their Magnitude

Determination of recurrence risks is an essential element of genetic counseling. Lifetime risk to mental disorders is not given as *present* or *absent* but rather is described in terms of percentages ("there is a 10% chance that your son will develop bipolar disorder at some point in his life") or odds ("there is a 1 in 10 chance that your son will develop schizophrenia at some point in his life"). Box 23-7 shows several factors that affect risk.

BOX 23-7

FACTORS THAT MAY INFLUENCE RISK TO A MENTAL DISORDER

Characteristics of relatives

Age of onset of affected relatives
Gender of affected relatives
Number of affected and unaffected relatives
Genetic relationship of affected relatives to the at-risk individual

Characteristics of the at-risk individual

Age
Gender

An individual with high liability to develop the illness will have an earlier onset than an individual with low liability; therefore relatives with earlier onset confer greater risk than relatives with later onset.

If a disorder is more common in one gender, risk is greater to a member of the gender more often afflicted. Risk tends to be higher for relatives of the less commonly affected gender. Therefore a female offspring of an affected man has a higher risk to severe depression (which occurs at a higher rate in women in the population) than her brothers do and also has a higher risk compared with the male or female offspring of an affected woman. A male offspring of an affected woman has lower risk than his sisters and also has lower risk compared with the male or female offspring of an affected man.

Recurrence risks increase (decrease) as the degree of genetic material shared between an affected relative and the riskee increases (decreases). Having an affected monozygotic twin confers the greatest risk, given that monozygotic twins have 100% of their genetic material in common. For example, in schizophrenia the recurrence risk given an affected nontwin sibling is 9%; this rises to 48% when the affected sibling is a monozygotic twin.

Risk also increases (decreases) as the number of affected relatives increases (decreases). A useful observation is that two affected second-degree relatives or several affected third-degree relatives (first cousins, great grandparents and great grandchildren, half-uncles and half-aunts, half-nephews and half-nieces) confer approximately the same risk as one affected first-degree relative.

The population prevalence and heritability of a disorder affect risk calculations. *Heritability* is the proportion of variation in risk of illness directly attributable to genetic differences among individuals. Heritability expresses the extent to which familial aggregation is due to genetic causes. Recurrence risks for a highly heritable but relatively less common disorder are lower than recurrence risks for another disorder that is less heritable but more prevalent.

None of the factors affecting risk estimation presented in Box 23-7 can be taken into account when using empirical risks (see Table 23-1). A useful approach is to individualize risk assessment by using a modified version of the computer program *RISKMF,* written by the animal-breeding geneticist Charles Smith for use with polygenic traits. RISKMF risk estimates depend on the number of affected and unaffected pedigree members, as well as on their gender and age (or age of onset).

RISKMF-generated lifetime recurrence risks to a child born into a typical two-generation five-member pedigree (one second-degree relative, two parents, and two siblings) are given in Table 23-2. The disorders shown are those that have been the most intensively studied in psychiatric genetic research. Risks were generated with knowledge of disease prevalence (see Table 23-1) and the following heritabilities: schizophrenia and bipolar disorder, high heritability (.8); severe depression, low heritability (.4); alcoholism, moderate heritability in men (.6) and low heritability (.4) in women.

These figures are meant to be used as a guide for a variety of genetic counseling scenarios, but they cannot replace individualized recurrence-risk estimation and face-to-face counseling for specific families. Figures were calculated ignoring the effect of age of onset on risk. When one risk is given, risks are identical for a male or female child. When one parent is affected, it is the mother, and risks are shown when the affected second-degree relative is either a maternal or paternal sibling. Risk is higher when the second-degree relative is a sibling of the unaffected parent (father); this is true because disease genes are coming from both sides of the family.

The use of Table 23-2 is straightforward. For example, the risk of bipolar disorder to either a male or female child with two unaffected siblings, an affected mother, and an affected aunt on the mother's side is 7%. If the affected aunt was on the father's side, the child's risk rises to 14%. Risk figures must always be discussed relative to population prevalence, as well as to the corresponding probability of not being affected (for example, "your son's chance of developing schizo-

TABLE 23-2

RISKS TO MENTAL DISORDERS FOR A CHILD BORN INTO A FIVE-MEMBER FAMILY

		Affected parents																				
		0						1									2					
		Affected siblings																				
		0		1		2		0			1			2			0		1		2	
		Affection status, second-degree relative*																				
		U	A	U	A	U	A	U	A		U	A		U	A		U	A	U	A	U	A
Disorder	**Population Rate**								SS	OS†		SS	OS†		SS	OS†						
Schizophrenia	1%	1	2	6	9	14	18	6	8	15	16	18	25	27	31	36	33	37	42	47	52	57
Bipolar disorder	.8%	1	2	5	8	13	17	6	7	14	15	17	24	26	29	35	32	36	41	46	51	56
Severe depression (male)	4%	3	4	6	8	10	12	6	7	8	10	12	13	15	18	19	13	15	18	21	24	28
(female)	8%	6	8	11	14	18	21	12	14	15	18	21	22	26	29	30	22	25	29	33	37	41
Alcoholism (male)	14%	10	16	22	29	35	42	24	30	32	38	43	45	50	56	57	45	52	57	63	67	72
(female)	3%	2	3	5	7	9	11	5	7	8	9	11	12	14	16	17	12	15	17	20	23	26

**U,* unaffected; *A,* affected; †*SS,* same side as affected parent; *OS,* opposite side as affected parent.
Risks are shown for a child born into a family with two female siblings, two parents, and one female second-degree relative. Risks to schizophrenia or bipolar disorder are the same for a male or female at-risk child; population rates are also the same in men and women. When one parent is affected, it is the mother.

phrenia is 10 times that of a child in the general population, but he also has a 90% chance of not being affected").

Burden of Illness

A common misunderstanding is that genetic counseling stops after recurrence-risk calculation. Without an understanding of the magnitude of the burden of illness, recurrence risk figures are essentially meaningless. It is important to specifically inform counselees that despite significant progress in research there is still no treatment to prevent or retard progression of serious mental disorders like schizophrenia and bipolar disorder. Careful consideration must be given to the financial, emotional, social, and legal burdens of illness that may be imposed on the patient and family members. The counselor must also help the patient realize that the burden of illness also varies both between and within families. This discussion is balanced with a description of current treatment options and the optimism for new drug treatments that is engendered by current pharmacological research.

When a counselee is affected and is planning to have a child, a great deal of the discussion should focus on consideration of the stresses associated with childbearing. The decision of someone affected with a mental disorder (particularly schizophrenia or bipolar disorder) to have a child cannot be based on a recurrence-risk figure alone. Rather, the decision must be based on an objective evaluation of the affected person's ability to cope with the stress of parenting. Counseling must be highly personalized to each situation.

Modifying Burden of Illness or Risk

After a recurrence risk has been calculated, many counselees ask what can be done to modify the burden of illness. Whereas mental disorders are not preventable or curable at the present time, considerable advances have been made in the development of new medications. For example, risperidone offers relief from many unwanted side effects and a higher quality of life for patients with schizophrenia. Valproic acid has improved the functioning of patients with a poor prior treatment response to lithium. Patients can be counseled that research provides hope for patients and their family members and that future identification of a specific genetic factor involved in disease transmission would lead to an understanding of pathophysiological mechanisms and potential development of preventive interventions.

Counselees often ask how risk to a mental disorder can be modified. Avoidance of prolonged, heavy abuse of alcohol and illicit substances is often recommended. Patients at high risk who are experiencing considerable occupational or interpersonal stress are counseled to develop more effective coping strategies for stress management; a referral for psychotherapy is often indicated. Patients who request advice regarding childbearing strategies are reminded that idiosyncratic stressors that are difficult to delineate may play a role in triggering illness. In these cases, especially when a child's lifetime risk is 10% or less, it is strongly recommended that parents not overreact to a child's behavior. Such overreactions can in fact lead to self-fulfilling prophecies. Prodromal signs (see the related discussion) are discussed with parents, and a cautious approach is often recommended, in which a psychiatric evaluation is obtained only if a child shows a clear pattern of persistent, pervasive behavioral disturbance and resulting deterioration and impairment in social or academic functioning. Such recommendations must be individualized to each family, based on recurrence-risk estimation and the emotional maturity of the parents.

The Decision-Making Process

The goal in counseling is never to make decisions but to provide as much information as possible about different available options. At all times the physician must balance his desire to provide medical advice with careful consideration for the patient's right to make an informed decision that may differ from the one recommended by the physician. Most importantly, the physician must fight the temptation to answer the question, "What would you do in this circumstance?" It is up to the counselee to develop answers to the complex questions engendered by counseling. It is in this regard that the counselor assumes a primary role in providing objective information and being empathically responsive to the counselee as she interprets genetic information and makes decisions. The need to reinforce the counselee's autonomous decision-making abilities is especially important in psychiatric genetic counseling; some affected individuals and their relatives view themselves as being victimized by the mental health care system and respond to paternalism and rigid directiveness with considerable resentment.

Prodromal Signs and Symptoms

Regardless of the patient's goal for obtaining genetic counseling, in many cases questions are asked about prodromal signs. This is motivated by the desire to provide a treatment intervention at the earliest possible sign of mental illness. Unfortunately, the onset of illness can be rapid and clear prodromal symptoms are absent. Another problem is that prodromal signs or symptoms for serious mental illness, when present, do not have high specificity for one particular illness. This is especially true in regard to schizophrenia and bipolar disorder. Given that the peak ages of onset for these disorders are in the late teens, behavioral disturbance during the tumultuous adolescent period often confounds accurate diagnosis; mood and other behavioral changes endemic to this period can be easily confused for prodromal signs or symptoms. Substance abuse can induce mood and possibly psychotic symptoms that can mimic prodromal signs of schizophrenia or bipolar disorder. On the other hand, an assumption of normal developmental upheaval can mask serious underlying psychopathological conditions.

These considerations must be carefully explained to counselees. When the physician is convinced that the counselee has sufficient grasp of the complexities of the unfolding course of illness, a set of prodromal signs and symptoms can be discussed. Clinical experience and review of the literature have identified the following prodromal signs for schizophrenia and mood disorders:

- **Schizophrenia:** marked social isolation or withdrawal, marked deterioration in functioning, markedly peculiar behavior (collecting garbage or talking to self), impairments in personal hygiene and grooming, blunted or inappropriate affect, digressive speech that "misses the point," odd beliefs (intense superstitiousness or ideas of reference), unusual perceptual experiences, marked lack of drive and initiative, irritability, hypersensitivity, emotional instability and immaturity, antisocial acts, sleep or appetite disturbances, distractibility, impulsivity, substance abuse, poor relatedness, suicide attempts, difficulties in concentrating, and irritability
- **Bipolar disorders:** hyperactivity, sleep or appetite disturbances, distractibility, rapid mood swings, aggression, antisocial acts, excitability, inappropriate affect, flagrant disregard for others, substance abuse, inflated self-esteem or grandiosity, rapid or pressured speech, flight of ideas or racing thoughts, increased goal-directed activities, sexual indiscretions, buying sprees, excessive gambling, and irritability
- **Severe depression:** depressed mood, loss of pleasure (anhedonia), suicide attempts, significant weight loss or gain, insomnia or hypersomnia, fatigue or loss of energy, feelings of worthlessness, excessive or inappropriate guilt, recurrent thoughts of death, difficulties concentrating, irritability, and tearfulness

No single sign or configuration of signs is pathognomonic. Likewise, transient expressions of many are commonly found during normal adolescence. One approach is to emphasize that persistent expression of several of the above signs and symptoms by a genetically predisposed individual, together with resulting deterioration or impairment in social or academic functioning, should raise concerns. Referral for a comprehensive psychiatric evaluation is often indicated in such cases.

Anticipated Developments

Counselees commonly ask if genetic testing for mental disorders is available. This provides a useful forum to discuss several highly complex issues in anticipation of the day when such tests will be available. Genetic testing is not an end in itself but rather a way to gather and interpret information that can help the provider in the differential diagnostic process and help counselees to make responsible choices. It is also a way to obtain more effective treatments. For example, a tested individual experiencing severe depression may discover that he has a bipolar genotype. Adjunctive lithium treatment may then be recommended.

For Mendelian disorders, genetic tests are highly predictive. Prediction will be far less certain in the case of mental disorders, given the involvement of multiple loci and idiosyncratic precipitating factors. Despite the advantages, a myriad of ethical, legal, and social issues will be engendered the day a genetic test is developed for any mental disorder. Although such tests will be in high demand and there will be intense pressure to make them rapidly available, caution must prevail. Legal and ethical safeguards are essential requirements in the era of managed care to protect the rights of the patient, his relatives, and society. The benefits of testing must be weighed against the anxiety that will be engendered. Most importantly, results must be handled with stringent attention to confidentiality.

The limitations of a genetic test for a multifactorial disorder must be clearly acknowledged to counselees, and any benefits of presymptomatic screening will have to be carefully weighed against potential abuses. If no highly effective treatments are available, testing in many individual cases may do more harm than good. Individuals with mental disorders and their relatives still often experience intense stigmatization that may be further augmented through use of genetic testing to confirm the presence of a "defective" gene. Social policies to "help" individuals with mental disorders in their reproductive planning would be patently eugenic and must be avoided at all costs. The availability of presymptomatic screening for mental disorders, which impose a heavy financial cost to society, would offer a strong temptation for well-meaning social planners to implement eugenic programs. Concerted efforts to resist such programs must develop from within the medical and scientific communities.

Another anticipated future development involves the use of information provided by traits correlated with liability to disease. Several biological or behavioral disturbances have been identified and studied. For example, disturbances in sustained attention and disturbances in ocular motor functioning are found in individuals with schizophrenia and also in their nonschizophrenic relatives. Examples of other diseases and associated traits used in genetic analysis include idiopathic hemochromatosis and a latent capacity of transferrin; colon cancer and adenomas; breast cancer and fibrocystic breast disease; and Graves' disease and thyroid autoantibody titer.

The efficiency and accuracy of recurrence-risk estimation would be greatly increased if correlated trait data on the at-risk individual could be taken into consideration. For example, an individual with deviant attention and a given family history would have a greater risk of developing schizophrenia than another with a similar family history but normal attention abilities. The future use of such information in psychiatric genetic counseling requires a better understanding of the precise genetic relationship between the traits identified and their respective diseases.

Follow-Up

An integral part of psychiatric genetic counseling is the follow-up discussion. This permits confirmation of an individual's understanding and recollection of genetic information provided during the counseling session, and it also provides the counselee with the opportunity to receive additional support and empathic understanding. At the WUCPGC, the follow-up procedure also includes sending a pedigree drawing and a letter summarizing the information provided during the genetic counseling session. A discussion of multifactorial transmission and the contributing role of genetic and environmental factors to disease susceptibility is provided, along with a summary of the recurrence-risk figures provided during the counseling session. A discussion of prodromal signs and caveats regarding diagnostic uncertainties and recurrence-risk estimation also typically are included.

Providing Psychiatric Genetic Counseling in the Era of Managed Care

This chapter provides information for primary care physicians who are not specialists in medical genetics or mental disorders. The expanding central role that primary care physicians will play in the delivery of health care services ensures that they will be responsible for an increasing number of patients who desire psychiatric genetic counseling services. Technologies that may emerge from ongoing psychiatric genetic research include genetic information services (such as screening, counseling, and testing), experimental technologies, and perhaps gene therapy. Service delivery in future predictive and presymptomatic screening programs for mental disorders will require a team of providers that include the primary care physician, a geneticist with a strong background in the principles of quantitative genetics and genetic epidemiology, a masters-level genetic counselor, and a psychiatrist or clinical psychologist with expertise not only in the clinical treatment and assessment of mental disorders but also with a strong background in the principles of psychiatric genetics.

It is likely that in the era of managed care a multi-tiered system of access will develop in which specialized psychiatric genetic services are available only on the basis of the patient's ability to pay. In such a system, fairness dictates that primary care physicians have a strong understanding of psychiatric diagnosis, psychiatric genetics, and other principles discussed in this chapter to provide psychiatric genetic counseling to those who cannot afford specialized services.

Clinical Vignettes

Cases 23-1, 23-2, and 23-3 are fictional case reports based on actual patient histories that illustrate typical psychiatric genetic counseling scenarios.

Conclusion

Considerable scientific evidence exists to support the role of genetic factors in the etiology of major mental disorders. As the USHGP nears its ambitious

CASE 23-1

A couple in their midtwenties came for genetic counseling with their adopted 3-month-old infant. Both were extremely hard-working and high-functioning professionals with well-developed coping skills. They had recently discovered from the adoption agency that both biological parents of the child had been hospitalized multiple times for serious mental disorders. Their goal in seeking psychiatric genetic counseling was to determine the risk of serious mental disorder to their child and to find out about precipitating environmental factors. The adoption case worker's notes indicated that the mother's diagnosis was most likely schizophrenia, but bipolar disorder could not be ruled out. The biological father was reported to have a diagnosis of schizophrenia. There is no available information about the family history of either biological parent. Unfortunately, neither biological parent would consent to a psychiatric examination, and they would not agree to release their medical records. Administration of the FIGS to the adoption case worker provided evidence for a diagnosis of schizophrenia with a rule-out diagnosis of bipolar disorder for the mother, and a diagnosis of schizophrenia for the father. Considerable time was spent with the adoptive couple describing potential prodromal signs and symptoms for both schizophrenia and bipolar disorder. The involvement of idiosyncratic environmental as potential precipitants was discussed, as was the potential of illicit drugs for precipitating psychotic symptoms. Recurrence risks were determined for several situations. Assuming both biological parents had schizophrenia, the lifetime risk of the child developing schizophrenia was 43%. If only the father had schizophrenia, the risk was 9%. If the mother had bipolar disorder, the risk of bipolar disorder to the child was 7%. The need to avoid parental behaviors that could lead to undo pressures and stresses (for example, overreacting to adolescent shyness, becoming controlling and intrusive to "protect" the child from any stress, and having the child placed in special classes to receive additional attention from teachers) were discussed, and empathic understanding was provided. The couple expressed an interest in obtaining genetic testing if this were to become available in the future. Limitations of testing, as well as the possible adverse effect on their child's future access to health, life, or disability insurance, were discussed.

CASE 23-2

A couple in their midforties wanted to know risks to mood disorder for their teenage daughter and preadolescent son. The father was diagnosed with major depression when he was in his thirties. Both his mother and a maternal uncle, who lived in other states, were diagnosed with bipolar disorder according to the FIGS and review of medical records. DIGS administration confirmed a diagnosis of severe recurrent depression in the male counselee; he had been hospitalized numerous times and had been treated with antidepressants and electroconvulsive therapy (ECT). At the present time he was psychiatrically stable, had not been hospitalized in over 2 years and had high social and occupational functioning. He appeared to have above average coping skills. The couple's goals for the genetic counseling session were to find out about prodromal signs of mood disorder and whether depression is always associated with mania. The relationship between bipolar disorder and unipolar depression was discussed extensively. The risk of major depression was 8% for the male child and 14% for the female. The risk for each child to develop bipolar disorder, assuming the father had a bipolar genotype, was 11%; assuming he did not have the bipolar genotype, the risk dropped to 4%. Particular emphasis in the counseling session was placed on the role that genes and environment play in the etiology of mental disorders, and prodromal signs were also discussed. The difficulty in distinguishing such signs from typical adolescent turmoil was discussed extensively.

CASE 23-3

A recently married man and woman in their late twenties desired children and requested psychiatric counseling to determine the possible risk of depression to their offspring. The husband has suffered three episodes of incapacitating depression that required inpatient hospitalization and antidepressant medication. Information provided by the couple during FIGS administration revealed that the husband's mother had multiple episodes of incapacitating depression that required hospitalization. She was treated with antidepressants and ECT, but she ultimately committed suicide. DIGS administration confirmed the husband's diagnosis of severe depression. When taking the family history, it was discovered that the wife, one of the wife's brothers, and a maternal uncle had been hospitalized for alcohol dependence. The DIGS confirmed the wife's diagnosis of alcohol dependence. Another brother and her mother were diagnosed according to the FIGS as having probable alcohol dependence. Both counselees were surprised to find out that alcohol dependence has a genetic component. The risk to depression was 10% for a male child and 17% for a female child. Assuming the wife, her brother, and her uncle were the only relatives with alcohol dependence, the risk to alcoholism for a male was 30%; for a girl it was 7%. Assuming that the wife's other brother and mother were also affected, lifetime risks rose to 42% for a male child and 11% for a female child. Focus was placed on discussing how heavy prolonged alcohol consumption is a risk factor for both alcohol dependence and depression. Although the risks of alcohol dependence were significantly higher, both counselees perceived this to be a more preventable condition than severe depression. Childrearing strategies to facilitate communication between the couple and the child were discussed, with specific emphasis on how and when to present information to their child regarding risks to depression and alcoholism.

goals of developing detailed genetic and physical maps of the human genome, the likelihood will increase of identifying specific genes that contribute to the susceptibility to mental disorders. The potential of generating complex genetic information about individuals' risks to mental disorders raises serious ethical, moral, social, and legal questions. Psychiatric genetic counseling services provide the means to communicate and explain such information to individuals with mental disorders and their relatives. This chapter is a guide for the clinical practice of psychiatric genetic counseling by primary care physicians who are not specialists in medical genetics or mental disorders. Information is provided about the epidemiology and familial transmission of mental disorders, clinical practice guidelines (with vignettes), the potential for future genetic discrimination, and the anticipated development of predictive genetic testing in the managed health care era.

Annotated Bibliography

Harper PS: *Practical genetic counseling,* Oxford, England, 1993, Butterworth-Heinemann.

This book provides an excellent introductory guide to genetic counseling for the practicing physician. The section on genetic counseling in non-Mendelian disorders is of particular relevance to psychiatric genetic counseling, and a useful glossary of genetic terms is included.

King RA, Rotter JI, Motulsky AG: *The genetic basis of common diseases,* New York, N.Y., 1992, Oxford University Press.

This outstanding textbook presents a scholarly and comprehensive description of the genetic features of common diseases. Chapters on immunological and infectious diseases, cardiovascular diseases, pulmonary disease, gastrointestinal and hepatic disorders, endocrine and metabolic diseases, genetic aspects of different cancers, neurological disorders, and mental disorders are included. Each chapter discusses genetic and epidemiological data, the biological basis of genetic susceptibility, and the clinical application of available data. Beginning chapters discuss molecular, population, and formal genetics, allowing the reader to understand unfamiliar terms.

McGuffin P et al: *Seminars in psychiatric genetics,* London, England, 1994, Royal College of Psychiatrists.

This concise text presents up-to-date information about the impact and utility of psychiatric genetics. Exceptionally well-written chapters present a considerable amount of information that the physician will find indispensable in the practice of psychiatric genetic counseling.

Moldin SO, Gottesman II: *Population genetics in psychiatry,* In Kaplan HI, Sadock B, editors: *Comprehensive textbook of psychiatry,* ed 6, Baltimore, Md., 1995, Williams and Wilkins.

This chapter provides an excellent overview to the principles of population genetics and genetic epidemiology as applied in the study of mental disorders. A clear discussion of genetic models, quantitative methods, and research designs provides the physician with a fundamental knowledge base for understanding research findings in psychiatric genetics and for providing psychiatric genetic counseling.

US Congress, Office of Technology Assessment: *Mental disorders and genetics: bridging the gap between research and society,* Washington, D.C., 1994, U.S. Government Printing Office.

This concise background paper relays information generated at a workshop cosponsored by the Office of Technology Assessment and the National Institute of Mental Health. This is the first comprehensive discussion focusing specifically on the implications of genetics and mental disorders research. Research findings and the impact of psychiatric genetic research on public policy decisions are discussed. The sections on ethics and research, genetic counseling, and social implications are well written and informative.

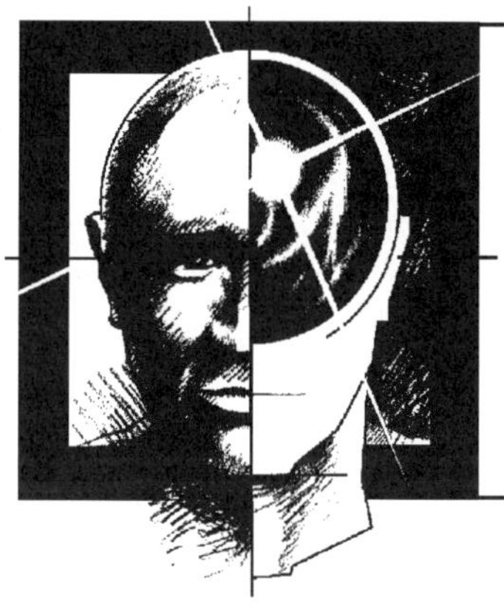

chapter 24

Adolescent Issues

Richard E. Mattison, MD and John N. Constantino, MD

Although many of the problems of adolescents are related to the developmental tasks of the adolescent period, primary care physicians should be cognizant of the rates of psychiatric disorders in this age group and of their associated serious dysfunction. The most recent epidemiological studies have found rates of psychiatric disorders in general adolescent populations of 15% to 20%. Furthermore, whereas some disorders, such as attention-deficit/hyperactivity disorder (ADHD), may persist from childhood, other diagnoses often have their onset during adolescence. These include affective disorders, anorexia nervosa, and substance abuse.

Adolescence is often assumed to be a time of major turmoil, and it was formerly thought that such turmoil is normal. However, research has demonstrated that the vast majority of teenagers negotiate this period of development with minimal social, academic, or familial disruption. Thus "turmoil" must be taken seriously. Given the 15% to 20% rate of psychiatric disorders, signs of serious life dysfunction during adolescence must be properly evaluated.

Accordingly, this chapter first briefly reviews for the primary care physician the major developmental tasks that teenagers must negotiate. Next, the physician's role in the assessment of adolescent psychopathological conditions is considered; this is followed by a discussion of other appropriate roles in the care of teenagers with psychiatric disorders. Information especially pertinent for general practitioners in the evaluation and care of major psychiatric disorders of adolescence is then presented. Finally, issues pertaining to teenagers with chronic medical disorders and accompanying psychopathological conditions, as well as issues related to teenagers with physical symptoms but no established medical basis, are also discussed.

Developmental Tasks and Problems in Adolescence

Struggles with issues of identity and self-esteem are common in adolescence. The physical and psychological transition from dependency on the family to autonomy and reproductive competency are the central developmental tasks of adolescence. The process seems to be driven by the increasing cognitive capacity for abstract thinking and by the physiological phenomenon of puberty.

Children develop their identities in the context of their families. Ideally they achieve a sense of uniqueness and importance as individuals and a sense that they are connected in stable relationships with family members. In adolescence, the individual develops his own standards to replace those of family members, and he forms an identity based on his perceived place in the societal context beyond the family. Adolescence is often seen as a time of conflict, and indeed it is only through conflict in the real world that many adolescents achieve sufficient understanding of themselves to develop their own standards.

The common problems of adolescents can often be related to basic issues of independence and the formation of a personal identity. For example, parents' intrusion into an adolescent's room is often met with resentment because it represents overt nonrecognition of such independence. Adolescents may withdraw or insist on being left alone when they perceive a threat to their autonomy. Conversely, adolescent delinquency often clashes with norms that represent authority and control.

Physicians can try to help parents understand their adolescent's transition into adulthood in such terms, and they can help parents understand their own reactions to what is happening. At the same time, parents must set limits that may help prevent disastrous consequences of judgment errors and strive to find a happy medium between too much freedom and too much restriction.

Recent research has pointed out that in high-risk environments (such as in impoverished urban communities with high rates of violent crime), it may be more difficult if not impossible for parents to walk the fine line of compromise. For example, efforts to protect adolescents from various forms of victimization or violence may necessitate difficult decisions about restrictions on social or peer-related activities that are crucial for normal development. Less-than-stable family structures add greatly to the difficulties associated with a reasonable balance.

Office Assessment

Appropriate assessment of any behavioral or emotional problems in an adolescent by a physician is important. Past research into this question has primarily focused on pediatricians and children. In both preschoolers and older children, pediatricians tend to underdiagnose psychiatric disorders, and they tend to underrefer appropriate cases to mental health professionals. Thus many children and adolescents with psychiatric problems are missed or are not properly referred despite their repeated presentations at the pediatrician's office. Several reasons are probable, such as the doctor's desire to prevent stigmatization, a lack of mental health resources, or the physician's perception of treatment as ineffective. Additionally, in the current managed-care environment, the physician has little time to explain a referral to a teenager and her family or to check that the mental health appointment is kept.

Given the primary care physician's common task of determining whether an adolescent has symptoms of a transient nature or of a more fully developed psychiatric disorder, how should a physician approach such evaluations? The reality for most physicians is that there is a limited amount of time per patient, certainly not the hour or more that is usually necessary to adequately assess a teenager's or a parent's complaints about possible psychopathological disorders. Some physicians solve this dilemma by setting aside a regularly scheduled evening with longer appointment times for adolescents about whom they are particularly concerned.

Another approach is the development of a screening battery of rating instruments to efficiently begin to evaluate an adolescent's or a parent's concerns. For younger children, Jellinek has developed a 35-item general behavior checklist (the Pediatric Symptom Checklist) to be completed by a parent for this purpose. A validated cut-off score indicates the potential seriousness of a young patient's problems and alerts the primary care physician to investigate more fully with an interview. Such an empirical approach can be practical and effective, and it uses the physician's limited time wisely.

Other checklists (such as the psychometrically sound battery that has been developed by Achenbach and his colleagues) are also available for the general screening of teenagers and can be completed by parents, teachers, and the teenagers themselves. Such batteries offer a comprehensive view of an adolescent's functioning and also use cut-off scores as levels of severity. Thus a physician can use simply gathered test scores to confirm her suspicions that an adolescent's problems are indeed serious enough to require referral to a psychiatrist or other mental health professional.

Primary care physicians should also develop an adequate, concise interview to assess adolescents about presenting behavioral or emotional problems. In such an interview, the physician must also ascertain an adolescent's general functioning at school as well as with friends and family. Specific probing questions must address the teenager's current states of anger, fear, sadness, and strange experiences. If such an interview has not been developed through training or sufficient clinical experience, then a physician might ask a child/adolescent psychiatrist to help in the realistic design of such an interview.

Finally, because a physician must determine his role in evaluating and caring for an adolescent's psychiatric problems, as well as develop relationships with local mental health resources, he must also be conscious of his referral techniques. Adolescents commonly fail to keep initial mental health appointments, so the doctor's referral process must be as effective as possible. The process of referring a teenager to another medical specialist is usually natural or well-practiced for general practitioners. In contrast, the referral of an adolescent to a psychiatrist often may not go as smoothly and is commonly compromised by awkwardness, doubt and hesitation, or negativity that the physician may communicate to the patient and family. To counter this potential problem, a child psychiatrist to whom a primary care physician refers can help by reviewing with the family doctor his referral technique for its strengths and weaknesses.

Specific Psychiatric Disorders in Adolescents

Attention-Deficit Hyperactivity Disorder

The knowledge base for ADHD continues to grow in several promising areas. This section on ADHD concentrates on the issues of course and treatment. More longitudinal studies of the course of ADHD have been accomplished and indicate that a majority of individuals with ADHD do not completely outgrow their symptoms (Box 24-1). Rather, the cardinal symptoms may often change. The symptom of hyperactivity may diminish to fidgetiness, which unfortunately in the past often led to the conclusion that adolescents were outgrowing the disorder (possibly related to the onset of puberty). Additionally, the childhood presentations of impulsivity and poor concentration may transform. Impulsivity in adolescence may reveal itself as poor frustration tolerance and wide mood swings with subsequent explosive anger. Poor attention and concentration may become exemplified by poor organization or planning abilities. Furthermore, accumulating complications, such as poor self-esteem, poor school performance, increasing conduct or drug problems, and strained relationships with peers and family, can add to the burden of a teenager living with ADHD.

Thus teenagers with ADHD and their families can be informed by primary care physicians that chances are good that a teenager who still has ADHD will probably have to contend with symptoms into adulthood. Some further prediction is also reasonable. The adolescent who has responded to treatment in a supportive, stable family and has not developed compromising secondary problems most likely has a good chance to continue an optimal course. In contrast, the teenager with ADHD who has obtained erratic treatment or lived in a stressful family environment, particularly one who has also developed symptoms of conduct disorder, most likely does not have a good prognosis. Indeed, such a patient would appear to have a course (followed by approximately 25% of individuals with ADHD) toward considerable life dysfunction and development of an antisocial personality disorder or complicating substance abuse. Clearly, when a physician encounters the latter struggling teenager with ADHD, the treatment plan must be intensified with appropriate warning to the parents about the poor predictors and the parents' need to sustain if not increase their treatment efforts. Consequently, a family physician must have an established network of mental health professionals who are especially skilled in the total care of youth with ADHD and in the support of these children's families (including, hopefully, access to a chapter of the excellent parent support network, Children and Adults with Attention Deficit Disorders or CHADD).

The primary care physician must also direct a different type of attention to the child with ADHD who appears to be entering adolescence successfully with her disorder; the approach is analogous to that for a child with diabetes who is entering adolescence with the disorder under good control and who is desiring the appropriate transfer of care to increased self-management. The teenager's understanding of her ADHD should be ascertained. Ideally, the adolescent will have reasonable knowledge that she has a chronic neurobiological disorder that is helped by medicine, and she will appreciate the cardinal symptoms of ADHD and the common secondary problems they may cause. The teenage patient may be able to use practical

DSM-IV DIAGNOSTIC CRITERIA

BOX 24-1 ATTENTION-DEFICIT/HYPERACTIVITY DISORDER

A. Either (1) or (2):

(1) six (or more) of the following symptoms of **inattention** have persisted for at least 6 months to a degree that is maladaptive and inconsistent with developmental level:

Inattention

(a) often fails to give close attention to details or makes careless mistakes in schoolwork, work, or other activities
(b) often has difficulty sustaining attention in tasks or play activities
(c) often does not seem to listen when spoken to directly
(d) often does not follow through on instructions and fails to finish schoolwork, chores, or duties in the workplace (not due to oppositional behavior or failure to understand instructions)
(e) often has difficulty organizing tasks and activities
(f) often avoids, dislikes, or is reluctant to engage in tasks that require sustained mental effort (such as schoolwork or homework)
(g) often loses things necessary for tasks or activities (e.g., toys, school assignments, pencils, books, or tools)
(h) is often easily distracted by extraneous stimuli
(i) is often forgetful in daily activities

(2) six (or more) of the following symptoms of **hyperactivity-impulsivity** have persisted for at least 6 months to a degree that is maladaptive and inconsistent with developmental level:

Hyperactivity

(a) often fidgets with hands or feet or squirms in seat
(b) often leaves seat in classroom or in other situations in which remaining seated is expected
(c) often runs about or climbs excessively in situations in which it is inappropriate (in adolescents or adults, may be limited to subjective feelings of restlessness)
(d) often has difficulty playing or engaging in leisure activities quietly
(e) is often "on the go" or often acts as if "driven by a motor"
(f) often talks excessively

Impulsivity

(g) often blurts out answers before questions have been completed
(h) often has difficulty awaiting turn
(i) often interrupts or intrudes on others (e.g., butts into conversations or games)

B. Some hyperactive-impulsive or inattentive symptoms that caused impairment were present before age 7 years.

C. Some impairment from the symptoms is present in two or more settings (e.g., at school [or work] and at home).

D. There must be clear evidence of clinically significant impairment in social, academic, or occupational functioning.

E. The symptoms do not occur exclusively during the course of a Pervasive Developmental Disorder, Schizophrenia, or other Psychotic Disorder and are not better accounted for by another mental disorder (e.g., Mood Disorder, Anxiety Disorder, Dissociative Disorder, or a Personality Disorder).

Code based on type:

Attention-Deficit/Hyperactivity Disorder, Combined Type: if both Criteria A1 and A2 are met for the past 6 months

Attention-Deficit/Hyperactivity Disorder, Predominantly Inattentive Type: if Criterion A1 is met but Criterion A2 is not met for the past 6 months

Attention-Deficit/Hyperactivity Disorder, Predominantly Hyperactive-Impulsive Type: if Criterion A2 is met but Criterion A1 is not met for the past 6 months

Coding note: For individuals (especially adolescents and adults) who currently have symptoms that no longer meet full criteria, "In Partial Remission" should be specified.

From American Psychiatric Association: *Diagnostic and statistical manual of mental disorders,* ed 4 (DSM-IV), Washington, D.C., 1994, American Psychiatric Press.

methods that she has already developed to deal with problems that the medicine cannot address. Commonly, such an adolescent is curious about other steps she can take to limit or decrease the use of medicine (much like children with other chronic medical disorders). Such a teenager should be referred to an appropriate mental health professional for a brief course in self-management of ADHD's symptoms; for example, the teenager must learn to identify situations where she is vulnerable to impulsive behavior and to develop techniques to prevent potentially embarrassing outbursts. If possible, the goal is to establish circumstances when self-management techniques could modify medication needs. This foundation will serve the adolescent well as she progresses into adulthood and assumes the full responsibility of managing her ADHD. As an adolescent reflects on the future, a healthy understanding of her strengths and weaknesses, as well as taking into account the symptoms of ADHD, also help in early career planning.

Advances in the treatment of ADHD are continuing. In general, medication is still considered necessary but not sufficient, with comprehensive treatment planning still needed as a constant consideration. Stimulants remain the first drug of choice. When indicated, they are now used more chronically (including into adulthood) and comprehensively (covering the entire day). The emphasis is on the constant maintenance of high-quality functioning to permit normal development. Adolescents, in particular, have increased homework and often need the benefit of increased concentration through a late-afternoon dose to successfully complete home assignments, which may in turn affect their overall school grades and overall success. Also, interpersonal relationships are vitally important, and an adolescent's uncontrolled impulsivity and hyperactivity may sabotage family and extracurricular peer activities. Thus any trial discontinuation of a teenager's medication must be carefully monitored, because an initially promising discontinuance may gradually relapse into a downward spiral with devastating effects on development.

More medications than the established stimulants methylphenidate, dextroamphetamine, and pemoline (adolescents often appreciate the long-acting stimulant preparations) are available to treat ADHD. Medicines such as desipramine and clonidine are better than placebo in treating ADHD, but they are generally not as effective for concentration as a stimulant. Desipramine may more help the adolescent who has ADHD with anxiety or depressive symptoms, whereas clonidine may particularly assist the adolescent who has ADHD with more serious overactivity or aggressivity. However, desipramine may produce cardiac complications (and even associated sudden death), and sedation can be troublesome with clonidine. The use of these drugs in combination with stimulants is not yet well understood. The possible efficacy of newer medications, such as fluoxetine, is not yet known.

What should a primary care physician do, given this array of medication selections, when monitoring an adolescent who was previously stable on methylphenidate but who is now destabilizing? In such cases beyond general maintenance, consultation is the best policy. For example, a teenager taking a stimulant who is stable may start to show some depressive signs, which in reality are situationally related and not at the magnitude of a major depression. Addition or substitution of the antidepressant desipramine could actually further complicate the teenager's condition (by destabilizing the ADHD or creating new side effects), but a brief course of therapy could correct the problem. The dictum of medication simplicity should always be followed instead of quick polypharmacy. Unless a physician has extensive experience with the wide range of medications for ADHD, consultation with a child psychiatrist for any new complication is indicated, much as it would be in the treatment of any other medical disorder with which the physician has experience primarily with monitoring the stable, uncomplicated condition. Often, when an adolescent who has previously uncomplicated ADHD changes, the issue is not medication but some other facet of the disorder that must be addressed in a nonmedication manner.

Finally, the monitoring of ADHD by primary care physicians has been improved by the development of good empirical rating instruments (such as the Conners rating scales), which help measure the status of a teenager's symptoms. Such information is especially important with regards to school. A parent typically cannot supply sufficient valid feedback about his child's school functioning, which must be obtained directly from teachers. Such teacher checklists (with either a general or ADHD-oriented focus) can be gathered twice a year—at the end of the first marking period and at the beginning of the fourth marking period—to monitor a teenager's initial adjustment and then to be sure that the stable status was maintained. Because of multiple teachers in secondary school, it is advisable to have a major subject teacher from the morning and one from the afternoon complete such forms.

Affective Disorders

The primary care physician commonly encounters depressive symptoms in adolescents, and she must be able to distinguish transient or situational depressive states from the more dysfunctional major depressive disorder (MDD) and dysthymic disorder (see Chapter 8). Early occurrence of a depressive disorder in childhood or adolescence may indicate the beginning of a more pernicious course of affective disorder than an initial onset in adulthood. For example, childhood dysthymic disorder may take an average of several years to dissipate, and youth with MDD (despite high rates of recovery from initial episodes) appear to be at high risk for recurrence or for the development of the disorder into bipolar disorder (which includes episodes of mania). Additionally, a youth with a depressive disorder is at higher risk for suicidal behavior. Thus early identification and intervention are important.

Unfortunately, effective treatments for affective disorders in youth are not well established. In comparison studies, children and adolescents with MDD do not respond to tricyclic antidepressants (TCAs) better than to placebo. Research is focusing on the establishment of characteristics that predict favorable a medication response, since some youth do appear to clearly benefit from the TCAs. However, these medicines are now used for only the most serious or treatment-resistant cases of depression. Studies have begun on the efficacy of the newer serotonin-selective reuptake inhibitors (SSRIs), such as fluoxetine, in teenagers and early results are promising. Similarly, little information has been established on the efficacy of any antidepressant in children or teenagers with dysthymic disorder. In contrast, lithium appears to be effective in teenagers who develop bipolar disorder (manic-depressive illness), but it also entails careful baseline and follow-up laboratory evaluations.

Research into the efficacy of nonmedication treatments for adolescents with depressive disorders has recently begun. In particular, cognitive behavior therapy (CBT) is showing promise. For example, an adolescent is taught to identify depressive thought patterns that he may automatically practice and then to develop new, more positive ways of thinking and acting; parents can then reinforce such advancements. Studies have also begun to contrast the effectiveness of antidepressant medication alone, CBT alone, and combined therapies, much as has already been accomplished for adults with major depression.

Thus physicians who suspect a depressive disorder in an adolescent should refer the youth to a psychiatrist for confirmation and any initiation of medication. Additionally, because a successful first course of an antidepressant in an adolescent is usually stopped after 6 to 12 months, careful monitoring for relapse must be done. More prolonged antidepressant use may be necessary, as is often the case in adults. This complexity in the management of depressive illness in adolescents indicates the need for close consultation between the family physician and a psychiatrist. If such communication occurs, the treatment outcome will most likely improve, similar to recent studies in which adults with major depression have been found to do better under the care of psychiatrists rather than general practitioners.

Intimately related to depressive illness in adolescents is the topic of suicide, since the two conditions are often associated (see Chapter 27). Suicide attempts and completions both markedly rise during adolescence, and completion rates in male teenagers have increased in recent years (overall, suicide is a leading cause of death in adolescents, along with AIDS, accidents, and violence). Male adolescents more commonly complete suicide; female adolescents more commonly attempt suicide; and completion is more common in the white population than in black people. The higher rate of male teenagers who complete suicide is probably related to the availability of firearms (their most common method) and drugs or alcohol (a common associated factor). Among adolescents who attempt suicide, up to 50% make a repeat attempt (especially during the 2 years after the initial attempt), and there may be an increased long-term risk for death by suicide.

In the instance of a suicide attempt by a teenager, immediate referral to a psychiatrist is indicated, even to the point of holding a teenager in an emergency room until his situation can be adequately assessed. Several factors raise the level of concern, including whether there has been a previous attempt, the seriousness of attempt, the presence of a recent disciplinary crisis or humiliation, access to drugs or firearms, a lack of family support, a history of violence, and the presence of a psychiatric disorder (not only depression, but also conduct disorder [CD] or substance abuse). After assessment, the primary care physician should make sure that a follow-up appointment with a mental health professional is kept (the chance of a repeat attempt is high, and follow-up appointments are notoriously not kept). Therapeutic programs for recent adolescent suicide attempts emphasize family involvement and increasing the youth's coping and problem-solving strategies.

Finally, whereas symptoms of depression and suicidal behavior cause family physicians to consider affective illness, one other common adolescent complaint—school refusal—should also raise a physician's concern about the possible presence of a depressive illness. Refusal to go to school may be related to pure truancy, to an ongoing struggle with a poorly treated learning disability, or to some stress at school, especially one involving peers. However, if a youth has previously been functioning reasonably well at school and then not only does not want to go to school but also declines usually enjoyable family or peer activities, further assessment for depression must be undertaken. In such cases, other depressive symptoms usually are readily elicited. It is important to prevent school absence from becoming chronic, because the secondary problems (teacher irritability with the student, embarrassment in explaining the situation to peers, and loss in steady course achievement) only compound the situation.

Anxiety Disorders

In the past, anxiety symptoms or disorders were often thought to be short-term. However, longitudinal studies have begun to indicate that anxiety disorders in youth can continue as adult anxiety disorders (see Chapters 9 and 10) or evolve into other adult disorders, especially depressive disorders. Thus child and adolescent anxiety disorders cannot be considered routine or short-lived and must at least be monitored.

Current treatment of childhood anxiety disorders primarily focuses on cognitive-behavioral management involving both the child and the family. The only firm treatment evidence thus far is for CBT with phobias, although this approach also holds promise for other anxiety disorders in children and teens. In this therapeutic approach with a teenager who has a phobia, the young patient is gradually exposed to the phobic situation first in thought and then in actuality. This process is supplemented by relaxation techniques and positive reinforcement by the family.

The only established pharmacotherapy for anxiety disorders in youth at this time is medication for obsessive-compulsive disorder (OCD). Otherwise, despite widespread use, no other medicine (neither anxiolytics nor TCAs) has been demonstrated effective in childhood anxiety disorders, except possibly benzodiazepines in acute, situational anxiety. More sustained use currently rests on little research support.

Psychiatry's understanding of OCD, especially its neurobiology (with focus on the basal ganglia), has recently grown considerably for both adults and children. Medications such as clomipramine and fluoxetine (and quite likely other SSRIs in the future) have been shown helpful in children and adolescents with OCD, although side effects such as sleepiness or behavioral disinhibition can be troublesome. OCD is proving to be a chronic disorder, even with medication that must also often be used chronically itself. Thus although medication can reduce symptoms of OCD, they are not always eliminated. Cognitive-behavioral intervention (which has proven helpful in adults with OCD) is now being studied in youth to complement medication. Teenagers are educated to understand symptoms of OCD as an intrusive process with accompanying anxiety that can be combated with a variety of symptom-reducing strategies. As with other adolescent psychiatric disorders, a primary care physician's role in OCD is probably best to monitor antiobsessional medication after a psychiatric consultant has stabilized the patient.

Finally, in the area of anxiety disorders, physicians must be aware of the symptoms of posttraumatic stress disorder (PTSD), or the reexperiencing of a traumatic event, avoidance of stimuli associated with the trauma, and general unresponsiveness, as well as symptoms of increased arousal. An adolescent may experience a trauma and then show an understandable initial reaction. However, symptoms of PTSD may then become intransigent after several months and are often related to the severity of the stressor or the reaction of the family. Thus if an adolescent has experienced a traumatic event, a physician should first ensure that the teenager is openly discussing the trauma with family members. Such open communication may reduce the risk of later development of a psychopathological disorder and is healthy for the family. If this does not occur, early referral to a mental health professional should be made. The physician then should monitor progress and make a referral if PTSD or some other psychopathological disorder appears to be developing. As with other anxiety disorders in youth, some type of CBT is typically implemented (focusing on gradual discussion of the trauma). No medication has been established to treat PTSD (but this may change as the impact of stress on a child's nervous system becomes better understood).

Additionally, in a related matter of long-term management, a teenager who has experienced a trauma (such as child abuse) and apparently recovered, still needs occasional brief reassessment for long-term symptoms of PTSD. Such an adolescent may still be at risk for PTSD or another psychopathological disorder, and abused children may show problems with mood control or interpersonal relationships.

Other Psychiatric Disorders

Youth with *CD* are problematic for all clinicians. Too often their courses are chronic and treatment-resistant. Consequently, a tendency for a primary care physician to give up early may often prevail; that is, any youth with symptoms of CD may too easily be thought to have a poor prognosis (Box 24-2). Therefore in adolescent patients with symptoms of CD physicians must be sure that certain basic steps have been accomplished early. Any success may help reduce the considerable morbidity—not only psychiatric but also medical—for which these children are at risk (premature death, injuries secondary to violence, sexually transmitted diseases, and substance-abuse sequelae).

An adolescent with an acute onset of symptoms of CD must be vigorously assessed, especially for physical or sexual abuse. Such a youth must also be evaluated for neurological disease, substance use, another experience of environmental violence, major depression or mania, and paranoia or psychosis. Swift diagnosis and proper intervention may lead to considerable improvement, as well as to the prevention of further progression and consolidation of the symptoms. Indeed, late-

DSM-IV DIAGNOSTIC CRITERIA

BOX 24-2 CONDUCT DISORDER

A. A repetitive and persistent pattern of behavior in which the basic rights of others or major age-appropriate societal norms or rules are violated, as manifested by the presence of three (or more) of the following criteria in the past 12 months, with at least one criterion present in the past 6 months:

Aggression to people and animals

(1) often bullies, threatens, or intimidates others
(2) often initiates physical fights
(3) has used a weapon that can cause serious physical harm to others (e.g., a bat, brick, broken bottle, knife, gun)
(4) has been physically cruel to people
(5) has been physically cruel to animals
(6) has stolen while confronting a victim (e.g., mugging, purse snatching, extortion, armed robbery)
(7) has forced someone into sexual activity

Destruction of property

(8) has deliberately engaged in fire setting with the intention of causing serious damage
(9) has deliberately destroyed others' property (other than by fire setting)

Deceitfulness or theft

(10) has broken into someone else's house, building, or car
(11) often lies to obtain goods or favors or to avoid obligations (i.e., "cons" others)
(12) has stolen items of nontrivial value without confronting a victim (e.g., shoplifting, but without breaking and entering; forgery)

Serious violations of rules

(13) often stays out at night despite parental prohibitions, beginning before age 13 years
(14) has run away from home overnight at least twice while living in parental or parental surrogate home (or once without returning for a lengthy period)
(15) is often truant from school, beginning before age 13 years

B. The disturbance in behavior causes clinically significant impairment in social, academic, or occupational functioning.

C. If the individual is age 18 years or older, criteria are not met for Antisocial Personality Disorder.

Specify type based on age at onset:
Childhood-Onset Type: onset of at least one criterion characteristic of Conduct Disorder prior to age 10 years
Adolescent-Onset Type: absence of any criteria characteristic of Conduct Disorder prior to age 10 years

Specify severity:
Mild: few if any conduct problems in excess of those required to make the diagnosis **and** conduct problems cause only minor harm to others
Moderate: number of conduct problems and effect on others intermediate between "mild" and "severe"
Severe: many conduct problems in excess of those required to make the diagnosis **or** conduct problems cause considerable harm to others

From American Psychiatric Association: *Diagnostic and statistical manual of mental disorders,* ed 4 (DSM-IV), Washington, D.C., 1994, American Psychiatric Press.

onset CD appears to have a better prognosis than early-onset CD. A teenager's history may also reveal that what appears to be acute is actually occurring in the context of another chronic psychiatric disorder, especially ADHD or a learning disorder. Such teenagers may have gone through grade school in precarious balance with these disorders, only to have their fragile equilibrium disrupted by entrance into the junior high or middle school atmosphere and its demands—especially those that are of a social nature or peer-related. Thus the updating of previous treatment plans may serve such youth well and also prevent early symptoms of CD from consolidating into a more troublesome condition.

More commonly, physicians have young patients who have chronic rather than acute conduct disturbances. Such youth and their families require constant support from family physicians and especially need to participate in available treatment programs. Emphasis should continue on structure and limits. The reexamination of school curriculum may reveal that a learning disorder in an adolescent is not being sufficiently addressed and must be further remedied by the school to diffuse the teenager's increasing frustration and anger. Some research has also shown the success and cost-effectiveness of after-school programs that emphasize prosocial activities for at-risk youth, such as sports promoting teamwork and good sportsmanship. No major pharmacotherapeutic advance has been made for the treatment of CD, and no medication should routinely be recommended.

Eating disorders have their peak ages of onset during adolescence, with anorexia nervosa's average age of onset at 14 and bulimia nervosa's at 19 (see Chapter 15). Both physicians and the public are quite aware of these illnesses, which combined with improved treatment approaches, appear to be making an impact on outcome. Longitudinal studies of anorexia nervosa (currently more substantial than studies of bulimia nervosa) can now provide primary care physicians with more information to advise families with teenagers who have anorexia nervosa. The majority of patients recover or improve, although approximately 20% develop a chronic course (and the course of about 5% leads to death). Eating habits return to normal in over 40% of patients, and weight is regained in 60%. The majority of all patients obtain normal educational and employment careers, but in contrast, only a minority achieve marriage or successful partnerships. Poor prognostic factors include bulimia nervosa, great loss of weight, and chronicity.

Specific medical issues of a patient with anorexia nervosa may confront the physician. At the initial examination, certain medical conditions must be ruled out (such as brain tumors, diabetes, adrenal disease, malabsorption syndrome, and regional enteritis), although the highly unusual eating habits and beliefs of anorexia nervosa are usually telltale. Additionally, the medical state of a teenager with anorexia nervosa may necessitate hospitalization for a number of serious complications, such as dehydration, electrolyte imbalance, or disturbances in cardiac condition. Hospitalization may also be necessary because of suicidal symptoms, failure to respond to outpatient treatment, or an unworkable family situation. An important first inpatient step is for the staff to make eating and exercising decisions for the patient until her weight has gradually restabilized.

Multifaceted outpatient treatment plans for adolescent eating disorders appear to be productive (after the initial goal of weight stabilization has been gradually achieved). The physician's important role is often to monitor weight and any medical complications that may have arisen. Other common components of comprehensive programs include individual CBT, group therapy, and family intervention tailored to specific needs. The contributions of the specific therapies are not yet clear. Finally, no medication is yet specific for anorexia nervosa, but fluoxetine may be helpful in bulimia nervosa. If major depression or OCD is present as a co-morbid disorder, the appropriate medication may prove helpful.

Drug and alcohol use by teenagers is common (see Chapter 14). For example, over 90% of high school seniors have used alcohol, and over 45% have used marijuana. Daily usage in this age group is 4% and 3%, respectively. Thus a primary care physician must be able to approach substance use much like sex education. Sensitive discussion and inquiry must be routine, and the physician should have a prevention protocol. The reduction of risk and harm is an important goal that can be achieved with emphasis on the vulnerability to dependence or the escalation to a more serious drug, contraction of human immunodeficiency virus (HIV) or sexually transmitted diseases, impulsive suicide, and death by car accident (40% of such deaths are associated with alcohol).

Screening is particularly important, because substance use is often missed. Although the instruments available for screening are reasonably sound, assessment by the individual physician is probably more productive. If use is acute, the observed changes are much like other acute behavioral and emotional changes in adolescents, and acute environmental problems or the early onset of another psychiatric disorder must be ruled out. The converse is also true; that is if there is any acute behavioral or emotional change in an adolescent, substance use must always be ruled out with a drug screen that assesses the suspected drugs. The possibility of dependence should also be ascertained; signs of dependence include daily use, withdrawal symptoms relieved by use, evidence of tolerance, subjective acknowledgment of lost control over use, and daily life revolving around drug activities and drug-using peers.

The adolescent's physician can make a difference in a teenager at-risk for or just beginning to use substances. Indeed, postponement of use until the late teens may reduce the chance of eventual addiction. Preusage warning factors should be noted, especially any history of substance use in the family and the presence of CD, and responded to with early education of the teenager and the family. Establishment of acute use should lead to aggressive intervention against causative situational problems or any psychiatric disorder. Identification of poor prognostic factors (that is early and frequent use) can lead to intensive individual and group intervention attempts by trained professionals. If use becomes more serious, with accompanying life dysfunction and resistance to outpatient intervention, then a residential treatment program may be necessary. Outcome studies show that success is now more possible with heroin and cocaine dependence among teenage users, whereas therapeutic impact is more limited against alcohol and marijuana dependence.

Issues in General Medical Disorders

Although the majority of children with chronic medical disorders do not have psychiatric disorders, they are twice as likely to have psychological problems as children without such medical disorders, especially when the more general concept of psychological distress is considered. Thus the primary care physician commonly (either directly or indirectly) observes anger, anxiety, or sadness in adolescents with chronic medical disorders. Such teenagers may be more at risk for anxiety and depressive disorders.

Psychological problems in adolescents with chronic medical disorders can partly be understood through consideration of the unique obstacles of their developmental stage. Teenagers with either longstanding or newly diagnosed medical conditions face increased struggles (compared with the average healthy teenager) as they negotiate independence, peer acceptance, sexual growth, establishment of self-identity, and the demanding future of adulthood. Thus a fluctuation in a previously stable child with a chronic medical illness must first be evaluated by the physician for its relationship to the encounter with any of several adolescent developmental tasks.

As a teenager and his family begin to face a chronic illness, thorough psychological assessment by the physician is important. Indeed, the initial participation of a psychiatrist may be even more advisable, since some research with asthma patients has shown the eventual reduction of long-term use of medical services when such a multidisciplinary approach is used. Additionally, recent research with newly diagnosed young patients with diabetes has demonstrated that past psychiatric illness or the development of an adjustment disorder within a few months of the initial diagnosis of diabetes increases the risk of patients for developing later psychiatric disorders. The following risk factors for psychological problems should also be considered in a teenager with a newly diagnosed medical disorder: relation of the illness to environmental exposure (such as trauma) or genetic factors, a prolonged diagnostic period or initial misdiagnosis, physical deformity or disability, and the degree of negative prognosis.

Thus in the initial psychological assessment, previous or ongoing psychopathological conditions in the adolescent and his family should be noted, as well as their patterns of coping with previous distress. Communication and education about the illness with the teenage patient and the family is essential at the beginning, as is thoroughly addressing their initial questions. Early misunderstanding or serious reactions must be dealt with expeditiously, especially to prevent the development of noncompliance. The patient and the family must be educated to recognize distress in themselves and to clearly assess their coping abilities. This establishment of a healthy working relationship with the adolescent and the family allows the medical care team, often led by a primary care physician, to provide for the psychological needs of the youth and the family swiftly and consistently.

With this appropriate baseline, specific future deviations may be more readily understood and addressed. That is, initial understanding of the "baseline" strengths and weaknesses of an adolescent with a medical disorder and his family, plus an appreciation of accompanying developmental tasks, helps a physician monitor and respond to any occurrence of psychological distress or temporary noncompliance. For example, brain involvement (secondary to either the disorder or the treatment) alerts the physician to more closely monitor school progress, because the occurrence of depressed performance or absenteeism may be related to neuropsychological impairment. The physician may have to assist the family in ensuring that the school staff understands and plans for a teenager with such a neurobiological compromise.

Finally, in addition to adolescents with chronic medical disorders, primary care physicians commonly face young patients with physical symptoms, such as recurrent abdominal pain, that are without an identifiable medical basis. The approach may be straightforward when an acute, stressful situation is identifiable along with relatively minor physical symptoms. However, more problematic is a prolonged or severe medical situation that has already generated an extensive and costly but negative workup and has also produced secondary psychological disruption that has progressively affected school, peer activities, and the family.

Research has not clearly shown how to handle such situations. However, close collaboration between a primary care physician and a psychiatrist appears important. As general principles, the physical symptoms are acknowledged, monitored, and reasonably treated by the family doctor, who also promotes the necessity of psychiatric consultation. At the same time, the mental health professional works to prevent further psycho-

PEARLS & PERILS

ADOLESCENT ISSUES

- Marked turmoil is not normal during adolescence; it is more likely related to the 15% to 20% prevalence rate of psychiatric disorders in this age group.
- Many of the less dysfunctional, common problems of adolescents can be understood through their relationships to the major developmental tasks of independence and identity formation.
- Primary care physicians both underdiagnose and underrefer teenagers with psychiatric disorders.
- Doctors who care for teenagers should emphasize their skills and techniques in the early detection, referral, and collaborative monitoring of adolescents with psychiatric disorders, rather than in the prescribing of psychiatric medications.
- The majority of children with ADHD do not outgrow the cardinal symptoms, and a large proportion continue to benefit from medication through adolescence (and quite likely adulthood) as part of their overall treatment plan.
- Antidepressants have not been shown to be more effective than placebo in teenagers with depressive disorders.
- Primary care physicians can often prevent the development of a conduct or addictive disorder through the aggressive evaluation of acute symptoms of CD or substance use in a teenager.
- In an adolescent with a newly diagnosed chronic medical disorder, a physician's thorough baseline understanding of and response to the youth's and the family's psychological states may eventually decrease the amount of subsequent needed medical service and the development of psychopathology.

logical deterioration as well as to identify and treat more basic individual or family psychopathological disorders. Frequent communication among the professionals is essential. Such a coordinated effort with these challenging young patients and families should begin as early as possible in the course of the youth's illness to prevent the development of secondary psychological sequelae that may over time become more debilitating than the original physical complaints.

Conclusion

Fortunately, the great majority of adolescents negotiate their developmental tasks well. When a primary care physician observes "turmoil" in a teenager, he must be suspicious of a psychiatric disorder, which occurs in about one fifth of this age group (see the Pearls & Perils box above). The crucial role for family physicians treating adolescents with psychopathological conditions is to properly screen and refer such teenagers to psychiatrists, a procedure that is currently not sufficiently accomplished. Physicians should emphasize their evaluation and referral techniques more than their practices of prescribing psychiatric medications, since the use of medicines in adolescent psychiatric disorders (with the possible exception of ADHD) is complicated and should be conservative. Primary care physicians should not underestimate their potential through aggressive initial inquiry and action to limit the growth of psychopathological disorders in teenagers who are abused, who come to them with acute symptoms of CD or substance use, or who develop a chronic medical disorder.

Annotated Bibliography

Barkley RA, editor: *Attention-deficit hyperactivity disorder: a handbook for diagnosis and treatment,* New York, 1990, Guilford.
This comprehensive book, especially the sections on assessment and treatment, can serve as a textbook on ADHD for primary care physicians.

McAnarney ER et al, editors: *Textbook of adolescent medicine,* Philadelphia, 1992, W.B. Saunders.
This textbook provides strong chapters on adolescent development and interviewing, as well as specific sections on psychological issues and disorders in adolescence.

Rudolph AM, Hoffman JIE, Rudolph CD, editors: *Rudolph's pediatrics,* ed 19, Norwalk, Conn., 1991, Appleton and Lange.
This book features aids for primary care physicians for distinguishing age-normal psychological problems from pathological symptoms and a discussion of specific assessment measures.

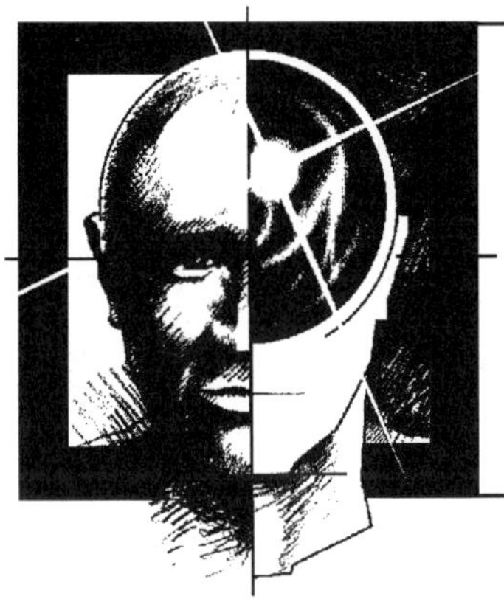

chapter 25

Psychiatry and Old Age

Eugene H. Rubin, MD, PhD

In the mid 1990s, there were 18 to 19 million Americans in the 65-to-74-year-old age group and 3 to 3.5 million Americans who were 85 years old and older. There will be about 31 million people age 65 to 74 in the year 2030 and 19 million people 85 and older by midcentury. This dramatic rise in the number of elderly people, coupled with increasing knowledge related to the specific problems and needs of this population, helped convince the American Board of Psychiatry and Neurology to approve geriatric psychiatry as a subspeciality. In 1991 the first certificates with "added qualifications" were issued. Board certification in general psychiatry, completion of 1 year of an approved geriatric psychiatric fellowship, and passing a written examination are prerequisites for this subspeciality. In this chapter, key geriatric principles and their application to psychopathology in the elderly are discussed.

Selected Demographics of Aging

There is no single definition of *old.* Currently (and subject to change), 65 is *old* in terms of eligibility for Medicare and full Social Security benefits. Although physicians attend to many ill people between the ages of 65 and 70, most people in this age range are reasonably healthy. Their health status more closely resembles people in their 50s than those in their 80s. An important indicator of geriatric health is the capability to function independently. This ability changes substantially between the ages of 65 and 85. For example, less than 20% of 65-year-old people have difficulty walking, compared to 40% of people who are 85 years old. Only 10% of 65-year-old people need help with bathing or showering, compared with 25% to 30% of 85-year-old people. Preparing meals is a problem for about 6% of the 65-year-old group, compared with more than 25% of the 85-year-old group. This difference between the "younger old" and the "older old" is further reflected in the percentage of people who reside in nursing homes; only 1% of people between the ages of 65 and 74 need this level of assistance, compared with 22% of those over 85. The elderly are a heterogenous group regarding most aspects of life from financial comfort to physical health; however, physical human frailities catch up with most people in their 80s. The size of this age group will increase more than sixfold during the next 50 years.

The older the patients a physician treats, the higher the percentage of women she will see. There are about 10 women for every 8 men in the 65-year-old population. Among people age 85, there are about 20 women for every 8 men. Older men are usually living with their spouses. Seventy-five percent of men age 65 and older still have living spouses, compared with 40% of women this age who have husbands alive and living at home (see the Pearls & Perils box to the right).

Money is a major concern for many older people. Some are wealthy; however, about 13% of people age 65 and older are at or below the poverty level, and another 7% are within 25% of this level. It becomes difficult for patients to purchase expensive medications when they can barely afford room and board. The financial concerns become all the more compelling when considering that a 65-year-old adult, on average, will live 15 to 19 more years and an 85-year-old person will live 5 to 6 more years.

PEARLS & PERILS

SELECTED DEMOGRAPHICS

- Over the next 50 years, there will be more than a sixfold increase in the number of people age 85 and older.
- One percent of people between the ages of 65 and 74 reside in nursing homes; about 22% of people age 85 and older reside in nursing homes.
- The ratio of women to men in the 85 and older age group is 2.5:1.

The Aging Body

Even though 70% of people age 65 and older describe their health as good, very good, or excellent, many are inconvenienced by painful or function-limiting conditions. About one half of those 65 and older have arthritis; about 40% have hypertension. Hearing and vision impairments are common and can disconnect people from human contact. Over 30% of people age 65 and older have hearing difficulties. High-frequency sounds become increasingly difficult to hear. Cataracts and other visual difficulties interfere with function in over 10% of the 65-and-over group, and this percentage is more than doubled in the 85-and-over group. Ischemic heart disease is symptomatic for over 10% of those over age 65. Cognitive impairment becomes increasingly common with age, and one third or more of those age 85 and older have dementia. All of these chronic conditions interfere with function. Heart disease is by far the most common cause of death in this age group, followed by cancer and cerebrovascular disease. These three groups of illness account for almost 70% of deaths in the elderly.

Anatomical and functional changes occur in every organ system with aging. Age-related changes in liver and kidney function, together with a decreasing percentage of muscle and increasing percentage of fat, change how the body handles drugs (discussed on pp 398-399). Visible changes occur in the skin. Pulmonary and cardiac reserves decrease. The aging of organs is probably related to several factors, including genetically programmed cell changes, acute and chronic environmental damage, and the influence of diseases.

Like other organs, the brain undergoes age-related changes, although the relative contribution of normal aging vs. disease is often unclear. Neurons in the central nervous system (CNS) do not replicate. Therefore when cells are destroyed or die, the remaining neurons must take over the functions of the dead tissue if recovery of those functions is to occur. Some brain atrophy occurs in old people who are cognitively intact, although the degree varies considerably among individuals. Neurons in different brain regions have varying degrees of susceptibility to genetic age-related changes or environmental damage. Various microscopic deposits accumulate in the aging brain. The amount of lipofuscin increases but currently has no clinical correlates. Other age-related neuroanatomical changes, such as Lewy bodies and Hirano bodies (cytoplasmic inclusions in certain neurons), granulovacuolar degeneration (intraneuronal vacuoles with dense cores), tangles, and plaques may occur in certain regions in small amounts in successful aging, but they occur in much larger amounts with diseases such as Alzheimer's disease or Parkinson's disease. The degree of accumulation of these changes in truly healthy aging is a subject of scientific debate. Aging is also associated with changes involving certain CNS transmitter systems. The degree to which such changes are a natural by-product of aging vs. the result of a pathological process is unknown. Neurotransmitter, neuroreceptor, and postreceptor age-related changes are important because they may explain why elderly people may be more sensitive to certain centrally active medications.

Obvious changes occur in physical and mental abilities with aging. Athletes in their 70s, although still capable of remarkable achievements, usually cannot compete with athletes in their 20s. Changes in brain function result in diminished maximal performance, although such changes do not usually interfere with most everyday activities. The degree to which these changes in brain performance are the result of inevitable aging processes vs. age-related diseases is difficult to determine. Certain skills change more than others. The ability to recall recent memories is more influenced than memory recognition. The ability to learn new information while simultaneously being distracted diminishes with age. Timed motor tasks requiring visuospatial processing are sensitive to age. It is common for elderly people to report increased difficulty in rapidly recalling names. Increasing dependency on notes and calendars occurs. These changes are usually reported to be a nuisance, but they do not interfere with the ability to be productive at work or home. If cognitive changes interfere with daily activities, the possibility of an incipient dementia needs to be entertained (see Chapter 12).

General Principles of Geriatric Psychiatry

One important principle of geriatrics is that diagnosis is more complicated with older patients; this principle also applies to geriatric psychiatry. Accurate psychiatric diagnosis is essential for maximizing successful treatment. Cognitive disorders are common in very old patients and can interfere with patients' remembering and reporting symptoms. Patients often have multiple medical illnesses with accompanying behavioral pathology which can complicate diagnosing primary psychiatric disorders. Lack of energy, poor appetite, and sleep difficulties are nonspecific symptoms associated with many chronic disorders such as renal failure, heart disease, arthritis, and diabetes. These symptoms can also occur as part of major depression, and deciding whether such symptoms result from a chronic medical illness or major depression can be difficult. Elderly patients may be taking multiple medications. Some agents have psychiatric side effects; little is known about the additive psychopathological toxicity of drug combinations. Confusion, anxiety, agitation, mood changes, personality changes, and psychotic symptoms are not uncommon side effects of polypharmacy in the elderly. People whose brain functions are already compromised from illnesses such as dementia or delirium are even more sensitive to CNS drug toxicity.

Diagnosis is further complicated by the possibility that psychiatric disorders may appear different in elderly patients than in younger patients. For example, young or middle-aged adults with depression are commonly symptomatic most of the day nearly every day. Symptoms of depression in the cognitively or medically impaired elderly person may not be as persistent; symptoms may persist only a few hours per day and may not occur every day. Although such a pattern of symptoms does not fulfill strict DSM-IV criteria for major depression, such a pattern of symptoms may be the way that depression occurs in the older, ill patient. The geriatric psychiatrist must be knowledgeable of the strict diagnostic criteria, but he also needs to use common sense when considering the possibilities of diagnostic interference caused by age, other medical illnesses, and drugs.

Some psychiatric disorders are strictly age-related. Dementia of the Alzheimer's type (DAT) is rare in people under age 50, but its incidence increases dramatically with age; it is one of the most common disorders of octogenerians. Such an age-associated pattern suggests a relationship between CNS aging and the pathophysiology of disease. Other psychiatric disorders generally have an age of onset in young or middle life. Some of these disorders with earlier onset are chronic or recurrent with symptoms continuing into old age. The elderly patient with a history of early onset recurrent depression is likely to continue to have depressive episodes in later life. In both chronic and recurrent disorders, symptoms may be influenced by age, concurrent medical disorders, and medications. Additionally, there may be age-related pharmacological changes in responsivity and side effects of treatments. Sometimes an illness that normally has a typical onset early in life appears for the first time in late life. Examples include late-onset major depression, bipolar disorder-manic episode, anxiety disorders, and schizophrenia. Interestingly, the pathophysiologies of such disorders may be different when symptoms occur for the first time late in life compared with initial presentation earlier in life. There may be age-related structural damage of CNS regions that results in the psychiatric symptoms. This is illustrated on pp. 400-401 in a discussion of late-onset depression.

Another common geriatric principle is the need to simplify the pharmacological regimen. Such simplification often leads to clinical improvement and allows for more accurate psychiatric diagnosis and treatment planning. Elderly patients are often under the care of several physicians and are ingesting a large number of medications. Additionally, elderly patients may continue to take medications prescribed years earlier without reevaluation for their need. Elderly people often self-medicate with powerful over-the-counter medications such as nonsteroidal antiinflammatory agents and antihistaminergic sleep enhancers. A patient's pharmacological history should be periodically reviewed, and whenever possible, gradual simplification of the pharmacological regimen should be attempted. Medications are often no longer necessary, or one agent can successfully serve the function of several. When eliminating medications, a gradual taper with careful monitoring is recommended. As medications are discontinued, psychiatric symptoms may disappear or patterns of symptoms may become clearer, allowing for more confidence in making diagnoses. Should psychopharmacological intervention be necessary, the simplification of drug regimens decreases the risks from medication interactions. When psychopharmacological agents are initiated, risk-to-benefit ratios need to be reevaluated often. Knowledge about the natural history of the disorder coupled with this risk-to-benefit evaluation is useful when deciding the duration of psychopharmacological treatment. Antipsychotic drugs are powerful and often necessary; however, susceptibility to acute and chronic side effects increases in the elderly, and it is imperative that these agents be used for the shortest appropriate time. Recent regulations in the nursing home industry require careful monitoring of such medications.

Another important principle that applies to geriatric psychiatry is the need to monitor patients' functional abilities (see the Pearls & Perils box to the right). Elderly patients can physically deteriorate rapidly if they are unnecessarily restricted to bed. If patients are not encouraged to be mobile, muscle atrophy can occur quickly. Elderly people can fall easily when they are weak. With falls come fractures. Patients with a history of falling or unsteadiness can develop a "fear of falling" syndrome that further restricts their mobility and may lead to further weakness and increased risk of fractures. Fractures can result in nursing home placement. Therefore it is important to maximize an elderly patient's mobility and to monitor the influence of psychiatric treatment on activities of daily living. Similarly, cognition can be adversely affected by medical illnesses and pharmacological treatment. Decreased function can also be secondary to hearing and vision difficulties, and even slight improvement helps patients regain their abilities to converse, listen, watch TV, and participate in activities. Simple interventions can improve function and can make major differences in the health of elderly patients. Improving a patient's blood pressure at the expense of diminishing function is not doing the patient justice. Patients should be monitored by brief assessments. For example, on the geropsychiatry unit at Barnes-Jewish Hospital in St. Louis, Missouri, every patient routinely receives assessments of cognition, affect, global psychopathological state, and function. It has been found that the Geriatric Depression Scale of Yesavage and colleagues is helpful in monitoring depressive symptoms. The Mini-Mental Status Examination (MMSE) of Folstein and the Short Blessed Test described by Katzman are useful instruments to monitor cognition.

PEARLS & PERILS

IMPORTANT GERIATRIC PRINCIPLES

- In elderly patients, psychiatric diagnoses are often complicated by behavioral symptoms associated with medical disorders and medications.
- Complicated drug regimens are common in the elderly and can confuse both the patient and the physician.
- The patient's ability to function in activities of daily living must be monitored closely when treating psychopathological conditions.

Pharmacological Principles of Geriatric Psychiatry

When using psychotropic medications in the elderly, the following four pharmacological areas require special attention: pharmacokinetic changes with age; pharmacodynamic changes with age; medication-illness interactions; and medication-medication interactions.

Pharmacokinetic Changes

Pharmacokinetics involves the physical handling of drugs by the body, including their absorption, distribution, metabolism, and elimination. Although pharmacokinetics can be complex, some basic, practical concepts that are helpful for everyday patient management are reviewed in this section. These concepts involve three pharmacokinetic terms: *half-life, volume of distribution (VOD),* and *clearance.*

Most psychotropic medications are handled by processes that follow first-order kinetics. This means that drugs accumulate or are eliminated in a manner proportional to the amount of drug present; that is, a proportion of drug is eliminated per unit of time regardless of the amount of drug. The time it takes to eliminate half the amount of the drug is called the *half-life* of the drug. For drugs following first-order kinetics, the half-life is the same for 1,000,000 units of drug to decrease to 500,000 and for 10 units to decrease to 5 units. Drugs such as alcohol are metabolized by processes following zero-order kinetics, which means that the same amount of agent is metabolized per unit of time independent of the initial amount; that is, the body processes the agent at the same rate independent of the amount of agent in the plasma.

The amount of time it takes an agent to accumulate to its steady-state plasma level depends on the agent's half-life. When a medication is taken repeatedly, approximately one half of the final steady-state level accumulates in the first half-life, 75% accumulates in two half-lives, 88% in three, 94% in four, and about 97% in five half-lives. Half-lives of many psychotropic drugs increase substantially with a patient's age. Agents with long half-lives, such as diazepam, desalkyl flurazepam (the active metabolite of flurazepam), or fluoxetine, can take weeks before plasma levels reach their final steady-state level.

All drugs are distributed to fat, muscle, and water. The proportion of a drug that accumulates in these different compartments depends on the chemical characteristics of the drug, such as its fat solubility. Most psychotropic drugs (with exceptions, such as lithium and risperidone) are highly fat soluble. At their steady state levels, fat-soluble drugs have relatively low concentrations in plasma and high concentrations in fat. The VOD is the volume that would be required to account for the total amount of drug in the body if the concentration were the same as it was in plasma. A compound that is highly fat soluble would have a low plasma concentration, and therefore a large volume of plasma (that is, a high VOD) would be required to account for the total amount of drug in the body. Conversely, a low VOD suggests that the agent is not highly concentrated in fat deposits but is more water soluble and would have higher concentrations in the plasma. With aging, the percentage of the body that is fat increases. This age-related change means that at the steady-state level, more agent accumulates in body fat. This increase in VOD of fat-soluble agents directly increases the half-life of the drug as discussed below.

Clearance is perhaps the most important pharmacokinetic parameter. It is defined as the volume of plasma that would be totally cleared of active drug per unit of time to account for the removal of the drug from plasma. Active drug is usually cleared by hepatic metabolism, renal elimination, or both. Clearance is the critical pharmacokinetic parameter in determining plasma steady-state levels. With aging, blood flow to the liver and kidneys can change. Also, certain liver enzymes work less efficiently in the elderly. Diminished clearance increases both a drug's half-life and its plasma steady-state concentrations.

The relationships between these three key pharmacokinetic parameters (half-life, VOD, and clearance) are illustrated in the following two clinically useful pharmacokinetic equations:

1. Half-life is proportional to VOD divided by clearance.
2. Steady-state plasma concentration is proportional to dose per time divided by clearance.

The influence of aging on the pharmacokinetics of psychotropic drugs can be understood using these two equations. Although the effect of aging on the pharmacokinetic parameters of each specific agent needs to be looked up in pharmacology references, most psychotropic drugs are highly fat soluble and are metabolized by liver enzymes that become less active with age. With such agents, the VOD increases and clearance decreases with age. From Equation 1, it is apparent that the half-life substantially increases. It can be seen from Equation 2 that the steady state plasma concentration of such agents increases to a degree inversely proportional to the clearance. Therefore patients develop higher steady-state plasma levels unless the dose is proportionately lowered. Neither half-life nor VOD directly influences the final steady-state plasma level; however, an increase in half-life means that it takes longer for steady-state levels to be reached. The practical consequences of these pharmacokinetic changes are that in the elderly, drugs may continue to accumulate for a long time, and that dosage may need to be substantially lowered to maintain an appropriate plasma level (see the Pearls & Perils box above).

PEARLS & PERILS

PHARMACOKINETICS AND AGING

- The accumulation and elimination of most drugs follow first-order pharmacokinetics.
- Clearance of many drugs decreases with patient age because of changes in hepatic and renal function.
- Since the percent of body fat increases with a patient's age, the volume of distribution of fat-soluble drugs increases with age.
- Half-life is proportional to the VOD divided by clearance.
- The half-life of a drug can increase substantially with a patient's age. Therefore both the time to reach steady-state level and the time to eliminate a drug can be much longer in older patients.
- Since the final steady-state level of a drug is inversely proportional to clearance, smaller doses are usually sufficient for elderly patients to attain similar plasma levels attained in younger patients.

Pharmacodynamic Changes

Pharmacodynamics deals with the responsivity of tissue to a given concentration of drug reaching that tissue. Tissue may be involved with the therapeutic effects of the agent or with its side effects. If with age, the sensitivity related to drugs' side effects increases and the responsivity of the brain systems related to therapeutic efficacy decreases, then the risk-to-benefit ratio changes in a disadvantageous direction. The mechanisms underlying pharmacodynamic changes may involve receptors, cell membranes, postreceptor coupling, or genomic control. Some psychotropic drugs (for example, diazepam) are characterized by increased effects at the same concentration with aging. Other agents, such as propranolol and furosomide, demonstrate decreased effects at equivalent concentration with aging. Increasing sensitivity to the development of long-term side effects can also occur, as exemplified by the increased incidence of tardive dyskinesia in elderly patients exposed to antipsychotic agents.

Medication-Illness Interaction

Elderly people are more likely than their younger counterparts to suffer from chronic illnesses. Such illnesses can influence the risks of psychiatric pharmacotherapy. For example, liver disease or renal disease may change the clearance of medications. The presence of arthritis may make it more difficult to tolerate antipsychotic-induced movement disorders. Patients with disorders influencing gait or balance may be less able to tolerate the orthostatic blood-pressure changes of certain antidepressants or antipsychotics. Some cardiac disorders increase the risk from tricyclic antidepressants (TCAs). Medications with sedative potential, including certain antianxiety agents, antidepressants, and antipsychotics, may increase confusion in patients who are cognitively impaired or falls in the frail elderly. Repeated reevaluation of risk-to-benefit ratios of psychopharmacological intervention is a key principle of geriatric psychiatry.

Medication-Medication Interaction

Many elderly people take multiple medications. Although a large number of drug interactions involving two agents have been reported, complexity expands when three or more drugs are prescribed. Specific polypharmacological interactions of complicated regimens are difficult to study, and therefore it is important to be aware of the possibility of such interactions. In general, it is preferable to use as few medications as possible. Medications accumulate for longer times in the elderly, and recently added medications can interfere with the clearance of the current drugs and change their steady-state levels. Risk can be kept to a minimum by being alert to these possibilities, carefully monitoring the patient, and measuring plasma levels when appropriate.

Psychopathology in the Elderly

The evaluation of psychiatric symptoms in the elderly is a several-step process and includes obtaining a complete history; performing physical, neurological, and psychiatric examinations; developing a differential diagnosis; and ordering appropriate laboratory, radiological, and psychological tests. With these data in hand, a working diagnosis can be made. Certain illnesses, such as dementia and delirium, commonly appear for the first time in old age. Other illnesses, such as major depression, mania, and schizophrenia, usually have an earlier onset, and it is important to know whether recent symptoms represent an initial episode or a relapse of prior episodes. Recurrent episodes often resemble earlier episodes after controlling for the potential age-related interactions discussed in the preceding paragraphs. Treatments that were effective with earlier episodes are likely to work again, as long as the appropriate pharmacokinetic and pharmacodynamic principles are considered to adjust the dose.

Different pathophysiological mechanisms may underlie disorders that typically have an early onset when the initial presentation occurs late in life. Patients who have early-onset illnesses usually have an increased family history of the illness, compared with elderly patients who have late onset of the same illness. This suggests that the mechanism in early-onset disease may involve genetic predilection. Initial presentation of the same illnesses late in life can be associated with increased anatomical abnormalities involving specific brain regions. In other words, genetics may lead to biochemical abnormalities in specific brain regions in young individuals, whereas the same symptoms may be produced by anatomical lesions in the same regions in the elderly.

Late-Onset Depression

Depression in the elderly illustrates many of the concepts discussed in the previous section. Depression can be an episodic or chronic illness. A person may experience only one or two episodes of depression during his life, or the illness may reoccur with painful frequency. Symptoms of depression may present at any age (see Chapter 8); however, attributing these symptoms to depression may be more difficult when other illnesses are present. Physiological symptoms of depression such as diminished appetite, poor sleep, and fatigue can occur as a result of many illnesses. A diagnosis of depression in the elderly requires both the physiological and psychological symptoms. Patients with recurrent depression often recognize their earliest symptoms and can accurately predict the return of the full syndrome. Early symptoms, such as a characteristic pattern of awakening or a specific type of low self-esteem, can be distinct to such patients. Somatic symptoms, such as a characteristic headache, may precede the onset of their depression. These early or prodromal symptoms are clinically important, since rapid pharmacological intervention may prevent the progression to more dangerous symptoms.

PEARLS & PERILS

EARLY VS. LATE ONSET ILLNESS

- Different pathophysiological mechanisms may cause the same clinical syndrome in older vs. younger patients.
- Anatomical lesions in specific parts of the brains of elderly patients can lead to a psychiatric syndrome, which in younger patients may be related to genetic or biochemical factors acting in the same brain regions.

When depression occurs for the first time late in life, especially when there is no family history of major mood disorders, it may be associated with pathological conditions in the brain, such as infarcts or white matter lucencies, particularly involving the left frontal lobe and striatum. These two regions have also been shown with positron emission tomography (PET) to have abnormal blood flow in young patients with familial depression. A careful neurological examination is important in the evaluation of elderly patients with new onset illness, and appropriate radiological tests may also be indicated (see the Pearls & Perils box on p. 400).

Depression is highly associated with specific CNS diseases such as Parkinson's disease. This association may be secondary to the involvement of the striatum in Parkinson's disease, since this region may also be involved in depression. When depression is associated with CNS illnesses or neuroanatomical damage, standard treatments are still often effective.

Major depression may also occur in patients suffering from chronic debilitating medical disorders (see Chapter 26). The mechanism of this association is not known. In some cases, the medical disorder may lower the threshold for developing depression in a person who is genetically predisposed. The major stress of a debilitating illness may also be involved in the development of a depressive syndrome. Major depression associated with diseases such as diabetes may be chronic unless treated. The majority of people with chronic medical illnesses do not develop major depression. It is a mistake to assume that major depression is an understandable response to the illness and therefore needs no treatment. Depressions associated with chronic illnesses usually respond to standard treatments, including pharmacotherapies and electroconvulsive therapy (ECT).

Depression and Dementia of the Alzheimer's Type

Several of the geriatric principles discussed earlier in this chapter are further illustrated by a review of the interaction of major depression and DAT. DAT is a common progressive illness of elderly people that gradually strips them of their memory, thinking abilities, orientation, personality, self-care abilities, and autonomy (see Chapter 12). Insight and understanding are often impaired early in the disease process. Patients with DAT may not be aware of any difficulties, whereas their families are distraught about their loved ones deteriorating before their eyes. Many patients with mild DAT exhibit no depressive symptoms. They describe themselves as being active, interested in life, and enjoying their senior years. They may report that their memory skills are not as good as before but that they are getting along just fine. Sleep is satisfactory, and their appetites are good, too. They appear content and have no thoughts of death or suicide. Their loved ones indicate that the patients are no longer active and have little ability to remember recent information but seem happy and unaware of what is happening. This type of history is consistent with DAT without major depression.

Other elderly patients exhibit the symptoms of a major depression without any evidence of cognitive difficulties. For example, a patient may have a history of excellent health until a marked change in behavior and activities develops. The patient becomes discouraged and disinterested in a busy schedule of activities. Crying and talking about being worthless and a failure become common. When the patient is reminded about being on many committees, running the lay ministry at church, and volunteering twice a week in the food pantry, these are dismissed as being insignificant. The patient seems convinced that family and friends are plotting. Sleep patterns change substantially. There is a loss of interest in food. The patient begins to talk about joining deceased relatives. When questioned about memory and thinking, the patient remembers past details too well. Details of a recent vacation, as well as all the travel arrangements to visit four European countries, are described accurately. On testing, recent and past details are remembered well. The patient balanced the checkbook the week before and brought a well-organized stack of papers to an accountant for tax-return preparation the previous month. This patient clearly has a major depression without evidence of DAT.

However, many patients fall in between these two extremes. Some patients develop not only clear-cut symptoms of classic depression over a month or two, but they also develop cognitive impairments that interfere with short-term and long-term memory and orientation. Such patients demonstrate diminished interest and abilities to take care of themselves. With this pattern of symptoms, it is important to obtain an accurate history of the patient's cognitive status before the development of the depressive syndrome. If after careful history gathering from knowledgeable collateral sources, it is evident that the patient did not have subtle signs of deterioration before the development of depression, it is likely that the patient is suffering from major depression and that the cognitive impairment is a result of the depressive disorder. This conclusion is strengthened if the history reveals that the patient had previous episodes of a cognition-impairing major depression. Aggressive treatment usually leads to improvement of both affective and cognitive symptoms. The cognitive impairment described in this type of patient has been referred to as *dementia of depression* and is usually a reversible dementia. There is nothing "pseudo" about the cognitive deficits, and the term *pseudodementia,* which is sometimes used to describe these cases, is inaccurate and should not be used. The long-term prognosis for such patients remains to be clarified, and it is possible that these patients have an increased risk for eventually developing DAT.

Another common scenario of cognitive and affective symptoms is illustrated by the following history. A 70-year-old patient and his family reported a 2-year history of increasing memory and thinking difficulties. Items were lost, messages were forgotton, and chores remained undone. Speech demonstrated increasing word-finding problems. Computational abilities were compromised. The patient became lost and no longer had the ability to perform tasks that were routine a few years earlier. Concentration and interest had gradually diminished in parallel with cognitive changes, and the patient had become increasingly more passive and withdrawn. Only during the last several months before the visit to the physician had the patient exhibited brief periods of crying and a low mood. These periods lasted for a few hours, and they responded to a change in activity such as going shopping with his spouse. Over the last month such symptoms occurred on about one half of the days. Such symptoms never had occurred earlier in his life. During these "bad days," the patient experienced feelings of worthlessness. Interest in activities, although gradually diminishing over the last several years, was significantly lower. Sleep was more disrupted during these bad periods, and the patient's appetite was diminished. The patient indicated increased thoughts about death if asked during such a day. This constellation of symptoms suggests the possibility of a depressive episode in addition to DAT. It is difficult to have complete confidence in diagnosing these symptoms as representing a concurrent major depression because DSM-IV criteria require symptoms to last for at least 2 weeks nearly every day for most of the day. It is likely that symptoms of major depression are modified by DAT, so it is difficult for patients with dementia to consistently maintain the psychological symptoms of depression over long periods. True symptoms of major depression in DAT may be fragmented and easier to interrupt by a change in activity. It is important to carefully inquire about a prior history of depression, because if such a history exists, the likelihood is increased that the symptoms described above represent a depression in addition to the dementia. If both the psychological and physiological symptoms of depression exist for the same several hours during a week or more in a month and such patterns did not exist several months previously, pharmacological and psychotherapeutic treatment of the depressive symptoms may be warranted. Before being confident that depression exists, it is important to be convinced that several of the following psychological symptoms of depression are present: dysphoria, crying spells, low self-esteem, guilt, death thoughts, and suicidal ideation. Diminished interest, decreased energy, and deteriorating concentration are symptoms common in DAT in the absence of concurrent depression. Assuming that these three symptoms alone suggest the presence of major depression could lead to overtreatment of depressive symptoms with the potential to harm patients by unnecessary use of antidepressants. Patients with cognitive impairment may be at increased risk for side effects from antidepressant medications. Careful use of the pharmacological principles discussed previously coupled with frequent patient monitoring is necessary. Longitudinal evaluation of specific target symptoms is useful in determining treatment efficacy. The relationship between symptoms of depression and dementia requires continued research to better define symptom specificity and responsivity. This becomes even more important as primary treatments of DAT become increasingly available.

Depression and Suicide in the Elderly

Major depression is associated with substantial morbidity and increased mortality. Even in medically healthy people, depression is associated with increased difficulties involving work, school, and family. Patients suffering from medical diseases together with concurrent depression have a more difficult course and poorer prognosis than patients with the same medical disorder without concurrent major depression. Additionally, depressed patients with or without concurrent medical illnesses have increased mortality because of an increased rate of suicide. Most people who take their own lives suffer from psychiatric illness at the time of death. Major depression is the most common psychiatric illness associated with suicide. Alcoholism, with or without concurrent major depression, also is associated with increased risk of suicide.

About 80% of elderly patients who commit suicide have an active major depression at the time of their deaths. The depressions often are not dramatic in presentation; common symptoms in the depressed elderly patient who is suicidal include recent decreases in activity, insomnia, and weight loss. The presence of a function-impairing medical illness is common in the elderly patient who is suicidal and depressed. Although prior depressive episodes occurred in the majority of those age 60 to 65 who take their own lives, only about 11% of depressed octogenerians who commit suicide have a prior history of depression.

Suicide rates vary as a function of both age and gender. Far fewer women commit suicide than men. The rate of suicide in women peaks at about age 50 and then gradually decreases. In contrast, suicide rates in men demonstrate a sharp increase beginning in the mid-60s. Elderly white men have the highest rate of suicide. White men age 85 and older have a suicide rate in excess of 65/100,000 per year in contrast to a rate of less than 10/100,000 per year in women of the same age. Elderly black men also have a much higher suicide rate than black women. The suicide rates in the white population are substantially higher than in the black population. The reasons why men and women have different patterns of suicide rates with aging or why there are race differences are unknown.

Elderly patients contemplating suicide often give hints that they are thinking about death. They usually admit to their thoughts when they are directly asked. Screening for depression, including specific inquiry regarding suicidal ideation, is an important part of every geriatric examination. A high percentage of both young and elderly patients who committed suicide had recently visited their primary care physician and were suffering from symptoms of major depression at the time of that visit. In fact, over 45% of those people had visited their primary care physicians the week before they committed suicide, and at least 70% did so within the month before they died.

When an elderly patient talks about suicide, this discussion needs to be responded to quickly. When an elderly man who is depressed talks about suicide, he may act without further warning. When elderly people with depression make suicide attempts, they are often successful. When they do not succeed, they are often seriously wounded both physically and psychologically. The preferred methods of completed suicide among the elderly are shooting, hanging, and overdosing. Most elderly who attempt suicide fully intend to die; their attempts are usually not cries for help (see the Pearls & Perils box above).

Some patients suffering from chronic debilitating medical disorders believe, for extended periods, that suicide makes sense for them. However, it is imperative for the physician to determine whether such thinking is being influenced by a concurrent depression. Even patients who are depressed and suicidal who also have terminal illnesses respond to antidepressant treatment and are usually pleased that they did not harm themselves when they were depressed. They appreciate an opportunity to take care of final tasks. Certainly there are also many patients suffering with painful, functionally debilitating disorders who consistently believe in their right to take their own lives and who are not depressed. The role of the physician with such patients can be difficult. Physicians need to let their patients know their own beliefs and allow another physician to take over a patient's care if such a request is made. Some patients request a physician's assistance in dying. Such assistance has complicated ethical, moral, and legal implications.

PEARLS & PERILS

SUICIDE AND THE ELDERLY

- Major depression is the most common illness associated with suicide.
- Elderly white men comprise a high-risk group for suicide.
- About 70% of people who complete suicide visited their physicians within the month before taking their lives; many were suffering from major depression at that time.

Chronic Psychosis and the Elderly

A discussion of chronic psychotic symptoms in the elderly presents another opportunity to demonstrate some of the principles discussed earlier in this chapter. Psychotic symptoms, including delusions, hallucinations, and formal thought disorders, are not uncommon in the elderly. Patients may also have negative symptoms, including passivity, withdrawal, poverty of thought content, and poverty of speech. The differential diagnoses of psychotic symptoms in older patients include psychotic depression, mania with psychosis, organic affective illness, dementias, deliria, and schizophrenia. When such symptoms persist in cognitively intact, medically stable patients without affective symptoms, the likelihood of schizophrenia increases.

Age of onset and family history contribute important diagnostic information. If a patient has had symptoms for decades, the illness is likely to be schizophrenia. Schizophrenia is commonly chronic, with symptoms lasting throughout middle and late life. Over time, some patients develop an increase in negative symptoms and a diminution of overt psychotic symptoms. Acute psychotic exacerbations can occur and can be associated with decreased compliance with antipsychotic medication. About one half of younger patients may have a favorable long-term outcome in terms of active psychotic symptoms, but only about one fourth of patients demonstrate improvement involving socialization skills.

When patients with early-onset schizophrenia reach old age, active pharmacological treatment needs to be reevaluated in terms of current symptoms. Antipsychotic medications can have side effects that are poorly tolerated in the elderly, including sedation, falls, orthostatic blood pressure changes, anticholinergic toxicity influencing peripheral organs (bladder, heart, eyes, and mouth) and central function (cognition), acute movement disorders, and chronic movement disorders. Elderly people are susceptible to parkinsonian side effects, including bradykinesia, tremor, and rigidity that can hamper mobilization and initiate a downward cycle of decreasing ability to function with activities of daily living. Tardive dyskinesias are common in elderly patients who have been chronically exposed to antipsychotic medications. Symptom severity can range from mild to severe. The social consequences of mild dyskinesias, such as lip smacking, can lead to decreased socialization. Severe dyskinesias can interfere with swallowing, communicating, walking, and breathing. Antipsychotic medications also have multiple pharmacokinetic and pharmacodynamic interactions with other medications.

Psychotic symptoms in the elderly are painful, debilitating, and potentially fatal. Despite the risk of significant side effects, antipsychotic medications are effective in the majority of patients. Lower doses may work well in the elderly, and the risk-to-benefit ratio needs close monitoring. Patients who reside in nursing homes should have doses titrated to the lowest effective amount. Patients with recurrent exacerbations of severe psychotic symptoms usually require continued therapy. Newer generations of antipsychotic medications have been and are being developed, and therefore the use of antipsychotic pharmacotherapy in the elderly may become safer and easier. Recently developed agents, such as clozapine and risperidone, have certain advantages compared with classic antipsychotics, but these agents do have specific risks.

Elderly patients can develop *de novo* symptoms that typically occur in early-onset schizophrenia. The prevalence of schizophrenia in the families of such elderly patients with this new onset schizophrenia-like disorder is about halfway between that occurring in families of the early-onset patients and families of the nonpsychiatrically ill. There are several interpretations of these data, including the possibility that elderly patients with the new onset disorder represent a heterogenous group, some with as high a genetic risk as patients with an earlier onset and others with a much lower genetic risk.

The premorbid history of elderly patients with new onset psychosis is also heterogenous. Some patients have no unusual premorbid features. However, about one half of these patients have a history suggestive of schizoid or schizotypal personality disorder. These patients are often loners, less likely to marry, and have had less socioeconomic success.

New onset psychotic disorder occurs much more often in elderly women than in elderly men, even after correction for the increased proportion of women in the elderly population. This is in sharp contrast to early-onset psychotic disorder in which the illness occurs at least as often in men as in women. The age of onset of paranoid schizophrenia may be later than it is for other subtypes of schizophrenia, and as age of onset increases, there is an increasing ratio of women to men with this form of schizophrenia. It is possible that the increased proportion of women in the elderly population with new onset illness may be a continuation of the gender-age relationship observed in the cases with earlier onset.

Recently, cognitive deficits associated with early-onset schizophrenias have been more fully examined. Cognitive changes in patients with early-onset schizophrenia appear not to be progressive. Although early reports indicated that elderly patients with new onset illness do not have major cognitive deficits, more recent studies challenge this notion. Between one third and one half of these patients may develop significant and progressive cognitive impairment during long-term follow-up.

Patients with DAT often demonstrate psychotic symptoms, especially during the middle stage of the illness (see Chapter 12). Psychotic symptoms can include delusions and hallucinations. These symptoms in DAT may be more fragmented than those observed in patients with schizophrenia. Some patients with early DAT can also demonstrate psychotic symptoms, and such symptoms may overshadow the more subtle difficulties with memory, orientation, and judgment. Since schizophrenia can also have cognitive deficits and DAT can on occasion have significant psychotic symptoms, it can be difficult to distinguish between these two disease entities. A careful longitudinal history from a knowledgeable collateral source is important in trying to determine whether subtle progressive cognitive deterioration preceded the psychotic symptoms. If so, DAT is more likely involved. Longitudinal follow-up with careful cognitive assessments may help to clarify the diagnosis. Since DAT is common in very old people, it is also possible for patients with late-onset schizophrenia to develop DAT as they age.

New onset psychoses in the elderly may actually represent a group of disorders that are phenotypically similar. A percentage of patients have "true" schizophrenia with later onset than usual. This subgroup should have the same genetic diathesis and family history as those with a younger onset of schizophrenia. Another group of patients may have a schizophrenia-like illness related to anatomical changes in certain brain regions. Abnormalities on magnetic resonance imaging (MRI) occur often in elderly patients with psychopathological conditions. It was suggested earlier that these MRI abnormalities can lead to depression when they are located in specific brain regions. Similarly, if these lesions interact with the circuitry that is related to schizophrenia, it is conceivable that schizophrenia-like symptoms can occur. A third group of elderly patients with late-onset psychosis includes those with DAT with psychotic symptoms out of proportion to the usual cognitive deficits.

Most patients with late-onset schizophrenia improve with the help of antipsychotic medications and attention to social intervention. Psychotic symptoms usually respond to pharmacotherapy. Elderly people have increased risks from these medications, and the physician needs to reevaluate the benefits vs. the side effects often. If late-onset psychoses have different etiologies, the natural history of these symptoms may vary depending on the pathophysiology. When the cause of symptoms is related to DAT, antipsychotic medications should be gradually decreased and stopped whenever possible. Psychotic symptoms secondary to DAT may not be as chronic as the psychotic symptoms caused by true late-onset schizophrenia.

Conclusion

Geriatric and pharmacological principles have been reviewed, and selected psychiatric topics that demonstrate certain of these principles have been presented. Several excellent geriatric psychiatry texts are available for further study and are listed in the reference section.

In terms of psychiatric treatment, it is important to make sure that the elderly patient with psychiatric illness is safe. If there is a risk of suicide, hospitalization can be life-saving. Consultation with a psychiatrist is important if the primary care physician is uncertain about evaluating safety issues pertaining to psychopathological disorders. Before pharmacological management, simplification of current treatment regimens can help clarify psychiatric symptoms and minimize risks from drug interactions. Many of the new psychiatric medications are simpler and safer to use than earlier generations of psychotropic medications. If the diagnosis is not clear or if there is concern about using psychotropic medications, psychiatric consultation should be made. If treatment has been implemented and a patient's mental status continues to deteriorate, a psychiatrist should be consulted. It is recommended that outpatient visits include assessments of suicidality, affect, function, and cognitive status. If the patient's condition does not begin to improve over several weeks, consultation with a psychiatrist experienced in psychopharmacological management is recommended.

Psychopathological disorders are common in elderly patients but are often not recognized. Cognitive impairment can be hidden behind a smile. Affective symptoms may not be detected unless the physician asks specific questions. Patients with multiple somatic complaints may have psychiatric illness exacerbating or mimicking medical disorders. Performing a brief mental status examination is important. When symptoms are discovered and appropriate diagnoses are made, treatments are typically effective. Recognizing and treating psychopathological symptoms decreases both morbidity and mortality.

Annotated Bibliography

Coffey CE, Cummings JL, editors: *Textbook of geriatric neuropsychiatry,* Washington, D.C., 1994, American Psychiatric Press.

This up-to-date, excellent text contains basic reviews of CNS function and assessment, as well as chapters addressing geriatric psychiatric disorders.

J Clin Psychiatry 54(9, suppl), 1993.

This is an excellent collection of articles reviewing psychopharmacological principles and practice.

Lazarus LW, editor: *Essentials of geriatric psychiatry: a guide for health professionals,* New York, 1988, Springer Publishing Company.

This short book is written in outline form and is packed with useful information about geriatric psychiatry.

Sadavoy J et al, editors: *Comprehensive review of geriatric psychiatry II,* ed 2, Washington, D.C., 1996, American Psychiatric Press.

This is a readable, high quality, general geriatric psychiatry text.

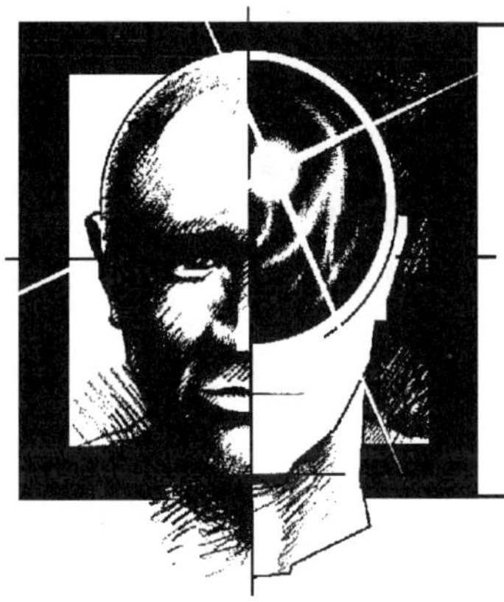

chapter 26

Psychiatric Disorders Associated with General Medical Conditions

Nuri B. Farber, MD and Kevin John Black, MD

In this chapter the focus turns from the consideration of any one psychiatric disorder to the complex issue of evaluating and treating psychiatric illness that appears in conjunction with other medical conditions. Given the continuing evolution of our understanding of the psychiatry-medicine interface, several key concepts are highlighted to establish a framework for understanding future developments. Special attention is given to the occurrence of psychiatric disorders in the context of neurological illness, endocrine disorders, or chronic medical illness. Additionally, puerperal disorders are discussed. The discussion starts with general guidelines.

General Guidelines

Importance of Diagnosing Psychiatric Disorders

In psychiatric parlance, patients who exhibit unexplained physical symptoms are said to be *somatizers*. As discussed in Chapter 16, in addition to being the main manifestation of somatization disorder, somatization can also be present in several other psychiatric disorders (for example, major depression, generalized anxiety disorder [GAD], and panic disorder). Although the occurrence of somatization in patients without medical illnesses has been recognized and diagnosed for decades, studies are just now beginning to show that certain physical complaints in patients with medical illness can be a reflection of a psychiatric disorder. For example, evidence is now accumulating that unsubstantiated complaints (that is, no confirming evidence from examination or laboratory studies) of lower extremity pain, gastrointestinal dysfunction (such as nausea, vomiting, diarrhea, constipation, pain, and bloating), and occasionally impotence in a patient with diabetes mellitus may be symptoms of a mood or anxiety disorder instead of being secondary to neuropathy.

Thus whenever the physician is confronted with the presence of a physical complaint that has an atypical symptom profile or is inconsistent with objective evidence, he should evaluate the patient for psychiatric illnesses associated with somatization. Establishing the presence of a psychiatric disorder in a somatizing patient is important for the following reasons.

BOX 26-1

IMPORTANCE OF DIAGNOSING PSYCHIATRIC DISORDERS IN PATIENTS WITH GENERAL MEDICAL CONDITIONS

- Somatization is common in several psychiatric disorders.
- Psychiatric disorders probably account for the majority of neuropathic symptoms in patients without objective indications of neuropathy.
- Psychiatric conditions can modify the clinical presentation of medical illness.
- Appropriate psychiatric diagnosis should result in decreased morbidity and mortality either from the effective treatment of the disorder or from the decreased use of unneeded diagnostic procedures.
- Appropriate psychiatric diagnosis leads to an overall decrease in the cost of heath care delivery.

Evaluation

The realization that the somatic complaints are a symptom of a psychiatric disorder and not an indicator of worsening physical health decreases the need to submit the patient to invasive tests that may subject the patient to significant risks and costs, and which often have only minimal beneficial consequences.

Treatment

Co-morbid psychiatric disorders can significantly affect the clinical treatment of general medical conditions. For example, hypoglycemic symptoms (such as dizziness or headaches) in a patient with diabetes who is currently symptomatic with major depression are an unreliable indicator of poor metabolic control. In this instance, the physician must rely on laboratory values (for example, serum glucose) instead of symptoms to determine the appropriate medical regimen for glucose control. In cases where major depression is unrecognized, the physician or the patient can make inappropriate medication changes that could have adverse consequences.

Appropriate diagnosis allows the institution of treatment directed at the underlying psychiatric illness. With treatment, improvement or resolution of the psychiatric syndrome and any associated somatic complaints is common. However, in cases where the psychiatric disorder goes undetected, the somatic symptoms typically persist, sometimes subjecting the patient to an unfavorable outcome.

Prognosis

Appropriate treatment of the psychiatric disorder often leads to its remission and the resolution of the associated signs and symptoms. With improvement in mental state, patients usually return to their previous level of functioning and are much better able to undergo appropriate medical treatment (for example, to comply with exercise or dietary regimens or to give informed consent for surgery). Not unexpectedly, the presence of a psychiatric illness can also have a substantial impact on the overall prognosis in patients with chronic medical illnesses. Recent studies suggest that in patients with coronary artery disease, the presence of major depression not only presages a worse cardiac outcome (that is myocardial infarction, angioplasty, coronary artery bypass graft, or death), but it is actually a better predictor of morbidity and mortality than traditional cardiac risk factors (such as degree of coronary artery occlusion or left ventricular ejection fraction). Although the reason for the increased morbidity and mortality in this subgroup of patients is not known, the higher prevalence of ventricular tachycardia in patients with major depression could account for their poorer outcome. Major depression appears to be associated with poorer outcomes in other chronic medical illnesses (end-stage renal disease, diabetes mellitus, and cancer) as well, but studies are still needed to better define the exact risk.

Financial

The recognition and treatment of psychiatric disorders with somatization in patients with chronic medical illness typically lead to a reduction in health care costs and an increase in productivity by avoiding unnecessary tests and medication and by improving the health of patients (Box 26-1).

If no psychiatric disorder can be found after a careful evaluation in such patients,* and if neither a neurological nor another medical disorder can be unearthed to account for the symptom, the clinical process responsible for the unexplained somatic symptom often eventually surfaces and turns out to be nonpsychiatric in nature. It is important that such patients be followed up carefully over time with an open mind regarding psychiatric vs. medical disorders. Finally, it should be emphasized that emerging clinical data indicate that the presence of a well-described and validated psychiatric disorder (such as major depressive disorder [MDD] or somatization disorder) probably accounts for the symptoms in a significant number of patients who were previously diagnosed with one of the several poorly validated syndromes (such as chronic fatigue syndrome or multiple chemical sensitivities).

Diagnosing Mental Disorders in Patients with General Medical Conditions

Throughout this book a medical model approach to the evaluation and treatment of the major psychiatric illnesses has been emphasized. Nowhere else is the medical model more important than in diagnosing and treating mental illness in medically ill patients. In this group of patients the physician must be adept in evaluating general medical and psychiatric illnesses and in determining whether given signs or symptoms are manifestations of a "medical" or a "psychiatric" process, or both. Whereas this determination is conceptually simple, in practice it can sometimes be exceedingly difficult to determine whether a symptom is part of a medical or psychiatric condition. For example, complaints of poor appetite in a patient with cancer could be secondary to a cachectic state, drug-induced nausea, or a major depressive episode. Similar difficulties can arise when evaluating poor energy, insomnia, or any of several other physical symptoms.

When evaluating a physical symptom that is part of a patient's general medical condition, the physician should first elicit in detail the characteristics of the symptom. Particular attention should be paid to timing of onset and offset of the symptom, aggravating and ameliorating factors, and the presence or absence of any associated symptoms. For example, complaints of insomnia in a patient with congestive heart failure could be secondary to paroxysmal nocturnal dyspnea, diuretics, or major depression. Awakening after a couple of hours of sleep is more consistent with the first two causes, whereas onset of insomnia in the early morning (for example, at 5:00 AM) with an inability to fall back asleep is more indicative of major depression. Special emphasis should be given to the physical signs or symptoms that are not manifestations of both the psychiatric and medical illness. In the above example, reports of orthopnea or the presence of edema would favor paroxysmal nocturnal dyspnea. However, poor appetite would suggest that major depression might be more likely. In difficult cases, interviewing outside sources and observing the patient over several weeks can prove helpful.

In contrast to physical signs and symptoms, psychological symptoms, since they are not typically a direct manifestation of medical illness, are much better indicators of the presence of a psychiatric disorder and do not pose as great a diagnostic dilemma. However, with psychological signs and symptoms, the physician is confronted with a new challenge: determining whether the psychological symptom is pathological or normal. For some psychological manifestations (for example, elevated mood, delusions, or hallucinations) the determination is relatively easy. In contrast, the depressive ones (such as poor mood and loss of interest) tend to pose conceptual problems for physicians and patients alike because they are understandable ("I'd be depressed too if . . ."). However, as in other fields of medicine, it is usually severity and duration and not understandability that are the critical factors in determining whether any given response is pathological or not. Although this concept is readily accepted when it is applied to the heart or other organs, it is not uncommon for physicians to have difficulty accepting its application to psychiatric illness. Instead, they insist on a brain-mind dichotomy—a dichotomy in which the brain follows the rules of nature, whereas the mind follows some unknown set of rules and operates as a black box. As discussed in Chapters 1 and 2, one of the fundamental principles of the medical model of psychiatry is that the nervous system (the "psychiatric" as well as "neurological" parts) follows the same rules as the rest of the body and that the practice of medicine should follow the same approach for both.

For example, the normal ("understandable") response to the stress of a cardiovascular treadmill test includes tachycardia and hyperventilation (to meet increased cardiac demand). However, in those patients with an abnormal cardiovascular system, the understandable response still occurs, but it appears typically at a lower level of cardiovascular stress. After the stress is discontinued it takes a longer time for the cardiovascular system to return to baseline. Furthermore, as the severity of the abnormality in the cardiovascular system increases, decreasing amounts of cardiovascular

*Given the potential ramifications, the physician should always resist the temptation of invoking a psychiatric disorder, such as major depression, to explain a somatic complaint without first having performed a complete and indepth psychiatric evaluation.

stress are needed to produce the same degree of cardiovascular response. Higher demands on the system lead to the appearance of other signs and symptoms (such as T-wave changes on the electrocardiogram [ECG], blood-flow changes on thallium scans, angina, chest pain, and diaphoresis) that are more obviously pathological, since they are not understandable. Thus the presence of signs and symptoms (that is, phenotype) of a pathological state in an organ (for example, the brain, heart, or lung) is a function of both the amount of stress placed on that organ (that is, current environment) and the current level of organ functioning. An organ's current level of functioning in turn is a property of the organ's initial capacity (that is, genotype) modified by past nongenetic events (for example, level of conditioning or previous ischemic events).

The same reasoning can be applied to the psychological responses to mental stress. Thus a complaint of sadness could be a normal reaction to a devastating illness (for example, a patient may be sad after being informed of a terminal illness). However, if the sadness continues unabated or worsens with time and becomes associated with dysfunction (such as severe distress or impairment in social or occupational functioning), it is considered abnormal. Depending on the presence or absence of other signs and symptoms, the pathological response is characterized as either an adjustment disorder or a major depressive episode (see Chapter 8).

In addition to poor mood, anxiety and worry are two other psychological responses that might be ignored because they are understandable. Psychological signs and symptoms such as suicidality, guilt feelings, and feelings of worthlessness, because of their severity, tend not to pose problems for most physicians and are readily accepted as pathological. However, in some circumstances (for example, in debilitating and progressive neurological illnesses) even suicidality may be considered a rational, normal, and understandable reaction by many. Although this is possible, physicians are urged to evaluate such patients carefully for psychiatric disorders such as major depression and to provide treatment if they are present.

After ascertaining the presence or absence of each diagnostic criterion, the physician should reevaluate the patient's medical status, including a review of the medical problems, medication, pertinent examination findings, and laboratory values. Following this approach should allow the physician to make the correct diagnosis in the majority of patients. However, even after extensive evaluations in which no stone has been left unturned, the diagnosis will remain unclear for some patients. In such instances the physician may elect to consider the presence or absence of a previous personal history or a family history of psychiatric illness. Given the strong familial pattern seen in most major psychiatric disorders and the knowledge that patients with previous psychiatric dysfunction are at higher risk for future psychiatric problems, medically ill patients with a positive family or past personal history of a psychiatric disturbance are probably at greatest risk for developing a co-morbid psychiatric condition. In cases where such an individual has several signs and symptoms suggestive of a psychiatric disorder but does not meet the specific syndromal criteria, close follow-up is warranted to ascertain whether the patient subsequently worsens. However, the physician might opt for empirical treatment in those patients with significant morbidity (for example, patients who are unable to function at work or having death thoughts) where conservative management might pose unwarranted risks.

By following this approach, physicians should be able to correctly evaluate most instances of psychiatric disorders that appear in the context of a general medical condition (see the Pearls & Perils box below). However, the inherent difficulty in determining the presence of specific criteria can sometimes result in the physician being unable, in spite of the expenditure of a substantial amount of effort, to either substantiate or rule out the presence of a psychiatric syndrome. Reevaluating these patients over time (for example, once every couple of weeks) often clarifies the diagnosis. However, some patients still might need to be treated empirically in the end.

PEARLS & PERILS

EVALUATING MEDICALLY ILL PATIENTS FOR PSYCHIATRIC DISORDERS

- Diagnosis is often complicated by the overlap of signs and symptoms between the two disorders.
- The presence or absence of each diagnostic criterion for the disorder under consideration should be ascertained.
- The severity of the medical illness should be ascertained to help guide interpretation of whether the somatic sign or symptom in question is psychiatric or medical in origin.
- The physician should look for the presence or absence of signs and symptoms that are not seen in the patient's medical illness but that occur in a psychiatric disorder (for example, psychological signs).
- Patients with a family or past personal history of psychiatric illness are typically those at highest risk for psychiatric illness.

Treatment

Studies indicate that antidepressants are effective for a major depressive episode, whether the cause is chronic medical illness, stroke, or the death of a spouse. Thus treatment is generally straightforward, with the rule being to treat the psychiatric disorder as if it did not occur in the context of a medical condition (see specific chapters in Section Two for treatment guidelines). However, the choice of a specific therapeutic agent and dose must take into account the patient's medical history and other medications. Since most patients with general medical conditions and comorbid psychiatric disorders are on at least two (and probably three or four) different medications, the potential for interaction between the different drugs exists. The general rule is to be vigilant for drug-drug interactions (pharmacokinetic and pharmacodynamic) and to simplify the medication regimen as much as possible to decrease the risk of a clinically significant interaction. Given the potential for drug-drug interactions, the physician should resist the temptation of prescribing additional medications that relieve specific signs or symptoms but do not treat the underlying psychiatric disorder (for example, benzodiazepines for insomnia* or for anxiety associated with major depression). Educating patients about their psychiatric illness and explaining that their troubling symptoms (such as insomnia or anxiety) will often start to improve after the first week or two of treatment and will resolve as their illness is treated will suffice and eliminate pressure from the patient for immediate symptom relief (Box 26-2).

BOX 26-2

TREATMENT GUIDELINES

- If the disorder is severe, or if the patient is suicidal or psychotic, refer the patient to a psychiatrist.
- In general, treat the patient as if the disorder occurred in isolation.
- Be vigilant of drug-drug and drug-illness interactions.
- If there is no response after 2 to 3 weeks, increase the dose if possible.
- If there is still no response, consider psychiatric referral.
- Avoid the use of other nonessential psychiatric medications (such as benzodiazepines for insomnia).

A major consideration in selecting a therapeutic agent for patients with coexisting medical illnesses concerns the metabolism of the agent and how the agent might interact with drugs being used to treat the medical disorder. The cytochrome P-450 (CYP) system is the main route of metabolism for most therapeutic agents. In humans, this enzyme system consists of 25 to 30 different enzymes (of which several are subject to genetic polymorphism) that are grouped into 12 different families. The approximately dozen enzymes responsible for drug oxidation belong to three families (CYP1, CYP2, and CYP3). Fortunately for the physician, most drugs are substrates for one of either two enzymes (CYP2D6 and CYP3A4). Several drugs can either induce or inhibit CYP enzymes, thus leading to the potential for drug-drug interactions. Whereas most interactions are not clinically significant, several (such as the now infamous terfenadine-ketoconazole interaction) can be disastrous if they occur. Table 26-1 is a listing of the major drug-metabolizing CYP enzymes, their known drug substrates, and their potential or known pharmacokinetic interactions. Currently, the ability to predict whether a clinically significant interaction will occur in any one individual is poor. However, in the not-too-distant future, laboratory tools will likely be available that allow for the identification of at-risk individuals. For now the physician can only be aware of the potential for an interaction and follow up the patient's clinical course, as well as the patient's serum drug levels whenever possible.

The physician must also be vigilant for the occurrence of pharmacodynamic interactions. The ability of psychiatric drugs to interact with several different receptor systems increases the chances that a significant pharmacodynamic interaction will occur. Monoamine oxidase inhibitors (MAOIs), tricyclic antidepressants (TCAs), and antipsychotics are the most notorious. Table 26-2 contains a listing of the more common pharmacodynamic interactions that occur with psychiatric medications.

Psychiatric Considerations in Patients with Neurological Illness

Many neurological illnesses have psychiatric sequelae, including psychosis, mania, major depression, and anxiety. However, reviewing all psychiatric complications of all neurological illnesses is beyond the scope of this chapter, and helpful reviews for specific conditions are listed in the bibliography and annotated bibliography. Here the focus is primarily on major depression, which (after delirium and dementia) is the

*Similar to the use of antipyretics to control the fever seen with infections, there are some data, albeit weak, showing that the use of sedatives to relieve the insomnia of major depression might even be counterproductive.

TABLE 26-1

SUBSTRATES AND INHIBITORS OF VARIOUS CYTOCHROME P-450 ENZYMES

Cytochrome P-450 Enzymes	Substrates	Inhibitors
CYP1A2	Caffeine* Haloperidol(?)* Phenacetin TCAs (demethylation)* Theophylline*	Fluvoxamine*
CYP2C	Citalopram Diazepam Hexobarbital Phenytoin(?)* TCAs (demethylation) Tolbutamide* Warfarin	Fluoxetine(?)* Fluvoxamine Sertraline(?)*

CYP2D6 (debrisoquine 4-hydroxylase)	Antiarrhythmics (Type 1c)*
	  Encainide
	  Flecainide
	  Propafenone
	Antidepressants
	  Brofaromine
	  Fluoxetine
	  Paroxetine
	  TCAs (hydroxylation)*
	  Venlafaxine
	Antihypertensives
	  Captopril
	  Debrisoquine
	Antipsychotics
	  Clozapine
	  Haloperidol
	  Phenothiazines
	  Risperidone
	Beta-blockers
	  Bufuralol
	  Metoprolol
	  Propranolol
	  Timolol
	Morphine derivatives
	  Codeine
	  Dextromethorphan
		Dextropropoxyphene
		Fluoxetine*
		Fluphenazine
		Haloperidol
		Paroxetine*
		Quinidine
		Sertraline*
		Thioridazine

*Potentially clinically significant; (?) = suspected.

most common psychiatric syndrome in these patients and a common reason for psychiatric referral.

Diagnostic Considerations

It has already been mentioned that considerable skill is required to distinguish depressive signs and symptoms from the effects of general medical illness and treatment. In hospitalized patients, *nil per os* (NPO) orders, nursing evaluations at midnight, and confinement to bed make it even more difficult to diagnose poor appetite, insomnia, and anhedonia, respectively. However, injury to the brain adds an additional level of diagnostic confusion. Although brain lesions can cause psychiatric illness, they can also directly cause other neurobehavioral syndromes that either mimic or hide signs of major depression. These include well-known syndromes such as aphasia, delirium, and amnesia, as well as lesser-known syndromes such as pure apathy, pathological crying, or akinetic mutism (also known as abulia). Two examples, aprosodia and anosognosia for depressive signs, are discussed to show how neurobehavioral syndromes can complicate psychiatric diagnosis after a stroke.

First, certain brain lesions can render patients unable to put emotional coloring (prosody) into their verbal communication by using pitch, inflection, ges-

TABLE 26-1

SUBSTRATES AND INHIBITORS OF VARIOUS CYTOCHROME P-450 ENZYMES—CONT'D

Cytochrome P-450 Enzymes	Substrates	Inhibitors
CYP3A4	Antihistamines (nonsedating)	Erythromycin
	Astemizole*	Fluoxetine(?)*
	Terfenadine*	Fluvoxamine*
	Benzodiazepines	Itraconazole*
	Alprazolam*	Ketoconazole*
	Midazolam*	Nefazodone*
	Triazolam	Sertraline(?)*
	Calcium channel blockers	
	Diltiazem	
	Felodipine	
	Nifedipine	
	Verapamil	
	Carbamazepine	
	Cortisol	
	Cyclosporine	
	Dapsone	
	Erythromycin	
	Lidocaine	
	Lovastatin	
	Nefazodone	
	Quinidine	
	Sertraline	
	Tamoxifen	
	TCAs (demethylation)	
	Warfarin	

*Potentially clinically significant; (?) = suspected.

TABLE 26-2

PHARMACODYNAMIC INTERACTIONS

Purported Mechanism	Interaction
α_1-Adrenergic receptor blockade	Potentiation of antihypertensives
Clozapine	Prazosin (especially)
Low-potency antipsychotics	
Risperidone	
TCAs	
Dopamine reuptake blockade	Interference of antipsychotic action
Bupropion	Dopamine receptor antagonists
Histamine receptor blockade	Potentiation of sedation
Clozapine	Alcohol
Low-potency antipsychotics	Antiepileptic agents
TCAs	Antihistamines
	Benzodiazepines
Inhibition of monoamine degradation	Serotonin syndrome
MAOIs	Meperidine
	Serotoninergic TCAs
	Serotonin-selective reuptake inhibitors (SSRIs)
	Tyramine
Membrane stabilization	Potentiation of arrythmias
TCAs	Type 1a antiarrythmics
Muscarinc receptor blockade	Potentiation of constipation, urinary retention
	Anticholinergic drugs
Clozapine	
Low-potency antipsychotics	
TCAs	

ture, and facial expression. This phenomenon has been seen with strokes in the right hemisphere corresponding to Broca's motor speech area and has been called *motor* (or *expressive*) *aprosodia*. Although there is some controversy as to the validity and localization of aprosodia, it is certainly present in some stroke patients. The importance for psychiatric diagnosis is that some patients are unable to look and sound sad even when they feel sad. Thus a patient with motor aprosodia may say that she is sad but not appear to be sad, and major depression may be underestimated by the physician. Or, "flat affect" in a patient with motor aprosodia may be mistaken for mild major depression when none is present. In short, the ability of stroke patients to show emotion must be specifically assessed before the physician can meaningfully interpret their affect (see the Pearls & Perils box below).

Second, anosognosia is a phenomenon in which patients lack awareness of a central nervous system (CNS) deficit. Although anosognosia is usually used in reference to hemiplegia, it can also describe unawareness of visual, tactile, cognitive, or emotional deficits after brain injury. Patients can have anosognosia for one type of deficit and remain aware of another. Concerning anosognosia for low mood, clearly it cannot be claimed that a patient feels sad if he denies it. However, major depression is a syndrome, not a symptom. In several cases, stroke patients show signs of major depression (for example, anhedonia, insomnia, anorexia, crying, and talk of suicide and hopelessness), but they deny both signs and symptoms. The responsible lesions tend to be in the right parietal lobe. Since a DSM-IV diagnosis of major depression can be made using observable signs of major depression even when there are no self-reported symptoms, these patients can be said to have anosognosia for major depression. It may be worth asking why a diagnosis of major depression need be made if the patient is unaware of the illness. However, major depression is a predictor of higher morbidity and mortality in stroke patients, and treatment may improve rehabilitation outcome even when patients do not recognize their major depression. Additionally, patients with this fascinating presentation have responded to antidepressant medications in a typical fashion. The importance of anosognosia for major depression can be summarized in this unsurprising way: patients with brain damage may not be able to reliably describe their own symptoms, including mood symptoms. Several other studies support this by showing poor correlation of self-reported symptoms and observable signs of major depression in stroke patients. Fortunately, the best solution is simply part of good medical practice—for confident diagnosis the physician must often gather diagnostic information not only from patients' self-reported symptoms but also from direct observation of their behavior, either by himself, other hospital personnel, family members, or other caregivers. The point is that the usual psychiatric examination must be expanded to adequately assess patients with known brain lesions. However, the additional effort required is modest.

Although a thorough psychiatric assessment is recommended in patients with neurological illness because of those cases in which diagnosis is difficult, there are many more patients in whom major depression is obvious. Prospective studies show that certain neurological illnesses have a high prevalence of major depression. In stroke, for instance, about 20% of patients have major depression (depending on the population studied), and another 20% show milder, subsyndromal depressive symptoms. The same proportions hold for Parkinson's disease. These numbers reflect cross-sectional prevalence; over the entire course of the illness the percentages are even higher. Huntington's disease, epilepsy, and multiple sclerosis are other neurological illnesses with a high prevalence of major depression.

As a rule, the symptom profile and the course of

PEARLS & PERILS

RECOMMENDATIONS FOR DIAGNOSING MAJOR DEPRESSION IN PATIENTS WITH FOCAL BRAIN LESIONS

- Before relying on depressive symptoms or signs from the patient interview, the physician should rule out fluent aphasia, rule out motor aprosodia, and assess memory.
- Diagnostic information should always be gathered from third parties (for example, family or nurses).
- The dexamethasone suppression test for melancholia may be helpful in carefully selected patients.
- The physician should be sure that the requirements for a full major depressive syndrome are present, including adequate duration. Specifically, individual symptoms or signs should not be counted toward the diagnosis of major depression if they are directly caused by the primary illness; crying or apathy alone should not be diagnosed as a major depression; and even a complete major depressive syndrome that is present on a single interview, or for only a week or so, should not be confidently considered to be major depression.

major depression in these patients are identical to those of idiopathic major depression.* This means that after careful clinical assessment and after ignoring symptoms or signs that are known to be caused by the primary illness even in the absence of major depression, standard diagnostic criteria can be used to diagnose major depression.

In several research studies of mood changes in neurological illness, the investigators have discussed "minor depression," referring to depressive symptoms that do not meet criteria for a major depressive episode. Minor depression defined in this way is more likely to develop in patients who are more neurologically impaired, and can persist for several years. However, there is little evidence to support the validity of this diagnostic label. Further studies are needed to determine its relationship to adjustment disorder, dysthymia, and major depression and to its response to treatment.

Major depression is a serious complication of neurological illness. Stroke patients with major depression have higher mortality than stroke patients who are not depressed. Additionally, they have a worse rehabilitation outcome compared with stroke patients who are not depressed and have similar lesions. Studies in stroke, multiple sclerosis, and Parkinson's disease all show that major depression strongly predicts cognitive impairment even after controlling for age, disability, and severity of neurological signs. Also, major depression can be responsible for somatic complaints. Furthermore, major depression carries with it its own risk of death and a great deal of suffering. One physician wrote that major depression "is probably more unpleasant than any disease except rabies" (Price, 1978). For all these reasons, effective treatment for major depression is important in patients with neurological illness.

Treatment Considerations

Fortunately, treatment studies have shown that major depression in neurologically impaired patients usually responds to antidepressant medication or electroconvulsive therapy (ECT). (Treatment studies with psychotherapy in this population are unfortunately lacking.) However, many neurologically impaired patients appear to be especially sensitive to treatment side effects. TCAs cause important side effects via their antagonism at α_1-adrenergic receptors (hypotension), muscarinic cholinergic receptors (confusion, dry mouth, impaired visual accommodation, urinary retention, and constipation), and H_1-histaminic receptors (sedation), among others. Among the TCAs, nortriptyline and desipramine are generally better tolerated. Serotonin-selective reuptake inhibitors (SSRIs) are generally well tolerated, although efficacy data are still limited. Because of its propensity to cause seizures, bupropion is relatively contraindicated in patients with known brain lesions, head trauma, or seizures. Newer drugs (such as venlafaxine and nefazodone) require further study. ECT can be safely used in most neurologically ill patients, often with gratifying results (see Chapter 22). However, since there are special considerations for ECT in several of these illnesses (Parkinson's disease, multiple sclerosis, epilepsy, brain tumors, and myasthenia gravis, among others), ECT in these patients should be performed by a psychiatrist with special expertise in using ECT in this population. In general, the recommendations of Box 26-2 apply to neurologically impaired patients with major depression. If patients do not respond within 6 to 8 weeks of treatment, consultation should be considered.

In spite of effective treatment, studies of major depression in patients with neurological disorders continue to show that only a fraction of the patients with major depression actually receive adequate antidepressant treatment. There seem to be two reasons for this inadequate treatment: (1) major depression is not diagnosed in many patients; and (2) major depression is not adequately treated when it is diagnosed. The following solutions are recommended.

To address the first problem, since major depression is so common in these patients, the physician should routinely screen for its presence. At a minimum, each patient with known brain disease should be asked about persistent sadness (this could even be accomplished by having the patient fill out a simple questionnaire like the Beck Depression Inventory; see Chapter 4). This screening method is imperfect, but it can be an important first step in preventing untreated major depression.

As to the second problem, undertreatment of diagnosed major depression may reflect an erroneous impression that major depression in these patients is somehow appropriate. It is unfortunate that major depression is named using the same word that more commonly refers to mild and transient sadness. Naturally no one is expected to feel happy about serious illness. However, when the full syndrome of major depression is present, physicians should actively treat it, no matter how understandable it may seem. Another cause of undertreatment of major depression after successful diagnosis is the common but erroneous use of small doses of TCAs (such as 25 mg of amitriptyline

*One exception is Parkinson's disease. Patients with Parkinson's disease and major depression are less likely to have self-reproach, delusions, hallucinations, or completed suicide than patients with idiopathic major depression alone, and they are more likely to have anxiety and a chronic course.

nightly). If a TCA is prescribed, it should be given in adequate doses (see Chapter 8). Low-dose TCAs offer only side effects and lethal risk without any proven benefit for major depression.

Special Issues with Psychiatric Treatment in Parkinson's Disease

In several neurological illnesses, such as stroke and multiple sclerosis, the available evidence suggests that patients with secondary psychiatric syndromes respond to the same pharmacological treatment used in psychiatric patients without a general medical illness (see the discussions on pp. 411 and 415). Parkinson's disease offers a number of exceptions to this general rule.

The most common psychiatric complication of Parkinson's disease is major depression. Persistent major depressive episodes (in the DSM-IV sense) generally do not respond to dopaminergic drugs typically used for the motor manifestations of parkinsonism (for example, levodopa [L-dopa] or bromocriptine). Psychostimulants (such as methylphenidate) are probably also ineffective. However, when mild major depression occurs in a patient who requires increases in antiparkinsonian medication to better treat motor signs, the institution of an antidepressant can sometimes be deferred briefly until the clinical picture is more stable. Close clinical follow-up is of course needed. This wait allows the physician to accurately interpret any treatment-emergent psychiatric side effects, and mood does improve during this interval in a few patients.

On the other hand, moderate to severe major depression is often the patient's most disabling problem, and vigorous treatment of major depression is indicated. Several antidepressants, in moderately high doses, have demonstrated superiority to placebo in the treatment of major depression in Parkinson's disease. Primarily serotoninergic drugs (such as SSRIs) appear to have a more pure effect on mood compared with antidepressants with prominent adrenergic or dopaminergic effects (such as desipramine or bupropion), which can also produce modest motor benefit. SSRIs have indirect antidopaminergic effects, but usually these are relatively insignificant clinically, compared with the effects of the primary disease and its treatment. Since anticholinergics have some efficacy in treating parkinsonism, physicians may be tempted to choose a tertiary amine TCA such as imipramine or amitriptyline. However, in most patients who are parkinsonian, doses adequate for antidepressant effect produce confusion or other significant anticholinergic side effects, and the risks outweigh the small motor benefit conferred. Newer antidepressants are usually better tolerated.

All antidepressants are relatively contraindicated in patients who are taking the MAOI selegiline (deprenyl); this is a result of the occasional occurrence of the so-called central serotonin syndrome, which can include confusion, rigidity, pyrexia, myoclonus, and autonomic instability and can be life-threatening. Often the antidepressant may be more important to the patient's overall health than the selegiline, and discontinuation of selegiline (with adjustment of other antiparkinsonian medication and an appropriate wait before beginning the antidepressant drug) can resolve the treatment dilemma. In other cases, ECT or psychotherapy may be used instead of an antidepressant medication, depending on the severity of the depression and other factors. If there is an exceptional clinical need to prescribe both selegiline and an antidepressant; this should be undertaken only with close monitoring by the physician after carefully weighing the risk-to-benefit ratio for the individual and obtaining informed consent. A relatively noradrenergic antidepressant with short half-life and useful serum levels, such as desipramine, may be more prudent in this situation, although this is speculative. Close collaboration with a psychiatrist may be wise in patients for whom continued monoamine oxidase inhibition is deemed necessary.

ECT can be helpful in selected patients with Parkinson's disease and major depression. In fact, ECT has been shown to produce short-lived improvements in motor signs even in patients who are nondepressed and parkinsonian (see Chapter 22). However, there is a high rate of interictal delirium in parkinsonian patients with depression who are undergoing ECT, so special care, possibly including a reduction of treatment frequency, is required when using ECT in this population. Interestingly, this complication of ECT is also commonly seen in patients with primary pathological disorders of the caudate nucleus.

One less common situation that should be distinguished from prolonged, steady major depression occurs in patients whose depressive symptoms are essentially limited to motor "off" periods. These patients have abrupt changes from a good response to L-dopa ("on") to a minimal response ("off"), and they also tend to have dopa-induced dyskinesias and a long history of L-dopa treatment. Off-period depression in these patients generally requires adjustment of dopaminergic treatment rather than traditional antidepressant therapy. The same appears to hold true for off-period anxiety (including panic attacks), although further studies are needed.

Psychosis is a common complication of dopaminergic therapy in patients with Parkinson's disease. The first step in treating psychosis is careful diagnosis. If attention, orientation, or level of consciousness are impaired, the usual diagnostic evaluation for delirium should be pursued (see Chapter 11). Unnecessary medications should also be eliminated, especially those with psychoactive effects. After ruling out delirium and reviewing all medications, anticholinergics should be eliminated, followed if necessary by elimination or reduction of amantadine and dopamine agonists. L-dopa generally has a better therapeutic index than these other agents. If these steps are ineffective, some patients with psychosis respond to a reduction in dosage of L-dopa. However, this response can take 2 weeks, and some patients cannot tolerate a lower dose because of their motor symptoms and signs, so the addition of an antipsychotic is often considered. Typical neuroleptics are generally unsatisfying, because they usually worsen parkinsonian signs and can lead to tardive movement disorders; lower-potency neuroleptics usually have excessive anticholinergic side effects. A more recent strategy is the prescription of low-dose clozapine (usually as little as 12.5 mg to 75 mg daily). Case reports and small studies indicate that this can adequately suppress psychosis while allowing more aggressive treatment of the motor signs. Clozapine for this indication has not been evaluated with double-blind methods; additionally, it implies significant expense, weekly blood draws, and a risk of agranulocytosis. However, clozapine still may represent the best treatment option for selected patients. The newer antipsychotic drug risperidone has been suggested for this purpose, but available data show no benefit over standard neuroleptics.

Etiological Considerations

So far the assessment and treatment of major depression have been discussed without answering the question of what causes the major depression. In several neurological diseases, there is enough evidence to help answer this question.

As discussed on p. 419, there is an increased prevalence of major depression in nearly all serious medical conditions. This is popularly attributed to expected sadness in the face of life difficulties, such as serious illness. However, the facts are not so simple as that. For instance, the majority of patients with a stroke feel some sadness and disappointment, but only a minority experience major depression. Thus the commonly heard statement, "I'd be depressed, too, if I had their illness" is only true for the symptom of depression (that is, low mood) and not for the major depressive syndrome. Additionally, although some might contend that major depression is a normal response to illness, this argument fails to explain the presence of poststroke mania and psychosis.

However, there is some evidence that life stress, including nonpsychiatric illness, may influence the timing of a major depressive episode in predisposed individuals. Along these lines, patients diagnosed with stroke or multiple sclerosis have a higher risk of major depression after their illness is diagnosed if they have a personal or family history of major depression before the diagnosis.

On the other hand, there is increasingly strong evidence that major depression in certain illnesses is directly caused by that illness (Box 26-3). These are illnesses that have direct physiological effects on the brain. It should not be surprising that injuring the organ of emotion can cause mood disorders, but many people react skeptically to this notion, probably because of the mind-body duality ingrained in our culture. Some of the evidence that some major depression is directly caused by certain illnesses is reviewed in Box 26-4.

The fact that some illnesses directly cause a major depressive episode is an unfortunate experiment of nature, but this experiment offers the hope of better understanding the pathophysiology and neuroanatomy of the more common idiopathic major depression. These secondary major depressions have been invaluable in motivating discoveries about the biology of idiopathic major depression. For instance, observations that major depression is common in Cushing's disease and hypothyroidism led to important studies of cortisol and thyroid dysregulation in severe idiopathic major depression. Secondary major depressions have also helped to validate new biological findings in idiopathic major depression. For instance, findings of decreased blood flow in the left caudate nucleus of patients with familial major depression are supported by the clinical observation that strokes in the left caudate nucleus often cause a secondary depression. The existence of psychiatric illnesses resulting from brain insults also supports other evidence that late-onset major depression is a different illness from early-onset familial major depression.

The etiological evidence reviewed in Box 26-4 is derived from studies in large groups of patients. However, it is usually impossible to definitely know the cause of a psychiatric illness in a single individual. For instance, there is no reason to think that having a stroke protects the patient from the usual risk factors for major depression, such as a personal or family history of major depression. Thus it is usually not possible to definitively state whether a particular episode of major depression, in a given patient with stroke, is the result of the direct physiological effects of the infarct. For this reason, several authors have argued that it is more defensible to simply diagnose a *major depressive episode* in these patients and note the possibility that it is directly caused by the stroke, without definitively specifying its cause. However, the DSM-IV committee felt that it was more clinically useful to diagnose either *major depressive disorder* (MDD), or *mood disorder due to a general medical condition,* using the physician's best judgment of etiology based

BOX 26-3

MEDICAL CONDITIONS ASSOCIATED WITH PSYCHIATRIC DISORDERS

Secondary anxiety

Adrenergic agonists
Alcohol/sedative withdrawal
Caffeine
Hypoglycemia
Hypoxia

Secondary catatonia

Bilateral infarcts of anterior cerebral arteries, globus pallidus, thalamus, or brainstem
Hypothalamic tumors
Neuroleptic toxicity
Phencyclidine (PCP) intoxication

Secondary depression

Human immunodeficiency virus (HIV) infection
Huntington's disease
Multiple sclerosis (especially temporal lobe plaques)
Parkinson's disease
Reserpine or alpha-methyl-dopa
Stroke
  Prefrontal cortex (left hemisphere)
  Basal ganglia (left hemisphere)
Wilson's disease

Secondary mania

Adrenergic agonists
Choreiform illnesses
Corticosteroids
Encephalitides
Orbitofrontal and brainstem tumors
Right orbitofrontal or subcortical brain injury

Secondary obsessive-compulsive disorder

Bilateral globus pallidus lesions
Carbon monoxide poisoning
Manganese poisoning
Encephalitis lethargica
Sydenham's chorea

Secondary panic disorder

Parkinsonism

Secondary personality change

Dementia of the Alzheimer's type (DAT)
Diffuse head injury
Epilepsy (limbic focus; controversial)
Focal head injury (frontal and temporal lobes)
General paresis (neurosyphilis)

Secondary psychosis

Acute intermittent porphyria
Dopamine agonist intoxication
Epilepsy (especially limbic focus)
Lysergic acid diethylamide (LSD) and other hallucinogen use
Lupus cerebritis
Metachromatic leukodystrophy
Neurosyphilis
PCP intoxication
Stroke
  Subcortical
  Right parietal cortex
Wilson's disease

BOX 26-4

EXAMPLES OF EVIDENCE FOR DIRECT CAUSATION OF MAJOR DEPRESSION IN CERTAIN NEUROLOGICAL ILLNESSES

1. In stroke and Parkinson's disease, major depression is more prevalent than in equally disabling conditions that do not affect the brain.
2. In stroke patients, lesion location is the strongest predictor of major depression, predicting over one half of the variance (left prefrontal and subcortical strokes have the highest likelihood of major depression).
3. In Huntington's disease, major depression is essentially confined to certain families, even though motor and cognitive disability is nearly universal.
4. Major depression has different demographics in Parkinson's disease (female to male ratio of 1:1) than in the general population (female to male ratio of 2:1).
5. Major depression can develop before physical symptoms or dementia in multiple sclerosis, Parkinson's disease, Huntington's disease, Alzheimer's disease, and Wilson's disease.
6. Patients with strokes, Huntington's disease, or Parkinson's disease who are depressed show orbitofrontal/cingulate/temporal/caudate hypometabolism compared with matched patients with the same neurological diagnosis who are not depressed.
7. Brain lesions also cause mania, which is hardly "understandable."

on the overall clinical picture. At least for the illnesses listed in Box 26-3, the latter diagnosis is probably defensible. However, liberal use of the more modest DSM-IV diagnosis *depressive disorder not otherwise specified* (NOS) is also recommended.

Summary

The main points made in this section are as follows. Major depressive episodes are common in illnesses that cause brain lesions, and they are probably largely a direct effect of lesioning the organ of emotional physiology, rather than an appropriate emotional response to illness. These patients require exceptionally careful, thorough clinical assessment by a physician to achieve accurate psychiatric diagnosis. Major depression in several neurological disorders confers a worse prognosis (at least if untreated) and generally has a rewarding treatment response, yet it is most commonly unnoticed or undertreated. Thus major depression should be actively sought and treated in these patients. Psychiatric consultation is recommended for any of the indications in Box 26-2.

Psychiatric Disorders in Patients with Chronic Medical Illness

Major Depression

The occurrence of major depression in patients with chronic medical illness has been the subject of much study. A good broad review is by Popkin and Tucker in 1992. For those interested in specific chronic illnesses, more focused reviews of major depression in specific conditions such as end-stage renal disease, diabetes mellitus,* and coronary artery disease are listed in the bibliography.

Major depression is now known to be a common co-morbid complication of several chronic medical illnesses (Box 26-5). Compared with a point prevalence of 3% to 5% for major depression in the general population,† patients with end-stage renal disease (5% to 8%), coronary artery disease (18% to 25%), and diabetes mellitus (15%) are all at an increased risk for major depression. Patients with malignancy or acquired immunodeficiency syndrome (AIDS) also have a similar risk of major depression. Although the risk for major depression in other chronic medical illnesses is not as clear, one might reasonably conclude that patients are at greater risk of developing major depression whenever any chronic medical illness is present. However, the picture is not all that simple, because certain chronic illnesses appear to have a substantially increased risk of major depression. Whereas malignancy in general probably has a prevalence of major depression similar to that seen in other chronic illnesses, fully 50% of patients with pancreatic cancer develop major depression. This predilection, combined with the observation that some patients develop major depression before the diagnosis of pancreatic cancer, suggests that major depression in some of these patients is not just a reaction to the illness but rather a part of it.

*Although diabetes mellitus is an endocrine disorder, it has been placed with the other chronic medical conditions and not with the section pertaining to endocrine disorders because the approach to evaluating and treating psychiatric illness in diabetes mellitus is much more similar to that of other medical conditions.

†Point prevalence is defined as the percentage of patients who will meet criteria for a given illness at *one point in time* and is different from lifetime prevalence, which is the percentage of patients who will meet criteria for a given illness *anytime* in their lives.

BOX 26-5

CHRONIC MEDICAL CONDITIONS COMMONLY ASSOCIATED WITH MAJOR DEPRESSION

Coronary artery disease
Diabetes mellitus
End-stage renal disease
Human immunodeficiency virus (HIV)
Malignancies, particularly pancreatic
Myocardial infarction

Treatment Issues in Patients with Coronary Artery Disease

In situations where major depression is present in patients with coronary artery disease, the physician must keep in mind that TCAs have Type 1a antiarrhythmic effects. Their ability to slow cardiac conduction combined with the higher prevalence of ventricular tachycardia in these patients argues for their relative contraindication in patients with coronary artery disease. However, TCAs have been safely used in this population, and in cases of severe major depression with suicidality they might be an appropriate front line treatment. For similar reasons, their use should be avoided in patients with a greater than grade I atrioventricular (AV) conduction block. SSRIs, since they lack type 1a effects, are more appropriate as front-line agents. However, SSRIs inhibit several enzymes of the cytochrome P-450 system, and the physician must be vigilant for pharmacokinetic interactions. For example, the dose of type 1c antiarrhythmics (such as encainide and flecainide), which are metabolized by CYP2D6, might need to be adjusted downward in patients taking a SSRI. Of the four available SSRIs (fluoxetine, fluvoxamine, paroxetine, and sertraline), sertraline appears to inhibit CYP2D6 the least and thus could be reasonably expected to affect the concentration of the antiarrhythmic the least. The ability of venlafaxine to cause a dose-dependent increase in heart rate, blood pressure, and cholesterol levels might limit its use in this patient group.

Treatment Issues in Patients with Diabetes Mellitus

With respect to the treatment of major depression in patients with diabetes mellitus, several studies have shown efficacy for antidepressants. In the past, TCAs have tended to be favored, especially for severe cases, but their hypotensive effects could make their use problematic in this patient group. It was originally thought that TCAs might exhibit antidiabetic effects through a direct drug effect on the adrenergic system, as well as through their indirect effects of ameliorating major depression. In the only double-blind placebo-controlled study to date, improvement in major depression by nortriptyline appears to lower glycosylated hemoglobin levels. However, nortriptyline also appears to directly elevate glycosylated hemoglobin and cancel out the indirect benefits from the improvement in major depression. Thus the use of TCAs in patients with major depression might have minimal overall effects on elevated glycosylated hemoglobin, despite effective treatment of major depression. In contrast, fluoxetine, an SSRI lacking appreciable adrenergic activity, does not elevate glycosylated hemoglobin when given for a year to patients with non-insulin-dependent diabetes mellitus who do not have major depression. Preliminary results from an ongoing study indicate that treatment of major depression with sertraline in patients with non–insulin-dependent diabetes mellitus is effective and leads to improved dietary compliance and glycosylated hemoglobin levels. Further studies are needed to confirm these initial findings. Given these effects on glucose control, TCAs are generally being supplanted as front-line agents by SSRIs. Based on pharmacokinetic concerns, sertraline is probably the preferred SSRI for this patient group. Studies are still needed to evaluate whether fluoxetine's greater tendency (as compared with other SSRIs) to cause anorexia and weight loss is clinically relevant in the routine treatment of major depression in patients with diabetes mellitus. MAOIs are relatively contraindicated in patients with diabetes mellitus, given their ability to cause severe hypoglycemia. Finally, the physician should not forget that diabetic patients with major depression need close monitoring of their glucose status, since caloric intake and physical activity vary depending on the depressive state of the patient.

Treatment Issues in Patients with End-Stage Renal Disease

The bulk of the literature on the treatment of major depression in patients with end-stage renal disease consists of case reports. Only one open trial has been reported, in which eight patients received desipramine at a decreased dose (ranging from 75 to 125 mg) or other antidepressants. Of the six patients who completed the study, five were in remission and one had significant improvement. In spite of receiving desipramine at doses approximately one half of those normally used, blood levels in the low therapeutic range were obtained in most of the patients. A similar result was found in patients on hemodialysis. These findings contradict the results of two other studies evaluating desipramine concentrations in patients with decreased renal function, as well as predictions of blood levels based on pharmacokinetic principles.* Until more definitive studies are done, it is safest to use a low dose initially and adjust upward if indicated by serum levels when prescribing desipramine in this patient population.

In contrast, most other antidepressants, including nortriptyline, follow pharmacokinetic predictions and do not require dose adjustment in patients with end-stage renal disease. Whereas the effective dose of most TCAs may not differ in patients with end-stage renal disease, the drugs should nevertheless be started at a lower dose and increased more slowly to prevent orthostatic hypotension in this patient group. As always, serum levels should be routinely monitored. Only two SSRIs have been studied in patients with renal dysfunction. Paroxetine, like desipramine, for unclear reasons does not follow pharmacokinetic predictions and it should also be used at one half the normal adult dose. The dose of fluoxetine does not need to be adjusted. In the case of sertraline and fluvoxamine, until clinical data are available, the physician should probably use lower doses and adjust upward if clinical status warrants it. Whereas patients with end-stage renal disease tolerate SSRIs better than TCAs, the ability to check serum levels and adjust the dose as needed suggests that TCAs might be the more appropriate agent in cases of moderate to severe major depression where a physician might not be able to wait 2 to 4 weeks to see whether a patient is responding to an SSRI before adjusting the dose upwards.

*If more than 95% of the drug is metabolized (that is, less than 5% is excreted unchanged by the kidney), then there is only a negligent decrease in the clearance of the drug in patients with compromised renal funtion. In such cases, serum levels do not change significantly and there should be no need for adjustment of dose.

Treatment Issues in Patients with Cancer

Although there is a relative dearth of studies on the use of antidepressants in patients with malignancy, the available evidence indicates that these drugs can be efficacious. TCAs are the best studied and are probably still front-line agents, given the propensity of SSRIs to cause nausea, anorexia, and weight loss. Nortryptiline or desipramine would probably be preferred agents because of their better side-effect profile. Venlafaxine might prove useful for those who cannot tolerate the side effects of TCAs. Bupropion should not be used in patients who are at risk for seizures (for example, those with CNS lesions).

Dysthymia

Dysthymia is a mood disorder in which the signs and symptoms are chronic and never reach the intensity of major depression (see Chapter 8). It can present as a co-morbid illness in patients with a chronic medical illness. In this context, dysthymia has been most thoroughly studied in patients with diabetes mellitus; however, even here the knowledge base is scant. Additionally, it is not entirely clear whether the term *dysthymia,* as applied to patients with medical conditions, represents a separate and distinct mood disorder, a mild variant of major depression, or a normal response to a stressful situation. In general, physicians should be suspicious of subclinical major depression in any patient with dysthymia and should consider instituting antidepressant treatment empirically in severe cases. Further conclusions and recommendations about dysthymia should be drawn with great care until the exact nature of dysthymia in medically ill patients is clearer.

Generalized Anxiety Disorder

Even though anxiety is the hallmark of GAD, it is also a common manifestation of major depression, and the physician must always rule out major depression as a cause (see Chapter 9). GAD has been most studied in association with diabetes mellitus, irritable bowel syndrome, and esophageal spasm syndrome. However, these avenues of research are in their infancy, and information is sparse at best. One interesting fact is that the symptoms of GAD usually precede the onset of intestinal symptoms in irritable bowel syndrome, suggesting that it might be etiologically related to this gastrointestinal disorder. As discussed later in this chapter, anxiety also is seen in several different endocrine disorders, although it is unclear whether its appearance occurs in isolation or in the context of GAD or major depression.

Treatment of GAD is the same as for when the disorder is not associated with a medical condition and consists of buspirone or benzodiazepines (see Chapter 9). Since the symptom of anxiety can be the initial presenting symptom of a major depressive episode, the physician should always continue to be vigilant for the potential manifestation of major depression. Such a change in diagnosis dictates a change in treatment.

Panic Disorder

Although anxiety can be commonly seen in medically ill patients, panic disorder, as defined by DSM-IV, does not often appear as a co-morbid process. It can be seen in diabetes mellitus, but it more commonly occurs in patients with irritable bowel syndrome and esophageal spasm syndrome. However, panic disorder typically is encountered by the primary care physician not as a true co-morbid process, but rather masquerading as angina in a person without coronary artery disease. Prompt recognition and appropriate treatment of panic disorder prevent the patient from undergoing potentially dangerous diagnostic procedures and being prescribed inappropriate medications. The treatment of panic disorder is the same as it is when the disorder is not associated with a medical condition (see Chapter 9).

Psychiatric Disorders in the Puerperium

The puerperium is a period of dramatic physiological changes that has long been associated with psychiatric disturbances. The following three syndromes are currently recognized: postpartum blues, postpartum depression, and postpartum psychosis (Box 26-6).

Postpartum Blues

Postpartum blues is a mild and transient syndrome. It typically begins in the first week after delivery. The major symptom is low mood, although mothers also

BOX 26-6

PUERPERAL DISORDERS

- Postpartum blues are normal and do not need specific treatment.
- Postpartum depression is pathological and must be treated as any major depression would be.
- Postpartum psychosis is a serious disorder and needs immediate psychiatric intervention.
- The postpartum period is considered to extend to the end of the fourth week after delivery.
- Typically the majority of patients will initially become symptomatic within the first 2 weeks after delivery.

report other affective symptoms (such as insomnia, anxiety, and fatigue). Given that the blues occur in 25% to 85% of mothers, the syndrome is usually considered a normal sequela of giving birth. It is assumed that abrupt changes in hormone levels occurring in the early postpartum period have a role in the syndrome. There is only minimal impact on the mother's ability to care for herself and her infant. No specific treatment is needed, and the syndrome resolves on its own within 2 weeks.

Postpartum Depression

Postpartum depression, like the postpartum blues, typically begins shortly after giving birth (50% of patients with postpartum depression develop symptoms within the first 2 weeks after delivery).* In contrast to the blues, the symptoms and signs of postpartum depression are not transient and worsen with time until a full major depressive syndrome occurs. The mothers (perhaps 10% to 20% of all postpartum women) whose signs and symptoms progress and who go on to develop postpartum depression might be those individuals who are at greatest risk for developing major depression in general. Much thought and study have been invested in determining the causes and risk factors of postpartum depression. Unfortunately the research is characterized by problems with diagnostic validity, definition, and design, and consistent results have been the exception rather than the rule.

Given the current state of knowledge, it would seem prudent that in the first month after delivery, the physician should follow closely any patients with a family history of major depression or a past history of either major depression or postpartum depression. Severe cases of postpartum depression, in which hopelessness or suicidality are present, should be referred to a psychiatrist. Mild to moderate depression usually can be treated by the primary physician with antidepressants, as long as the mother is not breast-feeding. Given that most antidepressants are excreted into milk, women suffering from postpartum depression who do not wish to discontinue breast-feeding should be referred to a psychiatrist who can aid in the assessment of benefits and risks of psychotherapeutic drug use and for the possible use of psychotherapy. Since data on the safety and pharmacokinetics of newer antidepressants (SSRIs, venlafaxine, nefazodone, and bupropion) are sparse, these should not be front-line agents in nursing mothers. Based on the data available, nortriptyline, because of its pharmacokinetic parameters, probably carries the least risk for the infant. When used, nortriptyline should be prescribed as a single dose at bedtime, and the mother should be instructed to skip the nighttime feeding. These two practices should minimize exposure to the infant by decreasing the amount of nortriptyline in the breast milk. For more specific information, the reader is referred to the article by Pons et al. that is listed in the bibliography.

Postpartum Psychosis

Postpartum psychosis, although occurring in only 0.1% to 0.2% of mothers who have given birth, is a severe sequela of pregnancy. Like other puerperal disorders it strikes typically within 2 weeks after delivery. The psychosis occurs usually in the setting of either depression or mania, and it is not unusual for a postpartum episode to be the initial presentation of bipolar disorder. Exacerbations of schizophrenia are rare in the immediate postpartum period. Instead, patients with schizophrenia tend to have psychotic exacerbations at least one month after giving birth and thus are not considered under DSM-IV to have postpartum psychosis. Given the severe nature of psychosis and its impact on mental functioning, immediate referral to a psychiatrist is almost always indicated. For the protection of the mother and the infant, patients who are psychotic typically need inpatient psychiatric treatment. Treatment and outcome depend on the underlying disorder, with most patients having a course similar to that of bipolar disorder. When lithium is indicated, the mother should be encouraged to forego breast-feeding, since lithium levels are measurable in the nursing infant and in some cases have been twice that of the mother's. With respect to prognosis, a substantial minority of patients (40% with a median follow-up period of 11 years in one study) have no further psychiatric sequelae. Twenty-five percent of patients suffer a relapse after a subsequent (but not necessarily the next) pregnancy, and the remaining 35% develop a recurrence of their psychiatric illness before their next pregnancy. Therefore patients with a history of postpartum psychosis (as well as those with a family history of bipolar disorder) should be observed closely in the first month after delivery for the emergence of this syndrome.

Given the documented risk of developing a postpartum psychosis in patients with bipolar disorder, psychiatric referral during pregnancy should be obtained for these patients to ensure close monitoring in the postpartum period. Additionally, since lithium, valproate, and carbamazepine all have teratogenic effects,

*Whereas a minority of patients develop a depressive syndrome up to 1 year after childbirth, it is doubtful that these cases are related to parturition. It seems wise for both investigative work and clinical care to adopt some arbitrary line to demarcate the end of the puerperal period. Although 6 weeks would be consistent with obstetrical practice, 4 weeks (as proposed in DSM-IV) is probably better, since it should improve the homogenity of the sample but still capture the vast majority of patients.

and strong consideration should be given to the discontinuation of these drugs during some parts of pregnancy. Consultation with a psychiatrist to better define the risk and benefits is preferable, with close monitoring by a psychiatrist for early signs of relapse in those cases where medication discontinuation is undertaken. Strong consideration should be given to the reinstitution of prophylactic treatment immediately after parturition. Finally, given the abrupt changes in volume status and drug clearance that occur in the immediate postpartum period, the physician needs to monitor the patient and follow drug levels closely, especially when prescribing lithium.

Psychiatric Manifestations of Endocrine Disorders

The ability of endocrine disorders to produce psychiatric disturbances has been recognized since the early days of medicine, and a further understanding of their associated psychiatric manifestations should enhance our understanding of idiopathic psychiatric disorders. Unfortunately little systematic research has been done recently, and thus this area has not benefited from the improved diagnostic and research techniques of modern psychiatry. Despite the lack of progress, the endocrine disorders have been placed into a separate section to highlight the following two points: (1) in contrast to psychiatric disorders in other medical conditions, psychiatric treatment initially is aimed at correcting the underlying endocrinological abnormality; and (2) except for neurological disorders, endocrine dysfunctions offer the best evidence for secondary psychiatric disorders and show great promise for further research.

The psychiatric manifestations of endocrine dysfunction include anxiety, major depression, mania, psychosis, dementia, and delirium (Table 26-3). Often the CNS effects of endocrine dysfunction can be the initial and most clinically obvious indicator of the hormonal disturbance. However, a complete discussion of the precise details in each endocrine disorder is beyond the scope of this chapter, and further details can be found in Reus' review from 1986 and Table 26-3. For discussion purposes, the focus of this section is on the thyroid gland.

Hyperthyroidism

The mental effects of hyperthyroidism can vary from mild (fatigue, anxiety, and irritability) to moderate (excitability and emotional instability) and severe (mania and psychosis). Delusions and hallucinations, typically visual, can also occur alone or in conjunction with a manic state. Typically, the severely affected patients also have physical signs of hyperthyroidism (for example, elevated pulse, a fine hand tremor, and hot dry hands), but their presence is often missed on the initial evaluation when the physician is confronted with the behavioral and cognitive signs of CNS dysfunction in a psychotic and hyperactive individual. In such cases the most obvious clue that the CNS dysfunction is caused by a general medical condition is age. The onset of psychosis or mania after the age 35 or 40 suggests that the psychosis may be secondary to a general medical condition. In such cases the physician should be vigilant for any features that indicate a nonpsychiatric cause and must pursue a complete

TABLE 26-3

PSYCHIATRIC MANIFESTATIONS ASSOCIATED WITH ENDOCRINE DISORDERS

Endocrine Abnormality	Psychiatric Manifestations
Adrenal	
Cushing's syndrome	Anxiety, delirium, major depression, mania, and psychosis
Addison's disease	Catatonia, delirium, dementia, major depression, and psychosis
Parathyroid	
Hyperparathyroidism	Anxiety, delirium, major depression, and psychosis
Hypoparathyroidism	Anxiety, delirium, dementia, major depression, mania, and psychosis
Pituitary	
Acromegaly	Major depression
Hyperprolactinemia	Major depression
Hypopituitarism	Delirium, dementia, and major depression
Thyroid	
Hyperthyroidism	Anxiety, delirium, major depression, mania, and psychosis
Hypothyroidism	Anxiety, delirium, dementia, major depression, mania, and psychosis

work-up to exclude other causes (see Box 26-3 and Table 26-3).

Although hyperthyroidism is typically associated with manic-like activated states, some patients develop a syndrome that consists of psychomotor retardation and apathy that is much more reminiscent of major depression. Still others have a syndrome akin to GAD. Delirium is a rare presentation of hyperthyroidism, occurring in less than 5% of cases, but given that delirium is an indicator of a medical emergency (in hyperthyroid patients, it typically heralds the impending onset of a thyroid storm), its presence must be considered in any patient with recent onset of CNS dysfunction. The presence of fluctuating impairments on bedside cognitive tests of orientation (person, place, and time) and attention (serial sevens and months backwards in order) suggests that a patient is delirious and that a general medical condition or medication side effect is likely to be the cause of the psychiatric signs and symptoms (see Chapter 11). Delirium can be thought of as "acute brain failure" akin to acute renal failure, in that both reflect organ dysfunction brought on either by the inability of the body to maintain the homeostatic environment needed for proper organ function (for example, decreased blood flow and hypoxia) or by a process intrinsic to the organ (for example, nephritis, trauma, meningitis, and seizures). Both are medical emergencies, since if the abnormality cannot be found quickly and corrected, death of the organ or individual may ensue.

Hypothyroidism

Typically the behavioral disturbances associated with *hyper*thyroidism (activated, manic-like) are envisioned as the opposite of those produced by *hypo*thyroidism (a hypoactive retarded state similar to that seen in major depression). Whereas decreased energy, poor concentration, weight gain, anhedonia, and poor mood are all common in hypothyroidism, a wide variety of signs and symptoms can be seen that overlap substantially with those seen in hyperthyroidism (such as anxiety, irritability, and agitation). If unrecognized and untreated, "myxedema madness" (in which delusions and hallucinations occur) can develop. In its final end state, dementia is present. Delirium is a rare consequence and usually only appears in those patients who develop hypothyroidism acutely, such as after thyroidectomy.

Thus the signs and symptoms of mental dysfunction of hypothyroidism and hyperthyroidism overlap significantly. This phenomenon extends to most other endocrine abnormalities, with a variety of different psychiatric disorders being associated with any one endocrine disorder. Whether the ability of an endocrine disorder to produce many different psychiatric syndromes reflects poor diagnostic techniques, genetic predisposition, the complex interaction between the neuronal and endocrine systems, or a combination of these is not known. Data emerging from basic research indicate that hormones, via several different mechanisms, can have direct effects on the functioning of neurons. The knowledge that mild endocrine abnormalities exist in patients considered to have a primary psychiatric disorder and that these abnormalities disappear with routine psychiatric treatment suggests that CNS function can alter endocrine systems. Thus the relationship between CNS and endocrine functioning is probably bidirectional. Furthermore, the anatomical evidence for a complex intertwined web of projection pathways between diverse limbic brain areas and the hypothalamus, combined with the location of hormone receptors in several areas of the CNS, indicate that the concept of a simple serial feedback mechanism for the control of endocrine function is probably oversimplistic. Instead there appears to be a highly complex relationship that governs the normal and abnormal functioning of these two systems and probably accounts for the diverse clinical pattern.

Diagnosis and Treatment

Until a clearer picture of this complex relationship is available, the general rule is to determine, to the extent possible, which system (endocrine or nervous) is the primary cause of the signs and symptoms. As is the case with diagnosing mental disorders in patients with chronic medical illnesses, clues such as age of onset, family history, and the presence or absence of nonoverlapping signs and symptoms can be used to determine whether the primary pathological condition is psychiatric or endocrinological. Treatment is aimed initially at correcting the primary disorder. Thus hypothyroid patients with secondary depressive-like sequelae are given thyroid supplementation and are not initially treated with antidepressants. The only definite exception is in the case of a patient who is agitated and psychotic but nondelirious where antipsychotics, benzodiazepines, and inpatient hospitalization are used to prevent physical harm. With appropriate endocrinological treatment, mental functioning typically improves over time as endocrine function returns to normal. However, it is not uncommon for patients to continue to have significant psychiatric symptoms in spite of normalized endocrine function. Whether the continuing presence of mental dysfunction in these cases represents persistent CNS dysfunction, a co-morbid psychiatric process, or a mild subclinical endocrine abnormality is unknown. Little can be done in the first scenario; however, further pharmacological manipulation might lead to additional improvement in the latter two scenarios. Although clinical data are lacking in such cases, it is reasonable to assume that the patient's past medical history or family history might offer clues as to whether the adjunctive use of psychiatric medications (such as antidepressants) or further endocrine manipulation (for example, additional thyroid supplementation in a previously hypothyroid patient who is biochemically euthyroid at the time of treatment) would be more likely to lead to further improvement.

Prognosis

Prognosis depends on the specific endocrine disorder, but physical stigmata usually resolve with the successful treatment of the endocrine abnormality. In contrast, the psychiatric manifestations tend to be more resistant to treatment and can persist even after the biochemical indexes have normalized. A definitive conclusion on whether there will be residual impairment cannot be reached for several months, since improvement in mental functioning can lag behind the successful treatment of the endocrine disorder. Additionally, the chance for a full recovery of CNS functioning decreases as the duration of symptoms increases. For example, in spite of delirium being a medical emergency, hypothyroid patients with delirium—when they are appropriately diagnosed and treated—have a high recovery rate (80%), probably because they are treated soon after the onset of hypothyroidism. In contrast, hypothyroid patients who have been symptomatic for over 2 years rarely show improvement in mental functioning (Box 26-7).

BOX 26-7

ENDOCRINE DISORDERS

- In general, any psychiatric presentation can be seen with any endocrine disorder.
- There is typically little correlation between the severity of the endocrine disorder or its physical signs and the presence or severity of the mental effects.
- It is not uncommon for the mental effects to be the first indication of endocrine dysfunction.
- Except in cases of psychosis, initial treatment is targeted at the underlying endocrine disorder.
- In cases of continued psychiatric symptoms where treatment of the endocrine disorder has been maximized, adjunctive psychiatric medications can be used.
- The longer the symptoms have been present, the poorer the prognosis.

Conclusion

In this chapter, several points have been made about psychiatric illness in patients with general medical illness. First, correct diagnosis is important because psychiatric illness in general medical patients is common and usually treatable. For instance, major depression is generally underdiagnosed, but effective treatment can relieve suffering, possibly improve medical outcomes, decrease medical costs, reduce physical complaints, and possibly prevent suicide. Delirium indicates a severe underlying general medical illness. Delirium can cause psychotic or depressive symptoms; if these symptoms are misdiagnosed as major depression, the physician has missed an important indication of the seriousness of the underlying medical condition. Second, diagnosis of psychiatric illness is sometimes straightforward in these patients but commonly requires significant clinical skill. A thorough psychiatric assessment is required, followed by careful consideration of the symptoms and signs. Deciding whether or not symptoms are the result of underlying nonpsychiatric illness requires knowledge of both the primary illness and the psychiatric side effects of medical treatment. Psychological symptoms can be especially important. Accurate psychiatric diagnosis can be especially difficult in patients with coarse brain disease. Third, treatment of psychiatric disorders in general medical patients typically follows established treatment recommendations for the disorder when it occurs in the absence of other medical conditions. However, drug-induced illness and drug-drug interactions can make treatment difficult. Referral to a psychiatric specialist is sometimes needed. Finally, the causes of psychiatric disorders in medically ill patients appear to be heterogeneous. For example, in many chronic illnesses, major depressive episodes might represent typical major depression, perhaps triggered by the loss of health and increase in life stress. Other conditions (such as certain endocrine and neurological illnesses, or the postpartum state) bring a markedly elevated risk of major mental illness. In some cases the reason for this high risk is still unknown, but in others there is substantial evidence that the psychiatric disorder is caused by direct pathological effects of the illness on brain functioning.

Psychiatric complications of nonpsychiatric illnesses are common and often add further suffering to an already difficult situation. They can also cause additional morbidity or even death, and they should not be considered normal responses. Accurate diagnosis and adequate treatment of delirium, major depression, GAD, panic disorder, or psychosis in this population can not only provide a rewarding challenge to the physician's skill but also greatly improve patients' quality of life.

Annotated Bibliography

Cummings JL, Trimble MR: *Concise guide to neuropsychiatry and behavioral neurology,* Washington, D.C., 1995, American Psychiatric Press.

This pocket guide includes brief discussions and valuable references for psychiatric complications of neurological diseases.

Cunningham LA: Depression in the medically ill: choosing an antidepressant, *J Clin Psychiatry* 55(9 Suppl A):90-97, 1994.

This article discusses the general approach to prescribing antidepressants in the medically ill. It also briefly reviews the treatment literature and makes specific recommendations about different antidepressants for four separate groups of illnesses (cancer, dementia, Parkinson's disease, and stroke).

Dobie SA, Walker EA: Depression after childbirth, *J Am Board Fam Pract* 5:303-311, 1992.

This article is a broad and excellent review of the literature on postpartum depression. The authors conclude that the literature supports the view that postpartum depression is the same disorder as major depression and that the postpartum period is a risk factor for its expression. It does not cover postpartum blues or psychosis.

Popkin MK, Tucker GJ: "Secondary" and drug-induced mood, anxiety, psychotic, catatonic, and personality disorders: a review of the literature, *J Neuropsychiatry Clin Neurosci* 4:369-385, 1992.

This article is a broad review of secondary psychiatric disorders undertaken by members of the DSM-IV task force. Although there has been substantial advancement in several areas since its writing, it still is probably the best brief review on this subject.

Reus VI: Behavioral disturbances associated with endocrine disorders, *Ann Rev Med* 37:205-214, 1986.

This review discusses briefly the psychiatric manifestations of Cushing's syndrome, Addison's disease, hyperparathyroidism, hyperthyroidism, hypothyroidism, hyperprolactinemia, and hypopituitarism. Its continued utility 10 years after publication is an indication of the scarcity of investigation that is occurring in this area.

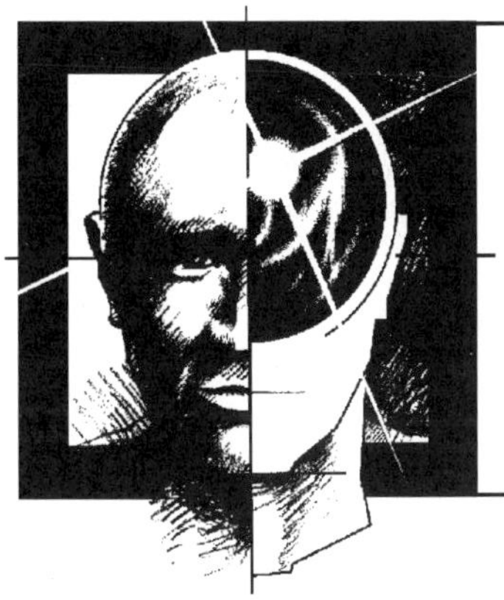

chapter 27

Suicide

George E. Murphy, MD

The Facts Regarding Suicide

Ninety-five percent of people who commit suicide around the world are suffering from a common and readily diagnosed psychiatric illness at the time of the fatal act. Two psychiatric illnesses account for two thirds of these deaths: major depressive disorder (MDD) for at least one half, and alcoholism and other substance abuse for one third. Two thirds of people who have committed suicide had communicated their suicidal thoughts to others in advance of the act. One half had consulted a physician within a month of their deaths. Most of those who had depression and killed themselves were underdiagnosed and/or undertreated by the physician. The potential is there for physicians to sharply reduce the suicide rate.

Who Is at Risk for Suicide?

Not everyone is equally at risk. All but a small fraction of people who commit suicide are psychiatrically ill, so such illness is for practical purposes a necessary condition, albeit not a sufficient one for self-destruction. Epidemiological studies show that only about one fourth of the adult population in the United States is at risk for psychiatric illness. Therefore for practical purposes, three fourths of the population are not candidates for suicide at any time. That narrows the field but not enough. Fortunately, the major contributors are few and readily recognizable. Depressive disorders (MDD and bipolar disorder) have been recognized as the primary illness in 25% to 70% of suicides worldwide (Table 27-1). Considering all suicides involving a depressive syndrome, whether primary or co-morbid (that is, occurring in the presence of another psychiatric illness), the range is from 30% to 86%. The mean for all studies is 52%. One half of all people who commit suicide are recognizably clinically depressed when they take their lives.

Alcohol abuse and dependence has been diagnosed in 15% to 54% of suicides, with a mean of 32% across 13 studies. Overall, substance abuse (including that of alcohol) was diagnosed in 37% of over 1900 suicides.

Schizophrenia has been identified in about 5% of cases in community studies. It is thus not a major

TABLE 27-1

SELECTED DIAGNOSES IN COMMUNITY SAMPLES OF SUICIDE

	N	Affective disorder %	Alcoholism %	Schizo-phrenia %	Substance abuse/ dependency %	No psychiatric illness %
Robins, Locke, and Regier United States (1959)	134	47 (56)*	24 (27)*	2	28*	6
Dorpat and Ripley United States (1960)	114	30	27	12	31*	0
Barraclough, et al. United Kingdom (1974)	100	70	15	3	19*	7
Beskow Sweden (1979)	270♂	28 (45)*	31 (44)*	3	37*	4
Hagnell and Rorsman Sweden (1979)	28	50	19	7	39*	7
Chynoweth, Tonge, and Armstrong Australia (1980)	135	38 (55)*	20	4	22 (34)*	2
Mitterauer Austria (1981)	94	63*	30*	5	45*	0
Kapamadžija, Biro, and Sovljanski Yugoslavia (1982)	100	75*	41*	3*	41*	0 (?)
Rich, Young, and Fowler United States (1986)	283	44*‡	54*‡	3*	56*§	5
Arató, et al. Hungary (1988)	200	58*	20*	8*	20*	19
Åsgård Sweden (1990)	104♀	25 (59)*	7 (16)*	3	12*	<5
Henriksson, et al. Finland (1993)	229	59*	17 (43)*	10	43	2
Cheng Taiwan (1995)	116	86*	44*	6*	45*	1.7

*Diagnoses inclusive, not hierarchical.
‡Rich et al. (1989).
§Rich et al. (1988).

player in the community, but the lifetime risk for suicide in those afflicted may be as high as that for affective disorder, 10% to 15%. It is the chief contributor to suicides among patients on psychiatric hospital rolls. Many of these suicides have occurred when the patients were on grounds passes or convalescent leave. Coarse brain dysfunction (delirium and dementia) contributes in a small way (1% to 2%).

In recent studies of suicides completed by people under age 30, investigators have diagnosed personality disorders in up to one third of cases. Antisocial and borderline personality disorders predominate. In nearly all cases, at least one co-morbid disorder is present as well. Substance abuse disorder (including alcohol abuse) is the most common Axis I complication, either with or without an affective disorder. The balance of co-morbidity is that of affective disorder alone.

A spate of recent follow-up studies has identified an excess of suicides in patients initially diagnosed with panic disorder. Curiously, that diagnosis has hardly appeared at all among 1900 suicides studied retrospectively. In its natural history, panic disorder commonly comes to be associated with other Axis I disorders, either as an antecedent or as a complication. Prominent among these Axis I disorders are affective disorder and substance abuse disorder, the symptoms of which are likely to be far more conspicuous if they are present at all. The explanation of the heightened risk for suicide in panic disorder appears to be in its co-morbidity with the otherwise "major" contributors. Alone, it is unlikely to lead to suicide.

Psychosocial Determinants of Suicide

Affective Disorders

Suicide in MDD occurs in response to internal cues. Recent disruptions in the social field do not significantly exceed the norms of the age-adjusted population. Suicide in widowhood is somewhat more common than expected, but a recent change to that state is not. Moreover, families appear to have remained sup-

PEARLS & PERILS

ALERTING CUES TO CONSIDER MDD

- Depression does not always walk in the door self-identified. It can develop insidiously in patients under treatment for other complaints.
- Psychomotor agitation and retardation are diagnostic signs. Medication effects (such as akathisia or oversedation) as well as major depression should be considered.
- Newly developing irritability, demandingness, and poor compliance with medication may be signs of depression as well.
- The facial appearance of sadness or tearfulness calls for directed inquiry regarding the depressive syndrome. Physicians readily recognize the mood, but they may miss the diagnosis.
- Likewise, unplanned weight loss or a complaint of poor appetite or insomnia should cue the physician to inquire about other symptoms of depression. Do not treat the symptom until depression has been ruled out.
- Not every depressed patient relates to feeling depressed. Synonyms include feeling sad, blue, down in the dumps, and "blah." Mood disturbance should not be ruled out without trying those probes.

portive. Ill health may be a more common contributor to suicide than expected in older people, but it is neither dramatically inflated nor especially pronounced in severity. The incidence of cancer increases with age and therefore is found with some frequency among the older people who commit suicide. However, equally common is an unwarranted conviction of harboring a malignancy. That should be understood as a symptom of depression.

Without salient external cues, the impetus to suicide can be seen as stemming chiefly from the combination of misery and hopelessness that are common features of depression. Sleepless nights bring neither rest nor escape from mental pain. Loss of interest and impaired concentration void escape through distraction. Guilt inflates worthlessness, and psychomotor agitation precludes rest. Hopelessness intrudes and then prevails, and the biological imperative of self-preservation is breached. Thoughts of death arise early in the course of most depressive episodes. Unchecked, they progress to consideration of self-destruction. The suicide notes of the depressed speak of internal rather than external concerns (see the Pearls & Perils box above).

Alcoholism

In contrast to those suffering from a primary depression, recent disruption in the lives of people afflicted with alcoholism characterizes their suicides. To be sure, personal, social, legal, and vocational troubles are the identifying consequences of the disorder. But the following fact should be considered: whereas one half of the people in three series of suicides completed by people with alcoholism had experienced the loss of a close interpersonal relationship in the last year of their lives, two thirds of these events had taken place in the last 6 weeks. That is different from the presuicidal experience of patients with depression. Moreover, the fear or expectation of such an event was equally as common as an actual loss among the people who were alcoholic.

These disruptions and threatened disruptions do not act alone. Nearly everyone (96%) in a series of 50 suicides by people suffering from alcoholism were still drinking excessively. More than four fifths had communicated suicidal thoughts or acts. Three fourths were experiencing a complicating major depressive episode. Nearly three fourths had little or no social support. More than one half had significant health problems; one half were unemployed; and more than one third were living alone. These findings were replicated in an earlier series of 32 suicides in which the people were alcoholic and strongly distinguished them from living alcoholics and from suicides completed by people suffering from depression. The recent loss experience of people who are alcoholic and commit suicide is precisely paralleled by that in abusers of other substances who commit suicide. Given the overall similarities of substance abusers of whatever preference, it is likely that the basis for suicide is the same in all of them.

Identifying Suicidal Risk

Major Depressive Disorder

Nearly all of the risk of suicide resides in that portion of the population that is identifiably psychiatrically ill. Risk assessment must therefore begin with accurate diagnosis. Studies have shown that physicians have been aware of the presence of depressed mood in their patients who took their own lives. However, they had not often pursued that lead to identify the syndrome of MDD. Instead they treated symptoms. To judge from the literature, this pattern is the rule among patients committing suicide who are under medical care. That is not to say that it is the rule regarding MDD in medical care. But the failure to recognize it allows the depression to go untreated, to worsen, and sometimes to eventuate in suicide.

It is one thing to recognize depression in a new patient complaining of insomnia, low energy, or weight loss. It is quite another to pick up an insidiously developing depression in a familiar patient. Even the patient may not be aware of the extent of the changes taking place. Psychological mindedness, the tendency to explain symptoms in psychosocial terms, leads to dismissing the significance of the symptoms. The more a physician knows about a patient's circumstances, the easier it is to assign causation. It is well to keep in mind Jan Fawcett's pithy dictum (1972): "The presence of a reason for depression is no reason to ignore the presence of the depression." The risk of suicide in depression runs with the episode and ceases when the depression fully remits. It returns when the depression returns.

The physician needs to maintain a high level of sensitivity to the ways a depression may appear. A mood change should trigger an inquiry after the other symptoms of depression. It takes only a minute. Unplanned weight loss is another clue. Uncooperativeness in a previously compliant patient may represent the apathy, irritability, or the marked pessimism of depression. Feeling one's spirit sink on seeing a certain patient's name on the day's appointment schedule can be a warning that that unpleasant or demanding patient is depressed.

Risk of suicide is not the only reason to be alert to the development of depression. It is a state of misery that can be relieved with appropriate intervention, and it is more common in medical practice than is generally appreciated. Its effective treatment benefits both the patient and the physician.

Alcohol and Substance Abuse

Physicians are reluctant to acknowledge character flaws in their patients and commonly equate substance abuse with weak character. Thus they avoid making the diagnosis. The behaviors that serve to identify substance abuse are often known to them but not named for what they are. Again, recognizing the disorder is primary.

Next comes the inquiry into the presence of factors associated with suicide. Loss or threatened loss of a close interpersonal relationship is important, especially when other social support is weak or absent. Subacute and chronic risk factors include continued substance abuse, a history of suicidal communication (including suicide attempts), a co-morbid depressive syndrome, poor or no social support, substantial health problems, unemployment, and living alone. They are easily tracked in an alcoholic patient, and their impact is cumulative. As the number of such factors climbs to three or more, risk of suicide becomes greater, and the need for intervention becomes more urgent. It is likely that these subacute and chronic risk factors for suicide in people suffering from alcoholism apply as well to abusers of other substances.

Schizophrenia

A majority of people with schizophrenia who take their lives are young, often better educated than the average, and previously had high expectations for their future. After one or two psychotic episodes, an awareness of a limited future dawns. Depression and suicide attempts become a part of the picture. The suicide usually appears to have been impulsive, if only in the lack of verbal warning. It often occurs when the patient is on leave from the hospital during a remission of psychotic symptoms. It is difficult to justify on humanitarian grounds continued restrictive hospitalization when the psychosis remits, although some small risk of suicide exists. Vigorous treatment of a complicating depressive syndrome may be protective and contribute something to the overall bearability of this unfortunate disorder.

Other Disorders

Panic Disorder and Generalized Anxiety Disorder

As indicated earlier, nearly all of the evidence implies that the risk of suicide in panic disorder and generalized anxiety disorder (GAD) is a function of comorbidity with the two major contributors, affective disorder and substance abuse disorder. Panic attacks or more general anxiety may increase when depression supervenes, but among actual cases of suicide it is the depression and not the anxiety that has taken the center of the stage. It is the depression that must be recognized and treated, although the panic disorder should not be neglected. When substance abuse complicates the picture, the risk factors are those described for substance abuse.

Delirium and Dementia

Distorted perceptions are the hallmark of delirium. Sometimes the visions (hallucinations) are terrifying. Perceiving the approach of a fearsome monster or the room to be wildly aflame, the patient who is delirious may leap through a window in a vain attempt to escape. If the ensuing fall proves fatal, it has more in common with accidental death than with suicide. Delirium is a dangerous state and calls for serious protective measures—impenetrable screens or unbreakable glass in the windows—while the source of the delirium is sought. An accumulation of medications, each by itself innocuous, is often the cause.

Poststroke dementia may be more depression than actual dementia. Depression is the risk factor.

Personality Disorders

Borderline personality disorder and antisocial personality disorder account for nearly all of the suicide mortality in this group, but they rarely are unaccompanied. Substance abuse (including alcohol) is the most common complication. It in turn may be complicated by a depressive episode. A history of suicide attempts is common in both antisocial personality disorder and in borderline personality disorder. Indeed, attempts and threats comprise one of the criterion symptoms of borderline personality disorder. Disruptions in the social sphere (such as rejection, abandonment, or arrest) may be the precipitant. But without the co-morbidity, the risk of a fatal outcome is slight.

Cancer and Other Life-Threatening Diseases

The rate of suicide in patients with cancer is unknown but finite. Some instances escape the medical examiner's attention. A lethal dose of a narcotic knowingly left at the bedside of a patient who is suffering greatly may terminate a life, but the death certificate shows the cause to be cancer. The physician and patient understand each other. Of course, a complicating depression affects the tolerability of the suffering and the attractiveness of the alternative. Depression should be treated vigorously, not only to relieve suicidal thoughts but also to make the patient more comfortable overall. Of equal or greater concern is the patient who mistakenly believes she has cancer. This conviction is nearly always a manifestation of a depressive episode, and it may be the presenting symptom. Risk assessment in depression has been discussed in this section under Major Depressive Disorder.

Acquired Immunodeficiency Syndrome

Among dreaded diseases, acquired immunodeficiency syndrome (AIDS) ranks at or near the top. Its diagnosis has been found to be associated with an increased risk of suicide—over 60 times that of the general population. Major depression commonly develops. Suicidal communication is common as well. Even receiving the diagnosis of human immunodeficiency virus (HIV) can precipitate suicide.

Other Disorders

Both Huntington's disease and chronic renal insufficiency carry an increased risk of suicide, most likely mediated by a co-morbid depression, a disorder to which sufferers from both illnesses are prone.

Preventing Suicide

The key to preventing suicide is to successfully treat the underlying psychiatric illness. That in turn calls for prompt and accurate diagnosis. Most people who have committed suicide while they were under medical care have been undiagnosed or underdiagnosed and undertreated as well. Depressed mood has been recognized but not translated into a diagnosis of the depressive disorder, of which it is but one symptom. Instead, symptoms have been treated—particularly those of insomnia and of anxiety. Hypnotics and anxiolytics do not relieve depression. Even in the cases where antidepressants have been prescribed, the dosage has been subtherapeutic by any standard. It is known that many depressions are diagnosed and treated aggressively. It is not those but the untreated and the undertreated who become suicide statistics.

After making the diagnosis, the next step is to assess the existence and level of suicidal thoughts. This is principally a matter of asking the questions such as those in the following list:

- Have you had thoughts of death?
- Have you wished you were dead?
- Have you thought of taking your life?
- What have you thought of doing?

Most patients who are suicidal report their thoughts if they are asked, but it does not occur to them to volunteer the information. Not only is it essential to ask, but it is also necessary to inquire again and again as long as the symptoms of depression persist. If the patient is evasive or unconvincing, ask the family as well. The physician should pay serious attention to any gut feelings. It is wrong to suppose that by inquiring, the physician can plant the idea of suicide. Thoughts of death are ubiquitous—nearly universal—in depression.

A majority of patients with suicidal thoughts can be safely treated in the office. It is a matter of clinical judgment. In choosing an antidepressant, the physician should consider its potential as an agent of self-destruction. All of the tricyclic antidepressants (TCAs) and doxepin are toxic. Even a week's supply at full therapeutic strength can prove fatal if taken in a single dose. If a responsible family member controls the medication, that risk is reduced. At subtherapeutic levels, the depression proceeds unchecked and the patient may find other means to achieve his end. It is important to remember that most depression-related suicides have been undertreated.

The serotonin-selective reuptake inhibitors (SSRIs) (fluoxetine, paroxetine, and sertraline) are less toxic than the TCAs and have fewer negative side effects in most patients. Idiosyncratic intolerance is a common cause of noncompliance with the prescribed medication regimen. Dosage must be monitored closely in the early weeks of treatment. Effective management of antidepressant therapy is not as difficult as many primary care physicians suppose. It is largely a matter of higher doses. Becoming familiar with two or three of the more popular antidepressants makes it much easier.

A 1990 report of six cases of emerging or reemerging suicidal preoccupation in patients receiving fluoxetine implied that this drug was solely responsible. Subsequent comment has been mostly nonconfirmatory. Fluoxetine is a useful and widely accepted antidepressant with a low side-effect profile. Its association with suicide is much lower than that of the TCAs. Early in the course of its administration, an occasional patient experiences marked anxiety or agitation. Patients should be warned to immediately discontinue the medication until they have discussed it with the physician if this or suicidal preoccupation should occur. Such a warning is equally appropriate with other antidepressants.

It is difficult for people who are mentally healthy to understand a person's decision to take his own life. It is not usually insanity in the customary sense. But with deepening depression, there often comes the conviction that life is futile and that suffering will never end. Rational arguments to the contrary may be reluctantly agreed to, but the half-life of that acquiescence is less than 5 minutes. A physician must not suppose for a minute that he has actually talked a patient out of suicidal thoughts.

At the same time, talking with a depressed patient is helpful. Some formal psychotherapies (cognitive, behavioral, and interpersonal) have demonstrated benefit in depressed outpatients. These may be beyond the scope or interest of the primary care physician, but referral to an experienced practitioner of one of these therapies is worth considering. In serious depression, psychotherapy alone is not to be relied on to prevent suicide.

The physician should keep informed as to the development and urgency of a plan. The intensity of suicidal thoughts waxes and wanes within an episode of depression. To some extent, it is a function of the severity of the symptoms, but it can increase even when other symptoms appear to be stationary or improving. At any level of death thoughts, the physician must insist that the family remove any and all firearms from the dwelling. The patient who has evolved a fully lethal plan and secured the means to its execution should be hospitalized forthwith under intensive psychiatric observation. A course of electroconvulsive therapy (ECT) is the quickest and surest way to reverse suicidal intent. When in doubt, always refer a depressed patient to a specialist in that disorder.

The frequency of suicide is sharply increased in the weeks immediately after discharge from inpatient psychiatric treatment. In part, this may simply represent premature discharge. Both hospital costs and policies discourage optimal length of stay. Too often the patient is given a follow-up appointment in a month or 6 weeks. That is not soon enough by far. The patient has been seen daily, or nearly daily, by the psychiatrist while in the hospital. Abruptly, there is a long hiatus. It feels to the patient like abandonment. Depressive symptoms often recur, and if the physician is hard to reach, despair may ensue. The primary care physician can provide the close professional support needed for the recently discharged patient.

The bottom line in preventing suicide in substance abusers is to stop the drinking or other substance abuse. Most of the social stressors that are found among the suicides are directly attributable to the consequences of substance abuse. With the exception of medical problems, the treatment of these conditions is outside the scope of all but a few primary care physicians. Most substance abuse treatment these days is outpatient treatment, and each physician should know of a treatment program to which she is comfortable referring patients. Alcoholics Anonymous (AA) is sometimes helpful and always worth trying. Patients should be advised to visit several chapters before deciding whether and where to continue. The tone, social level,

PEARLS & PERILS

TO REEMPHASIZE:

- Although most patients with thoughts of suicide tell the physician if they are asked, they rarely volunteer that information. The physician should ask gently, but it is most important to *ask*.
- The patient with a fully lethal plan and the means at her disposal is at high risk and should be hospitalized without delay in a secure psychiatric facility.
- Even at low levels of suicidal ideation, the physician should insist that the family remove all firearms from the home.
- Too many physicians look for an explanation for the depression, and having found one, they fail to treat the depression. The diagnosis is the diagnosis and calls for vigorous treatment.
- Having another psychiatric diagnosis is not protective. Depression can and does complicate any of them (for example, substance abuse or panic disorder) and brings with it the risk of suicide.

and orthodoxy vary considerably, and a good social fit is necessary for continued participation.

The acute, subacute, and chronic risk factors identified thus far for suicide in people who are alcoholic were described in this chapter's section on alcoholism. There is reason to believe that substance abusers of all preferences share the same vulnerability. When social support is poor or absent, loss or threats of loss (equally as potent) may be decisive. The period of greatest danger probably lasts no more than 2 months around the event, so hospitalization, day hospital, or other supportive measures may buy the needed protection. The depressive syndrome commonly encountered in people with severe alcoholism often remits spontaneously with detoxification. When it does not, it must be treated vigorously. Substance abusers are so often uncooperative and noncompliant that protective efforts do not always prevail. However, it is far better to try and fail than to fail to try (see the Pearls & Perils box at the bottom of p. 432).

Attempted Suicide

A suicide attempt is usually not that at all. What was attempted is rarely suicide. Rather, a suicide attempt is a drastic form of communication—a cry for help. But the behavior sometimes signals more serious trouble, including the wish to die. Nine out of ten identified acts of deliberate self-harm are by overdose of medication. Wrist cutting is in second place. Sublethal, often trivial, amounts of medication are the rule, as are provisions for rescue. More than one half of these events come to a physician's attention later or not at all. But the lifetime risk of suicide in people who attempt suicide is 12% to 15%, about that of suicide in major depression.

All suicide attempts should be taken seriously, in the sense that they provide the opportunity to examine for psychiatric illness. What to look for is mainly evidence of major depression or substance abuse, alone or co-morbid with a personality disorder. Age is a risk factor, too. Suicide attempts after the age of 40 must be regarded with great caution. By that age, most people have found better ways to handle all but the weightiest problems. The acts become more dangerous both physically and psychiatrically. Survival may be by accident or unplanned intervention. However, even a medically trivial act may be a practice run for the real thing. The physician must take no chances. If the physician is not sure—*really* sure—the patient is safe, a psychiatric opinion should be secured. One third of suicides have a history of deliberate self-harm.

Annotated Bibliography

Murphy GE: *Suicide in alcoholism,* New York, 1992, Oxford University Press.

The case histories of 50 people with alcoholism who committed suicide comprise the core of this book. Each story is different, but there are many features in common. The methodology of the research is described, as are the risk factors for suicide derived from this study and compared with other populations.

Robins E: *The final months: a study of the lives of 134 persons who committed suicide,* New York, 1981, Oxford University Press.

This is the first systematic study of suicide in the community and the first case histories of its victims. The findings of this work, completed in 1958, have been replicated over and over. None has ever been disputed.

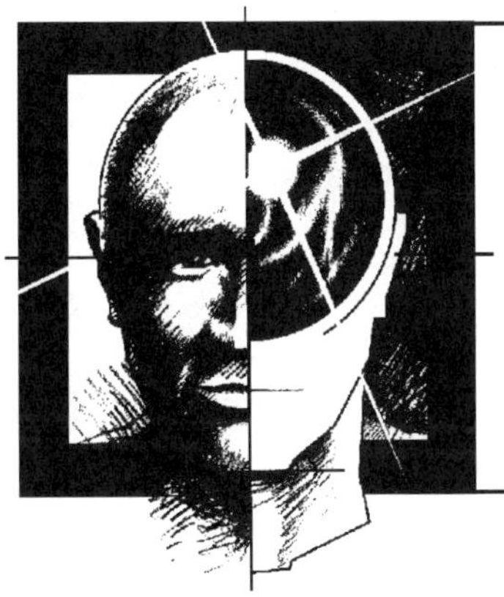

chapter 28

Forensic Issues

Sean H. Yutzy, MD and Stephen H. Dinwiddie, MD

Although the primary care physician's exposure to the legal system is limited, the occurrence of psychiatric illness in patients broadens the scope of potential medicolegal issues for the treating physician. Although many physicians regard any intrusion of law into medicine as being at best an inconvenience and at worst a disaster, the physician who adheres to the principles of good medical practice using a pure advocacy model of patient care will have little trouble meeting any challenges that the adversarial system produces.

Identified in this chapter are five issues that commonly precipitate consultation with a general psychiatrist or, perhaps sometimes more appropriately, a subspecialty psychiatrist who focuses on issues at the interface among medicine, psychiatry, and the law. This area, known as *forensic psychiatry,* has been in existence for a number of years, but only recently has the American Board of Psychiatry and Neurology begun to offer additional certification in this area.

The case studies, principles, and discussions detailed in this chapter should not be taken as legal advice but as a guide to considering the facts, circumstances, and issues of the physician's case. The practitioner should also be aware that the legal principles outlined are broadly described in the medicolegal literature, but statutory and case laws vary between jurisdictions. When indicated, medicolegal or legal consultation should be undertaken.

When Psychiatric Consultation is "Required" by Law

Principle

The legal standard that guides practice in particular against improper acts of commission or omission is the unintentional tort of professional negligence (malpractice) (Case 28-1). To best understand this rule of law, a brief description of the general concept is nec-

CASE 28-1

A 64-year-old, part-time employed, recently widowed man with abdominal pain was admitted to the hospital. The patient had come to the hospital with alcohol on his breath, and when questioned about his drinking, he indicated that he did not have a history of significant intake until his wife died 4 months before. Regarding the abdominal pain, he stated that approximately 3 weeks before admission he developed vague central abdominal pain that eventually shifted to the right lower quadrant. He described the pain as intermittent, vague, and diffuse. He denied all other upper or lower gastrointestinal symptoms. He stated that over-the-counter pain medications did not seem to help but that the alcohol completely alleviated the problem temporarily. He related that he had no significant past medical history. He recalled that his only surgical history was the removal of his tonsils as a child and the removal of two .45 slugs from his abdomen as a result of self-inflicted gunshot wounds when he was in his mid-40s. At that time he had been evaluated and transferred to the psychiatric ward for treatment. He recalled that he had been depressed over the loss of his son and treated with "some sort of shock treatment." He did not see a psychiatrist after discharge. His family medical history was significant only for a brother who had intentionally electrocuted himself. The patient had been married for 44 years until his wife died earlier that year. They had one child who had died in an accident at age 15. He indicated that he was employed part-time and that he was concerned about being able to pay for hospitalization. When asked whether he had other problems or concerns, he described not sleeping for months and loss of appetite with an approximate 15-pound weight loss. He complained that he consistently felt down in the dumps and just did not seem to have his "usual amount of energy." He also stated that he had an occasional "crying jag," which he could not stop or understand. He volunteered that he had some thoughts about not wanting to be around since he was "the only one left." At this juncture, the physician asked him whether he had any plans to intentionally hurt himself, to which he appeared somewhat surprised and stated, "Yes, before coming in but . . . no, not while I am here in the hospital." The physical examination revealed the patient to be under his ideal body weight and to have vague, diffuse lower and right-lower quadrant abdominal pain without point or rebound tenderness. There was an old laparotomy scar from the bullet removal, but the examination was otherwise negative. Working diagnoses were rule-out appendicitis; rule-out pancreatitis; rule-out gastritis; and rule-out depression with somatic pain (abdominal pain). The nursing entries in the record on the first evening of hospitalization described the patient as crying on several occasions. After the first full hospital day, the routine laboratory work returned negative. Clinical examination of the patient continued to reveal unchanged abdominal pain. The nurses documented that he appeared sullen and withdrawn.

On the second full hospital day, a barium enema was performed and was negative. Clinical examination by the physician's covering internal medicine partner revealed that the physical examination was essentially unchanged, and the partner documented his opinion that the patient was "melancholically depressed and must have psychiatric consultation because of suicidal thoughts before being discharged." Nursing notes on that day documented that the patient talked about missing his wife and stated that there was really little point in his continued living with this pain. Additionally, they documented that he stated he felt "hopeless and completely fatigued." Surgical consultation was requested for the next day.

On the third day, an upper GI with small bowel follow-through examination was performed and found to be negative. The surgical consultation revealed the opinion that the pain was probably not from an appendicitis and that the more likely explanation was "depression with somatic abdominal pain." The attending physician documented that the patient "will need formal psychiatric evaluation for depression and suicidality before discharge." Additionally the doctor's working diagnosis was changed to "probably not an appendicitis, but most likely a depression-related problem." On returning to his office late that day, the attending physician was contacted by the patient's insurer, who informed the physician that they had read his most recent note and were wondering whether the patient could be discharged the next day. The physician informed them that he intended to perform a colonoscopy in the morning and that this would complete the evaluation. The insurer asked whether the patient could then be discharged. The physician indicated that he was not sure; he would have to discuss this with the patient. The insurer indicated firmly that the patient's benefits would not extend beyond the next day.

On the morning of the fourth day, a colonoscopy was performed and revealed no organic pathological condition. The physician went by to see the patient in the afternoon after the anesthesia had worn off and informed him of the lack of pathological findings.

The patient accepted the positive news that there was nothing "physically wrong" with him but appeared reluctant to be discharged. The physician indicated that there was nothing further the internist could do for him in the hospital, and he was released. He was to be seen in the internist's office in 1 week.

The next day the internist received a visit from local homicide detectives regarding his patient. During the initial part of the interview the physician asked what had happened, and the detectives indicated that his patient had been discovered dead early that morning and that they were performing a routine investigation. On further inquiry, the detectives indicated that the scene did not suggest foul play but that they were charged with investigating any death in which a physician was not in attendance—even if it was just a suicide.

essary. There are four required elements that must be present in a potential legal case, and they are best illustrated through the "four *D*s" shown in the following list (Simon, 1987):

1. ***Duty:*** once a doctor-patient relationship has been established, the physician has a fiduciary obligation to treat his patient in all aspects of medical care as defined by the prevailing standards of good medical practice.
2. ***Dereliction:*** during the performance of his duties, a physician may deviate from the generally accepted standard of good medical practice through an act of commission or omission.
3. ***Directly:*** as a direct result of the deviation (dereliction) of an owed duty, the patient may be injured.
4. ***Damage:*** if the injury directly flowed from the deviation (dereliction) from the owed duty, it may be a compensable legal damage.

All four elements must be present to a preponderance of the evidence ("more likely than not," or anything greater than a 50.1% likelihood) for a legal case to be potentially successful.

Discussion

Most people are aware that in a free society, the law (criminal and civil) only proscribes conduct for a limited number of behaviors (or potential behaviors). Interestingly, civil tort theory applies a rather broad duty to every person in society to conduct himself in all his diverse activities so as to not create an unreasonable risk of harm to others. In professional matters, one adheres to this same duty (although now contractual as well), which in essence "requires" a physician to conduct himself medically in a manner that does not place a patient at unreasonable risk; failure to do so risks civil litigation consequences.

In medical theory and practice, initiation of formal psychiatric consultation is a medical decision undertaken at the discretion and request of the attending physician. The driving forces for consultation are the facts and circumstances of the case, as well as what is in the best medical interest of the patient as determined by good medical practice. When the totality of the evidence is considered, and a formal psychiatric consultation is not only indicated and necessary but to not obtain consultation would be below the prevailing standard of good medical practice (in the view of a similarly trained and reasonably prudent medical practitioner), then there exists a formal legal duty to obtain appropriate consultation. If it is not obtained and if as a direct result of this deviation below the standard of good medical practice a legal damage results, then the case may be legally actionable.

The following medical facts in Case 28-1 support psychiatric consultation: (1) the current diagnosis of depression made by the physician, supported by a history of depression, serious suicide attempt, and electroconvulsive therapy (ECT); (2) an overall high-risk suicide profile; (3) recent suicidal ideas; and (4) the physician's documented opinion that the patient will need formal psychiatric evaluation for depression and suicidality before discharge, as well as his partner's documentation of a definite need for psychiatric consultation before discharge. Whereas the legal case is relatively clear, defense counsel might consider taking (among other counterarguments) the position that just because the two physicians stated psychiatric consultation was indicated, necessary, and must (or should) be performed before discharge, that still does not mean that failure to obtain it was below the prevailing community standard. Such a question of fact becomes an issue for a jury.

Competency to Refuse Treatment

Principle

The legal concept underlying a decision to accept (or refuse) an offered procedure or medication is the principle of informed consent (Case 28-2). It is sometimes referred to as competency to consent to accept (or refuse) a procedure (or medication).

The following three elements are considered to compromise informed consent: (1) information, (2) voluntariness, and (3) competency. The element of information has several interpretations, and the precise language varies among the jurisdictions. A significant number of jurisdictions adhere to a professional standard wherein the sufficiency of the information provided to the patient to make a decision is judged by what most physicians provide their patients. However, one of the more widely accepted paradigms of this element is known as the "reasonable person" (or patient) test and described as the information that a reasonable person would need to know to make an informed decision. The necessary points of information are generally considered to include the following: (1) precisely what the medication (or procedure) consists of along with its risks and benefits, (2) alternative medications (or procedures) along with their risks and benefits, (3) the risks and benefits of no medication (or procedure), and (4) time to ask any questions that the patient deems necessary.

The second element of informed consent is voluntariness. Patients must voluntarily make a decision for

CASE 28-2

A 55-year-old man with a long history of diabetes, alcoholism, and schizophrenia came to the emergency room with severe pain related to a large soft tissue abscess on his neck. Physical examination revealed the individual to be in overall deteriorated condition. On the right lateral aspect of his neck he had a 3 cm by 3 cm fluctuant mass immediately adjacent to the trachea but posterior to the jugular vein. His entire neck was tender to palpation and any movement. He was febrile (103° F), and he had a white blood cell count of 17,000, indicating acute infection, as well as an elevated blood sugar of 250. The patient reported that he routinely gave himself two shots of insulin a day and his blood sugar usually ranged between 85 and 175. When asked where he had been living, the patient became evasive and refused to answer the question. When observed sitting alone, the patient was noted to carry on a conversation with himself. When the physician inquired about incising and draining the lesion, the patient responded with the following comment: "No way I'm letting you near me with a knife so that you can kill me for my money." The patient further stated that he had only come to the emergency room at the behest of the voices. A request was made for the consulting psychiatrist to come to the emergency room and declare the patient incompetent so the treatment refusal could be overridden.

the process to be valid. Coercion, even subtle, may invalidate the process of consent.

The third element is competency, and here a brief aside is necessary. In law there is a fundamental presumption that all individuals are competent to conduct their affairs unless there is a special consideration present, such as juvenile status or a previous formal adjudication of incompetency (by a judge and not a physician). Physicians may consider the issue of mental competency when reviewing a medical situation, but they are in fact opining on an individual's medical capacity to provide valid (or invalid) informed consent. That is, they will consider whether a mental illness interferes with the patient's capacity to comprehend the risks and benefits of the proposed treatment, alternatives, or no treatment and to voluntarily make a decision.

Discussion

Although most physicians are generally aware of the elements of informed consent, not all are aware that when the patient refuses a procedure (or medication) the same basic elements apply. Therefore if the individual understands the information (from a reasonable-person perspective, where applicable) related to a particular procedure (or medication) and voluntarily declines, and if there is no question as to the individual's competency (medical capacity), in legal theory the refusal is valid and should be honored. When nonserious issues are disposed of by informed refusal, few problems arise. However, when serious or life-saving treatments are being considered and potentially refused, a thorough review of the situation by all interested parties, including family, second-opinion physicians, various committees, lawyers, and judges, may be undertaken.

In Case 28-2, a question is raised as to the individual's competency (medical capacity) to provide a valid informed refusal, since he appears to be refusing the procedure because of a paranoid psychotic misperception. Consultation with psychiatry is most appropriate, even though the psychiatrist will *not* be able to declare the patient incompetent. However, the consultant will be able to perform a psychiatric examination of the individual and evaluate for the presence of mental illness that may impair the patient's mental capacity to arrive at an informed decision. If the consultant opines psychiatric (medical) incapacity, steps to override this refusal should be initiated based on consideration of the regulations and laws of the state and on the best medical interest of the patient. In some states, emergency situations may be reviewed by judges via telephone, and authorization to override an incompetent legal refusal can be adjudicated without significant delay. In other states, a temporary guardian must be appointed at a formal court proceeding, and this person can make the decision to override an incompetent legal refusal; however, this usually necessitates significant delay.

Guardianship and Conservatorship

Principle

The concepts of guardianship and conservatorship are often confused, and the precise statutory language (and case law) varies among the states. Generally, a guardianship can be established if as a result of a medical or mental condition the individual is unable to receive and process information to the extent that he cannot adequately provide for the basic necessities of life (for example, food, shelter, safety, and emergency procedures) (Case 28-3). Similarly, conservatorship can be established if as a result of a medical or mental condition the individual is unable to receive and process information such that he cannot adequately address their basic financial affairs.

CASE 28-3

A 65-year-old, widowed woman, living independently with a history of coronary artery disease, hypertension, and a family history of Alzheimer's disease had been medically stable taking multiple medications over the last year, except for a minor complaint about forgetfulness. The physician had noted some minor problems with memory, but the patient had been able to articulate her need for medication, as well as list doses and complicated schedules. One month ago she voiced a concern that somebody had broken into her house and stolen or "rearranged" her furniture. The police were summoned but did nothing. During a more recent office visit she related that she had confirmed that people were rearranging her furniture by placing a hair between various pieces of furniture and the wall. On reassessment the next day, the hair had fallen to the floor. Mrs. X could still articulate her need for medication, but she appeared suspicious of her "need for all that medication."

The physician expressed concern about the patient living alone and asked to be allowed to contact her family, who lived in another state. The patient agreed. The patient's daughter voiced a surprising amount of concern and stated that she would be in town the next day to assess the situation; 2 days later an attorney contacted the physician's office, saying that he had been retained by the family. He explained that the family was going to file a petition to have Mrs. X declared incompetent and wanted to know if the physician would be kind enough to execute some paperwork that the attorney could either hand deliver or fax to the office that day. The physician divulged no information about the patient but agreed to consider the material. On review, the physician noted that in addition to a guardianship affidavit there was a conservatorship affidavit.

The next day Mrs. X called the physician and was quite distraught. She explained that her family had descended on her and was trying to take control of her person and assets. She related to the physician that she thought the family could hardly wait to get their hands on her $500,000 held in the bank. The patient pleaded with her physician to assist her in her plight.

Discussion

All physicians are aware that they have an obligation to advocate for their patient's best medical interest. In Case 28-3, this obligation properly impelled the physician to initiate a process that inadvertently upset her patient. One way to approach the situation would be to strongly suggest that the patient obtain legal counsel to advocate for her interests. Furthermore, the physician should inform the patient that the physician has an obligation to advocate for the patient's best medical interest and that she will, of course, continue to fulfill this obligation.

Once the patient has attained proper legal representation, the physician's role may subsequently take several different pathways. The patient's attorney might ask the physician's assistance in considering whether guardianship (and conservatorship) is indicated under the applicable laws of the state. The physician may refuse this offer, stating that she wishes to remain completely neutral in this matter and not risk jeopardizing the physician-patient relationship.

Alternatively, if the physician considers proffering a medical opinion she should be cognizant of a number of issues. First, she should be aware of the precise statutory language and relevant case law for the applicable jurisdiction. Second, she may wish to consult the available literature for models or medicolegal tests to guide these sometimes intricate and complicated evaluations. Third, the patient needs to release the physician to discuss fully and freely the medical considerations (as well as formal medicolegal opinions) with the attorney. Fourth, the patient should be aware that the physician will be formulating a narrow opinion on what is in the patient's best medical interest and that this opinion may or may not be the same as what the patient feels is in her overall best interest. In fact there is no guarantee that the potential formal medicolegal opinions will be helpful, and there is the possibility that the opinions may be harmful to the legal case. Fifth, *before* the formalization of opinions (on guardianship and conservatorship), the patient should be made aware that she will be waiving confidentiality and testimonial privilege if she wishes her physician to testify with formal opinion, although the obligation (confidentiality) and duty (privilege) may be dispensed by the legal process. Sixth, once formal opinions are formulated and expressed (helpful or not), they will be subject to the applicable discovery process (for example, affidavit, interrogatories, report, deposition, hearing, trial, and other procedures). Seventh, the physician's formulated medical opinions are usually considered by the judge in the broad context of a general guardianship determination. In fact, the physician should be aware that her medical testimony may completely drive an adjudication that full guardianship is needed, which would be a finding by the court that the patient is incompetent to handle all her affairs except financial matters.

The conservatorship issue is narrower but often more aggressively litigated because of the substantial monies involved.

Civil Commitment

Principle

Civil commitment is a legal mechanism whereby patients who are mentally ill and dangerous to themselves or others may be detained and forcibly treated at an appropriate receiving facility (Case 28-4).

Historically the foundation for this mechanism has been in the concepts of *parens patriae* and the states' police power. *Parens patriae* is a concept rooted in English law that enabled the king to act as "general guardian of incapacitated classes, including infants and the mentally disordered" (Developments, 1974). In theory, when the state takes steps exercising the *parens patriae* power, the actions are considered benevolent. The police power enables the state to act as a protector of society through the generation and enforcement of laws for the protection of general societal health and safety. Actions taken to promote these societal interests as opposed to furthering the interest of an individual constitute an exercise of police power.

Review of civil commitment laws in the United States before 1960 at the appellate level revealed that the courts identified the basis for detention laws within the states' *parens patriae* power. However, in the 1970s the laws were challenged and substantially modified to address the issue of *parens patriae* and a newfound concern about the police power of the state. Statutory changes relevant to the following discussion included judicial review of a codified civil commitment test, as well as affording the potential detainee a number of constitutional safeguards normally guaranteed a criminal defendant.

Although the precise statutory language regulating civil commitment varies among the states, the substan-

CASE 28-4

A 54-year-old single man with a lengthy history of rheumatic heart disease, hyperthyroidism, and paranoid schizophrenia was involuntarily detained at the petition of the attending psychiatrist. The medical history showed that the patient had had rheumatic heart disease as a child with mild aortic and mitral valve regurgitation as a young adult. Around age 30 he had onset of hyperthyroidism, which had been relatively well controlled medically with propylthiouracil. He had refused medical and surgical ablation. On the only two occasions when he stopped his antithyroid medication, he rapidly became hyperthyroid. His hyperthyroidism precipitated frank congestive heart failure, necessitating admission to the intensive care unit for life-threatening illness.

The psychiatric history was significant for a 35-year history of schizophrenia with six previous psychiatric hospitalizations. The last five hospitalizations occurred shortly after the patient stopped taking his antipsychotic medication because he felt "fine." Subsequently, he had a rapid onset of paranoia and command auditory hallucinations telling him to strike out at strangers because they were part of a conspiracy to kill him. He had attempted this once before 10 years earlier.

Approximately 1 week before this admission the patient disposed of his antipsychotic and antithyroid medication, informing his family that he no longer had any medical problems. The patient began to develop signs of suspiciousness and paranoia after several days. The family contacted the attending psychiatrist, who instructed them to bring the patient to the emergency room as soon as possible. He was brought to the emergency room and was initially noted to be calm and cooperative. He admitted hearing voices commanding him to hurt people in red shirts because they were part of the plot to kill him. He acknowledged that he did not know whether he could continue to control himself because the voices were so loud. He was offered admission to the hospital, which he refused. He was offered medication in the emergency room, which he refused, and he became angry. A brief detention order was executed at the direction of the attending psychiatrist, and the patient was transferred to the secure psychiatric unit.

After admission, the patient was calm and cooperative during all aspects of the evaluation process. He was suspicious and rather paranoid but demonstrated no overtly hostile behavior. To the intake nurses and attending physician he denied auditory hallucinations and indicated that he was not suicidal or homicidal. He further stated that he was in control of his emotions, thoughts, and impulses. Physical examination and laboratory testing revealed the patient to have a mild tremor and moderately elevated free T_4. He refused both antipsychotic and antithyroid medication.

Over several observation days on the ward, the patient was noted to be withdrawn from the other patients. He was noted by the staff to argue in a loud manner with himself on several occasions. He was sleeping and eating well, and he demonstrated only mild agitation when offered his medication. The patient continued refusing his medicines, stating that there was nothing wrong with him medically or psychiatrically. He also related that he was not going to take the medications because he was convinced that the pharmaceutical company had "adulterated the medicine with rat feces." The psychiatrist was aware of the lack of comments or overt behavior suggestive of suicidal or homicidal intent, but because of the impending medical illness decided to ask the patient's internist to testify at the formal civil commitment hearing to bolster the petition for extended judicial detention.

tive requirements are similar. First, there must be a mental illness present. Second, the mental illness must be "serious," a term that is variably defined, although some jurisdictions require the illness result in an impaired capacity to recognize the need for treatment. Third, the mental illness must "cause" or result in the individual representing a danger to self or others. Fourth, alternatively, most states permit civil commitment if the mental illness renders the individual unable to care for himself and there is a concern about harm if the illness is not treated.

Discussion

In Case 28-4, the psychiatrist recognizes that his patient has a major mental illness that interferes with his ability to recognize the need for treatment. Unfortunately for the legal case (civil commitment), after several days of inpatient observation, the mental illness and lack of insight did not appear to cause the individual to meet the third element of the test; namely, the patient was not suicidal or homicidal. However, a strong case can be made that because of the patient's paranoia and incapacity to recognize his need for medical (and psychiatric) treatment he will not be able to care for himself if released, because he will likely deteriorate to a potentially life-threatening state (hyperthyroidism leading to congestive heart failure). Whereas the psychiatrist, as a physician, can testify to this medical opinion, judicial decision-makers often prefer (and weigh more heavily) testimony from medical experts with specific expertise in the area being considered. The general practitioner will probably have the option of choosing whether to appear in court, but he should always be cognizant of his fiduciary obligation to advocate for his patient's best medical interest. Before appearing at the civil commitment hearing, the physician should educate himself about the relevant issues, rules, and laws. Review of all facets of this type of proceeding is beyond the scope of this chapter, but a more than adequate general level of sophistication can easily be achieved by reviewing the matter with the interested and experienced parties, including the treating psychiatrist (petitioner) and the lawyer taking the case.

However, several narrow but important points need to be reviewed. First, many physicians are concerned about a potential breach of confidentiality or violation of testimonial privilege. The civil commitment process is an exception to both as long as the action taken is in the furtherance of the detention. Second, it is always helpful to review the specific language applicable to the jurisdiction. Third, the potential opinions that the physician may offer can be broad (or narrow), and they will be based on the physician's level of comfort and expertise (as determined by the court) with the medical facts, as well as on the attorney's strategy for the legal case. In the broadest scenario, the physician may form and render to the court opinions on any (or all) of the following issues: (1) the presence or absence of a mental illness (as defined by the jurisdiction in statutory language or case law); (2) the potential for exacerbation or reoccurrence of an underlying mental illness; (3) the presence or absence of a medical illness; (4) the potential for exacerbation or reoccurrence of an underlying medical illness; (5) the seriousness of the medical illness (and the mental illness); (6) the interplay (or potential) between the mental and medical illness; (7) the patient's capacity to recognize need for treatment; (8) opinions on any other medical issues; and (9) hypothetical testimony using the facts of this case or other cases to base opinions on potential outcomes.

Insanity

Principle

Although the statutory language and case law regulating the insanity defense varies among the states, the substantive elements are relatively uniform. The individual must suffer from a mental disease or defect, which at the time of the criminal behavior interfered with the person's capacity to perceive wrongfulness (of the behavior) or interfered with the individual's capacity to conform his conduct to the requirements of law (this last element has been struck from the federal statutes as well as in many states) (Case 28-5). Of particular interest is the fact that the underlying mental illness labeled as a *mental disease or defect* is not explicitly defined by law and is therefore subject to interpretation by the user with review by judge and jury in court.

The basis for the insanity defense can be found in two fundamental medicolegal principles. First, there is a moral imperative in society to not hold blameworthy or culpable those people who do not merit application of these concepts because of their impaired psychiatric or neurological condition. Minors and people who are severely mentally retarded have traditionally been identified as individuals who should not be held responsible, but the mentally ill have always been in a more precarious position on this issue. Second, society is best served if there is a perception of fairness in the adjudications by the courts. This sense may be undermined if, as one judge stated, "Drooling idiots are treated as responsible defendants" (Gutheil, 1995).

Discussion

Although the charges described in Case 28-5 may be disposed by several more expedient avenues, pros-

CASE 28-5

A 50-year-old widower with a long history of porphyria and no criminal record was in an automobile accident while vacationing in a neighboring state. The patient was unconscious when taken to the hospital, and surgery was performed to pin his broken leg. A barbiturate was used as part of the anesthetic induction regimen. The patient convalesced in the hospital for a day and was noted to complain about abdominal discomfort at discharge. He subsequently resided with his deceased wife's family, and he complained of abdominal pain and demonstrated erratic behavior and frank paranoia. His urine turned dark. The family tolerated his unusual behavior even though it was grossly inappropriate. One day he wandered away from the house and went to a local park. He sat down on a bench and fell asleep. A park ranger came by and notified him that he could not sleep on the bench. The patient was noted to be well dressed but incoherent in his conversation and bizarre in his interaction. The conversation escalated into an argument, and the patient took a swing at the park ranger, who pulled his gun. The patient advanced on the park ranger, who fled. The police were summoned and after an extended brawl, the patient wound up in custody and five policemen went to the emergency room for bruises and bites. The patient was legally processed and five counts of first-degree assault were brought. He was transferred from the jail to the hospital as a prisoner because of his unstable medical condition. He was eventually discharged and noted by the family to seem "normal." The patient retained counsel to defend him. The attorney contacted the patient's treating physician in his home state about his long history of porphyria. The lawyer then informed the physician that he would like him to review the state statutes on sanity, case law, medical records, and police reports and consider offering an opinion on insanity.

ecutorial discretion occasionally requires a full sanity evaluation and sometimes trial. In potential sanity cases where an underlying medical illness can be documented by laboratory testing and the disease is outside the usual evaluation and treatment role of a psychiatrist, a general medical physician may be invited to proffer an opinion. Often attorneys avoid using the patient's treating physician for a variety of reasons, including the inherent bias to advocate for his patient's best interest, lack of medicolegal sophistication, possible hidden concern on the part of the treating physician that he may be the eventual target of a malpractice suit (because of the original incident), causing perversion of subsequent testimony, and other reasons. However, in cases where the presence of an unusual medical "mental illness" is central, the attorney may feel strongly that not only should an independent medical expert testify but that the treating physician should also play a significant role in assisting the trier-of-fact (judge or jury) in deciding the case. Although the treating physician usually has the option not to participate (citing possible interference with physician-patient relationship), he should always consider the fiduciary obligation to advocate for the patient's best medical interest.

In cases where the treating physician elects to become involved, he should expend every effort to gain as complete an understanding of the entire process as possible. After obtaining a formal release from his patient to speak to the attorney, the physician can begin this educational process. The attorney will be able to provide the physician with all the available relevant information, including the statutory language and case law. However, the physician should be aware that the attorney represents the best legal interest of the patient and not the interests of the physician. Should the physician develop any concern or question about any issue related to his role, he may wish to retain his own counsel. Working with the patient's attorney will probably give rise to a number of potential issues of interest, but the core request by the attorney is for the production of medical (clinical) and perhaps medicolegal opinions. Medical opinion is considered here to be all the medical knowledge, information, and inferences that a physician can offer to assist the trier-of-fact in understanding the medical issues related to the case but not including a direct statement containing the ultimate medicolegal opinion on insanity (that is, the examiner's opinion as to whether patient was insane at the time of the crime). In the majority of cases, medical opinions represent the entire request of the treating physician. However, before arriving at any "formal" medicolegal opinions to be expressed and rendered to the court, the physician may find review of the considerations detailed in the following paragraph helpful.

In certain cases, the attorney may request a medicolegal opinion on insanity (criminal responsibility). The following discussion represents an outline of the general issues to be considered, but the physician should be aware that this is not a comprehensive list (because every case has its own specific issues). First, the patient should be made aware that the treating physician is interested and willing to consider offering an opinion about the medical and perhaps medicolegal aspects of the case for a legal determination regarding responsibility (insanity). Generally, the patient needs to agree for the physician to proceed after consideration is given to the following subset of preliminary issues by those involved. Confidentiality has to be waived either directly by the patient, through court appointment, or by other methods applicable in the jurisdiction. Testimonial privilege has to be waived either directly by the patient, directly through judicial order, directly through the fact that it is a criminal proceeding, or by methods applicable in the jurisdiction. The patient should be aware that there is no guarantee that the physician will be helpful. The patient should be aware of the usual avenues that formal opinions (helpful, neutral, or harmful to their interests) may become part of the public record. The physician should consider the possible deleterious effects of harmful legal opinions on the overall physician-patient relationship. Second, the physician needs to review and understand the applicable statutory language and case law. This may be involved and entail learning legal interpretation of special language as opposed to routine medical knowledge. Third, the physician usually needs to review all available written materials pertaining to his patient's longitudinal medical illness (and behavior) before the alleged assault, as well as the patient's medical status and behavior immediately before, during, and after the incident. Fourth, the physician may need to interview individuals who observed the patient's behavior at the time of the incident and when he had prior exacerbations of porphyria. Fifth, subsequent to considering the legal test and reviewing all collateral information, an examination of the patient is usually undertaken. The patient's complete history is usually reviewed, but the bulk of the examination is spent considering the patient's medical and psychiatric status at the time of the incident and whether or not the legal test was met. Sixth, arrival at formal medicolegal opinions should be driven by careful consideration (and weighing) of every relevant medical, legal, and psychiatric fact, such that the physician proffers an opinion at the level of certitude articulated by the legal profession as "reasonable medical certainty"—a phrase that has been variably defined by the courts and must be ascertained for that particular jurisdiction at the beginning of the case.

Conclusion

The principles identified by the case studies and discussed in this chapter represent the major issues that precipitate consultation with a psychiatric specialist. The primary care physician should be aware that the principles of professional negligence (malpractice), informed consent, and competence are the same as applied to other medical decisions where no psychiatric issue is raised. Whereas the principles of civil commitment and insanity do not routinely necessitate input from the general practitioner, the principle of patient advocacy (considering certain caveats) may demand assistance in legal determinations.

Finally, the physician should always be cognizant of the theme underlying these issues and guiding the physician-patient relationship: the fiduciary obligation of the physician to advocate for the patient's best medical interest in every aspect of care.

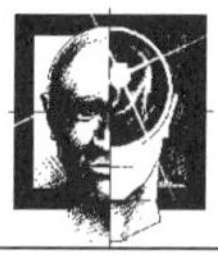

Annotated Bibliography

Appelbaum PS, Gutheil TG: *The clinical handbook of psychiatry and the law*, ed 2, Baltimore, 1991, Williams and Wilkins.

Kaplan HI, Sadock BJ: *Comprehensive textbook of psychiatry*, vol 2, ed 6, Baltimore, 1995, Williams and Wilkins.

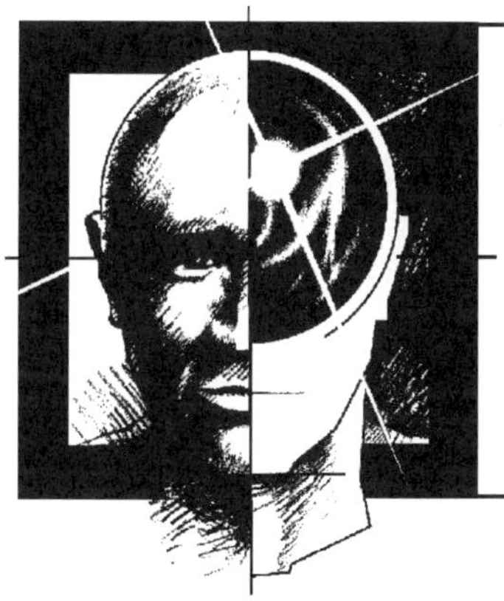

chapter 29

Ethical Issues in Psychiatric Practice

Stephen H. Dinwiddie, MD and Sean H. Yutzy, MD

Conflict between ethical principles and the necessity of resolving such conflicts are inherent in the practice of medicine. As practitioners of a medical specialty, psychiatrists must deal with many of the same ethical problems and challenges that face physicians in any other field of medicine. However, clinical dilemmas may gain another layer of complexity when the patient suffers from a significant psychiatric disorder that may affect her judgment, decision-making capability, and desires.

The Medical Model of Psychiatry

The medical model of psychiatry, discussed in greater detail in Chapter 1, is an approach to the care of patients that emphasizes attention to reliable diagnosis and careful evaluation of treatment effectiveness. Adherents of the medical model emphasize that accurate knowledge of the cause, course, and optimal treatment of psychiatric illness, as for any disorder, is central to the role of the physician and is best obtained by rigorous, well-designed study without deference to any particular psychological theory in the absence of experimental proof of its validity and utility. Although such "toughmindedness" has on occasion been criticized as being uncaring and unsympathetic, Guze (1970) has pointed out:

> Scientific skepticism is in no way incompatible with compassion for the sick or disabled. In fact, it is the desire

> to help patients that causes one to be frustrated by the lack of definite knowledge about what really helps and what does not. There are few things more humanitarian than the effective use of knowledge to relieve suffering . . . .

Although ethical questions are rarely amenable to simple answers, the decisions most likely to be beneficial to the patient are those that are most accurately informed, and that are made with a clear understanding of the nature and extent of the physician's obligation to the patient.

Paternalism, Autonomy, and Beneficence

The patient-physician relationship historically has been a fiduciary one, with substantial constraints placed on the physician's behavior. By virtue of training and experience the physician has superior access to information about the patient's condition and is better able to understand the implications of the disease and treatments to be offered. Professional standards also impose an obligation on the physician to act in the patient's best medical interest. The patient, on the other hand, does not have equivalent restrictions and is free to accept or reject the physician's advice or treatment, even though disregarding it may lead to continuing health problems or even death.

The freedom to make health care decisions for oneself is considered to be a more important social value than optimal medical treatment. But the concept of autonomy in making medical decisions presupposes at least that the patient is able to rationally choose between treatment alternatives; the prospect of a patient basing decisions about his health care on delusional material would certainly be disturbing to most physicians. Thus *autonomy* cannot mean merely that decision-making power must be completely vested in the patient; it also implies that the decision-making process should be logical and the outcome consistent with the patient's usual beliefs and values. Rather than simply dictating treatment decisions to the patient or ceding all responsibility for decision-making, to be assured that treatment decisions are appropriately made it would seem that the physician has some responsibility to be sure that the patient's decision was arrived at rationally, even if the ultimate decision is one with which the physician might disagree. Deferring to the patient's choice without regard to the way it was made may not be sufficient, and psychiatric consultation may be sought if the patient appears to be acting against values previously expressed or demonstrated and if there is the possibility that such action stems from a mental illness.

In extreme cases (such as demonstrated danger to self or others) there are social mechanisms (such as civil commitment or guardianship proceedings) that allow for involuntary treatment of individuals so mentally ill that they are judged unable to make medical decisions. But whereas impairment of ability to consent to treatment can be quite dramatic—as in the case of a psychotic individual who responds to hallucinatory commands forbidding him to cooperate—more subtle degrees of impairment are certainly possible. Where is the line drawn? Should the consent of a patient with depression who assents to electroconvulsive therapy (ECT) because she is convinced it will cause her death be honored? Has a cancer patient who agrees to chemotherapy only because his spouse insists he do so truly acted voluntarily? Does it matter if he has always been a passive, easily led individual? Autonomy in making medical (or any other) decisions is not an all-or-none characteristic. Based on a variety of factors that may include the presence or absence of psychiatric illness (and symptoms thereof), personality style, store of knowledge, information-processing ability, and preexisting attitudes, patients show a range of ability to actively participate in the process of deciding to undergo treatment. Even when the psychiatric condition is not severe enough to warrant commitment, the physician may have an obligation to vigorously advocate for a course of treatment judged to be in the patient's best medical interest.

Irrational treatment refusal, of course, is only one side of the coin. Although concern about impaired competency arises most often when the patient refuses treatment that the physician firmly feels to be indicated, it is no less an issue when a patient assents to treatment without being able to truly participate in the decision-making process. In either case, the patient's autonomy has been abrogated.

If the patient is suffering acutely, the physician is inclined to act. Is such an exercise in medical paternalism justifiable? If treatment is imposed, how can the physician be sure that the patient's goals and not the physician's that are being furthered? Conversely, is it reasonable to believe that a patient whose decision-making ability is obviously impaired by medical or psychiatric illness can truly act autonomously? Greater harm may result from an exaggerated and unrealistic deference to the patient's stated wishes than by an infringement of that autonomy on the part of the physician. It can be argued that adequate treatment of psychotic states or severe mood disorders, even if instituted without all the elements of informed consent, ameliorate the patient's irrational thought processes, enhancing rather than detracting from the patient's freedom.

Such difficulties have led to the suggestion that rather than conceptualizing the physician-patient relationship in terms of paternalism or autonomy, the physician's duty to the patient is instead one of beneficence; it is a requirement to act in a way that will most benefit the patient. Whereas acting in a beneficent manner often involves fostering and strengthening the patient's autonomy, it is certainly conceivable that there are circumstances requiring the physician to act in a paternalistic way.

But whereas overt psychiatric illness may affect the patient's ability to consent to treatment, its mere presence does not negate competence, nor does its absence guarantee valid consent. A patient's competency to consent may vary over time and is influenced by a multitude of emotional and intellectual factors. The effect, if any, of mental illness can be determined only by careful examination. Ultimately, the decision as to how forcefully to persuade a reluctant patient (or to decline to treat an incompetently assenting one) must, in this view, be based on the physician's assessment of likelihood, imminence, and severity of harm with or without treatment, combined with an understanding of the patient's values and goals.

More importantly, the obligation to act beneficently requires that the physician also be aware of his own preconceptions and understand his own motives when recommending treatment. Respect for the individual requires sufficient self-knowledge that there is a reasonable assurance that the physician's recommendation stems from a balanced, objective reasoning process rather than being an automatic imposition of the physician's values without reference to those of the patient.

This objectivity is needed especially in the case of the patient who may develop an unrealistically favorable view of the physician, discount any risks or reservations about treatment, and passively comply with the physician's advice. Conversely, whereas the physician should try not to use the patient's dependency to coerce her into agreeing to a course of action of which the physician approves (for his own reasons), there is nothing wrong with a physician explicitly stating his belief (and the bases for that belief) concerning the best treatment. Especially in a pluralistic society where many strongly-held personal beliefs may influence the patient's attitude toward a procedure, a partnership dedicated to the patient's well-being, where both parties are actively informed of each other's values and goals, appears to be the most efficient vehicle for protecting and furthering the patient's interests.

Balancing Risk and Benefit

One of the duties of beneficence is highlighted when considering treatment options for psychiatric illness. Arguably the most drastic intervention, involuntary hospitalization and treatment, should carry with it a clear benefit, potentially setting the stage for treatment of a life-threatening disease state when lesser interventions fail. Of course, the risks are also great; overt violation of the patient's refusal of treatment (though presumably irrational) carries the possibility of serious repercussions, including discrimination by employers and insurers, and limitation of civil rights ranging from restriction on ability to purchase firearms to restriction of freedom of movement.

It is well recognized that somatic treatments—as in other areas of medicine—carry with them potential risks and side effects, including tardive dyskinesia from antipsychotics, dependence on many anxiolytics, memory loss from ECT, and so on. Less widely recognized are potential adverse outcomes of psychotherapy, which may include significant changes in attitude and behavior toward family members and other significant figures in the patient's life. For example, one not uncommon outcome of marital therapy is the conclusion (by one or both members of the couple) that dissolution of the relationship is preferable to its continuation. Although presumably in most cases such changes are seen as positive, or at least the losses (in terms of changed relationships) appear to be counterbalanced by improvement in other areas of the patient's life, the possibility of an overall worse outcome nonetheless exists.

Even the act of diagnosis, a necessary and fundamental aspect of treatment and prognosis, can potentially lead to harm. Obviously, a misdiagnosis may lead to inadequate or harmful treatment; but even a correct diagnosis may be associated with discrimination from insurers or employers and stigmatization by society. Reliance solely on diagnostic classification may also lead to routinized forms of care (or denial of care), with insufficient attention paid to the individual patient's manifestations of illness and response to treatment. More subtle forms of harm may also arise from misuse of diagnostic categories, such as absolving a patient of responsibility for her acts based solely on the presence of a given diagnosis.

As in any other area of medicine, the fact that therapeutic efforts may be ineffective or even cause more rather than less suffering does not mean that the treatment must be ineffective or fundamentally flawed. However, it is the physician who is most informed about the nature and likelihood of any risks and who therefore is best able (with due regard for the patient's attitudes and values) to choose the optimum balance between risk and benefit. In the case of diagnosis, it is particularly important to realize that assigning a diagnosis may have unintended effects; the patient, family, or society may focus on the diagnostic label rather than on the individual's own characteristics.

Dual Agentry and Exploitation of Patients

Because of the demands and expectations placed on them by society, psychiatrists, perhaps more than other medical professionals, run the risk of dual agentry. That is, the psychiatrist, although professing that she is acting solely in the patient's interests, may have another, inapparent motive, as well. The psychiatrist's ability to commit patients to the hospital involuntarily, for example, has been criticized for this reason. The argument is that this ability means that the psychiatrist, rather than acting as a physician, is actually acting as an agent of the state to control a citizen's behavior, or as a sort of unofficial policeman. Obviously, supporters of such a position claim that individual autonomy (in the sense of behavioral freedom, without regard to rationality) should not be abrogated on the basis of mental illness. However, although there has been a significant shift toward greater judicial oversight of the commitment process and a requirement that the mental illness must manifest in some form of dangerousness, there is general agreement that the ability to detain some mentally ill individuals is a legitimate and indeed necessary part of psychiatry.

Other forms of dual agentry are potentially more problematic. Individuals may be interviewed by psychiatrists for a wide variety of reasons other than treatment—for evaluation of criminal responsibility, competency to stand trial, and other civil and criminal competencies, for example. The nature of the psychiatric interview, which requires establishment of a significant degree of interpersonal rapport with the interview subject, may be misinterpreted as a therapeutic intervention. Thus there is an obligation on the part of the psychiatrist to inform the individual ahead of time of the nature and purpose of the interview, and to state that the information obtained may be used in a way that will not further the individual's interests.

There has also been a trend toward more conflicting loyalties as mechanisms for the delivery of health care evolve. Physicians are increasingly regulated and reviewed, with payment for certain classes of procedures limited. Particularly for physicians employed by or contracting with organizations that use managed care arrangements, there is increasing pressure to withhold rather than provide care; thus whereas the patient may be led to believe that his medical interests are paramount, the physician may experience pressure to minimize costs (to the patient's detriment).

A more egregious violation of the physician's fiduciary duty is sexual exploitation of patients (or former patients). Although it is almost universally believed that such relationships, based on intense feelings arising from the therapeutic situation, are a violation of trust, exploitive, and inherently unethical, it is estimated that between 5% and 10% of therapists engage in sexual contact with a patient at some time. This rate accords with estimates of the incidence of sexual contact between patients and other primary-care physicians.

A number of other forms of exploitation exist as well. Short of sexual abuse, probably the most egregious violations of the patient-physician relationship include taking financial advantage of the patient, such as entering into business relationships or using "insider" information to play the stock market. Other forms of financial exploitation may include the physician's using his influence with the patient to help a relative get a job, accepting large gifts or bequests, or providing medically unnecessary services.

The treating physician may also be tempted to be overly controlling with patients who are easily influenced, justifying such intrusiveness on the basis of benevolence, or overly punitive of patients who are noncompliant or are seen as uncooperative. In some cases, merely revealing the existence of a treatment relationship, if done for purposes of self-aggrandizement (for example, a physician letting it be known that he is treating a celebrity), may be a form of exploitation.

Confidentiality

"What I may see or hear in the course of the treatment or even outside of the treatment . . . I will keep to myself . . ." goes the Hippocratic oath. Particularly in psychiatry, where in the course of treatment information that is painful, shameful, or illegal may be brought out, the need to safeguard patients' privacy is great on practical as well as ethical grounds. The patient who withholds information relevant to the therapeutic process out of fear of further dissemination obviously undermines the therapeutic relationship.

Although it is an important aspect of the treatment relationship, confidentiality between the patient and the physician is not absolute (see the Pearls & Perils box on p. 449). It is generally accepted that it may appropriately be breached in some situations, such as when a patient presents a substantial likelihood of harming himself or another person; under other circumstances, such as the discovery of certain communicable diseases or child abuse, reporting may be legally required.

Not addressing with the patient issues of when or if confidentiality should be breached can seriously imperil the therapeutic relationship. If the possibility is not addressed early in the course of treatment and before any such issues might arise, when the physician is impelled to disclose information (for example, to warn

PEARLS & PERILS

WHEN CONFIDENTIALITY IS A CONCERN

- During communication with peers (presentations, case conferences, "curbside consults") sensitive information may be inadvertently disclosed.
- In cases where treatment is provided by several practitioners, information may be inappropriately shared, thus increasing risk of further disclosure.
- Only minimum necessary information should be disclosed to third-party payers and reviewers.
- Treatment of minors is particularly problematic in that parents (or guardians) may feel entitled to information the patient does not wish to share.
- In child custody evaluations and/or courtroom testimony, there is the risk that sensitive or damaging information may be publicly disclosed.
- Although testimony in court may require confidentiality to be abridged, care should be taken to restrict disclosure to the minimum necessary degree.
- Concerned family members may legitimately wish to know details of the patients diagnosis, prognosis, and treatment, but their wishes cannot supersede the patient's desire for confidentiality.
- Electronic databases may be vulnerable to unauthorized access, thus placing privacy of patient information at risk.
- Warning any endangered third party may require that patient confidentiality be breached to ensure the potential victim's safety.
- The duty to protect confidentiality does not end with the patient's death.

an identifiable third party of threats made by the patient), the physician may be seen as having represented herself as an ally of the patient and then betraying him. Of course, if a situation arises where the patient's privacy must be compromised, the situation can be further worsened by concealing (or attempting to conceal) the fact of a breach after a report is made.

In addition to situations where breach of privacy is legally or ethically mandated, patient confidentiality continues to be eroded by economic forces, as third-party payers become increasingly intrusive in scrutinizing care and requiring more and more specific information be disclosed before authorizing treatment. Even though it is perhaps true that disclosure in such situations is not technically coerced, it is clear that a choice between maintaining confidentiality and having payment for necessary and otherwise unaffordable care denied is not much of a choice. Moreover, how this information is electronically stored, as well as what safeguards are in place to check its accuracy, protect it from unauthorized access, and ensure that it is not released inappropriately may vary between insurers and is a mystery to most patients and physicians. Neither the physician nor the patient may know the specifics of what has been recorded nor to whom and under what conditions the information may be released. Particularly if the patient is being treated for behaviors or conditions that often result in social condemnation (such as acquired immunodeficiency syndrome [AIDS], pedophilia, or alcoholism), it may be necessary for the physician to inform the patient before release that although failure to comply may result in treatment not being covered, disclosure may also be harmful.

A related issue involves provision of treatment by multiple caregivers. This is often true in psychiatry, where the patient may be seen for pharmacological treatment by a psychiatrist, for individual psychotherapy by a different professional, and perhaps for group or family therapy provided by yet a third therapist. Even if treatment is facilitated by free exchange of information, there is still a need for each treating professional to maintain confidentiality unless it is specifically waived by the patient. Moreover, the greater the number of people with access to the information (and who have recorded it in progress notes), the greater the likelihood is of its inadvertent disclosure. With the increasing prevalence of managed care "carve-outs" of mental health treatment and increasing reliance on primary care physicians for prescription of psychopharmacological agents, it is likely that the fragmentation of mental health care will be exacerbated with consequent risk to confidentiality.

A similar conflict may arise when the same individual functions in more than one role, such as providing individual and family therapy to the same patient. In this case, steps must be taken to safeguard against the possibility that information provided in individual sessions might be disclosed to family members.

It is also possible for the duty to maintain confidentiality to conflict with what is perceived to be civic duty. For example, there is a common misperception that in line with the duty to protect potential victims there is a corresponding duty to report past crimes. In fact, quite the opposite is true; not only is there no such legal requirement, but such a breach of confidentiality clearly violates a duty to the patient. A practice of such disclosure, if commonplace, could potentially affect the entire profession, undermining any trust in the therapist's assurances of privacy.

Perhaps the most difficult situations arise in dealing with family members who may wish to know details of the patient's illness, treatment, and prognosis. Providing information may be of great benefit by reducing the family's worries, and it may help the patient as well; the patient often has no objections. However, if the patient objects, the family's wants or needs cannot supersede the patient's wishes. This duty to maintain confidentiality holds even after the patient's death; whereas disclosing information may help to assuage grief by family members, there is always the possibility that the knowledge will later be misused.

Of course in the case of minors, under most circumstances the patient cannot legally consent or refuse the release of information about his treatment. Particularly in the case of the adolescent patient, the issue of dual agentry may arise, with the patient wishing the physician to conceal information to which parents feel they have a right. An even more complex situation may arise in the setting of a custody dispute, where parents may disagree about releasing treatment information or may wish it released to harm the other parent's legal position rather than to further the child's interests. In such a case, the various obligations the physician has to the patient and to both parents may be irreconcilable. Once again, rather than having clear rules to follow in such cases, the physician is left to try to balance on a case-by-case basis the obligations to maintain confidentiality, to advocate for the best medical interests of the child against conflicting duties, and to try to estimate the likelihood and probable magnitude of harm caused by any course of action undertaken.

The Difficult Patient

Patients may provoke a number of feelings in the treating physician. When those feelings are of anger or frustration, care may suffer because the physician wishes to avoid seeing the patient or becoming more involved in her treatment. Conversely, some patients (particularly celebrity patients or family members of colleagues) may evoke in the treating physician a desire to provide exceptionally good or solicitous care (the "VIP Syndrome"). Whether the physician strives too much or not enough, objectivity may be eroded, with consequent impairment in the physician's ability to provide optimal care.

Particularly in the case of patients perceived as resistant, antagonistic, or otherwise overtly uncooperative with treatment, delivery of care may be hindered by the physician's reluctance to become or stay closely involved in the patient's treatment. In such cases the possible contribution of psychiatric illness cannot be ignored. This is not to suggest that lack of cooperation with treatment is a mental illness, but feelings of frustration, disappointment, or anger at a patient are not necessarily illegitimate and should be considered a clinical indication for more careful psychiatric assessment (see Chapter 18). For example, patients with somatization disorder may be quite demanding (of both time and patience), and patients with substance-related problems may feign pain syndromes or complain of anxiety. Individuals with obsessive-compulsive disorder (OCD) may require a great deal of reassurance about trivial physical complaints. Less commonly, patients with unusual physical complaints may on closer examination prove to be suffering from delusional illnesses.

Once a diagnosis is made, treatment may be substantially improved not only because the underlying psychiatric illness can be addressed (thus simplifying the clinical situation), but also because the reason for the previous conflict in treatment is clarified for both parties. Ideally, at that point the patient and the physician can then explicitly agree on the nature of subsequent treatment.

Physician-Assisted Suicide

Over the last several years, a great deal of debate has been stimulated both in the lay press and in medical journals over the issue of physician-assisted suicide. Referenda on the issue have underlined the importance of the issue to the public.

Generally, those who support physician-assisted suicide frame the case in terms of autonomy, arguing that rational patients are allowed to refuse life-sustaining treatment and should be allowed to make the choice to end their lives more directly. They further note that physicians traditionally have been able to withhold futile treatment and that any distinction between hastening death by withholding treatment and actively assisting in the process is at best a subtle one.

Those who oppose this intervention argue that although patients may accept or decline treatment (even of a fatal illness), this principle of self-determination is not equivalent to a right to demand assistance in terminating one's life. Whereas it is permissible to provide treatment that also increases the risk of death, purposefully taking a life is a contravention of a basic principle of the practice of medicine. Moreover, legitimizing this activity might serve to undermine trust in the medical profession by obscuring the motives of the physician, who might be seen as interested in taking—rather than preserving—life. Opponents also argue that once physician-assisted suicide is allowed, a "slippery slope" could result, with greater and greater latitude allowed in determining who should be assisted in dying (with or without adequate consent), and point to historical examples to justify such concern.

Proponents argue that with sufficient safeguards, respect for individual autonomy dictates that patients should be allowed this option, despite such concerns. However, as noted earlier, the physician's duty to the patient requires active engagement with the patient rather than simply passive acceptance of her treatment desires. In the case of physician-assisted suicide, medical judgment could be required to determine the following circumstances: (1) that the underlying medical condition could cause intolerable pain, (2) that no less drastic intervention would relieve such suffering, and (3) that the patient's reported anguish is in fact the result of the underlying condition and not related to a potentially treatable intercurrent process. Thus the physician asked to assist in a patient's suicide would be faced with the task of determining the degree of the patient's suffering, its cause (including the absence of intercurrent, treatable disorders), and its prognosis to a high standard of accuracy and without external validators such as laboratory tests to exclude psychiatric illness. Under such circumstances, physicians might be tempted either to justify their misgivings about the procedure by overdiagnosing psychiatric illness (and thus subjecting the patient to unneeded and possibly intrusive treatment) or to act on feelings (either the physician's, the family's, or the patient's) of hopelessness and frustration and agree too precipitously.

There are other requirements, as well. Even among supporters of physician-assisted suicide, there is general agreement that the procedure should be restricted to patients who are competent to make the choice and who repeatedly and voluntarily request assisted death. Given the long-recognized association between suicide and psychiatric illness (particularly depression), as well as the difficulty in definitively diagnosing depressive illness in medically ill patients, it seems that if physician-assisted suicide were to become generally accepted, psychiatric referral for evaluation of the patient's mental competency to request death would become routine.

What would psychiatrists have to offer in such cases? Less, perhaps, than one might think. Leaving aside issues of whether consultation would (or should) include psychiatric opinion about the treating physician's feelings toward the patient (or the procedure), there has been no study of what it means to be "competent" to request assistance in suicide, nor are there data on accuracy or interrater agreement of psychiatric or other assessment in such cases. Conversely, there is evidence that depressive illness in severely medically ill patients is commonly overlooked, thus raising the possibility that an eminently treatable intercurrent illness might be missed quite often. If mental competency and absence of contribution from treatable, intercurrent diseases are, as proponents suggest, necessary conditions if physician-assisted suicide is to be allowed, it would seem that until there is adequate study of the accuracy and reliability of clinical judgement about issues such as mental competency to request assisted suicide, absences of treatable intercurrent mental or physical illness, and palliability of pain, debate over its status is premature unless it is acknowledged that the risk of clinical error on these points is unknown.

Organ Transplantation

The substantial improvement in organ transplantation technique and outcome has raised a number of ethical issues, primarily centering around the problem of allocation of increasingly scarce resources. How should an expensive procedure that carries with it the potential for saving lives and substantially improving the quality of life be offered to those who need it, when it is known that the demand far outstrips the supply? On what basis should patients be chosen to receive transplants? Should psychosocial factors be weighed in such decisions, and if so, what role should psychiatrists play in the determination of suitability for transplantation?

If psychiatric evaluation does in fact play a role in the determination of suitability for transplantation, the psychiatrist must be careful to avoid the perception of acting as a double agent. That is, before the psychiatric interview the patient should be informed of the nature and purpose of the interview and made aware that the information elicited might be used in determining whether or not he will be accepted on the transplant service. Such disclosure should eliminate the possibility that the patient misperceives the consultation as being purely therapeutic in nature and without impact on the decision of whether to transplant.

More importantly, as with the issues surrounding physician-assisted suicide, basic empirical issues with direct bearing on questions of biomedical ethics remain unaddressed. Whether or not basic fairness allows one to deny organ transplantation to patients with severe, treatment-resistant mental illness (a purely ethical issue), mental illness has often been proposed as a relative contraindication to transplantation because of associated risk of noncompliance with necessary treatment (a reasonable question but little examined despite being amenable to empirical study). The issue is that under circumstances of scarcity, resources should be allocated on the basis of likelihood of successful transplantation. However, further examination shows that success is not always clearly defined. Do we mean immediate survival, long-term functional outcome, quality of life, length of survival after transplantation, or an amalgam of all of these?

In fact, few studies have examined the impact of specific psychiatric conditions on outcome; even less attention has been paid to the effect of personality traits on compliance and psychosocial outcome (see Chapter 18), even though such factors might be expected to play at least as great a role as an overt psychiatric disorder. Indeed, there appears to be surprisingly little agreement between transplant centers regarding importance of prior history of mental disorder, with some centers regarding schizophrenia (even if controlled), mental retardation, or a history of affective disorder to be absolute contraindications for certain types of transplants.

The impact of alcohol dependence on whether a patient is judged suitable for liver transplantation is of particular interest, since the psychiatrist may play a more central role in the transplant decision. A brief analysis of the debate shows how empirical data may shape ethical debate.

Individuals with a history of alcoholic cirrhosis represent one of the largest groups of those requesting liver transplantation. The case has been made that people who have developed cirrhosis because of abusive drinking should be held responsible for their illness and assigned a lower priority for transplantation. Such ranking appears to have the advantage of fairness, penalizing those who have significantly contributed to their health problems over a prolonged period vs. those whose behavior did not lead to their hepatic failure. However, such a formulation ignores the substantial variability in the natural history of alcoholism, which is one of relapse and remission and not uncommonly characterized by spontaneous improvement and subsequent abstinence. Despite concerns about the recurrence of abusive drinking, there is little evidence to show that transplant outcome in this group is significantly worse than in other conditions, particularly if the individual has demonstrated the ability to abstain from alcohol for a time (typically 6 months) before the transplant. Moreover, if poor prognosis (because of alcoholism) were used to deny transplantation, in fairness other groups with comparably poor prognoses because of other medical or psychiatric conditions should be denied this procedure as well.

Ethics and Research

The need for high-quality, carefully-designed research in psychiatry, as in other medical specialties, is obvious. The tremendous suffering and disability entailed by severe psychiatric illness mandates ongoing efforts to improve our understanding of mental illness and its causes, mechanisms, and treatment.

Research into mental illness entails special pitfalls. Patients undergoing drug trials for many conditions must be withdrawn from medications that are often of some benefit, and they may relapse either before starting a trial of the new agent or while taking it; this dilemma is hardly unique to psychiatry. However, for many psychiatric conditions, relapse may alter not only the subject's mental capacity to further participate in research but his ability to consent to treatment once participation in the study is ended.

More likely to be peculiar to psychiatric research is the problem that highly sensitive, personal information—possibly involving behaviors that are illegal or otherwise socially condemned—may need to be gathered, with consequent concerns about confidentiality. But patients with severe mental illnesses—the ones most in need of improvements in treatment—are often the ones most lacking the ability to truly understand the risk involved, whether it is breach of confidentiality or substantial worsening of illness, and least able to validly consent to research protocols.

Competency to participate in research, as in other settings, has no clear threshold. It seems clear that at a minimum, to be allowed to participate, research subjects should demonstrate a level of competency at least equivalent to that required for consent to treatment. But the dilemma noted in the previous paragraph, that those most in need of improved treatment are those least likely to demonstrate high levels of insight or grasp of the risks involved, suggests that the stringency of the competency requirement might be altered depending on the nature, severity, and likelihood of the risks involved, as well as on the potential value of the knowledge gained. Thus in some settings, after being informed of the nature of the project, the ability to evidence a choice as to whether or not to participate might be sufficient. Next most stringent would be a requirement that the individual has a factual understanding of the issues involved. An even stricter requirement would be that the individual not only has adequate factual information but can rationally manipulate it. Finally, the most restrictive standard of competency to consent to research would require that the individual not only could rationally process the information given but could demonstrate the ability to relate it to her own situation; that is, that she is aware of the personal implications of consenting or refusing, can rationally explicate the reasons for consent or refusal, and so forth. Although the individual may benefit from participation in a research trial, in this setting the benefit is to a class of individuals (possibly at the expense of the research subject) rather than an issue involving the best medical interest of the individual patient.

Conclusion

In this brief overview, a few of the ethical issues that may arise in the practice of psychiatry, either in the office or via consultation with other professionals, have been delineated. Such an analysis may be of interest from the perspective of primary care physicians faced with similar dilemmas. From the standpoint of psychiatry, an understanding of the varied manifestations of mental illness, as well as an appreciation for the clinical and epistemological limitations of psychiatric knowledge, can play a substantial role in the way ethical questions are framed and decisions are made. Whereas empirical research cannot take the place of rigorous ethical analysis of the issues and duties involved when such questions arise, where available, such information can substantially add to the soundness of the choices made. Better decisions about the allocation of scarce resources (such as in organ transplantation) might be made if good information is available about the natural history and likelihood of relapse of alcoholism in a patient needing a liver transplant. Similarly, knowledge about the sensitivity and specificity of a clinical diagnosis of depression in medically ill patients may become important when the physician is faced with the decision of whether or not to respect a patient's request to terminate renal dialysis or life support.

In most cases, these empirical questions remain unanswered. However, even in the absence of data, by asking such questions the unexamined assumptions on which ethical decisions are founded may be considered more broadly, and thereby lead to more judicious choices.

Annotated Bibliography

Guze SB: *Why psychiatry is a branch of medicine*, New York, 1992, Oxford University Press.

This is an excellent, concise, and clearly written explication of the medical-model approach to psychiatry.

Pellegrino ED, Thomasma DC: *For the patient's good*, Oxford, England, 1988, Oxford University Press.

This book delves more deeply into the ethical basis of the physician-patient relationship.

Bibliography

Chapter 1

American Psychiatric Association: *Diagnostic and statistical manual of mental disorders,* ed 3, Washington, D.C., 1980, American Psychiatric Association.

Beck AT, Freeman AM: *Cognitive therapy of personality disorders,* New York, 1990, Guilford Press.

Black KJ: Helicopters and Aunt Minnie, *N C Med J* 53:175-177, 1992.

Black KJ: The scientific method in clinical psychiatry (or, Research for the rest of us), *Psychiatric Research Report* 9:10-11, 1994.

Brown GW, Harris T: *Social origins of depression,* London, 1978, Tavistock Publications.

Cheyette SR, Cummings JL: Encephalitis lethargica: lessons for contemporary neuropsychiatry, *J Neuropsychiatry Clin Neurosci* 7:125-134, 1995.

Csernansky JG, Black KJ, Faustman WO: *The interface between standard psychiatric and neuropsychological diagnoses.* In Maruish ME, Moses JA Jr, editors: *Theoretical foundations of clinical neuropsychology for clinical practitioners,* Hillsdale, N.J., Lawrence Erlbaum Associates (in press).

Damasio AR: *Descartes' error: emotion, reason, and the human brain,* New York, 1994, G.P. Putnam.

Feighner JP et al: Diagnostic criteria for use in psychiatric research, *Arch Gen Psychiatry* 26:57-63, 1972.

Gabbard GO: *Psychodynamic psychiatry in clinical practice,* Washington, D.C., 1990, American Psychiatric Press.

Gazzaniga MS, editor: *The cognitive neurosciences,* Cambridge, Mass., 1994, MIT Press.

Gelenburg AJ: The catatonic syndrome, *Lancet* 2:1339-1341, 1976.

Goodwin DW, Guze SB: *Psychiatric diagnosis,* New York, 1989, Oxford University Press.

Guze SB: The need for toughmindedness in psychiatric thinking, *South Med J* 63:662-671, 1970.

Guze SB: Research and psychiatric training, *Biol Psychiatry* 11:265-266, 1976.

Guze SB: Can the practice of medicine be fun for a lifetime? *JAMA* 241:2021-2023, 1979.

Headache Classification Committee of the International Headache Society: Classification and diagnostic criteria for headache disorders, cranial neuralgias and facial pain, *Cephalalgia* 8(Suppl 7):1-96, 1988.

Hudgens RW: The turning of American psychiatry, *Mo Med* 90:283-291, 1993.

Meyer A: A short sketch of the problems of psychiatry [1897], *Am J Psychiatry* 151(Suppl):43-47, 1994.

Murphy GE: The physician's responsibility for suicide. I. An error of commission, *Ann Intern Med* 82:301-304, 1975.

Murphy GE: The physician's responsibility for suicide. II. Errors of omission, *Ann Intern Med* 82:305-309, 1975.

Myerson A: The attitude of neurologists, psychiatrists and psychologists towards psychoanalysis [1939], *Am J Psychiatry* 151(Suppl):48-54, 1994.

Myerson A: Some trends of psychiatry [1944], *Am J Psychiatry* 151(Suppl):55-63, 1994.

National Advisory Mental Health Council: Health care reform for Americans with severe mental illnesses: report of the National Advisory Mental Health Council, *Am J Psychiatry* 150:1447-1465, 1993.

Popkin MK, Tucker GJ: "Secondary" and drug-induced mood, anxiety, psychotic, catatonic, and personality disorders: a review of the literature, *J Neuropsychiatry Clin Neurosci* 4:369-385, 1992.

Szasz TS: *The myth of mental illness,* New York, 1961, Hoeber-Harper.

Weiner WJ, Lang AE, editors: *Behavioral neurology of movement disorders (advances in neurology vol 65).* New York, 1995, Raven Press.

Woodruff RA Jr., Clayton PJ, Guze SB: Hysteria: studies of diagnosis, outcome, and prevalence, *JAMA* 215:425-428, 1971.

Chapter 2

Akiskal HS: *The mental status examination.* In Winokur G, Clayton PJ, editors: *The medical basis of psychiatry,* Philadelphia, 1994, W.B. Saunders.

Akiskal HS et al: Switching from "unipolar" to bipolar II: an 11-year prospective study of clinical and temperamental predictors in 559 patients, *Arch Gen Psychiatry* 52:114-123, 1995.

American Psychiatric Association: *Diagnostic and statistical manual of mental disorders,* ed 4, Washington, D.C., 1994, American Psychiatric Press.

Arntz A et al: The interrater reliability of a Dutch version of the Structured Clinical Interview for DSM-III-R personality disorders, *Acta Psychiatr Scand* 85:394-400, 1992.

Barsky AJ, Wyshak G, Klerman GL: Psychiatric comorbidity in DSM-III-R hypochondriasis, *Arch Gen Psychiatry* 49:101-108, 1992.

Bauer MS, Dunner DL: Validity of seasonal pattern as a modifier for recurrent mood disorders for DSM-IV, *Compr Psychiatry* 34:159-170, 1993.

Bauer MS et al: Multisite data reanalysis of the validity of rapid cycling as a course modifier for bipolar disorder in DSM-IV, *Am J Psychiatry* 151:506-515, 1994.

Brown TA, Barlow DH, Liebowitz MR: The empirical basis of generalized anxiety disorder, *Am J Psychiatry* 151:1272-1280, 1994.

Bryant KJ et al: Reliability of dual diagnosis: substance dependence and psychiatric disorders, *J Nerv Ment Dis* 180:251-257, 1992.

Buysse DJ et al: Clinical diagnoses in 216 insomnia patients using the International Classification of Sleep Disorders (ICSD), DSM-IV and ICD-10 categories: a report from the APA/NIMH DSM-IV Field Trial, *Sleep* 17:630-637, 1994.

Buysse DJ et al: Diagnostic concordance for DSM-IV sleep disorders: a report from the APA/NIMH DSM-IV field trial, *Am J Psychiatry* 151:1351-1360, 1994.

Cloninger CR: *Establishment of diagnostic validity in psychiatric illness: Robins and Guze's method revisited.* In Robins LN, Barrett JE, editors: *The validity of psychiatric diagnosis,* New York, 1989, Raven Press.

Corty E, Lehman AF, Myers CP: Influence of psychoactive substance use on the reliability of psychiatric diagnosis, *J Consult Clin Psychol* 61:165-170, 1993.

Dahl AA: The validity of the Scandinavian concept of reactive psychoses, *Seishin Shinkeigaku Zasshi* 96:660-675, 1994.

Dunner DL, Tay LK: Diagnostic reliability of the history of hypomania in bipolar II patients and patients with major depression, *Compr Psychiatry* 34:303-307, 1993.

Faraone SV, Tsuang MG: Measuring diagnostic accuracy in the absence of a "gold standard," *Am J Psychiatry* 151:650-657, 1994.

Feighner JP et al: Diagnostic criteria for use in psychiatric research, *Arch Gen Psychiatry* 26:57-63, 1972.

Fennig S et al: Best-estimate versus structured interview-based diagnosis in first-admission psychosis, *Compr Psychiatry* 35:341-348, 1994.

Gauron EF, Dickinson JK: Diagnostic decision making in psychiatry. I. information usage, *Arch Gen Psychiatry* 14:225-232, 1966.

Goldstein MG, Niaura R: Psychological factors affecting physical condition: cardiovascular disease literature review. I. Coronary artery disease and sudden death, *Psychosomatics* 33:134-145, 1992.

Guze SB: The need for toughmindedness in psychiatric thinking, *South Med J* 63:662-671, 1970.

Guze SB: *Diagnosis.* In *Why psychiatry is a branch of medicine,* New York, 1992, Oxford.

Hatcher S: Decision analysis in psychiatry, *Br J Psychiatry* 166:184-190, 1995.

Heun R, Maier W: The distinction of bipolar II disorder from bipolar I and recurrent unipolar depression: results of a controlled family study, *Acta Psychiatr Scand* 87:279-284, 1993.

Hyler SE, Williams JBW, Spitzer RL: Reliability in the DSM-III field trials: interview v case summary, *Arch Gen Psychiatry* 39:1275-1278, 1982.

Jensen P et al: Test-retest reliability of the Diagnostic Interview Schedule for Children (DISC 2.1): parent, child, and combined algorithms, *Arch Gen Psychiatry* 52:61-71, 1995.

Keller MB: Dysthymia in clinical practice: course, outcome and impact on the community, *Acta Psychiatr Scand* 383(Suppl):24-34, 1994.

Keller MB et al: Results of the DSM-IV Mood Disorders Field Trial, *Am J Psychiatry* 152:843-849, 1995.

Marten PA et al: Evaluation of the ratings comprising the associated symptom criterion of DSM-III-R generalized anxiety disorder, *J Nerv Ment Dis* 181:676-682, 1993.

McGorry PD et al: Spurious precision: procedural validity of diagnostic assessment in psychotic disorders, *Am J Psychiatry* 152:220-223, 1995.

Meyer A: A short sketch of the problems of psychiatry [1897], *Am J Psychiatry* 151(Suppl):43-47, 1994.

Mellsop GW et al: Reliability of the draft diagnostic criteria for research of ICD-10 in comparison with ICD-10 and DSM-III-R, *Acta Psychiatr Scand* 84:332-335, 1991.

Muñoz RA, Amado H, Hyatt S: Brief reactive psychosis, *J Clin Psychiatry* 48:324-327, 1987.

Myerson A: Some trends of psychiatry [1944], *Am J Psychiatry* 151(Suppl):55-63, 1994.

North CS et al: *Multiple personalities, multiple disorders: psychiatric classification and media influence,* New York, 1993, Oxford University Press.

Noyes R Jr et al: The validity of DSM-III-R hypochondriasis, *Arch Gen Psychiatry* 50:961-970, 1993.

Okubo Y et al: Collaborative multicenter field trial of the Draft of ICD-10 in Japan—interdiagnostician reliability and disagreement: a report from the WHO project on "field trials of ICD-10, Chapter V," *Jpn J Psychiatry Neurol* 46:23-35, 1992.

Parker G et al: Defining melancholia: properties of a refined sign-based measure, *Br J Psychiatry* 164:316-326, 1994.

Pilgrim JA et al: Inter-rater and temporal reliability of the Standardized Assessment of Personality and the influence of informant characteristics, *Psychol Med* 23:779-786, 1993.

Regier DA et al: The ICD-10 clinical field trial for mental and behavioral disorders: results in Canada and the United States, *Am J Psychiatry* 151:1340-1350, 1994.

Reynolds CF III et al: Subtyping DSM-III-R primary insomnia: a literature review by the DSM-IV Work Group on Sleep Disorders, *Am J Psychiatry* 148:432-438, 1991.

Rhea SA, Nagoshi CT, Wilson JR: Reliability of sibling reports on parental drinking behaviors, *J Stud Alcohol* 54:80-84, 1993.

Rounsaville BJ et al: Cross system agreement for substance use disorders: DSM-III-R, DSM-IV and ICD-10, *Addiction* 88:337-348, 1993.

Rush AJ: Recurrent brief depression: a DSM-IV perspective, *Clin Neuropharmacol* 15(Suppl 1):15A, 1992.

Schatzberg AF, Rothschild AJ: Psychotic (delusional) major depression: should it be included as a distinct syndrome in DSM-IV? *Am J Psychiatry* 149:733-745, 1992.

Skre I et al: High interrater reliability for the Structured Clinical Interview for DSM-III-R Axis I (SCID-I), *Acta Psychiatr Scand* 84:167-173, 1991.

Spitzer RL: An outsider-insider's view about revising the DSMs, *J Abnormal Psychol* 100:294-296, 1991.

Spitzer RL, Endicott J, Robins E: *Research diagnostic criteria (RDC) for a selected group of functional disorders,* New York, 1975, Biometrics Research, New York State Psychiatric Institute.

Verne, J: *Twenty thousand leagues under the sea,* 1869, (Translated by WJ Miller), New York, 1966, Washington Square Press.

Williams JB et al: The structured clinical interview for DSM-III-R (SCID). II. Multisite test-retest reliability, *Arch Gen Psychiatry* 49:630-636, 1992.

Wittchen HU: Reliability and validity studies of the WHO Composite International Diagnostic Interview (CIDI): a critical review, *J Psychiatr Res* 28:57-84, 1994.

Yutzy SH et al: DSM-IV field trial: testing a new proposal for somatization disorder, *Am J Psychiatry* 152:97-101, 1995.

Zanarini MC et al: The face validity of the DSM-III and DSM-III-R criteria sets for borderline personality disorder, *Am J Psychiatry* 148:870-874, 1991.

Zimmerman M et al: DSM-IV: a nosology sold before its time? *Am J Psychiatry* 148:463-467, 1991.

Zimmerman M et al: DSM-III and DSM-III-R: what are American psychiatrists using and why? *Compr Psychiatry* 34:365-374, 1993.

Chapter 3

American Psychiatric Association: *The American psychiatric glossary,* ed 7, Washington, D.C., 1994, author.

Folstein MF et al: Mini-mental state: a practical method for grading of the cognitive state of patients for the clinician, *J Psychiatr Res* 12:189, 1975.

Goldberg DP et al: The ability of trainee general practitioners to identify psychological distress among their patients, *Psychol Med* 23:185, 1993.

Hamilton M, editor: *Fish's clinical psychopathology: signs and symptoms in psychiatry,* ed 2, Bristol, U.K., 1985, John Wright & Sons Ltd.

Katzman R et al: Validation of a short orientation-memory-concentration test of cognitive impairment, *Am J Psychiatry* 140:734, 1983.

Pfeiffer E: A short portable mental status questionnaire for the assessment of organic brain deficit in elderly patients, *J Am Geriatr Soc* 23:433, 1975.

Wells KB et al: Detection of depressive disorder for patients receiving prepaid or fee-for-service care: results from the medical outcomes study, *JAMA* 262:3298, 1989.

Chapter 4

American Psychiatric Association: *Diagnostic and statistical manual of mental disorders,* ed 4, Washington, D.C., 1994, author.

Ben-Porath YS, Butcher JN, Graham JR: Contribution of the MMPI-2 content scales to the differential diagnosis of schizophrenia and major depression, *Psychol Assessment* 3:634-640, 1991.

Boring EG: Intelligence as the tests test it, *New Republic* 35:35-37, 1923.

Cohen FW, Phelp RE: Incest markers in children's artwork, *Arts in psychotherapy* 12:265-283, 1985.

Dahlstrom WG, Welsh GS, Dahlstrom LE: *An MMPI handbook: clinical interpretation,* vol 1, revised, Minneapolis, Minn., 1972, University of Minnesota Press.

Exner JE Jr: *The Rorschach: a comprehensive system,* ed 3, New York, 1993, Wiley Interscience.

Eyde LD et al: *Responsible test use: case studies for assessing human behavior,* Washington, D.C., 1993, American Psychological Association.

Franzen MD, Robbins DE, Sawicki RF: *Reliability and validity in neuropsychological assessment,* New York, 1989, Plenum Press.

Greene, RL: *Assessment of malingering and defensiveness by objective personality inventories.* In Rogers R, editor: *Clinical assessment of malingering and deception,* New York, 1988, Guilford Press.

Grossman HJ, editor: *Classification in mental retardation,* 1983 revision, Washington, D.C., 1983, American Association on Mental Deficiency.

Hagood MM: Diagnosis or dilemma: drawings of sexually abused children, *Br J Projective Psychol* 37:22-33, 1992.

Holtzman WH, Swartz JD: The Holtzman inkblot technique: a review of 25 years of research, *Zeitschrift für differentielle und diagnostische Psychologie* 4:241-259, 1983.

Klein RG: *Questioning the clinical usefulness of projective psychological tests for children.* In Chess S, Thomas A, Hertzig M, editors: *Annual progress in child psychiatry and child development,* New York, 1987, Brunner and Mazel.

Kline P: *Intelligence, the psychometric view,* New York, 1991, Routledge.

Lyons JA, Keane TM: Keane PTSD scale: MMPI and MMPI-2 update, *J Trauma Stress* 5:111-117, 1992.

Matarazzo JD: *Wechsler's measurement and appraisal of adult intelligence,* ed 5, Baltimore, 1972, Williams and Wilkins.

Nihara K et al: *AAMR adaptive behavior scale,* Washington, D.C., 1974, American Association on Mental Deficiency.

North CS et al: *Multiple personalities, multiple disorders: psychiatric classification and media influence,* New York, 1993, Oxford University Press.

Rapaport D, Gill MM, Schafer R: *Diagnostic psychological testing,* rev ed, Holt RR, editor, Bern, 1968, International Universities Press.

Rorschach H: *Psychodiagnostik.* Bern, 1942, Hans Huber Verlag. Cited in Exner JE Jr: *The rorschach: a comprehensive system,* ed 3, New York, 1993, Wiley Interscience.

Sparrow SS, Balla DA, Cicchetti DV: *Vineland adaptive behavior scales,* Circle Press, Minn., 1984, American Guidance Service.

Sparrow SS, Carter AS: *Mental retardation: current issues related to assessment.* In Rapin I, Segalowitz SJ, editors: *Handbook of neuropsychology* vol 6, Amsterdam, 1992, Elsevier Science Publishing Co.

Sparrow SS, Cicchetti DJ: *The Vineland adaptive behavior scales.* In Newmark C, editor: *Major psychological assessment instruments,* vol 2, Needham, Mass., 1989, Allyn & Bacon.

Welsh GS, Dahlstrom WG, editors: *Basic readings on the MMPI in psychology and medicine,* Minneapolis, Minn., 1956, University of Minnesota Press.

Ziskin J, Faust D: *Coping with psychiatric and psychological testimony,* ed 4, Los Angeles, 1988, Law and Psychology Press.

Chapter 5

Andreasen NC: *The scale for assessment of negative symptoms (SANS),* Iowa City, Iowa, 1983, The University of Iowa.

Andreasen NC: *The scale for assessment of positive symptoms (SAPS),* Iowa City, Iowa, 1984, The University of Iowa.

Barnes TRE: A rating scale for drug-induced akathisia, *Br J Psychiatry* 154:672-676, 1989.

Beck AT et al: An inventory for measuring depression, *Arch Gen Psychiatry* 4:561-571, 1961.

Beigel A, Murphy DL, Bunney WE Jr: The Manic-State Rating Scale: scale construction, reliability, and validity, *Arch Gen Psychiatry* 25:256-262, 1971.

Csernansky JG et al: Clinical factors that may confound the assessment of drug efficacy, *Psychopharmacol Bull* 27:231-235, 1991.

Faustman WO, Moses JA Jr, Csernansky JG: Limitations of the Mini-Mental State Examination in predicting neuropsychological functioning in a psychiatric sample, *Acta Psychiatr Scand* 81:126-131, 1990.

Folstein MF, Folstein SE, McHuch PR: Mini-Mental State: a practical method for grading the cognitive state of patients for the clinician, *J Psychiatr Res* 12:189-198, 1975.

Goodwin FK, Jamison KF: *Assessment of manic and depressive states.* In *Manic-depressive illness,* New York, 1990, Oxford University Press.

Goodman WK, Price LH: Assessment of severity and change in obsessive compulsive disorder, *Psychiatr Clin North Am* 14:861-869, 1992.

Goodman WK et al: The Yale-Brown Obsessive Compulsive Scale (Y-BOCS). I. Development, use, and reliability, *Arch Gen Psychiatry* 46:1006-1011, 1989.

Goodman WK et al: The Yale-Brown Obsessive Compulsive Scale (Y-BOCS). II. Validity, *Arch Gen Psychiatry* 46:1012-1016, 1989.

Grebb JA: *Psychiatric rating scales.* In Kaplan HI, Sadock BJ, editors: *Comprehensive textbook of psychiatry,* ed 5, Baltimore, 1989, Williams & Wilkins.

Guy W: *NCDEU assessment manual for psychopharmacology,* U.S. Department of Health, Education, and Welfare Publication (ADM)-76-338, Rockville, Md., 1976, Alcohol, Drug Abuse, and Mental Health Administration.

Hamilton M: The assessment of anxiety states by rating, *Br J Med Psychol* 32:50, 1959.

Hamilton M: A rating scale for depression, *J Neurol Neurosurg Psychiatry* 23:56-62, 1960.

Honigfeld G, Klett C: The Nurses' Observation Scale for Inpatient Evaluation (NOSIE): a new scale for measuring improvement in chronic schizophrenia, *J Clin Psychol* 21:65-71, 1965.

Levine J, Schooler NR: SAFTEE (systematic assessment for treatment emergent events): a new technique for detecting side effects in clinical trials, *Clin Neuropharmacol* 7:856-857, 1984.

MacKinnon RA, Yudofsky SC: *The psychiatric evaluation in clinical practice,* Philadelphia, 1986, J.B. Lippincott.

Malla AK, Norman RMG, Williamson P: Stability of positive and negative symptoms in schizophrenia, *Can J Psychiatry* 38:617-621, 1993.

Mungas D: In-office mental status testing: a practical guide, *Geriatrics* 46:54-66, 1991.

Newcomer JW et al: Distinguishing depression and negative symptoms in unmedicated patients with schizophrenia, *Psychiatry Res* 31:243-250, 1990.

Overall JE, Gorham DR: The brief psychiatric rating scale, *Psychol Rep* 10:799-812, 1962.

Overall JE: The brief psychiatric rating scale in psychopharmacology research, *Mod Probl Pharmacopsychiatry* 7:67-78, 1974.

Petterson U, Fyrö B, Sedvall G: A new scale for the longitudinal rating of manic states, *Acta Psychiatr Scand* 49:248-255, 1973.

Rabkin JG, Klein DF: *The clinical measurement of depressive disorders.* In Marsella AJ, Hirschfeld RMA, Katz MM, editors, *The measurement of depression,* New York, 1987, The Guilford Press.

Rhoades HM, Overall JE: The Hamilton Depression Scale: factor scoring and profile classification, *Psychopharmacol Bull* 19:91-96, 1983.

Simpson GM, Angus JWS: A rating scale for extrapyramidal side effects, *Acta Psychiatr Scand (Suppl)* 212:11-19, 1970.

Wing JK: *A standard form of psychiatric present state examination and a method for standardizing the classification of symptoms.* In Hare EH, Wing JK, editors: *Psychiatric epidemiology: an international symposium,* London, 1970, Oxford University Press.

Wise MG, Rundell JR: *Mental status examination.* In Hales RE, Series editor: *Consultation psychiatry,* ed 2, Washington DC, 1994, American Psychiatric Press.

Chapter 6

Altschuler LL et al: Reduction of temporal lobe volume in bipolar disorder: a preliminary report of magnetic resonance imaging, *Arch Gen Psychiatry* 48:482-483, 1992.

Barta P et al: Auditory hallucinations and smaller superior temporal gyrus volume in schizophrenia, *Am J Psychiatry* 147:1457-1462, 1990.

Baxter LR et al: Cerebral metabolic rates for glucose in mood disorders, *Arch Gen Psychiatry* 42:441-447, 1985.

Baxter LR et al: Local cerebral glucose metabolic rates in obsessive-compulsive disorder, *Arch Gen Psychiatry* 44:211-218, 1987.

Baxter LR et al: Reduction of prefrontal cortex glucose metabolism common to three types of depression, *Arch Gen Psychiatry* 46:243-250, 1989.

Bench CH et al: The anatomy of melancholia: focal abnormalities of cerebral blood flow in major depression, *Psychol Med* 22:607-615, 1992.

Benes FM: Is there a neuroanatomic basis for schizophrenia? An old question revisited, *The Neuroscientist* 1:104-115, 1995.

Biver F et al: Frontal and parietal metabolic disturbances in unipolar depression, *Biol Psychiatry* 36:381-388, 1994.

Botteron KN et al: Magnetic resonance imaging in childhood and adolescent bipolar affective disorder: a pilot investigation, *J Am Acad Child Adolesc Psychiatry* 34:742-749, 1995.

Buchsbaum MS et al: Frontal cortex and basal ganglia metabolic rates assessed by positron emission tomography with [^{18}F]2-deoxyglucose in affective illness, *J Affect Disord* 10:137-152, 1986.

Calabrese G et al: Phosphorus magnetic resonance spectroscopy of the temporal lobes in schizophrenia, *Biol Psychiatry* 32:26-32, 1992.

Castellanos FX et al: Quantitative morphology of the caudate nucleus in attention deficit hyperactivity disorder, *Am J Psychiatry* 151:1791-1796, 1994.

Cazzullo CL et al: Cerebral ventricular size and age of onset in major depression, *IRCS Med Sci* 12:917-918, 1984.

Coffey CE et al: White matter hyperintensity on magnetic resonance imaging: clinical and neuroanatomic correlates in the depressed elderly, *J Neuropsychiatry* 1:135-144, 1989.

Coffey CE et al: Quantitative cerebral anatomy in depression, *Arch Gen Psychiatry* 50:7-16, 1993.

Cohen RM et al: Evidence for common alterations in cerebral glucose metabolism in major affective disorders and schizophrenia, *Neuropsychopharmacology* 2:241-254, 1989.

Courchesne E et al: The brain in infantile autism, *Neurology* 44:214-223, 1994.

Crawley JCW et al: Uptake of 77Br-spiperone in the striata of schizophrenic patients and controls, *Nucl Med Commun* 7:599-607, 1986.

DeLisi L et al: Positron emission tomography in schizophrenic patients with and without neuroleptic medication, *J Cereb Blood Flow Metab* 5:201-206, 1985.

Dewan MJ et al: Bipolar affective disorder. I. Comprehensive quantitative computed tomography, *Acta Psychiatr Scand* 77:670-676, 1988.

DiRocco RJ et al: The relationship between CNS metabolism and cytoarchitecture: a review of ^{14}C-deoxyglucose studies with correlation to cytochrome oxidase histochemistry, *Comput Med Imaging Graph* 13:81-92, 1989.

Drevets WC et al: A functional anatomical study of unipolar depression, *J Neurosci* 12:3628-3641, 1992.

Drevets WC, Spitznagel E, Raichle ME: Functional anatomical differences between major depressive subtypes, *J Cereb Blood Flow Metab* 15:S93, 1995a.

Drevets WC et al: Regional blood flow changes in response to phobic anxiety and habituation, *J Cereb Blood Flow Metab* 15:S856, 1995b.

Early TS et al: Left globus pallidus abnormality in never-medicated patients with schizophrenia, *Proc Natl Acad Sci USA* 84:561-563, 1987.

Ebert D, Feistel H, Barocka A: Effects of sleep deprivation on the limbic system and the frontal lobes in affective disorders: a study with Pc-99m-HMPAO SPECT, *Psychiatry Res Neuroimaging* 40:247-251, 1991.

Farde L et al: D_2 dopamine receptors in neuroleptic-naive schizophrenic patients, *Arch Gen Psychiatry* 47:213-219, 1990.

Farde L et al: Positron emission tomographic analysis of central D_1 and D_2 dopamine receptor occupancy in patients treated with classical neuroleptics and clozepine: relation to extrapyramidal side effects, *Arch Gen Psychiatry* 49:538-544, 1992.

Figiel GS et al: Subcortical hyperintensities on brain magnetic resonance imaging: a comparison of normal and bipolar subjects, *J Neuropsychiatry* 3:18-22, 1991.

Fox PT et al: Nonoxidative glucose consumption during focal physiologic neural activity, *Science* 241:462-464, 1988.

Hauser P et al: Temporal lobe measurement in primary affective disorder by magnetic resonance imaging, *J Neuropsychiatry* 1:128-134, 1989.

Husain MM et al: A magnetic resonance imaging study of putamen nuclei in major depression, *Psychiatry Res* 40:95-99, 1991.

Hynd GW et al: Corpus callosum morphology in attention deficit-hyperactivity disorder: morphometric analysis of MRI, *J Learn Disab* 24:141-146, 1991.

Kellner C et al: Brain MRI in obsessive-compulsive disorder, *Psychiatry Res* 36:45-49, 1991.

Kellner H et al: Relationship of cortisol hypersecretion to brain CT scan alters in depressed patients, *Psychiatry Res* 8:191-197, 1983.

Krishnan KRR et al: Magnetic resonance imaging of the caudate nuclei in depression, *Arch Gen Psychiatry* 49:553-557, 1992.

LaPlane D et al: Obsessive-compulsive and other behavioural changes with bilateral basal ganglia lesions, *Brain* 112:699-725, 1989.

Martinot J et al: Striatal D_2 dopaminergic receptors assessed with positron emission tomography and [^{76}Br] bromospiperone in untreated schizophrenic patients, *Am J Psychiatry* 147:44-50, 1990.

Mazziotta JC et al: Quantitation in positron emission computed tomography. 5. Physical-anatomical effects, *J Comput Assist Tomogr* 5:734-743, 1981.

Mentis MH et al: Cerebral glucose metabolism in late onset depression without cognitive impairment, *Soc Neurosci Abstracts* 21:1736, 1995.

Nasrallah HA et al: Structural brain-imaging findings in affective disorders: an overview, *J Neuropsychiatry* 1:21-26, 1989.

Pearlson GD et al: In vivo D_2 dopamine receptor density in psychotic and nonpsychotic patients with bipolar disorder, *Arch Gen Psychiatry* 52:471-477, 1995.

Petersen SE et al: Positron emission tomographic studies of the processing of single words, *J Cogn Neurosci* 1:153-170, 1989.

Peterson B et al: Reduced basal ganglia volumes in Tourette's syndrome using three-dimensional reconstruction techniques from magnetic resonance images, *Neurology* 43:941-949, 1993.

Pettegrew JW et al: Alterations in brain high-energy phosphate and membrane phospholipid metabolism in first-episode, drug-naive schizophrenics, *Arch Gen Psychiatry* 48:563-568, 1991.

Prichard JW: The nuclear magnetic resonance revolution in basic and clinical neuroscience, *The Neuroscientist* 1:84-94, 1995.

Reiman EM et al: Neuroanatomical correlates of a lactate-induced anxiety attack, *Arch Gen Psychiatry* 46:493-500, 1989.

Schlegel S, Kretzschmar K: Computed tomography in affective disorders. 1. Ventricular and sulcal measurements, *Biol Psychiatry* 22:4-14, 1987.

Schwartz JM et al: The differential diagnosis of depression: relevance of positron emission tomography studies of cerebral glucose metabolism to the bipolar-unipolar dichotomy, *JAMA* 258:1368-1373, 1987.

Semrud-Clikeman M et al: Attention-deficit hyperactivity disorder: magnetic resonance imaging morphometric analysis of the corpus callosum, *J Am Acad Child Adolesc Psychiatry* 33:875-881, 1994.

Shenton ME et al: Abnormalities of the left temporal lobe and thought disorder in schizophrenia, *New Engl J Med* 327:604-612, 1992.

Sheppard G et al: ^{15}O-Positron emission tomographic scanning predominantly never-treated acute schizophrenic patients, *Lancet* ii:1448-1452, 1983.

Shima S et al: Depression and ventricular enlargement, *Acta Psychiatr Scand* 70:275-277, 1984.

Singer HS et al: Volumetric MRI changes in basal ganglia of children with Tourette's syndrome, *Neurology* 43:950-956, 1992.

Suddath R et al: Anatomical abnormalities in the brains of monozygotic twins discordant for schizophrenia, *New Engl J Med* 322:789-794, 1990.

Swayze VW et al: Subcortical and temporal structures in affective disorder and schizophrenia: a magnetic resonance imaging study, *Biol Psychiatry* 31:221-240, 1992.

Swedo SE et al: Cerebral glucose metabolism in childhood-onset obsessive-compulsive disorder, *Arch Gen Psychiatry* 46:518-523, 1989.

Tamminga CA et al: Limbic system abnormalities identified in schizophrenia using positron emission tomography with fluorodeoxyglucose and neocortical alterations with deficit syndrome, *Arch Gen Psychiatry* 49:522-530, 1992.

Trivedi MH, Devous MD, Rush AJ: RCBF findings in major depression: pre- and post-treatment with fluoxetine, *ACNP Abstracts*, p. 149, 1994.

Uytdenhoef P et al: Regional cerebral blood flow and lateralized hemipheric dysfunction in depression, *Br J Psychiatry* 143:128-132, 1983.

Volkow ND et al: Brain metabolism in patients with schizophrenia before and after acute neuroleptic administration, *J Neurol Neurosurg Psychiatry* 49:1199-1202, 1986.

Volkow ND et al: Effects of chronic cocaine abuse on postsynaptic dopamine receptors, *Am J Psychiatry* 147:719-724, 1990.

Weinberger DR et al: Physiologic dysfunction of dorsolateral prefrontal cortex in schizophrenia. I. Regional cerebral blood flow evidence, *Arch Gen Psychiatry* 43:114-124, 1986.

Williamson P et al: Localized phosphorus 31 magnetic resonance spectroscopy in chronic schizophrenic patients and normal controls, *Arch Gen Psychiatry* 48:578, 1991.

Wong DF et al: Positron emission tomography reveals elevated D_2 dopamine receptors in drug-naive schizophrenics, *Science* 234:1558-1563, 1986.

Wu JC et al: Effect of sleep deprivation on brain metabolism of depressed patients, *Am J Psychiatry* 149:538-543, 1992.

Chapter 7

Crum RM, Cooper-Patrick L, Ford DE: Depressive symptoms among general medical patients: prevalence and one-year outcome, *Psychosom Med* 56:109-117, 1994.

Depression Guideline Panel: *Clinical practice guideline no 5: depression in primary care,* vol 1: *Detection and diagnosis,* vol 2: *Treatment of major depression,* Agency for Health Care Policy and Research Publication 93-0551, Rockville, Md., 1993, U.S. Department of Health and Human Services, Public Health Service.

Katon W et al: Methodological issues in randomized trials of liaison psychiatry in primary care, *Psychosom Med* 56:97-103, 1994.

Lefley HP, Wasow M, editors: *Helping families cope with mental illness,* Langhorne, Penn., 1994, Harwood Academic Publishers.

Mueser KT, Gingerich S: *Coping with schizophrenia,* Oakland, Calif., 1994, New Harbinger Publications.

Regier DA, Goldberg ID, Taube CH: The defacto U.S. mental health service system, *Arch Gen Psychiatry* 45:977-986, 1988.

Robins LN, Regier DA, editors: *Psychiatric disorders in America,* New York, 1991, The Free Press.

Smith MD, Hong BA, Robson AM: Diagnosis of depression in patients with end-stage renal disease, *Am J Med* 79:160-166, 1985.

Wetzel RD: The diagnosis and treatment of patients with poor compliance to medical regimen, Unpublished manuscript, 1995.

Chapter 8

American Psychiatric Association: *Diagnostic and statistical manual of mental disorders,* ed 4, Washington, D.C., 1994, American Psychiatric Press.

Arango V et al: Autoradiographic demonstration of increased serotonin 5-HT_2 and β-adrenergic receptor binding sites in the brain of suicide victims, *Arch Gen Psychiatry* 47:1038-1047, 1990.

Barden N, Reul J, Holsboer F: Do antidepressants stabilize mood through actions on the hypothalamic-pituitary-adrenocortical system? *Trends Neurosci* 18:6-11, 1995.

Baxter LR et al: Reduction of prefrontal cortex glucose metabolism common to three types of depression, *Arch Gen Psychiatry* 46:243-250, 1989.

Biver F et al: Frontal and parietal metabolic disturbances in unipolar depression, *Biol Psychiatry* 36:381-388, 1994.

Bohn J, Jefferson JW: *Lithium and manic depression: a guide,* ed 2, Madison, Wis., 1993, Lithium Information Center, Dean Foundation.

Bowden CL et al: Efficacy of divalproex vs lithium and placebo in the treatment of mania: the Depakote mania study group, *JAMA* 271:918-924, 1994.

Bradwejn J et al: Double blind comparison of the effects of clonazepam and lorazepam in acute mania, *J Clin Psychopharmacol* 10:403-408, 1990.

Coryell W et al: The enduring psychosocial consequences of mania and depression, *Am J Psychiatry* 150:720-727, 1993.

Drevets WC: Geriatric depression: brain imaging correlates and pharmacologic considerations, *J Clin Psychiatry* 55:71-81, 1994.

Drevets WC, Raichle ME: Neuroanatomical circuits in depression: implications for treatment mechanisms, *Psychopharmacol Bull* 28:261-274, 1992.

Drevets WC, Raichle ME: *PET imaging studies of human emotional disorders.* In Gazzaniga MS, editor: *The Cognitive Neurosciences,* Cambridge, Mass., 1994, MIT Press.

Drevets WC et al: A functional anatomical study of unipolar depression, *J Neurosci* 12:3628-3641, 1992.

Elkin I et al: National Institute of Mental Health treatment of depression collaborative research program, *Arch Gen Psychiatry* 46:971-982, 1989.

Feighner JP et al: Diagnostic criteria for use in psychiatric research, *Arch Gen Psychiatry* 26:57-63, 1972.

Folstein SE et al: *Subcortical triad of Huntington's disease: a model for a neuropathology of depression, dementia, and dyskinesia.* In Carroll BJ, Barrett, editors: *Psychopathology and the brain,* New York, 1991, Raven Press.

Francis PT et al: Brain amino acid concentrations and Ca^{2+}-dependent release in intractable depression assessed antemortem, *Brain Res* 494:314-324, 1989.

Goodwin DW, Guze SB: *Psychiatric diagnosis,* ed 4, New York, 1989, Oxford University Press.

Graybiel AM: Neurotransmitters and neuromodulators in the basal ganglia, *Trends Neurosci* 13:244-254, 1990.

Iverson SD, Mishkin M: Perserverative interference in monkeys following selective lesions of the inferior prefrontal convexity, *Exp Brain Res* 11:376-386, 1970.

Jefferson JW, Greist JH: *Valproate and manic depression: a guide,* ed 2, Madison, Wis., 1993, Lithium Information Center, Dean Foundation.

Jeste DV, Lohr JB, Goodwin FK: Neuroanatomical studies of major affective disorders: a review and suggestions for further research, *Br J Psychiatry* 153:444-459, 1988.

Kathol RG et al: Diagnosis of major depression in cancer patients according to four sets of criteria, *Am J Psychiatry* 147:1021-1024, 1990.

Kupfer DJ et al: Five-year outcome for maintenance therapies in recurrent depression, *Arch Gen Psychiatry* 49:769-773, 1992.

LeDoux JE: *Emotion.* In Mills J et al, editors: *Handbook of physiology: the nervous system,* Baltimore, Md., 1987, Williams & Wilkins.

Lenox RH et al: Adjunctive treatment of manic agitation with lorazepam versus haloperidol: a double-blind study, *J Clin Psychiatry* 53:47-52, 1992.

Lesch KP, Manji HK: Signal-transducing G proteins and antidepressant drugs: evidence for modulation of α subunit gene expression in rat brain, *Biol Psychiatry* 32:547-579, 1992.

Mayeux R: *Emotional changes associated with basal ganglia disorders.* In Heilman KM, Satz P, editors: *Neuropsychology of human emotion,* New York, 1983, Guilford.

McEwen BS: *Stressful experience, brain, and emotions: developmental, genetic and hormonal influences.* In Gazzaniga M, editor: *The cognitive neurosciences,* Cambridge, Mass., 1995, MIT Press.

McHugh PR: The neuropsychiatry of basal ganglia disorders, *Neuropsych Neuropsychol Behav Neurol* 2:239-247, 1989.

Medenwald JR, Greist JH, Jefferson JW: *Carbamazepine and manic depression: a guide,* ed 2, Madison, Wis., 1993, Lithium Information Center, Dean Foundation.

Miller NA, Gold MS: Abuse, addiction, tolerance and dependence to benzodiazepines in medical and nonmedical populations, *Am J Drug Alcohol Abuse* 17:27-37, 1991.

Moldin SO, Reich T, Rice JP: Current perspectives on the genetics of unipolar depression, *Behav Genet* 21:211-242, 1991.

Mukherjee S, Sackeim HA, Schnurr DB: Electroconvulsive therapy of acute manic episodes: a review, *Am J Psychiatry* 151:169-176, 1994.

Müller-Oerlinghausen B, Muser-Causemann B, Volk J: Suicides and parasuicides in a high risk patient group on and off lithium long-term medication, *J Affect Disord* 25:261-269, 1992.

Müller-Oerlinghausen B, et al: The effect of long-term lithium treatment on the mortality of patients with manic-depressive and schizoaffective illness, *Acta Psychiatr Scand* 86:218-222, 1992.

Musselman DL, Nemeroff CB: The role of corticotropin-releasing factor in the pathophysiology of psychiatric disorders, *Psychiatr Ann* 23:676-681, 1993.

Peet M: Induction of mania with selective serotonin re-uptake inhibitors and tricyclic antidepressants, *Br J Psychiatry* 164:549-550, 1994.

Post RM: Transduction of psychosocial stress into the neurobiology of recurrent affective disorder, *Am J Psychiatry* 149:999-1010, 1992.

Post RM et al: Lithium-discontinuation-induced refractoriness: preliminary observations, *Am J Psychiatry* 149:1727-1729, 1992.

Price JL, Carmichael ST, Drevets WC: Networks related to the orbital and medial prefrontal cortex: a substrate for emotional behavior? *Prog Brain Res* 107:523-536, 1996.

Rice J et al: The familial transmission of bipolar illness, *Arch Gen Psychiatry* 44:441-447, 1987.

Robins L et al: Lifetime prevalence of specific psychiatric disorders in three sites, *Arch Gen Psychiatry* 41:949-958, 1984.

Roose SP et al: Comparative efficacy of selective serotonin reuptake inhibitors and tricyclics in the treatment of melancholia, *Am J Psychiatry* 151:1735-1739, 1994.

Sackeim HA, Steif BL: *Neuropsychology of depression and mania.* In Georgota A, Cancro R, editors: *Depression and mania,* New York, 1988, Elsevier.

Schou M: Effects of long-term lithium treatment on kidney function: an overview, *J Psychiatr Res* 22:287-296, 1988.

Schou M: *Lithium treatment of manic-depressive illness: a practical guide,* ed 5, New York, 1993, S Karger.

Suppes T et al: Risk of recurrence following discontinuation of lithium treatment in bipolar disorder, *Arch Gen Psychiatry* 48:1082-1088, 1991.

Starkman MN, Schteingart DE: Neuropsychiatric manifestations of patients with Cushing's Syndrome: relationship to cortisol and adrenocorticotropic hormone levels, *Arch Intern Med* 141:215-219, 1981.

Starkstein SE, Robinson RG: Affective disorders and cerebral vascular disease, *Br J Psychiatry* 154:170-182, 1989.

Starkstein SE et al: Manic-depressive and pure manic states after brain lesions, *Biol Psychiatry* 29:149-158, 1991.

Swerdlow NR, Koob GF: Dopamine, schizophrenia, mania and depression: toward a unified hypothesis of cortico-striato-pallido-thalamic function, *Behav Brain Sci* 10:197-245, 1987.

Thase ME, Simons A, Reynolds C: Psychobiological correlates of poor response to cognitive behavior therapy: potential indications for antidepressant pharmacotherapy, *Psychopharmacol Bull* 29:293-301, 1993.

Weissman MM et al: Affective disorders in five United States communities, *Psychol Med* 18:141-153, 1988.

Weller BW, Weller RA: *Mood disorders.* In Lewis M, editor: *child and adolescent psychiatry: a comprehensive textbook,* Baltimore, 1991, Williams and Wilkins.

Winokur G: The development and validity of familial subtypes in primary unipolar depression, *Pharmacopsychiatry* 15:142-146, 1982.

Winokur G: *Unipolar depression.* In Winokur G, Clayton P, editors: *The medical basis of psychiatry,* ed 2, Philadelphia, 1994, Saunders.

Zisook S: *Biopsychosocial aspects of bereavement,* Washington, D.C., 1987, American Psychiatric Press.

Chapter 9

Ballenger JC et al: Alprazolam in panic disorder and agoraphobia: results from a multicenter trial. I. Efficacy in short-term treatment, *Arch Gen Psychiatry* 45:413-422, 1988.

Brown TA et al: The empirical basis of generalized anxiety disorder (review), *Am J Psychiatry* 151:1272-1280, 1994.

Burke KC et al: Age at onset of selected mental disorders in five community populations, *Arch Gen Psychiatry* 47:511-518, 1990.

Fyer AJ et al: A direct interview family study of social phobia, *Arch Gen Psychiatry* 50:286-293, 1993.

Gelernter CS et al: Cognitive-behavioral and pharmacological treatments of social phobia: a controlled study, *Arch Gen Psychiatry* 48:938-945, 1991.

Kahn RJ et al: Imipramine and chlordiazepoxide in depressive and anxiety disorders. II. Efficacy in anxious outpatients, *Arch Gen Psychiatry* 43:79-85, 1986.

Kahn RJ et al: Tricyclic treatment of generalized anxiety disorder, *J Affect Disord* 13:145-151, 1987.

Kendler KS et al: Generalized anxiety disorder in women: a population-based twin study, *Arch Gen Psychiatry* 49:267-272, 1992.

Kendler KS et al: The genetic epidemiology of phobias in women: the interrelationship of agoraphobia, social phobia, situational phobia, and simple phobia, *Arch Gen Psychiatry* 49:273-81, 1992.

Kessler RC et al: Lifetime and 12-month prevalence of DSM-III-R psychiatric disorders in the United States, *Arch Gen Psychiatry* 51:8-19, 1994.

Liebowitz MR et al: Treatment of social phobia with drugs other than benzodiazepines, *J Clin Psychiatry* 52(11, Suppl):10-15, 1991.

Liebowitz MR et al: Phenelzine vs atenolol in social phobia: a placebo-controlled comparison, *Arch Gen Psychiatry* 49:290-300, 1992.

Lipman RS et al: Imipramine and chlordiazepoxide in depressive and anxiety disorders. I. Efficacy in depressed outpatients, *Arch Gen Psychiatry* 43:68-77, 1986.

Marks I, Lader M: Anxiety states (anxiety neurosis): a review, *J Nerv Ment Dis* 156:3-18, 1973.

Marshall RD et al: Medication therapy for social phobia (review), *J Clin Psychiatry* 55(Suppl):33-37, 1994.

Nagy LM et al: Clinical and medication outcome after short-term alprazolam and behavioral group treatment in panic disorder: 2.5 year naturalistic follow-up study, *Arch Gen Psychiatry* 46:993-999, 1989.

Noyes R Jr et al: Relationship between panic disorder and agoraphobia: a family study, *Arch Gen Psychiatry* 43:227-232, 1986.

Noyes R Jr et al: Alprazolam in panic disorder and agoraphobia: results from a multicenter trial. II. Patient acceptance, side effects, and safety, *Arch Gen Psychiatry* 45:423-428, 1988.

Noyes R Jr et al: Follow-up study of patients with panic disorder and agoraphobia with panic attacks treated with tricyclic antidepressants, *J Affect Disord* 16:249-257, 1989.

Noyes R Jr et al: Outcome of panic disorder: relationship to diagnostic subtypes and comorbidity, *Arch Gen Psychiatry* 47:809-818, 1990.

Pecknold JC et al: Alprazolam in panic disorder and agoraphobia: results from a multicenter trial. III. Discontinuation effects, *Arch Gen Psychiatry* 45:429-436, 1988.

Pecknold JC et al: Serotonin uptake in panic disorder and agoraphobia, *Neuropsychopharmacology* 1:173-176, 1988.

Pecknold JC et al: Evaluation of buspirone as an antianxiety agent: buspirone and diazepam versus placebo, *Can J Psychiatry* 34:766-771, 1989.

Regier DA et al: Comorbidity of mental disorders with alcohol and other drug abuse, *JAMA* 264:2511-2518, 1990.

Schneier FR et al: Fluoxetine in panic disorder, *J Clin Pharmacol* 10:119-121, 1990.

Schneier FR et al: Social phobia: comorbidity and morbidity in an epidemiologic sample, *Arch Gen Psychiatry* 49:282-288, 1992.

Schneier FR et al: Buspirone in social phobia, *J Clin Psychopharmacol* 13:252-256, 1993.

Torgersen S: Genetic factors in anxiety disorders, *Arch Gen Psychiatry* 40:1085-1089, 1983.

Versiana M et al: Pharmacotherapy of social phobia: a controlled study with moclobemide and phenelzine, *Br J Psychiatry* 161:353-360, 1992.

Weissman MM et al: Suicidal ideation and suicide attempts in panic disorder and attacks, *N Engl J Med* 321:1209-1214, 1989.

Chapter 10

American Psychiatric Association: *Diagnostic and statistical manual of mental disorders,* ed 4, Washington, D.C., 1994, American Psychiatric Press.

Baxter LR et al: Cerebral glucose metabolic rates in nondepressed patients with obsessive-compulsive disorder, *Am J Psychiatry* 145:1560-1563, 1988.

Baxter LR et al: Caudate glucose metabolic rate changes with both drug and behavior therapy for obsessive-compulsive disorder, *Arch Gen Psychiatry* 49:681-689, 1992.

Bellodi L et al: Psychiatric disorders in the families of patients with obsessive-compulsive disorder, *Psychiatry Res* 42:111-120, 1992.

Berrios GE: Obsessive-compulsive disorder: its conceptual history in France during the 19th century, *Compr Psychiatry* 30:283-295, 1989.

Black DW et al: A family study of obsessive-compulsive disorder, *Arch Gen Psychiatry* 49:362-368, 1992.

Carey G, Gottesman II: *Twin and family studies of anxiety, phobic and obsessive disorders.* In Klein DG, Rabkin J, editors: *Anxiety: new research and changing concepts,* New York, 1981, Raven Press.

Christopher PL et al: Fluvoxamine versus clomipramine in the treatment of obsessive compulsive disorder: a multicenter, randomized, double-blind, parallel group comparison, *J Clin Psychiatry* 55:301-305, 1994.

Clomipramine Collaborative Study Group: Clomipramine in the treatment of patients with obsessive-compulsive disorder, *Arch Gen Psychiatry* 48:730-738, 1991.

Cummings JL, Cunningham K: Obsessive-compulsive disorder in Huntington's disease, *Biol Psychiatry* 31:263-270, 1992.

Foa EB, Steketee GS, Azarow BJ: *Behavior therapy with obsessive compulsives.* In Mavissakalian M, Turner SM, Michelson L, editors: *Obsessive-compulsive disorder:* psychological and pharmacological treatment, New York, 1985, Plenum.

Foa EB et al: DSM-IV field trial: obsessive-compulsive disorder, *Am J Psychiatry* 152:90-96, 1995.

Freeman CPL et al: Fluvoxamine or clomipramine in the treatment of obsessive compulsive disorder: a multicenter, randomized, double-blind, parallel group comparison, *J Clin Psychiatry* 55:301-305, 1991.

Goodman WK et al: The Yale-Brown obsessive compulsive scale, *Arch Gen Psychiatry* 46:1012-1016, 1989.

Goodman WK et al: Specificity of serotonin reuptake inhibitors in the treatment of obsessive compulsive disorder: a comparison of fluvoxamine and desipramine, *Arch Gen Psychiatry* 47:577-585, 1990.

Goodwin DW, Guze SB, Robins E: Follow-up studies in obsessional neurosis, *Arch Gen Psychiatry* 20:182-187, 1969.

Griest JH et al: Efficacy and tolerability of serotonin transport inhibitors in obsessive-compulsive disorder, *Arch Gen Psychiatry* 52:53-60, 1995.

Hewlett WA et al: Clomipramine, clonazepam, and clonidine in the treatment of obsessive-compulsive disorder, *J Clin Psychopharmacol* 12:420-430, 1992.

Insel TR: Toward a neuroanatomy of obsessive-compulsive disorder, *Arch Gen Psychiatry* 49:739-744, 1992.

Jenike MA et al: Cingulotomy for refractory obsessive-compulsive disorder, *Arch Gen Psychiatry* 48:548-555, 1991.

Laplane D et al: Obsessive-compulsive and other behavioral changes with bilateral basal ganglia lesions: a neuropsychological, magnetic resonance imaging and positron tomography study, *Brain* 112:699-725, 1989.

Leonard HL et al: Treatment of obsessive-compulsive disorder with clomipramine and desipramine in children and adolescents: a double-blind crossover comparison, *Arch Gen Psychiatry* 46:1088-1092, 1989.

Mavissakalian MR, Jones B, Olson S: Absence of placebo response in obsessive-compulsive disorder, *J Nerv Ment Dis* 178:268-270, 1990.

McDougle CJ et al: Neuroleptic addition in fluvoxamine-refractory obsessive-compulsive disorder, *Am J Psychiatry* 147:652-654, 1990.

McGuire PK et al: Functional anatomy of obsessive-compulsive phenomena, *Br J Psychiatry* 164:459-468, 1994.

Mindus P, Nyman H: Normalization of personality characteristics in patients with incapacitating anxiety disorders after capsulotomy, *Acta Psychiatr Scand* 83:283-291, 1991.

Pato MT et al: Return of symptoms after discontinuation of clomipramine in patients with obsessive-compulsive disorder, *Am J Psychiatry* 145:1521-1525, 1988.

Pauls DL et al: Gilles de la Tourette's syndrome and obsessive-compulsive disorder: evidence supporting a genetic relationship, *Arch Gen Psychiatry* 43:1180-1182, 1986.

Piccinelli M et al: Efficacy of drug treatment in obsessive-compulsive disorder: a meta-analytic review, *Br J Psychiatry* 166:424-443, 1995.

Piggot TA et al: Controlled comparisons of clomipramine and fluoxetine in the treatment of obsessive-compulsive disorder: behavioral and biological results, *Arch Gen Psychiatry* 47:926-932, 1990.

Rasmussen SA: Genetic studies of obsessive-compulsive disorder, *Ann Clin Psych* 5:241-248, 1993.

Rasmussen SA, Eisen JL: The epidemiology of obsessive compulsive disorder, *J Clin Psych* 51(suppl 6):10-13, 1990.

Rasmussen SA, Tsuang MT: DSM-III obsessive compulsive disorder: clinical characteristics and family history, *Am J Psychiatry* 143:317-322, 1986.

Rasmussen et al: Fluvoxamine in the treatment of obsessive compulsive disorder: a multi-center, double-blind, placebo-controlled study, *Am J Psychiatry* (in press).

Rauch SL et al: Regional cerebral blood flow measured during symptom provocation in obsessive-compulsive disorder using oxygen 15-labeled carbon dioxide and position emission tomography, *Arch Gen Psychiatry* 51:62-70, 1994.

Ricciardi JN et al: Changes in DSM-III-R Axis II diagnoses following treatment of obsessive-compulsive disorder, *Am J Psychiatry* 149:829-831, 1992.

Riddle MA et al: Obsessive compulsive disorder in children and adolescents: phenomenology and family history, *J Am Acad Child Adolesc Psychiatry* 29:766-772, 1990.

Robins LN et al: Lifetime prevalence of specific psychiatric disorders in three sites, *Arch Gen Psychiatry* 41:949-958, 1984.

Shapiro AK, Shapiro E: Evaluation of the reported association of obsessive-compulsive symptoms or disorder with Tourette's disorder, *Compr Psychiatry* 33:152-165, 1992.

Swedo SE et al: Cerebral glucose metabolism in childhood-onset obsessive-compulsive disorder, *Arch Gen Psychiatry* 46:518-523, 1989.

Swedo SE et al: High prevalence of obsessive-compulsive symptoms in patients with Sydenham's chorea, *Am J Psychiatry* 146:246-249, 1989.

Swedo SE et al: Cerebral glucose metabolism in childhood-onset obsessive-compulsive disorder: revisualization during pharmacotherapy, *Arch Gen Psychiatry* 49:690-694, 1992.

Tollefson GD et al: A multicenter investigation of fixed-dose fluoxetine in the treatment of obsessive-compulsive disorder, *Arch Gen Psychiatry* 51:559-567, 1994.

Vallejo J et al: Clomipramine versus phenelzine in obsessive-compulsive disorder: a controlled clinical trial, *Br J Psychiatry* 161:665-670, 1992.

Chapter 11

Alluisi EA et al: Behavioral effects of tularemia and sandfly fever in man, *J Infect Dis* 128:710, 1973.

Ammoni JM, Beer S, Kesselring J: Severe traumatic brain injury: epidemiology and outcome after 3 years, *Disabil Rehabil* 14:23, 1992.

Arcia E, Gualtieri CT: Association between patient report of symptoms after mild head injury and neurobehavioral performance, *Brain Inj* 7:481, 1993.

Baigrie RJ et al: Oxybutynin: is it safe? *Br J Urol* 62:319, 1988.

Berk M: Indications for computed tomographic brain scanning in psychiatric inpatients, *S Afr Med J* 82:338, 1992.

Binder LM: Persisting symptoms after mild head injury: a review of the postconcussive syndrome, *J Clin Exp Neuropsychol* 8:323, 1986.

Blansjaar BA, Horjus MC, Nijhuis HGJ: Prevalence of the Korsakoff syndrome in The Hague, The Netherlands, *Acta Psychiatr Scand* 75:604, 1987.

Breitbart W: Psycho-oncology: depression, anxiety, delirium, *Semin Oncol* 21:754, 1994.

Butters N, Delis DC, Lucas JA: Clinical assessment of memory disorders in amnesia and dementia, *Annu Rev Psychol* 46:493, 1995.

Butterworth RF, Krill JJ, Harper CG: Thiamine-dependent enzyme changes in the brains of alcoholics: relationship to the Wernicke-Korsakoff syndrome, *Alcohol Clin Exp Res* 17:1084, 1993.

Callender TJ et al: Three-dimensional brain metabolic imaging in patients with toxic encephalopathy, *Environ Res* 60:295, 1993.

Cole MG et al: Systematic intervention for elderly inpatients with delirium: a randomized trial, *Can Med Assoc J* 151:965, 1994.

Crippen DW: Pharmacologic treatment of brain failure and delirium, *Crit Care Clin* 10:733, 1994.

Dikmen S, McLean A, Temkin N: Neuropsychological and psychosocial consequences of minor head injury, *J Neurol Neurosurg Psychiatry* 49:1227, 1986.

Duus BR et al: Prognostic signs in the evaluation of patients with minor head injury, *Br J Surg* 80:988, 1993.

Englander J et al: Mild traumatic brain injury in an insured population: subjective complaints and return to employment, *Brain Inj* 6:161, 1992.

Fleming JM, Maas F: Prognosis of rehabilitation outcome in head injury using the disability rating scale, *Arch Phys Med Rehabil* 75:156, 1994.

Fontaine DK: Nonpharmacologic management of patient distress during mechanical ventilation, *Crit Care Clin* 10:695, 1994.

Francis J, Kapoor WN: Prognosis after hospital discharge of older medical patients with delirium, *J Am Geriatr Soc* 40:601, 1992.

Francis J, Martin D, Kapoor WN: A prospective study of delirium in hospitalized elderly, *JAMA* 263:1097, 1990.

Frankowski RF: Descriptive epidemiologic studies of head injury in the United States: 1974-1984, *Adv Psychosom Med* 16:153, 1986.

Frederiks JAM: Transient global amnesia, *Clin Neurol Neurosurg* 95:265, 1993.

Gallassi R et al: Transient global amnesia: neuropsychological findings after single and multiple attacks, *Eur Neurol* 33:297, 1993.

Goldstein LH et al: The effect of anticonvulsants on cognitive functioning following a probable encephalitic illness, *Br J Psychiatry* 160:546, 1992.

Good MI: Substance-induced dissociative disorders and psychiatric nosology, *J Clin Psychopharmacol* 9:88, 1989.

Goodwin DW: Alcohol amnesia, *Addiction* 90:315, 1995.

Gottlieb GL et al: Delirium in the medically ill elderly: operationalizing the DSM-III criteria, *Int Psychogeriatr* 3:181, 1991.

Gustafson Y et al: A geriatric-anesthesiologic program to reduce acute confusional states in elderly patients treated for femoral neck fractures, *J Am Geriatr Soc* 39:655, 1991.

Hanrahan JP, Gordon MA: Mushroom poisoning: case reports and a review of therapy, *JAMA* 251:1057, 1984.

Harper C et al: The Wernicke-Korsakoff syndrome in Sydney: a prospective necropsy study, *Med J Aust* 149:718, 1988.

Harper CG, Kril JJ: Neuropathology of alcoholism, *Alcohol Alcohol* 35:207, 1990.

Hodges JR: Semantic memory and frontal executive function during transient global amnesia, *J Neurol Neurosurg Psychiatry* 57:605, 1994.

Hodges JR, Warlow CP: The aetiology of transient global amnesia, *Brain* 113:639, 1990.

Hodges JR, Warlow CP: Syndromes of transient amnesia: towards a classification, *J Neurol Neurosurg Psychiatry* 53:834, 1990.

Inouye SKS et al: A predictive model for delirium in hospitalized elderly medical patients based on admission characteristics, *Ann Intern Med* 119:474, 1993.

Johnson JC et al: Using DSM-III criteria to diagnose delirium in elderly general medical patients, *J Gerontol* 45:M113, 1990.
Johnson R, Gleave J: Counting the people disabled by head injury, *Injury* 18:7, 1987.
Kapur N: Amnesia in relation to fugue states: distinguishing a neurological from a psychogenic basis, *Br J Psychiatry* 159:872, 1991.
Kopelman MD: Amnesia: organic and psychogenic, *Br J Psychiatry* 150:428, 1987.
Koski KJ, Marttila RJ: Transient global amnesia: incidence in an urban population, *Acta Neurol Scand* 81:358, 1990.
Levine RL: Pharmacology of intravenous sedatives and opioids in critically ill patients, *Crit Care Clin* 10:709, 1994.
Levkoff S et al: Epidemiology of delirium: an overview of research issues and findings, *Int Psychogeriatr* 3:149, 1991.
Marcantonio ER et al: A clinical prediction rule for delirium after elective noncardiac surgery, *JAMA* 271:134, 1994.
Marcantonio ER et al: The relationship of postoperative delirium with psychoactive medications, *JAMA* 272:1518, 1994.
McCartney JR, Boland RJ: Anxiety and delirium in the intensive care unit, *Crit Care Clin* 10:673, 1994.
Melo TP, Ferro JM, Ferro H: Transient global amnesia, *Brain* 115:261, 1992.
Miller W et al: Transient global amnesia: clinical characteristics and prognosis, *Neurology* 37:733, 1987.
Millis SR: Assessment of motivation and memory with the recognition memory test after financially compensable mild head injury, *J Clin Psychol* 50:601, 1994.
Murray AM et al: Acute delirium and functional decline in the hospitalized elderly patient, *J Gerontol* 48:M181, 1993.
Nanji AA: Drug-induced electrolyte disorders, *Drug Intelligence Clin Pharm* 17:175, 1983.
Nejo TA, Pitt BM: Delirium in elderly people, *Curr Opin Psychiatry* 8:246, 1995.
Newcombe F, Rabbitt P, Briggs M: Minor head injury: pathophysiological or iatrogenic sequelae? *J Neurol Neurosurg Psychiatry* 57:709, 1994.
Newton NL, Janati A: Delirium, a study of 100 cases, *Stress Med* 2:267, 1986.
Noronha-Blob L, Kachur JF: Enantiomers of oxybutynin: in vitro pharmacological characterization at M_1, M_2 and M_3 muscarinic receptors and in vivo effects on urinary bladder contraction, mydriasis and salivary secretion in guinea pigs, *J Pharmacol Exp Ther* 256:562, 1991.
O'Neill D: Brain stethoscopes: the use and abuse of brief mental status schedules, *Postgrad Med J* 69:599, 1993.
Pompeii P et al: Delirium in hospitalized older persons: outcomes and predictors, *J Am Geriatr Soc* 42:809, 1994.
Preskorn SH, Jerkovich GS: Central nervous system toxicity of tricyclic antidepressants: phenomonology, course, risk factors, and the role of therapeutic drug monitoring, *J Clin Psychopharmacol* 10:88, 1990.
Price J et al: The Wernicke-Korsakoff syndrome: a reappraisal in Queensland with special reference to prevention, *Med J Aust* 147:561, 1987.
Pritchard PB et al: Epileptic amnesic attacks: benefit from antiepileptic drugs, *Neurology* 35:1188, 1985.
Purdie FR, Honigman B, Rosen P: Acute organic brain syndrome: a review of 100 cases, *Ann Emerg Med* 10:455, 1981.
Richardson JTE: Imagery mnemonics and memory remediation, *Neurology* 42:283, 1992.
Saravay SM, Lavin M: Psychiatric comorbidity and length of stay in the general hospital: a critical review of outcome studies, *Psychosomatics* 35:233, 1994.
Schor JD et al: Risk factors for delirium in hospitalized elderly, *JAMA* 267:827, 1992.
Shih WJ, Hyatt M: Volume and surface three-dimensional displays of Tc-99m HMPAO brain SPECT imaging in a chronic hypnosedative abuser, *Clin Nucl Med* 18:506, 1993.
Sirois F: Delirium: 100 cases, *Can J Psychiatry* 33:375, 1988.
Smith AJ et al: The effects of experimentally induced respiratory virus infections on performance, *Psychol Med* 18:65, 1988.
Squire LR, Amaral DG, Press GA: Magnetic resonance imaging of the hippocampal formation and mammillary nuclei distinguish medial temporal lobe and diencephalic amnesia, *J Neurosci* 10:3106, 1990.
Stracciari A et al: Post-traumatic retrograde amnesia with selective impairment of autobiographical memory, *Cortex* 30:59, 1994.
Sullivan EV et al: Anterior hippocampal volume deficits in nonamnesic, aging chronic alcoholics, *Alcohol Clin Exp Res* 19:110, 1995.
Sullivan TE et al: Closed head injury assessment and research methodology, *J Neurosci Nurs* 26:24, 1994.
Sumner D, Simons RJ: Delirium in the hospitalized elderly, *Cleve Clin J Med* 61:258, 1994.
Taheri PA et al: Can patients with minor head injuries be safely discharged home? *Arch Surg* 128:289, 1993.
Triebig G, Lang C: Brain imaging techniques applied to chronically solvent-exposed workers: current results and clinical evaluation, *Environ Res* 61:239, 1993.
Tucker GJ: DSM-IV: proposals for revision of diagnostic criteria for delirium, *Int Psychogeriatr* 3:197, 1991.
Verfaellie M, Cermak LS: Acquisition of generic memory in amnesia, *Cortex* 30:293, 1994.
Victor M: Alcoholic dementia, *Can J Neurol Sci* 21:88, 1994.
Williams DH, Levin HS, Eisenberg HM: Mild head injury classification, *Neurosurgery* 27:422, 1990.

Chapter 12

American Psychiatric Association: *Diagnostic and statistical manual of mental disorders,* ed 4 (DSM-IV), Washington, D.C., 1994, American Psychiatric Press.
Barinaga M: Missing Alzheimer's gene found, *Science* 269:917-918, 1995.
Berg L et al: Mild senile dementia of the Alzheimer type. 2. Longitudinal assessment, *Ann Neurol* 23:477-484, 1988.
Berg L et al: Mild senile dementia of the Alzheimer type. 4. Evaluation of intervention, *Ann Neurol* 31:242-249, 1992.
Blass JP: Pathophysiology of the Alzheimer's syndrome, *Neurology* 43(suppl 4):S25-S38, 1993.
Bloom FE, Kupfer DL, editors: *Psychopharmacology: the fourth generation of progress,* New York, 1995, Raven Press.
Clark RF, Goate AM: Molecular genetics of Alzheimer's disease, *Arch Neurol* 50:1164-1172, 1993.
Corey-Bloom J et al: Diagnosis and evaluation of dementia, *Neurology* 45:211-218, 1995.
Drevets WC, Rubin EH: Psychotic symptoms and the longitudinal course of senile dementia of the Alzheimer type, *Biol Psychiatry* 25:39-48, 1989.
Ebly EM et al: Prevalence and types of dementia in the very old: results from the Canadian study of health and aging, *Neurology* 44:1593-1600, 1994.
Folstein ME, Folstein SE, McHugh PR: Mini-mental state: a practical method for grading the cognitive state of patients for the clinician, *J Psychiatr Res* 12:189-198, 1975.
Friedland RP: Alzheimer's disease: clinical features and differential diagnosis, *Neurology* 43(suppl 4):S45-S51, 1993.
Games D et al: Alzheimer-type neuropathology in transgenic mice overexpressing V717F β-amyloid precurser protein, *Nature* 373:523-527, 1995.
Graves AB, Kukull WA: *The epidemiology of dementia.* In Morris JC, editor: *Handbook of dementing illnesses,* New York, 1994, Marcel Dekker.

Hebert LE et al: Age-specific incidence of Alzheimer's disease in a community population, *JAMA* 273:1354-1359, 1995.

Katzman R: *Apoliprotein E4 as the major genetic susceptibility factor for Alzheimer disease.* In Terry RD, Katzman R, Bick KL, editors: *Alzheimer's disease,* New York, 1994, Raven Press, Ltd.

Katzman R, Kawas C: *The epidemiology of dementia and Alzheimer's disease.* In Terry RD, Katzman R, Bick KL, editors: *Alzheimer's disease,* New York, 1994, Raven Press, Ltd.

Katzman R et al: Validation of a short orientation-memory-concentration test of cognitive impairment, *Am J Psychiatry* 140:734-739, 1983.

Koller WC, Megaffin BB: *Parkinson's disease and parkinsonism.* In Coffey CE, Cummings JL, editors: *Textbook of geriatric neuropsychiatry,* Washington, D.C., 1994, American Psychiatric Press.

Levy-Lahad E et al: Candidate gene for the chromosome 1 familial Alzheimer's disease locus, *Science* 269:973-977, 1995a.

Levy-Lahad E et al: A familial Alzheimer's disease locus on chromosome 1, *Science* 269:970-973, 1995b.

Max W: The economic impact of Alzheimer's disease, *Neurology* 43(suppl 4):S6-S10, 1993.

McKeith IG et al: The clinical diagnosis and misdiagnosis of senile dementia of Lewy body type (SDLT), *Br J Psychiatry* 165:324-332, 1994.

Miller BL et al: *Alzheimer's disease and frontal lobe dementias.* In Coffey CE, Cummings JL, editors: *Textbook of geriatric neuropsychiatry,* Washington, D.C., 1994, American Psychiatric Press.

Mirra SS, Gearing M: *The neuropathology of dementia.* In Morris JC, editor: *Handbook of dementing illnesses,* New York, 1994, Marcel Dekker.

Morris JC: The Clinical Dementia Rating (CDR): current version and scoring rules, *Neurology* 43:2412-2414, 1993.

Morris JC: *Evaluation of the demented patient.* In Morris JC, editor: *Handbook of dementing illness,* New York, 1994, Marcel Dekker.

Morris JC, Rubin EH: Clinical diagnosis and course of Alzheimer's disease, *Psychiatr Clin North Am* 14(2):223-236, 1991.

Pearlson GD, Petty RG: *Late-life onset psychoses.* In Coffey CE, Cummings JL, editors: *Textbook of geriatric neuropsychiatry,* Washington, D.C., 1994, American Psychiatric Press.

Rubin EH: *Psychopathology of senile dementia of the Alzheimer Type.* In Wurtman RJ, Corkin S, Growdon JH, editors: *Advances in neurology: Alzheimer's disease,* vol 51, New York, 1990, Raven Press.

Rubin EH: *Depression and dementia.* In Morris JC, editor: *Handbook of dementing illnesses,* New York, 1994, Marcel Dekker.

Rubin EH: Differentiating of dementia of the Alzheimer type and healthy aging, *Clinical Geriatrics and Issues in Long Term Care* 3:30-46, 1995.

Rubin EH et al: Influence of age on clinical and psychometric assessment of subjects with very mild or mild dementia of the Alzheimer type, *Arch Neurol* 50:380-383, 1993.

Salzman C, editor: *Clinical geriatric psychopharmacology,* ed 2, Baltimore, 1992, Williams and Wilkins.

Schatzberg AF, Nemeroff CB, editors: *Textbook of psychopharmacology,* Washington, D.C., 1995, American Psychiatric Press.

Schneider EL, Guralnik JM: The aging of America, *JAMA* 263:2335-2340, 1990.

Sherrington R et al: Cloning of a gene bearing missense mutations in early-onset familial Alzheimer's disease, *Nature* 375:754-760, 1995.

Tariot PN, Blazina L: *The psychopathology of dementia.* In Morris JC, editor: *Handbook of dementing illnesses,* New York, 1994, Marcel Dekker.

Torack RM, Morris JC: Mesolimbocortical dementia: a clinical case study of a putative disorder, *Arch Neurol* 43:1074-1078, 1986.

Torack RM, Morris JC: The association of ventral tegmental area histopathology with adult dementia, *Arch Neurol* 45:497-501, 1988.

Chapter 13

Allebeck P, Wistedt B: Mortality in schizophrenia, *Arch Gen Psychiatry* 43:650, 1986.

Andreasen NC et al: Thalamic abnormalities in schizophrenia visualized through magnetic resonance image averaging, *Science* 266:294-298, 1994.

Andreasen NC et al: Symptoms of schizophrenia: methods, meanings, and mechanisms, *Arch Gen Psychiatry* 52:341-351, 1995.

Andreasen NC, Carpenter WT: Diagnosis and classification of schizophrenia, *Schizophr Bull* 19:199-214, 1993.

Arnold SE et al: Smaller neuron size in schizophrenia in hippocampal subfields that mediate corticol-hippocampal interactions, *Am J Psychiatry* 152:738-748, 1995.

Baldessarini RJ, Viguera AC: Neuroleptic withdrawal in schizophrenic patients, *Arch Gen Psychiatry* 52:189, 1995.

Berman KF, Weinberger DR: *Schizophrenia: brain structure and function.* In Kaplan HI, Sadock BJ, editors: *Comprehensive textbook of psychiatry/V,* Baltimore, 1989, Williams and Wilkins.

Berman KF, Zec RF, Weinberger DR: Physiological dysfunction of dorsolateral prefrontal cortex in schizophrenia. II. Role of neuroleptic treatment, attention, and mental effort, *Arch Gen Psychiatry* 43:126, 1986.

Bleuler E: *Dementia praecox or the group of schizophrenias,* New York, 1950, International Universities Press.

Caldwell CB, Gottesman II: Schizophrenics kill themselves too: a review of risk factors for suicide, *Schizophr Bull* 16:571-589, 1990.

Cloninger CR: *Schizophrenia: genetic etiological factors.* In Kaplan HI, Sadock BJ, editors: *Comprehensive textbook of psychiatry/V,* Baltimore, 1989, Williams and Wilkins.

Cloninger CR et al: Diagnosis and prognosis in schizophrenia, *Arch Gen Psychiatry* 42:15-25, 1985.

Cohen LJ, Test MA, Brocon RL: Suicide and schizophrenia: data from a prospective community treatment study, *Am J Psychiatry* 147:602-607; correction: 147:1110, 1990.

Cooper JE et al: Cross-national study of diagnosis of the mental disorders: some results from the first comparative investigation, *Am J Psychiatry* 125:21, 1969.

DeLisi LE: *Viral and immune hypotheses for schizophrenia.* In Meltzer HY, editor: *Psychopharmacology: third generation of progress,* New York, 1987, Raven Press.

Docherty JP et al: Stages of onset of schizophrenic psychosis, *Am J Psychiatry* 135:4, 1978.

Drake RE et al: Suicide among schizophrenics: a review, *Compr Psychiatry* 26:90, 1985.

Flaum M et al: Effects of diagnosis, laterality, and gender on brain morphology in schizophrenia, *Am J Psychiatry* 152:5, 1995.

Gilbert PL, Harris MJ, Jeste DV: Neuroleptic withdrawal in schizophrenic patients, *Arch Gen Psychiatry* 52:173-188, 1995.

Gottesman II: *Schizophrenia genesis: the origins of madness,* New York, 1991, W.H. Freeman and Company.

Grebb JA, Cancro R: *Schizophrenia: clinical features.* In Kaplan HI, Sadock BJ, editors: *Comprehensive textbook of psychiatry/V,* Baltimore, 1989, Williams and Wilkins.

Hafner H: *Der Krankheitsbegriff in der Psychiatrie.* In Degkwitz R, Siedow H, editors: *Standorte der Psychiatrie,* vol 2, *Zum umstrittenen psychiatrischen Krankheitsbegriff,* Munich, 1981, Urban and Schwarzenberg.

Hafner H, Gattaz WF, Janzarik W: *Search for the causes of schizophrenia,* Berlin, 1987 Springer-Verlag.

Harris MJ, Cullum CM, Jeste DV: Clinical presentation of late-onset schizophrenia, *J Clin Psychiatry* 49:356-360, 1988.

Haywood TW et al: Predicting the "revolving door" phenomenon among patients with schizophrenic, schizoaffective, and affective disorders, *Am J Psychiatry* 152:856-861, 1995.

Heston LL: Psychiatric disorders in foster home reared children of schizophrenic mothers, *Br J Psychiatry* 112:819-825, 1966.

Huse MA et al: The economic costs of non-insulin-dependent diabetes mellitus, *JAMA* 262:2708, 1989.

Jeste DV et al: Clinical and neuropsychological characteristics of patients with late-onset schizophrenia, *Am J Psychiatry* 152:722-730, 1995.

Kane JM: *Schizophrenia: somatic treatment.* In Kaplan HI, Sadock BJ, editors: *Comprehensive textbook of psychiatry/V,* Baltimore, 1989, Williams and Wilkins.

Karno M, Norquist GS: *Schizophrenia: epidemiology.* In Kaplan HI, Sadock BJ, editors: *Comprehensive textbook of psychiatry/V,* Baltimore, 1989, Williams and Wilkins.

Kay SR: *Positive and negative syndromes in schizophrenia: assessment and research,* New York, 1991, Brunner/Mazel.

Kendler KS et al: The Roscommon family study. I. Methods, diagnosis of probands, and risks of schizophrenia in relatives, *Arch Gen Psychiatry* 50:527-540, 1993.

Kendler KS et al: The Roscommon family study. II. The risk of nonschizophrenic nonaffective psychoses in relatives, *Arch Gen Psychiatry* 50:645-652, 1993.

Kessler RC, et al: Lifetime and 12-month prevalence of DSM-III-R psychiatric disorders in the United States, *Arch Gen Psychiatry* 51:8-19, 1994.

Kety SS et al: *Mental illness in the biological and adoptive families of adopted individuals who have become schizophrenic: a preliminary report based on psychiatric interviews.* In Fieve R, Rosenthal D, Brill H, editors: *Genetic Research in Psychiatry,* Baltimore, 1975, Johns-Hopkins Press.

Koreen AR et al: Depression in first-episode schizophrenia, *Am J Psychiatry* 150:1643-1648, 1993.

Kraepelin E: *Dementia praecox and paraphrenia,* New York, 1971, RE Krieger Publishing Co.

Kramer MS et al: Antidepressants in "depressed" schizophrenic inpatients: a controlled trial, *Arch Gen Psychiatry* 46:922-928, 1989.

Levinson DF et al: Fluphenazine plasma levels, dosage, efficacy, and side effects, *Am J Psychiatry* 152:5, 1995.

Manschreck TC: Delusional (paranoid) disorders. In Kaplan HI, Sadock BJ, editors: *Comprehensive textbook of psychiatry/V,* Baltimore, 1989, Williams and Wilkins.

Mellor CS: First rank symptoms of schizophrenia, *Br J Psychiatry* 117:15-23, 1970.

Meltzer HY et al: Cost-effectiveness of clozapine in neuroleptic-resistant schizophrenia, *Am J Psychiatry* 150:1630-1638, 1993.

Miller NE, Cohen GD: *Schizophrenia and aging,* New York, 1987, The Guilford Press.

National Advisory Mental Health Council: Health care reform for Americans with severe mental illnesses: report of the national advisory mental health council, *Am J Psychiatry* 150:1447-1465, 1993.

Pearlson GD, Marsh L: *Magnetic resonance imaging in psychiatry.* In *American psychiatric press review of psychiatry,* vol 12, Washington D.C., 1993, American Psychiatric Press.

Petty RG et al: Reversal of asymmetry of the planum temporale in schizophrenia, *Am J Psychiatry* 152:5, 1995

Pope HG, Lipinski JF: Diagnosis in schizophrenia and manic-depressive illness, *Arch Gen Psychiatry* 35:811, 1978.

Regier DA et al: The NIMH epidemiologic catchment area program, *Arch Gen Psychiatry* 41:934, 1984.

Robins E, Guze SB: Establishment of diagnostic validity in psychiatric illness: its application to schizophrenia, *Am J Psychiatry* 126:7, 1970.

Robins LN et al: Lifetime prevalence of specific psychiatric disorders in three sites, *Arch Gen Psychiatry* 41:949, 1984.

Schneider K: *Clinical Psychopathology,* New York, 1939, Grune and Stratton.

Siris SF et al: Adjunctive imipramine in the treatment of post-psychotic depression: a controlled study, *Arch Gen Psychiatry* 44:533-539, 1987.

Spitzer RL et al: *DSM-IV casebook,* Washington, D.C., 1994, American Psychiatric Press.

Sydenham T: *Observations medicare (1676).* In J Swan, editor: *The entire works of Thomas Sydenham newly made English from the originals,* London, 1742, Cave.

Weinberger DR: Brain disease and psychiatric illness: when should a psychiatrist order a CAT scan? *Am J Psychiatry* 141:1521, 1984.

Weinberger DR, Berman KF, Torrey EF: Correlations between abnormal hippocampal morphology and prefrontal physiology in schizophrenia, *Clin Neuropharmacol* 15:393A-394A, 1992.

Weinberger DR, Berman KF, Zec RF: Physiological dysfunction of dorsolateral prefrontal cortex in schizophrenia. I. Regional cerebral blood flow (rCBF) evidence, *Arch Gen Psychiatry* 43:114, 1986.

Weinberger DR, Wagner R, Wyatt RJ: Neuropathological studies of schizophrenia: a selective review, *Schizophr Bull* 9:193, 1983.

Westermeyer JF, Harrow M, Marengo JT: Risk for suicide in schizophrenia and other psychotic and non-psychotic disorders, *J Nerv Ment Dis* 179:259-266, 1991.

Wing JK, Cooper JE, Sartorius N: *Measurement and classification of psychiatric symptoms: an instruction manual for the present state examination and CATEGO program,* Cambridge, 1974, Cambridge Press.

Wong DF et al: Positron emission tomography reveals elevated D_2 dopamine receptors in drug-naive schizophrenics, *Science* 234:1558, 1986.

World Health Organization: *Report on the International Pilot Study of Schizophrenia,* Geneva, 1973, World Health Organization.

Wyatt RJ, Kirch DG, DeLisi LE: *Schizophrenia: biochemical, endocrine, and immunological studies.* In Kaplan HI, Sadock BJ, editors: *Comprehensive textbook of psychiatry/V,* Baltimore, 1989, Williams and Wilkins.

Wyatt RJ et al: Schizophrenia, just the facts: what do we know, how well do we know it? *Schizophr Res* 1:1, 1988.

Yesavage JA: Correlates of dangerous behavior by schizophrenics in hospital, *J Psychiatr Res* 18:225, 1984.

Zubin J, Magaziner J, Steinhauer SR: The metamorphosis of schizophrenia: from chronicity to vulnerability, *Psychol Med* 13:551-571, 1983.

Chapter 14

Anglin MD, Hser Y, Booth MW: Sex differences in addict careers, *Am J Drug Alcohol Abuse* 13:253-280, 1994.

Anton RF: *Pharmacology of alcohol withdrawal: an update,* Miami, 1995, Annual Meeting of the American Psychiatric Association.

Babor TF: *Alcohol: customs and rituals,* London, 1988 Burke Publishing.

Babor TF et al: *Audit: the Alcohol Use Disorders Identification Test: guidelines for use in primary health care,* Geneva, 1992, World Health Organization Programme on Substance Abuse.

Bohman M, Sigvardsson S, Cloninger CR: Maternal inheritance of alcohol abuse: cross-fostering analysis of adopted women, *Arch Gen Psychiatry* 38:965-969, 1981.

Cadoret RJ, Cain CA, Grove WM: Development of alcoholism in adoptees raised apart from alcohol biologic relatives, *Arch Gen Psychiatry* 37:561-563, 1979.

Cadoret RJ, Troughton E, O'Gorman TW: Genetic and environmental factors in alcohol abuse and antisocial personality, *J Stud Alcohol* 48:1-8, 1987.

Cloninger CR, Bohman M, Sigvardsson S: Inheritance of alcohol abuse: cross-fostering analysis of adopted men, *Arch Gen Psychiatry* 36:861-868, 1981.

Compton WM et al: Inhalant use: characteristics and predictors, *Am J Addictions* 3:263-272, 1994.

Compton WM et al: Is antisocial personality disorder associated with increased HIV risk behaviors in cocaine users? *Drug Alcohol Depend* 37:37-37-43, 1995.

Cotton NS: The familial incidence of alcoholism: a review, *J Stud Alcohol* 40:89-116, 1979.

D'Aunno T, Vaughn TE: Variations in methadone treatment practices: results from a national study. *JAMA* 267:253-258, 1992.

Edwards G et al: Alcohol-related disabilities, Geneva, 1977, World Health Organization.

Goodwin DW: Alcoholism and genetics: the sins of the fathers, *Arch Gen Psychiatry* 42:171-174, 1985.

Goodwin DW, Crane JB, Guze SB: Felons who drink: an 8-year follow-up, *Q J Stud Alcohol* 32:136-147, 1971.

Goodwin DW et al: Alcohol problems in adoptees raised apart from alcoholic biological parents, *Arch Gen Psychiatry* 28:238-243, 1973.

Grove WM et al: Heritability of substance abuse and antisocial personality of monozygotic twins reared apart, *Biol Psychiatry* 27:1293-1304, 1990.

Guze SB: Why psychiatry is a branch of medicine, New York, 1992, Oxford University Press.

Helzer JE et al: The extent of long-term moderate drinking among alcoholics discharged from medical and psychiatric treatment facilities, *N Engl J Med* 312:1678-1682, 1985.

Helzer JE et al: Alcoholism: North America and Asia, *Arch Gen Psychiatry* 47:313-319, 1990.

Hrubec Z, Omenn GS: Evidence of genetic predisposition to alcoholic cirrhosis and psychosis: twin concordances for alcoholism and its biological end points by zygosity among male veterans, *Alcohol Clin Exp Res* 5:207-215, 1981.

Hyman MM: Alcoholics 15 years later, *Ann NY Acad Sci* 273:613-623, 1976.

Jellinek EM: Phases of alcohol addiction, *Q J Stud Alcohol* 13:673-684, 1952.

Jellinek EM: *The disease concept of alcoholism,* New Haven, Conn., 1960, College and University Press.

Kaij L: *Studies on the etiology and sequels of abuse of alcohol,* Lund, Sweden, 1960, University of Lund.

Keller M: On defining alcoholism: with comment on some other relevant words. In *Alcohol, science and society revisited,* Ann Arbor, Mich., 1982, University of Michigan Press.

Kendler KS et al: A population-based twin study of alcoholism in women, *JAMA* 268:1877-1882, 1992.

Kessler RC et al: Lifetime and 12-month prevalence of DSM-III-R psychiatric disorders in the United States, *Arch Gen Psychiatry* 51:8-19, 1994.

Kranzler HR: *Serotonergic agonists in alcoholism treatment,* Miami, 1995, Annual Meeting of the American Psychiatric Association.

Liebman JM, Cooper SJ, editors: *The neuropharmacological basis of reward,* Oxford, 1989, Oxford University Press.

O'Malley SS et al: Naltrexone and coping skills therapy for alcohol dependence, *Arch Gen Psychiatry* 49:881-887, 1992.

Pemberton DA: A comparison of the outcome of treatment in female and male alcoholics, *Brit J Psychiatry* 113:367-373, 1967.

Pickens RW et al: Heterogeneity in the inheritance of alcoholism, *Arch Gen Psychiatry* 48:19-28, 1991.

Regier DA et al: Comorbidity of mental disorders with alcohol and other drug abuse, *JAMA* 264:2511-2518, 1990.

Robins LN: Vietnam veterans' rapid recovery from heroin addiction: a fluke or normal expectation? *Addiction* 88:1041-1054, 1993.

Robins LN, Regier DA, editors: *Psychiatric disorders in America,* New York, 1991, The Free Press.

Robins LN et al: NIMH diagnostic interview schedule: version III, Rockville, Md, 1981, National Institute of Mental Health.

Rouche B: *Alcohol,* New York, 1960, Grove Press.

Saitz R et al: Individualized treatment for alcohol withdrawal, *JAMA* 272:519-523, 1994.

Schuckit MA: Drug and alcohol abuse, New York, 1989, Plenum Press.

Skinner HA: A multivariate evaluation of the MAST, *J Stud Alcohol* 40:831-844, 1979.

Skinner HA: The drug abuse screening test, *Addictive Behav* 7:363-371, 1982.

Spragg SDS: Morphine addiction in chimpanzees, *Comp Psychol Monogr* 15:1-132, 1940.

Sullivan JT et al: Assessment of alcohol withdrawal: the revised clinical institute withdrawal assessment for alcohol scale (CIWA-Ar), *Br J Addic* 84:1353-1357, 1989.

Vaillant GE: A 20-year follow-up of New York narcotic addicts, *Arch Gen Psych* 19:237-241, 1973.

Vaillant GE: *The natural history of alcoholism: causes, patterns, and paths to recovery,* Cambridge, Mass, 1983, Harvard University Press.

Volpicelli JR et al: Naltrexone in the treatment of alcohol dependence, *Arch Gen Psychiatry* 49:876-880, 1992.

Warner LA et al: Prevalence and correlates of drug use and dependence in the United States: results from the National Comorbidity Survey, *Arch Gen Psychiatry* 52:219-229, 1995.

Chapter 15

American Dietetic Association: Position on nutrition intervention in the treatment of anorexia nervosa, bulimia nervosa, and binge eating, *J Am Diet Assoc* 94:902-907, 1994.

American Psychiatric Association: *Diagnostic and statistical manual of mental disorders,* ed 4, Washington, D.C., 1994, American Psychiatric Association.

American Psychiatric Association: Practice guideline for eating disorders, *Am J Psychiatry* 150:207-228, 1993.

Antony MM et al: Psychopathology correlates of binge eating and binge eating disorder, *Compr Psychiatry* 35:85-92, 1994.

Bliss EL, Branch CHH: *Anorexia nervosa: its history, psychology, and biology,* New York, 1960, Hoeber.

Brewerton TD et al: β-Endorphin and dynorphin in bulimia nervosa, *Am J Psychiatry* 149:1086-1090, 1992.

Bruch H: *Eating disorders: obesity, anorexia nervosa, and the person within,* New York, 1973, Basic Books.

Cariem AK et al: Severe hypophosphataemia in anorexia nervosa, *Postgrad Med J* 70:825-827, 1994.

Collings S, King M: Ten-year follow-up of 50 patients with bulimia nervosa, *Br J Psychiatry* 164:80-87, 1994.

Dally P: *Anorexia nervosa,* New York, 1969, Grune and Stratton.

De Simone G et al: Cardiac abnormalities in young women with anorexia nervosa, *Br Heart J* 71:287-292, 1994.

Deter HC, Herzog W: Anorexia nervosa in a long-term perspective: results of the Heidelberg-Mannheim Study, *Psychosom Med* 56:20-27, 1994.

Drewnowski A et al: Eating pathology and DSM-III-R bulimia nervosa: a continuum of behavior, *Am J Psychiatry* 151:1217-1219, 1994.

Ferguson JM: The use of electroconvulsive therapy in patients with intractable anorexia nervosa, *Int J Eat Disord* 13:195-201, 1993.

Giannini AJ, Slaby AE, editors: *The eating disorders,* New York, 1993, Springer-Verlag.

Gillberg IC, Rastam M, Gillberg C: Anorexia nervosa outcome: six-year controlled longitudinal study of 51 cases including a population cohort, *J Am Acad Child Adolesc Psychiatry* 33:729-739, 1994.

Goldbloom DS, Olmsted MP: Pharmacotherapy of bulimia nervosa with fluoxetine: assessment of clinically significant attitudinal change, *Am J Psychiatry* 150:770-774, 1993.

Greenfeld D et al: Hypokalemia in outpatients with eating disorders, *Am J Psychiatry* 152:60-63, 1995.

Gull W: Anorexia nervosa, *Lancet* 1:516-517, 1888.

Halmi KA, editor: *Psychobiology and treatment of anorexia nervosa and bulimia nervosa,* Washington, D.C., 1992, American Psychiatric Press.

Haus G et al: Key modifiable factors in weight maintenance: fat intake, exercise, and weight cycling, *J Am Diet Assoc* 94:409-413, 1994.

Holden JH et al: Long-term follow-up of patients attending a combination very-low calorie diet and behaviour therapy weight loss programme, *Int J Obes Relat Metab Disord* 16:605-613, 1992.

Holderness CC, Brooks-Gunn J, Warren MP: Co-morbidity of eating disorders and substance abuse review of the literature, *Int J Eat Disord* 16:1-34, 1994.

Hsu LKG, Lee S: Is weight phobia always necessary for a diagnosis of anorexia nervosa? *Am J Psychiatry* 150:1466-1471, 1993.

Jimerson DC et al: Low serotonin and dopamine metabolite concentrations in cerebrospinal fluid from bulimic patients with frequent binge episodes, *Arch Gen Psychiatry* 49:132-138, 1992.

Kalodner CR, DeLucia JL: The individual and combined effects of cognitive therapy and nutrition education as additions to a behavior modification program for weight loss, *Addict Behav* 16:255-263, 1991.

Kaplan AS, Garfinkel PE, editors: *Medical issues and the eating disorders: the interface,* New York, 1993, Brunner/Mazel.

Kendler KS et al: The genetic epidemiology of bulimia nervosa, *Am J Psychiatry* 148:1627-1637, 1991.

Kennedy SH: Melatonin disturbances in anorexia nervosa and bulimia nervosa, *Int J Eat Disord* 16:257-265, 1994.

Kuehnel RH, Wadden TA: Binge eating disorder, weight cycling, and psychopathology, *Int J Eat Disord* 15:321-329, 1994.

Laségue C: De l'anorexie hystérique, *Archives Générales de Médecine* 1:385-403, 1873.

Lydiard RB et al: CSF cholecystokinin octapeptide in patients with bulimia nervosa and in normal comparison subjects, *Am J Psychiatry* 150:1099-1101, 1993.

Marcé LV: On a form of hypochondriacal delirium occurring consecutive to dyspepsia, and characterized by refusal of food, *J Psychol Med Ment Pathol* 13:264-266, 1860.

Olmsted MP, Kaplan AS, Rockert W: Rate and prediction of relapse in bulimia nervosa, *Am J Psychiatry* 151:738-743, 1994.

Pagsberg AK, Wang AR: Epidemiology of anorexia nervosa and bulimia nervosa in Bornholm County, Denmark, 1970-1989, *Acta Psychiatr Scand* 90:259-265, 1994.

Pera V, Clark MM, Abrams DB: Current treatment of obesity: a behavioral medicine perspective, *R I Med* 75:477-481, 1992.

Rastam M: Anorexia nervosa in 51 Swedish adolescents: premorbid problems and comorbidity, *J Am Acad Child Adolesc Psychiatry* 31:819-829, 1992.

Russell GFM: Bulimia nervosa: an ominous variant of anorexia nervosa, *Psychol Med* 9:429-449, 1979.

Sharp CW et al: Clinical presentation of anorexia nervosa in males: 24 new cases, *Int J Eat Disord* 15:125-134, 1994.

Schork EJ, Eckert ED, Halmi KA: The relationship between psychopathology, eating disorder diagnosis, and clinical outcome at 10-year follow-up in anorexia nervosa, *Compr Psychiatry* 35:113-123, 1994.

Silber TJ: Eating disorders and health insurance, *Arch Pediatr Adolesc Med* 148:785-788, 1994.

Spitzer RL et al: Binge eating disorder: its further validation in a multisite study, *Int J Eat Disord* 13:137-153, 1993.

Stunkard AJ: Eating patterns and obesity, *J Behav Ther Exp Psychiatry* 12:333-336, 1959.

Theander S: Anorexia nervosa: a psychiatric investigation of 94 female patients, *Acta Psychiatr Scand Suppl* 214:1-94, 1970.

Theil A et al: Obsessive-compulsive disorder among patients with anorexia nervosa and bulimia nervosa, *Am J Psychiatry* 152:72-75, 1995.

Wallin MS, Rissanen AM: Food and mood: relationship between food, serotonin and affective disorders, *Acta Psychiatr Scand Suppl* 377:36-40, 1994.

Walters EE, Kendler KS: Anorexia nervosa and anorexic-like syndromes in a population-based female twin sample, *Am J Psychiatry* 152:64-71, 1995.

Wolfe BL: Long-term maintenance following attainment of goal weight: a preliminary investigation, *Addict Behav* 17:469-477, 1992.

Yanovski SZ et al: Association of binge eating disorder and psychiatric comorbidity in obese subjects, *Am J Psychiatry* 150:1472-1479, 1993.

Chapter 16

Abbey SE, Garfinkel PE: Neurasthenia and chronic fatigue syndrome: the role of culture in the making of a diagnosis, *Am J Psychiatry* 148:1638-1646, 1991.

Bass C, Benjamen S: The management of chronic somatization, *Br J Psychiatry* 162:472-480, 1993.

Bibb RC, Guze SB: Hysteria (Briquet's syndrome) in a psychiatric hospital: the significance of secondary depression, *Am J Psychiatry* 129:224-228, 1972.

Black DW: Somatoform disorders, *Prim Care* 14:711-723, 1987.

Boffeli TJ, Guze SB: The simulation of neurologic disease, *Psychiatr Clin North Am* 15:301-310, 1992.

Brown FW, Golding JM, Smith GR Jr: Psychiatric comorbidity in primary care somatization disorder, *Psychosom Med* 52:445-451, 1990.

Brown FW, Smith GR Jr: Somatization disorder in general medical settings, *Psychiatr Ann* 18:353-356, 1988.

Brown FW, Smith GR Jr: Diagnostic concordance in primary care somatization disorder, *Psychosomatics* 32:191-195, 1991.

Cadoret RJ: Psychopathology in adopted-away offspring of biologic parents with antisocial behavior, *Arch Gen Psychiatry* 35:176-184, 1978.

Cadoret RJ et al: Studies of adoptees from psychiatrically disturbed biological parents. III. Medical symptoms and illnesses in childhood and adolescence, *Am J Psychiatry* 133:1316-1318, 1976.

Cloninger CR, Guze SB: Psychiatric illness and female criminality: the role of sociopathy and hysteria in the antisocial woman, *Am J Psychiatry* 127:303-311, 1970.

Cloninger CR, Reich T, Guze SB: The multifactorial model of disease transmission. II. Sex differences in the familial transmission of sociopathy (antisocial personality), *Br J Psychiatry* 127:11-12, 1975.

Cloninger CR et al: A prospective follow-up and family study of somatization in men and women, *Am J Psychiatry* 143:873-878, 1986.

Creed F, Guthrie E: Techniques for interviewing the somatizing patient, *Br J Psychiatry* 162:467-471, 1993.

deGruy F et al: Somatization disorder in a family practice, *J Fam Pract* 25:579-584, 1987.

DeSouza C et al: Major depression and somatization disorder: the overlooked differential diagnosis, *Psychiatr Ann* 18:340-348, 1988.

Engel GL: *Conversion symptoms.* In MacBryde CM editor: *Signs and symptoms: applied pathologic physiology and clinical interpretation,* ed 5, Philadelphia, 1970, Lippincott.

Ford CV, Folks DG: Conversion disorders: an overview, *Psychosomatics* 26:371-373, 1985.

Gatfield PD, Guze SB: Prognosis and differential diagnosis of conversion reactions (a follow-up study), *Dis Nerv Sys* 23:1-8, 1962.

Guze SB: The diagnosis of hysteria: what are we trying to do? *Am J Psychiatry* 124:77-84, 1967.

Guze SB: The role of follow-up studies: their contribution to diagnostic classification as applied to hysteria, *Semin Psychiatry* 2:392-402, 1970.

Guze SB: The validity and significance of the clinical diagnosis of hysteria (Briquet's syndrome), *Am J Psychiatry* 132:138-141, 1975.

Guze SB: Genetics of Briquet's syndrome and somatization disorder, *Ann Clin Psychiatry* 5:225-230, 1993.

Guze SB, Perley MJ: Observations on the natural history of hysteria, *Am J Psychiatry* 119:960-965, 1963.

Guze SB, Woodruff RA, Clayton PJ: Hysteria and antisocial behavior: further evidence of an association, *Am J Psychiatry* 127:133-136, 1971.

Guze SB, Woodruff RA, Clayton PJ: A study of conversion symptoms in psychiatric outpatients, *Am J Psychiatry* 128:135-138, 1971.

Guze SB, et al: A follow-up and family study of Briquet's syndrome, *Br J Psychiatry* 149:17-23, 1986.

Holt RE, LeCann AF: Use of an integrative interview to manage somatization, *Psychosomatics* 25:663-665; 668-669, 1984.

Lazare A: *Hysteria.* In Hackett TP, Cassem NH, editors: *Massachusetts General Hospital handbook of general hospital psychiatry,* St. Louis, 1978, Mosby.

Lazare A: Conversion symptoms, *N Engl J Med* 305:745-748, 1981.

Lipowski ZJ: Somatization: the concept and its clinical application, *Am J Psychiatry* 145:1358-1368, 1988.

Liskow B et al: Is Briquet's syndrome a heterogeneous disorder? *Am J Psychiatry* 143:626-629, 1986.

Ljungberg L: Hysteria, a clinical, prognostic, and genetic study, *Acta Psychiatr Neurol Scand Suppl* 112:1-62, 1957.

Mai FM, Merskey H: Briquet's treatise on hysteria, *Arch Gen Psychiatry* 37:1401-1405, 1980.

Martin RL: Problems in the diagnosis of somatization disorder: effects on research and clinical practice, *Psychiatr Ann* 18:357-362, 1988.

Martin RL et al: Excessive surgery in hysteria, *JAMA* 151:977-986, 1953.

Monson RA, Smith GR Jr: Somatization disorder in primary care, *N Engl J Med* 308:1464-1465, 1983.

Morrison JR: Management of Briquet syndrome (hysteria), *West J Med* 128:482-487, 1978.

Morrison JR: Managing depression in a woman with somatization disorder, *Ann Clin Psychiatry* 1:255-257, 1989.

Murphy GE: The clinical management of hysteria, *J Am Med Assoc* 247:2559-2564, 1982.

North CS et al: *Multiple personalities, multiple disorders: psychiatric classification and media influence,* New York, 1993, Oxford University Press.

Othmer E: Somatization disorder, *Psychiatr Ann* 18:330-331, 1988.

Pendergrast M: *Victims of memory: incest accusations and shattered lives,* Hinesburg, Vt., 1995, Upper Access Books.

Pennebaker JW, Watson D: The psychology of somatic symptoms. In Kirmayer LJ, Robbins JM, editors: *Current concepts of somatization: research and clinical perspectives,* Washington, D.C., 1991, American Psychiatric Press.

Perley MJ, Guze SB: Hysteria: the stability and usefulness of clinical criteria, *N Engl J Med* 266:421-426, 1962.

Purtell JJ, Robins E, Cohen ME: Observations on clinical aspects of hysteria, *JAMA* 146:902-909, 1951.

Quill TE: Somatization disorder: one of medicine's blind spots, *JAMA* 252:3075-3079, 1985.

Rost KM et al: The comorbidity of DSM-III-R personality disorders in somatization disorder, *Gen Hosp Psychiatry* 14:322-326, 1992.

Simon GE, VonKorff M: Somatization and psychiatric disorder in the NIMH epidemiologic catchment area study, *Am J Psychiatry* 148:1494-1500, 1991.

Smith GR Jr: The epidemiology and treatment of depression when it coexists with somatoform disorders, somatization or pain, *Gen Hosp Psychiatry* 14:265-272, 1992.

Smith GR Jr: The course of somatization and its effects on utilization of health care resources, *Psychosomatics* 35:263-267, 1994.

Smith GR Jr, Miller LM, Monson RA: Consultation-liaison intervention in somatization disorder, *Hosp Commun Psychiatry* 37:1207-1210, 1986.

Smith GR Jr, Monson RA, Livingston RL: Somatization disorder in men, *Gen Hosp Psychiatry* 7:4-8, 1985.

Smith GR Jr, Monson RA, Ray DC: Psychiatric consultation in somatization disorder, *N Engl J Med* 314:1407-1413, 1986.

Stewart DE: The changing faces of somatization, *Psychosomatics* 31:153-158, 1990.

Swartz M et al: Somatization disorder. In Robins LN, Regier DA, editors: *Psychiatric disorders in America: the epidemiologic catchment area study,* New York, 1991, The Free Press.

Tomasson K, Kent D, Coryell W: Somatization and conversion disorders: comorbidity and demographics at presentation, *Acta Psychiatr Scand* 84:288-293, 1991.

Torgerson S: Genetics of somatoform disorders, *Arch Gen Psychiatry* 43:502-505, 1986.

Wetzel RD et al: Briquet's syndrome (hysteria) is both a somatoform and a "psychoform" illness: a Minnesota Multiphasic Personality Inventory study, *Psychosom Med* 56:564-569, 1994.

Woerner PI, Guze SB: A family and marital study of hysteria, *Br J Psychiatry* 114:161-168, 1968.

Woodruff RA, Clayton PJ, Guze SB: Hysteria: studies of diagnosis, outcome, and prevalence, *JAMA* 215:425-428, 1971.

Young SJ et al: Psychiatric illness and the irritable bowel syndrome, *Gastroenterology* 70:162-166, 1976.

Zoccolillo M, Cloninger CR: Somatization disorder: psychologic symptoms, social disability and diagnosis, *Compr Psychiatry* 27:65-73, 1986.

Chapter 17

Aduan RP et al: Factitious fever and self-induced infection: a report of 32 cases and review of the literature, *Ann Intern Med* 90:230-242, 1979.

Asher R: Munchausen's syndrome, *Lancet* 1:339-341, 1951.

Barker JC: The syndrome of hospital addiction (Munchausen syndrome): a report on the investigation of seven cases, *J Ment Sci* 108:167-182, 1962.

Bliss EL: Multiple personalities: a report of 14 cases with implications for schizophrenia and hysteria, *Arch Gen Psychiatry* 37:1388-1397, 1980.

Bliss EL: *Multiple personality, allied disorders, and hypnosis,* New York, 1986, Oxford University Press.

Bowers MK, Brecher-Marer S, Newton BW: Therapy of multiple personality, *Int J Clin Exp Hypn* 19:57-65, 1971.

Braun BG: Hypnosis creates multiple personality: myth or reality? *Int J Clin Exp Hypn* 32:191-197, 1984.

Braun BG: Towards a theory of multiple personality and other dissociative phenomena, *Psychiatr Clin North Am* 7:171-193, 1984.

Bursten B: On Munchausen's syndrome, *Arch Gen Psychiatry* 13:261-268, 1965.

Carney MWP: Artefactual illness to attract medical attention, *Br J Psychiatry* 136:542-547, 1980.

Chapman JS: Peregrination problem patients—Munchausen's syndrome, *JAMA* 165:927-933, 1957.

Clarke E, Melnick SC: The Munchausen syndrome or the problem of hospital hoboes, *Am J Med* 25:6-12, 1958.

Coons PM: Multiple personality: diagnostic considerations, *J Clin Psychiatry* 41:330-336, 1980.

Coons PM: The differential diagnosis of multiple personality: a comprehensive review, *Psychiatr Clin North Am* 7:51-67, 1984.

Coons PM: The prevalence of multiple personality disorder, *Newsletter International Society of Study of Multiple Personality Dissociation* 4:6-7, 1986.

Coons PM, Bowman ES, Milstein V: Multiple personality disorder: a clinical investigation of 50 cases, *J Nerv Ment Dis* 175:519-527, 1988.

Coryell W: Single case study: multiple personality and primary affective disorder, *J Nerv Ment Dis* 171:388-390, 1983.

Cutler B, Reed J: Multiple personality: a single case study with a 15-year follow-up, *Psychol Med* 5:18-26, 1975.

Decker HS: The lure of nonmaterialism in materialist Europe: Investigations of dissociative phenomena, 1880-1915. In Quen JM, editor: *Split minds/split brains: historical and current perspectives,* New York, 1986, New York University Press.

Dinwiddie SH, North CS, Yutzy SH: Multiple personality disorder: scientific and medicolegal issues, *Bull Am Acad Psychiatry Law* 21:69-79, 1993.

Eisendrath SJ: *Factitious disorder with physical symptoms.* In American Psychiatric Association: *Treatments of psychiatric disorders: a task force report of the American Psychiatric Association,* Washington, D.C., 1989, American Psychiatric Press.

Enoch MD, Trethowan WH: *Uncommon psychiatric syndromes,* ed 2, Bristol, England, 1979, John Wright and Sons.

Fahy TA, Abas M, Brown JC: Multiple personality: a symptom of psychiatric disorder, *Br J Psychiatry* 154:99-101, 1989.

Feighner JP et al: Diagnostic criteria for use in psychiatric research, *Arch Gen Psychiatry* 26:57-62, 1972.

Ford CV: The Munchausen syndrome: a report of four new cases and a review of psychodynamic considerations, *Int J Psychiatry Med* 4:31-45, 1973.

Fras I, Coughlin BE: The treatment of factitial disease, *Psychosomatics* 12:117-122, 1971.

Ganaway GK: Historical versus narrative truth: clarifying the role of exogenous trauma in the etiology of MPD and its variants, *Dissociation* 2:205-220, 1989.

Gorman CA, Wahner HW, Tauxe WN: Metabolic malingerers: patients who deliberately induce or perpetrate a hypermetabolic or hypometabolic state, *Am J Med* 48:708-714, 1970.

Greaves GB: Multiple personality: 165 years after Mary Reynolds, *J Nerv Ment Dis* 168:577-596, 1980.

Gruenewald D: Multiple personality and splitting phenomena: a reconceptualization, *J Nerv Ment Dis* 164:385-393, 1977.

Hacking I: Two souls in one body, *Crit Inquir* 17:838-867, 1991.

Hawkings JR et al: Deliberate disability, *Br Med J* 1:361-367, 1956.

Hollender MH, Hersh SP: Impossible consultation made possible, *Arch Gen Psychiatry* 23:343-345, 1970.

Horevitz RP, Braun BG: Are multiple personalities borderline? An analysis of 33 cases, *Psychiatr Clin North Am* 7:69-87, 1984.

Ireland P, Sapira JD, Templeton B: Munchausen's syndrome: review and report of an additional case, *Am J Med* 43:579-592, 1967.

Jonas JM, Pope HG: The dissimulating disorders: a single diagnostic entity? *Compr Psychiatry* 26:58-62, 1985.

Kasl SV, Chisholm RE, Eskenazi B: The impact of the accident at Three Mile Island on the behavior and well-being of nuclear workers, *Am J Pub Health* 71:472-495, 1981.

Kluft RP: Varieties of hypnotic interventions in the treatment of multiple personality, *Am J Clin Hypn* 24:230-240, 1982.

Kluft RP: An introduction to multiple personality disorder, *Psychiatr Ann* 14:19-24, 1984.

Kluft RP: Treatment of multiple personality disorder: a study of 33 cases, *Psychiatr Clin North Am* 7:9-29, 1984.

Kluft RP: Making the diagnosis of multiple personality disorder (MPD), *Dir Psychiatry,* 5:1-12, 1985.

Kluft RP: The postunification treatment of multiple personality disorder: first findings, *Am J Psychother* 42:212-228, 1988.

Kluft RP: Clinical presentations of multiple personality disorder, *Psychiatr Clin North Am* 14:605-629, 1991.

Kohlenberg RJ: Behavioristic approach to multiple personality: a case study, *Behav Ther* 4:137-140, 1973.

Meadow R: Munchausen's syndrome by proxy: the hinterland of child abuse, *Lancet* 2:343-345, 1977.

Nadelson T: The Munchausen spectrum: borderline character features, *Gen Hosp Psychiatry* 1:11-17, 1979.

Pankratz L: A review of the Munchausen syndrome, *Clin Psychol Rev* 1:65-78, 1981.

Patterson R: The Münchausen syndrome: Baron von Münchausen has taken a bum rap, *Can Med Assoc J* 139:566-569, 1988.

Piper A Jr: Treatment for multiple personality disorder: at what cost? *Am J Psychother* 48:392-400, 1994.

Putnam FW: The scientific investigation of multiple personality disorder. In Quen JM, editor: *Split minds/split brains: historical and current perspectives,* New York, 1986, New York University Press.

Putnam FW: *Diagnosis and treatment of multiple personality disorder,* New York, 1989, Guilford Press.

Putnam FW: Recent research on multiple personality disorder, *Psychiatr Clin North Am* 14:489-502, 1991.

Putnam FW et al: The clinical phenomenology of multiple personality disorder: review of 100 recent cases, *J Clin Psychiatry* 47:285-293, 1986.

Raspe RE et al: *Singular travels, campaigns and adventures of Baron Munchausen,* London, 1948, Cresset Press.

Reich P, Gottfried LA: Factitious disorders in a teaching hospital, *Ann Intern Med* 99:240-247, 1983.

Robins E, Guze SB: Establishment of diagnostic validity in psychiatric illness: its application to schizophrenia, *Am J Psychiatry* 126:983-987, 1970.

Rosenberg DA: Web of deceit: a literature review of Munchausen syndrome by proxy, *Child Abuse Negl* 11:547-563, 1987.

Ross CA: *Multiple personality disorder: diagnosis, clinical features, and treatment,* New York, 1989, Wiley.

Ross CA: Epidemiology of multiple personality disorder and dissociation, *Psychiatr Clin North Am* 14:503-517, 1991.

Ross CA, Miller SD, Reagor P: Structured interview data on 102 cases of multiple personality from four centers, *Am J Psychiatry* 147:596-601, 1990.

Roth M: The desire to be ill, *Univ Durham Med Gaz* 57:1-18, 1962.

Saltman V, Solomon RS: Incest and the multiple personality, *Psychol Rep* 50:1127-1141, 1982.

Serban G: Multiple personality: an issue for forensic psychiatry, *Am J Psychother* 46:269-280, 1992.

Sergi JS, Murray M, Cotanch PH: An understudied population: the homeless, *Oncol Nurs Forum* 16:113-114, 1989.

Simpson MA: Multiple personality disorder (letter), *J Nerv Ment Dis* 176:535, 1988.

Sneed RC, Bell RF: The dauphin of Munchausen: factitious passage of renal stones in a child, *Pediatrics* 58:127-130, 1976.

Spanos NP, Weekes JR, Bertrand LD: Multiple personality: a social psychological perspective, *J Abnorm Psychol* 94:362-376, 1985.

Spiegel D: Multiple personality as a post-traumatic stress disorder, *Psychiatr Clin North Am* 7:101-110, 1984.

Spiro HR: Chronic factitious illness: Munchausen's syndrome, *Arch Gen Psychiatry* 18:569-579, 1968.

Stafne WA, Moe AE: Hypoprothrombinemia due to Dicumarol in a malingerer: a case report, *Ann Intern Med* 35:910-911, 1951.

Stone MH: Factitious illness: psychological findings and treatment recommendations, *Bull Menninger Clin* 41:239-254, 1977.

Taylor WS, Martin MF: Multiple personality, *J Abnorm Soc Psychol* 39:281-300, 1944.

Thigpen CH, Cleckley HM: On the incidence of multiple personality disorder: a brief communication, *Int J Clin Exp Hypn* 32:63-66, 1984.

Wallach J: Laboratory diagnosis of factitious disorders, *Arch Intern Med* 154:1690-1696, 1994.

Chapter 18

American Psychiatric Association: *Diagnostic and statistical Manual of mental disorders,* ed 4 (DSM-IV), Washington, D.C., 1994, American Psychiatric Press Inc.

Cloninger CR: *Antisocial behavior.* In Smith-Grahame DG, Hippius H, Winokur G, editors: *Psychopharmacology,* vol 1, Amsterdam, 1983, Excerpta Medica.

Cloninger CR: A systematic method for clinical description and classification of personality variants, *Arch Gen Psychiatry* 44:573, 1987.

Cloninger CR, Svrakic DM, Przybeck TR: A psychobiological model of temperament and character, *Arch Gen Psychiatry* 50:975, 1993.

Cloninger CR et al: Predisposition to petty criminality in Swedish adoptees. II. Cross-fostering analysis of gene-environment interaction, *Arch Gen Psychiatry* 39:1242, 1982.

Cowdry RW: Psychopharmacology of borderline personality disorder: a review, *J Clin Psychiatry* 48(Suppl):15-22, 1987.

Cowdry RW, Gardner DL: Pharmacotherapy of borderline personality disorder, *Arch Gen Psychiatry* 45:111-119, 1988.

Deltito J, Stam M: Psychopharmacological treatment of avoidant personality disorder, *Compr Psychiatry* 30:498-504, 1989.

Derksen J: Personality disorders: clinical and social perspectives, New York, 1995, John Wiley and Sons.

Ekselius L: Personality disorders in the DSM-III-R, *Acta Univ Uppsala,* Dissertation 484, 1994.

Faltus FJ: The positive effects of alprazolam in the treatment of three patients with borderline personality disorder, *Am J Psychiatry* 141:802-803, 1984.

Gardner DL, Cowdry RW: Pharmacotherapy of borderline personality disorder: an overview, *Psychopharmacol Bull* 25:515-523, 1989.

Heath AC, Cloninger CR, Martin NG: Testing a model for the genetic structure of personality: a comparison of the personality systems of Cloninger and Eysenck, *J Pers Soc Psychology* 66:762, 1994.

Heatherton TF, Weinberger JL, editors: Can personality change? Washington, D.C., 1994, American Psychological Press.

Hedberg DL, Houck JH, Glueck BC: Tranylcypromine-trifluoperazine combination in the treatment of schizophrenia, *Am J Psychiatry* 127:1141-1146, 1971.

Joyce PR, Mulder RT, Cloninger CR: Temperament and hypercortisolemia in depression, *Am J Psychiatry* 151:195, 1994.

Joyce PR, Mulder RT, Cloninger CR: Temperament predicts clomipramine and desipramine response in major depression, *J Affect Disord* 30:35, 1994.

Klar H, Siever L: The psychopharmacologic treatment of personality disorders, *Psychiatr Clin North Am* 7:791-801, 1984.

Klein D: Psychiatric diagnosis and a typology of clinical drug effects, *Psychopharmacologia* 13:359-386, 1968.

Klein D et al: *Clinical management of affective disorders.* In Klein D, Davis J, editors: *Diagnosis and drug treatment of psychiatric disorders,* Baltimore, 1980, Williams and Wilkins.

Liebowitz MR: Discussions arising from Cloninger CR: a unified biosocial model of personality and its role in the development of anxiety states, *Psychiatric Developments* 4:385-387, 1987.

Liebowitz M, Klein D: Hysteroid dysphoria, *Psychiatr Clin North Am* 2:555-575, 1979.

Liebowitz M et al: Phenelzine in social phobias, *J Clin Psychopharmacol* 6:93-98, 1986.

Liebowitz M et al: Pharmacotherapy of social phobia: an interim report of a placebo-controlled comparison of phenelzine and atenolol, *J Clin Psychiatry* 49:252-257, 1988.

Links P et al: Lithium therapy for borderline patients: preliminary findings, *Journal of Personality Disorders* 4(3):173-181, 1990.

Menza MA et al: Dopamine-related personality traits in Parkinson's disease, *Neurology* 43:505, 1993.

Myers JK, Weissman MM: Use of a self-report symptom scale to detect depression in a community sample, *Am J Psychiatry* 137:1081, 1980.

Nelson EC, Cloninger CR: The tridimensional personality questionnaire as a predictor of response to nefazodone treatment of depression, *J Affect Disord* 35:51-57, 1995.

Nelson EC et al: Platelet serotonergic markers and tridimensional personality questionnaire measures in a clinical sample, *Biol Psychiatry* (in press).

Norden MJ: Fluoxetine in borderline personality disorder, *Prog Neuropsychopharmacol Biol Psychiatry* 13:885-893, 1989.

Parsons B et al: Phenelzine, imipramine, and placebo in borderline patients meeting criteria for atypical depression, *Psychopharmacol Bull* 25:524-534, 1989.

Radloff LS: The CES-D scale: a self-report depression scale for research in the general population, *Appl Psychol Meas* 1:385, 1977.

Reich J, Yates W: A pilot study of treatment of social phobia with alprazolam, *Am J Psychiatry* 145:590-594, 1988.

Reyntjens AM: A Series of multicentric pilot trials with pimozide in psychiatric practice. I. Pimozide in treatment of personality disorders, *Acta Psychiatr Belg* 72:653-661, 1972.

Rifkin A et al: Lithium carbonate in emotionally unstable character disorders, *Arch Gen Psychiatry* 27:519-523, 1972.

Robins L: *Deviant children grown up: a sociological and psychiatric study of sociopathic personality,* Baltimore, 1966, Williams and Wilkins.

Selzer ML, Vinokur A, van Rooijen L: A self-administered short Michigan alcoholism screening test (SMAST), *J Stud Alcohol* 36:117, 1975.

Sheard MH: Lithium in the treatment of aggression, *J Nerv Ment Dis* 160:108-112, 1976.

Sheard MH et al: The effect of lithium on impulsive aggressive behavior in man, *Am J Psychiatry* 133:1409-1412, 1976.

Sheehan DV, Ballenger J, Jacobson G: Treatment of endogenous anxiety with phobic hysterical and hypochondriacal symptoms, *Arch Gen Psychiatry* 37:51-59, 1980.

Siassi I: Lithium treatment of impulsive behavior in children, *J Clin Psychiatry* 43:482-484, 1982.

Soloff P: *Psychopharmacologic therapies in borderline personality disorder.* In Tasman A, Hales E, Frances A, editors: *American Psychiatric Press Review of Psychiatry,* 8:65-83, 1989.

Soloff P: What's new in personality disorders? An update on pharmacologic treatment, *Journal of Personality Disorders* 4:233-243, 1990.

Soloff PH et al: Paradoxical effects of amitriptyline in borderline patients, *Am J Psychiatry* 143:1603-1605, 1986.

Soloff P et al: Amitriptyline versus haloperidol in borderlines: final outcomes and predictors of response, *J Clin Psychopharmacol* 9:238-246, 1989.

Stallings MC et al: Genetic and environmental structure of the tridimensional personality questionnaire: three or four primary temperament dimensions, *J Pers Soc Psych* 70:127-140, 1996.

Stewart AL, Hays RD, Ware JE Jr: The Medical Outcome Study (MOS) short-form General Health Survey: reliability and validity in a patient population, *Med Care* 26:724, 1988.

Stringer AY, Josef NC: Methylphenidate in the treatment of aggression in two antisocial personality disorders, *Am J Psychiatry* 140:1365-1366, 1983.

Svrakic NM, Svrakic DM, Cloninger CR: A general quantitative theory of personality development: fundamentals of a self-organizing psychobiological complex, *Dev Psychopathol* 8:247-272, 1996.

Svrakic DM et al: Differential diagnosis of personality disorders by the seven-factor model of temperament and character, *Arch Gen Psychiatry* 50:991, 1993.

Thapar A, McGuffin P: Is personality disorder inherited? An overview of the evidence, *J Psychopathol Behav Assess* 15:325, 1993.

Vaillant GE, Perry JC: *Personality disorders.* In Kaplan HI, Freedman AM, Sadock BJ editors: *Comprehensive textbook of psychiatry,* ed 3, Baltimore, 1980, Williams and Wilkins.

Chapter 19

Abenhaim L: Study of civilian victims of terrorist attacks (France 1982-1987), *J Clin Epidemiol* 45:103-109, 1992.

Archibald HC, Tuddenham RD: Persistent stress reaction after combat, *Arch Gen Psychiatry* 12:475-481, 1965.

Bass E, Davis L: *The courage to heal: a guide for women survivors of child sexual abuse,* New York, 1992, Harper Perennial.

Bremner JD et al: Dissociation and post-traumatic stress disorder in Vietnam combat veterans, *Am J Psychiatry* 149:328-332, 1992.

Breslau N, Davis GC: Posttraumatic stress disorder in an urban population of young adults: risk factors for chronicity, *Am J Psychiatry* 149:671-675, 1992.

Breslau N et al: Traumatic events and posttraumatic stress disorder in an urban population of young adults, *Arch Gen Psychiatry* 48:216-222, 1991.

Briere A et al: Controllable and uncontrollable stress in humans: alterations in mood and neuroendocrine and psychophysiological function, *Am J Psychiatry* 144:1419-1425, 1987.

Buydens-Branchey L, Noumair D, Branchey M: Duration and intensity of combat exposure and posttraumatic stress disorder in Vietnam veterans, *J Nerv Ment Dis* 178:582-587, 1990.

Centers for Disease Control: Health status of Vietnam veterans. I. psychosocial characteristics, *JAMA* 259:2701-2708, 1988.

Cottler LB et al: Posttraumatic stress disorder among substance users from the general population, *Am J Psychiatry* 149:664-670, 1992.

Davidson J et al: A diagnostic and family study of posttraumatic stress disorder, *Am J Psychiatry* 142:90-93, 1985.

Dobbs D, Wilson WP: Observations on persistence of war neurosis, *Dis Nerv Sys* 21:686-691, 1960.

Dodge KA, Bates JE, Pettit GS: Mechanisms in the cycle of violence, *Science* 250:1678-1683, 1990.

Engdahl BE et al: Comorbidity of psychiatric disorders and personality profiles of American World War II prisoners of war, *J Nerv Ment Dis* 179:181-187, 1991.

Epstein RS: Posttraumatic stress disorder: a review of diagnostic and treatment issues, *Psychiatr Ann* 19:556-563, 1989.

Friedman MJ: Toward rational pharmacotherapy for posttraumatic stress disorder: an interim report, *Am J Psychiatry* 145:281-285, 1988.

Green BL: Defining traumas: terminology and generic stressor dimensions, *J Appl Soc Psychol* 20:1632-1641, 1990.

Green BL et al: Buffalo Creek survivors in the second decade: stability of stress symptoms, *Am J Orthopsychiatry* 60:43-54, 1990.

Helzer JE, Robins LN, McEvoy L: Post-traumatic stress disorder in the general population, *N Engl J Med* 317:1630-1634, 1987.

Horowitz MJ: Disasters and psychological responses to stress, *Psychiatr Ann* 15:161-167, 1985.

Javitt DC, Zukin SR: Recent advances in the phencyclidine model of schizophrenia, *Am J Psychiatry* 148:1301-1308, 1991.

Kolb LC: A neuropsychological hypothesis explaining posttraumatic stress disorders, *Am J Psychiatry* 144:989-995, 1987.

Kolb LC: The psychobiology of PTSD: perspectives and reflections on the past, present, and future, *J Trauma Stress* 6:293-304, 1993.

Kramer M, Kinney L: Is sleep a marker of vulnerability to delayed posttraumatic stress disorder? *Sleep Res* 14:181, 1985.

Kramer N, Kinney L, Scharf M: Sleep in delayed stress victims, *Sleep Res* 11:113, 1982.

Krause N: Exploring the impact of a natural disaster on the health and psychological well-being of older adults, *J Hum Stress* 13:61-69, 1987.

Krystal JH et al: *Effects of the NMDA antagonist, ketamine, in humans.* In *1992 New research program and abstracts, 145th annual meeting.* Washington, D.C., 1992, American Psychiatric Press.

Kulka RA et al: *Trauma and the Vietnam war generation,* New York, 1990, Bruner/Mazel.

Lavie P et al: Long-term effects of traumatic war-related events on sleep, *Am J Psychiatry* 136:175-178, 1979.

Madakasira S, O'Brien KF: Acute posttraumatic stress disorder in victims of a natural disaster, *J Nerv Ment Dis* 175:286-290, 1987.

Mason JW et al: Elevation of urinary norepinephrine-cortisol ratio in post-traumatic stress disorder, *J Nerv Ment Dis* 176:498-502, 1988.

McCaffrey RJ, Hickling EJ, Marrazo MJ: Civilian-related post-traumatic stress disorder: assessment-related issues, *J Clin Psychol* 45:72-76, 1989.

McCarroll JE et al: Handling bodies after violent death: strategies for coping, *Am J Orthopsychiatry* 63:209-214, 1993.

Mitchell JT: *Comprehensive traumatic stress management in the emergency department,* American Critical Incident Stress Foundation, Cooperative Extension Service, 1994, University of Illinois at Urbana-Champaign.

Mullen PE, et al: Childhood sexual abuse and mental health in adult life, *Br J Psychiatry* 163:721-732, 1993.

Norris FH: Epidemology of trauma: frequency and impact of different potentially traumatic events on different demographic groups, *J Consult Clin Psychol* 60:409-418, 1992.

North CS: Human response to violent trauma, *Ballieres Clin Psychiatry* 1:225-245, 1995.

North CS, Smith EM, Spitznagel EL: Posttraumatic stress disorder in survivors of a mass shooting, *Am J Psychiatry* 151:82-88, 1994.

North CS, Smith EM: Post-traumatic stress disorder in disaster survivors, *Compr Ther* 16:3-9, 1990.

North CS et al: Acute post-disaster coping and adjustment, *J Trauma Stress* 2:353-360, 1989.

North CS et al: *Multiple personalities, multiple disorders: psychiatric classification and media influence,* New York, 1993, Oxford University Press.

Piper A: Multiple personality disorder, *Br J Psychiatry* 164:600-612, 1994.

Pitman RK et al: Naloxone-reversible analgesic response to combat-related stimuli in posttraumatic stress disorder: a pilot study, *Arch Gen Psychiatry* 47:541-544, 1990.

Ramsay R: Post-traumatic stress disorder: a new clinical entity? *J Psychosom Res* 34:355-365, 1990.

Robert JA et al: MCMI characteristics of DSM-III posttraumatic stress disorder in Vietnam veterans, *J Pers Assess* 49:226-230, 1985.

Robins LN: Steps toward evaluating post-traumatic stress reaction as a psychiatric disorder, *J Appl Soc Psychol* 20:1674-1677, 1990.

Rubonis AV, Bickman L: Psychological impairment in the wake of disaster: the disaster-psychopathology relationship, *Psychol Bull* 109:384-399, 1991.

Schlossberg A, Benjamin M: Sleep patterns in three acute combat fatigue cases, *J Clin Psychiatry* 39:546-549, 1978.

Shaliv A: *Impaired habitation of the autonomic component of the acoustic startle response in post traumatic stress disorder.* Paper presented at the annual American Psychiatric Association meeting, 1991. Washington, D.C.

Shore JH, Tatum EL, Vollmer WM: *The Mount St. Helens stress response syndrome.* In Shore JH, editor: *Disaster stress studies: new methods and findings,* Washington, D.C. 1986, American Psychiatric Press.

Sierles FS et al: Concurrent psychiatric illness in non-Hispanic outpatients diagnosed as having posttraumatic stress disorder, *J Nerv Ment Dis* 174:171-173, 1986.

Smith EM, North CS: *Post-traumatic stress disorder in natural disasters and technological accidents.* In Wilson JP, Raphael B, editors: *International handbook of traumatic stress syndromes,* New York, 1993, Plenum Press.

Smith EM, North CS, Spitznagel EL: *Post-traumatic stress in survivors of three disasters.* In Allen RD, editor: *Handbook of post disaster interventions, J Soc Behav Pers* 8:353-368, 1993.

Smith EM et al: *Psychosocial consequences of a disaster.* In Shore JH, editor: *Disaster stress studies: new methods and findings,* Washington, D.C., 1986. American Psychiatric Press.

Smith EM et al: Acute postdisaster psychiatric disorders: identification of persons at risk, *Am J Psychiatry* 147:202-206, 1990.

Solomon SD, Canino GJ: Appropriateness of DSM-IIIR criteria for post-traumatic stress disorder, *Compr Psychiatry* 31:227-237, 1990.

Solomon SD et al: Social involvement as a mediator of disaster-induced stress, *J Appl Soc Psychol* 17:1092-1112, 1987.

Southwick SM, Yehuda R, Giller EL: Personality disorders in treatment-seeking combat veterans with posttraumatic stress disorder, *Am J Psychiatry* 150:1020-1023, 1993.

Southwick SM, et al: *Yohimbine and m-chlorophenylipiperazine in* PTSD. Paper presented at the annual American Psychiatric Association meeting, 1991, Washington, D.C.

Spiegel D: Multiple personality as a post-traumatic stress disorder, *Psychiatr Clin North Am* 7:101-110, 1984.

Sutker PB, Allain AN, Winstead DK: Psychopathology and psychiatric diagnoses of World War II Pacific theater prisoner of war survivors and combat veterans, *Am J Psychiatry* 150:240-245, 1993.

Terr LC: Childhood traumas: an outline and overview, *Am J Psychiatry* 148:10-20, 1991.

Van der Kolk BA et al: Inescapable shock, neurotransmitters, and addiction to trauma: toward a psychobiology of post traumatic stress, *Biol Psychiatry* 20:314-325, 1985.

Watson IPB, Hoffman L, Wilson GV: The neuropsychiatry of post-traumatic stress disorder, *Br J Psychiatry* 152:164-173, 1988.

Yehuda R et al: Lymphocyte glucocorticoid receptor number in post-traumatic stress disorder, *Am J Psychiatry* 148:499-504, 1991.

Chapter 20

American Heritage Dictionary of English Language, ed 3, Boston, 1996, Houghton Mifflin.

Dorland's Illustrated Medical Dictionary, ed 28, Philadelphia, 1994, W.B. Saunders.

Guze SB: *Why psychiatry is a branch of medicine*, New York, 1992, Oxford University Press.

Oxford English Dictionary, ed 2, Oxford, 1989, Oxford University Press.

Chapter 21

Ballenger JC: The use of anti-convulsants in manic-depressive illness, *J Clin Psychiatry* 49(Suppl 11):21-24, 1988.

Bech P: Acute therapy of depression, *J Clin Psychiatry* 54(Suppl 8):18-27, 1993.

Berwish N, Amsterdam J: An overview of investigational antidepressants, *Psychosomatics* 30:1-17, 1989.

Biederman J, Lerner Y, Belmaker RH: Combination of lithium carbonate and haloperidol in schizo-affective disorder, *Arch Gen Psychiatry* 36:327-333, 1979.

Brady HR, Horgan JH: Lithium and the heart: unanswered questions, *Chest* 92:166-169, 1988.

Braude WM, Barnes TRE, Gore SM: Clinical characteristics of akathisia, *Br J Psychiatry* 143:134-150, 1983.

Cade JFJ: *The story of lithium.* In Ayd RJ Jr, Blackwell B, editors: *Biological psychiatry,* Philadelphia, 1970, J.B. Lippincott.

Calabrese JR et al: Mixed states and bipolar rapid cycling and their treatment with VPA, *Psychiatr Ann* 23:70-78, 1993.

Calabrese JR et al: Predictors of valproate response in bipolar rapid cycling, *J Clin Psychopharmacol* 13:280-283, 1993.

Chouinard G, Young SN, Annable L: Antimanic effect of clonazepam, *Biol Psychiatry* 18:451-466, 1983.

Cowan PJ: A role for 5-HT in the action of antidepressant drugs, *Pharmacol Ther* 46:43-51, 1990.

Creese I, Burt DR, Snyder SH: DA receptor binding predicts clinical and pharmacological potencies of antischizophrenic drugs, *Science* 192:481-483, 1976.

Fieve RR, Platman SR, Plutchik RR: The use of lithium in affective disorders. I. Acute endogenous depression, *Am J Psychiatry* 125:487-491, 1968.

Frank E et al: Comparison of full-dose versus half-dose pharmacotherapy in the maintenance treatment of of recurrent depression, *J Affect Disord* 27:139-145, 1993.

Frank E et al: Three-year outcomes for maintenance therapies in recurrent depression, *Arch Gen Psychiatry* 47:1093-1099, 1990.

Haefely W, Martin JR, Schoch P: Novel anxiolytics that act as partial agonists at benzodiazepine receptors, *Trends Pharmacol Sci* 11:452-456, 1990.

Hollister LE, Csernansky JG: *Clinical pharmacology of psychotherapeutic drugs,* New York, 1990, Harcourt Brace and Janovich.

Jann MW: Buspirone: an update on a unique anxiolytic agent, *Pharmacotherapy* 8:100-116, 1988.

Jones KL et al: Pattern of malformation in the children of women treated with carbamazepine during pregnancy, *N Engl J Med* 320:1661-1666, 1989.

Kane JM: et al: Clozapine for the treatment-refractory schizophrenic: a double-blind comparison with chlorpromazine, *Arch Gen Psychiatry* 45:789-796, 1988.

Kane JM et al: A one-year comparison of four dosages of haloperidol decanoate, *Schizophr Res* 9:239-240, 1993.

Keepers GA, Clappison VJ, Casey DE: Initial anticholinergic prophylaxis for neuroleptic-induced extrapyramidal syndromes, *Arch Gen Psychiatry* 40:1113-1117, 1983.

Lerer B et al: Carbamazepine versus lithium in mania: a double-blind study, *J Clin Psychiatry* 48:89-93, 1987.

Levinson DF et al: Fluphenazind dose, clinical response, and extrapyramidal symptoms during acute treatment, *Arch Gen Psychiatry* 47:761-768, 1990.

Lieberman JA et al: Time course and biologic correlates of treatment response in first-episode schizophrenia, *Arch Gen Psychiatry* 50:369-376, 1993.

Lieberman JA: Understanding the mechanism of action of atypical antipsychotic drugs, *Br J Psychiatry* 163(Suppl 22):7-18, 1993.

Linden S, Rich CL: The use of lithium during pregnancy and lactation, *J Clin Psychiatry* 44:358-361, 1983.

Marder SR, Meibach RC: Risperidone in the treatment of schizophrenia, *Am J Psychiatry* 151:825-835, 1994.

Meltzer HY: Clinical studies on the mechanism of action of clozapine: the dopamine-serotonin hypothesis of schizophrenia, *Psychopharmacol* 99:S18-S27, 1989.

Meltzer HY: *Atypical antipsychotic drugs.* In Bloom FE, Kupfer DJ, editors: *Psychopharmacology: the fourth generation of progress,* New York, 1994, Raven Press.

Newcomer JW et al: Correlations between akathisia and residual psychopathology: a by-product of neuroleptic-induce dysphoria, *Br J Psychiatry* 164:834-838, 1994.

Nierenberg AA, White K: What next? A review of pharmacologic strategies for treatment resistant depression, *Psychopharmacol Bull* 26:429-460, 1990.

Noyes R, Garvey MJ, Cook BL: Follow-up study of patients with panic disorder and agoraphobia with panic attacks treated with tricyclic antidepressants, *J Affective Dis* 16:249-256, 1989.

Pope HG et al: Valproate in the treatment of acute mania: a placebo controlled study, *Arch Gen Psychiatry* 48:62-68, 1991.

Post RM et al: Correlates of anti-manic response to carbamazepine, *Psychiatry Res* 21:71-83, 1987.

Prosser ES et al: Depression, parkinsonian symptoms, and negative symptoms in schizophrenics treated with neuroleptics, *J Nerv Ment Dis* 175:100-105, 1987.

Richelson E: Pharmacology of antidepressants: characteristics of the ideal drug, *Mayo Clin Proc* 69:1069-1081, 1994.

Rickels K et al: Long-term therapeutic use of benzodiazepines. I. Effects of abrupt discontinuation, *Arch Gen Psychiatry* 47:899-907, 1990.

Schweizer E et al: Long-term therapeutic use of benzodiazepines. II. Effects of gradual taper, *Arch Gen Psychiatry* 47:908-915, 1990.

Seeman P: Dopamine receptor sequences: therapeutic levels of neuroleptics occupy D2 receptors, clozapine occupies D4, *Neuropsychopharmacology* 7:261-284, 1992.

Shader RI, Greenblatt DJ: Use of benzodiazepines in anxiety disorders, *New Engl J Med* 328:1398-1405, 1993.

Sokoloff P et al: Molecular cloning and characterization of a novel dopamine receptor (D3) as a target for neuroleptics, *Nature* 347:146-151, 1990.

Stancer HC, Forboth N: Hyperparathyroidism, hypothyroidism and impaired renal function after 10 to 20 years of lithium treatment, *Arch Intern Med* 149:1042-1045, 1989.

Stewart J et al: Atypical depression: a valid clinical entity? *Psychiatr Clin North Am* 16:479-495, 1993.

Takezaki H, Hanaoka M: The use of carbamazepine (Tegretol) in the control of manic depressive psychosis and other manic depressive states, *J Clin Psychiatry* 13:173-183, 1971.

Tallman JF, Dahl SG: *New drug design in psychopharmacology: the impact of molecular biology.* In Bloom FE, Kupfer DJ, editors: *Psychopharmacology. the fourth generation of progress,* New York, 1994, Raven Press.

Thase ME, Rush AJ: *Treatment-resistant depression.* In Bloom FE, Kupfer DJ, editors: *Psychopharmacology: the fourth generation of progress,* New York, 1994, Raven Press.

Van Putten T, Marder SR, Mintz J: A controlled dose comparison of haloperidol in newly admitted schizophrenic patients, *Arch Gen Psychiatry* 47:754-758, 1990.

Van Putten T et al: Haloperidol plasma levels and clinical response: a therapeutic window relationship, *Am J Psychiatry* 49:500-505, 1992.

Van Tol HHM et al: Cloning of the gene for a human dopamine D4 receptor with high affinity for the antipsychotic clozapine, *Nature* 350:610-614, 1991.

Wilkinson G et al: Meta-analysis of double-blind placebo-controlled trials of antidepressants and benzodiazepines for patients with panic disorders, *Psychol Med* 21:991-998, 1991.

Zeller EA: Amine oxidase inhibitors, *Ann N Y Acad Sci* 80:551-1045, 1959.

Chapter 22

Abrams R: *Electroconvulsive therapy,* ed 2, New York, 1992, Oxford University Press.

Abrams R, Swartz C, Vedak C: Antidepressant effects of high-dose right unilateral electroconvulsive therapy, *Arch Gen Psychiatry* 48:746-748, 1991.

American Psychiatric Association: Practice guideline for major depressive disorder in adults, *Am J Psychiatry* 150(Suppl):4, 1993.

American Psychiatric Association: Practice guideline for the treatment of patients with bipolar disorder, *Am J Psychiatry* 151(Suppl):12, 1994.

American Psychiatric Association Task Force: *The practice of electroconvulsive therapy: recommendations for treatment, training and privileging,* Washington D.C., 1990, American Psychiatric Press.

Calev A et al: *ECT and memory.* In Coffey CE, editor: *The clinical science of electroconvulsive therapy,* Washington D.C., 1993, American Psychiatric Press.

Castelli I et al: Comparative effects of esmolol and labetalol to attenuate hyperdynamic states after electroconvulsive therapy, *Anesth Analg* 80:557-561, 1995.

Coffey CE et al: Brain anatomic effects of electroconvulsive therapy: a prospective magnetic resonance imaging study, *Arch Gen Psychiatry* 48:1013-1021, 1991.

Devanand DP, Sackeim HA, Prudic J: Electroconvulsive therapy in the treatment-resistant patient, *Psychiatr Clin North Am* 14:905-924, 1991.

Devanand DP et al: Does ECT alter brain structure? *Am J Psychiatry* 151:957-970, 1994.

Figiel GS et al: Combined use of labetalol and nifedipine in controlling the cardiovascular response from ECT, *J Geriatr Psychiatry Neurol* 1:20-24, 1993.

Fink M: Meduna and the origins of convulsive therapy, *Am J Psychiatry* 141:1034-1041, 1984.

Grunhaus L, Pande AC: *Electroconvulsive therapy for severe depressive disorders.* In Grunhaus L, Greden JF, editors: *Severe depressive disorders,* Washington, D.C., 1994, American Psychiatric Press.

Hicks F: ECT modified by atracurium, *Convuls Ther* 3:54-59, 1987.

Hinkle PE et al: Use of caffeine to lengthen seizures in ECT, *Am J Psychiatry* 144:1143-1148, 1987.

Janicak PG et al: Efficacy of ECT: a meta-analysis, *Am J Psychiatry* 142:297-302, 1985.

Kellner CH, Bernstein HJ: *ECT as a treatment for neurological illness.* In Coffey CE, editor: *The clinical science of electroconvulsive therapy,* Washington, D.C., 1993, American Psychiatric Press.

Kramer BA, Allen RE, Friedman B: Atropine and glycopyrrolate as ECT preanesthesia, *J Clin Psychiatry* 47:199-200, 1986.

Lerer B, Weiner RD, Belmaker RH, editors: *ECT: basic mechanisms,* Washington D.C., 1986, American Psychiatric Press.

Manning M: *Undercurrents,* San Francisco, 1994, Harper San Francisco.

Mattingly G et al: Prospective uses of ECT in the presence of intracranial tumors, *J Neuropsychiatry Clin Neurosci* 3:459-463, 1991.

Monroe RR: Maintenance electroconvulsive therapy, *Psychiatr Clin North Am* 14:947-960, 1991.

Mukherjee S, Sackeim HA, Schnur DB: Electroconvulsive therapy of acute manic episodes: a review of 50 years' experience, *Am J Psychiatry* 151:169-176, 1994.

Nutt DJ, Glue P: *The neurobiology of ECT: animal studies.* In Coffey CE, editor: *The clinical science of electroconvulsive therapy,* Washington D.C., 1993, American Psychiatric Press.

Packman PM, Meyer DA, Verdun RM: Hazards of succinylcholine administration during electrotherapy, *Arch Gen Psychiatry* 35:1137-1141, 1978.

Rasmussen K, Abrams R: Treatment of Parkinson's disease with electroconvulsive therapy, *Psychiatr Clin North Am* 14:925-934, 1991.

Rasmussen K, Zorumski CF: Electroconvulsive therapy in patients taking theophylline, *J Clin Psychiatry* 54:427-431, 1993.

Rohland BM, Carroll BT, Jacoby RG: ECT in the treatment of the catatonic syndrome, *J Affect Disord* 29:255-261, 1993.

Sackeim H: Central issues regarding the mechanisms of electroconvulsive therapy: directions for future research, *Psychopharmacol Bull* 30:281-308, 1994.

Sackeim H et al: Seizure threshold in electroconvulsive therapy: effects of sex, age, electrode placement, and number of treatments, *Arch Gen Psychiatry* 44:355-360, 1987.

Sackeim HA et al: Effects of stimulus intensity and electrode placement on the efficacy and cognitive effects of electroconvulsive therapy, *N Engl J Med* 328:839-846, 1993.

Sackheim HA et al: Physical properties and quantification of the ECT stimulus. I. Basic principles, *Convuls Ther* 10:93-123, 1994.

Salzman C: The use of ECT in the treatment of schizophrenia, *Am J Psychiatry* 137:1032-41, 1980.

Schwarz T, Loewenstein J, Isenberg KE: Maintenance ECT: indications and outcome, *Convuls Ther* 11:14-23, 1995.

Shapira B, Kindler S, Lerer B: Medication outcome in ECT-resistant depression, *Convuls Ther* 4:192-198, 1988.

Small JG, Milstein V: Lithium interactions: lithium and electroconvulsive therapy, *J Clin Psychopharmacol* 10:346-350, 1990.

Weiner RD: Does electroconvulsive therapy cause brain damage? *Behav Brain Sci* 7:1-53, 1984.

Weiner RD: Treatment optimization with ECT, *Psychopharmacol Bulletin* 30:313-320, 1994.

Welch CA: *ECT in medically ill patients.* In Coffey CE, editor: *The clinical science of electroconvulsive therapy,* Washington D.C., 1993, American Psychiatric Press.

Welch CA, Drop LJ: Cardiovascular effects of ECT, *Convuls Ther* 5:35-43, 1989.

Zorumski CF, Rubin EH, Burke WJ: Electroconvulsive therapy for the elderly: a review, *Hosp Commun Psychiatry* 39:643-647, 1988.

Zorumski CF et al: ECT in primary and secondary depression, *J Clin Psychiatry* 47:298-300, 1986.

Chapter 23

Ad Hoc Committee on Genetic Testing/Insurance Issues: Background statement: genetic testing and insurance, *Am J Hum Genet* 56:319-326, 1995.

Andrews LB et al: *Assessing genetic risks: implications for health and social policy,* Washington, D.C., 1994, National Academy Press.

Benjamin CM et al: Proceed with care: direct predictive testing for Huntington Disease, *Am J Hum Genet* 55:606-617, 1994.

Bennett RL et al: Recommendations for standardized human pedigree nomenclature, *Am J Hum Genet* 56:745-752, 1995.

Berg K, Kirch DG: *Genetic counseling.* In Kaplan H, Sadock B, editors: *Comprehensive textbook of psychiatry,* ed 6, Baltimore, Md., 1995, Williams and Wilkins.

Billings PR et al: Discrimination as a consequence of genetic testing, *Am J Hum Genet* 50:476-482, 1992.

Blacker D, Tsuang MT: Unipolar relatives in bipolar pedigrees: are they bipolar? *Psychiatr Genet* 3:5-16, 1993.

Blendon RJ et al: How white and African Americans view their health and social problems: different experiences, different expectations, *JAMA* 273:341-346, 1995.

Bulyzhenkov V, Christen Y, Prilipko L: *Genetic approaches in the prevention of mental disorders,* New York, 1990, Springer-Verlag.

Cox DR et al: Assessing mapping progress in the Human Genome Project, *Science* 265:2031-2036, 1994.

Davies JL et al: A genome-wide search for human type 1 diabetes susceptibility genes, *Nature* 371:130-136, 1994.

Erlenmeyer-Kimling L: *Biological markers for the liability to schizophrenia.* In Helmchen H, Henn FA, editors: *Biological perspectives of schizophrenia,* New York, 1987, Wiley and Sons.

Gershon ES, Cloninger CR: *Genetic approaches to mental disorders,* Washington, D.C., 1994, American Psychiatric Press.

Goodwin FK, Jamison KR: *Manic-depressive illness,* New York, N.Y., 1990, Oxford University Press.

Gottesman II: *Schizophrenia genesis: the origins of madness,* New York, 1991, W.H. Freeman and Company.

Gottesman II, Moldin SO: *Schizophrenia and genetic risks: a guide to genetic counseling,* Arlington, Va., 1992, National Alliance for the Mentally Ill.

Hagnell O et al: Are we entering an age of melancholy? Depressive illnesses in a prospective epidemiological study over 25 years: the Lundby Study, Sweden, *Psychol Med* 12:279-289, 1982.

Helzer JE, Burnam A, McEvoy LT: *Alcohol abuse and dependence.* In Robins LN, Regier DA, editors: *Psychiatric disorders in America: the epidemiologic catchment area study,* New York, N.Y., 1991, Free Press.

Kendler KS, Diehl SR: The genetics of schizophrenia: a current, genetic-epidemiologic perspective, *Schizophr Bull* 19:261-285, 1993.

Kendler KS et al: A population-based twin study of alcoholism in women, *JAMA* 268:1877-1882, 1992.

Kendler KS et al: A population-based twin study of major depression in women: the impact of varying definitions of illness, *Arch Gen Psychiatry* 49:257-266, 1992.

Kessler S: Psychological aspects of genetic counseling. VII. Thoughts on directiveness, *Genet Couns* 1:9-17, 1992.

Lander ES, Schork NJ: Genetic dissection of complex traits, *Science* 265:2037-2048, 1994.

Mann C: Behavioral genetics in transition, *Science* 264:1686-1689, 1994.

Marshall E: Highs and lows on the research roller coaster, *Science* 264:1693-1695, 1994.

McGuffin P, Murray R: *The new genetics of mental illness,* Oxford, 1991, Butterworth-Heinemann.

McKusick VA: *Mendelian inheritance in man: catalogs of autosomal dominant, autosomal recessive, and x-linked phenotypes,* Baltimore, Md., 1990, Johns Hopkins University Press.

Mehlman MJ et al: Coverage of genetic technologies under national health reform, *Am J Hum Genet* 55:1054-1060, 1995.

Moldin SO: Indicators of liability to schizophrenia: perspectives from genetic epidemiology, *Schizophr Bull* 20:169-184, 1994.

Moldin SO, Reich TR: The genetic analysis of depression: future directions, *Clin Neurosci* 1:139-145, 1993.

Moldin SO, Reich T, Rice JP: Current perspectives on the genetics of unipolar depression, *Behav Genet* 21:211-242, 1991.

Morejon-Punales D, Rapp R: Ethnocultural diversity and genetic counseling training: the challenge for a twenty-first century, *Genet Couns* 2:155-158, 1993.

Nurnberger JI et al: Diagnostic interview for genetic studies: rationale, unique features, and training, *Arch Gen Psychiatry* 51:849-859, 1994.

Reveley A: Genetic counseling for schizophrenia, *Br J Psychiatry* 147:107-112, 1985.

Rice JP, Moldin SO, Neuman R: *Age, period, and cohort effects on rates of mental disorders: summary of data and implications for genetic analysis.* In Tsuang MT, Kendler KS, Lyons MJ, editors: *Genetic issues in psychosocial epidemiology,* New Brunswick, N.J. 1991, Rutgers University Press.

Rice JP, Reich T: Familial analysis of qualitative traits under multifactorial inheritance, *Genet Epidemiol* 2:301-315, 1985.

Rice JP et al: The familial transmission of bipolar illness, *Arch Gen Psychiatry* 44:441-447, 1987.

Risch N: Genetic linkage and complex diseases, with special reference to psychiatric disorders, *Genet Epidemiol* 7:3-16, 1990.

Robins LN, Regier DA: *Psychiatric disorders in America: the epidemiologic catchment area study,* New York, N.Y., 1991, Free Press.

Schulz PM et al: Patient and family attitudes about schizophrenia: implications for genetic counseling, *Schizophr Bull* 8:504-513, 1982.

Shore D et al: Legal and ethical issues in psychiatric genetics research, *Am J Med Genet* 48:17-21, 1993.

Suarez BK, Hampe CL, Van Eerdewegh P: *Problems of replicating linkage claims in psychiatry.* In Gershon ES, Cloninger CR, Barrett JE, editors: *Genetic approaches to mental disorders,* Washington, D.C., 1994, American Psychiatric Press.

Targum SD et al: The Family Attitudes Questionnaire: patients' and spouses' views of bipolar illness, *Arch Gen Psychiatry* 38:562-568, 1981.

Tsuang MT: Genetic counseling for psychiatric patients and their families, *Am J Psychiatry* 135:1465-1475, 1978.

Tsuang MT, Faraone SV: *The genetics of mood disorders,* Baltimore, Md., 1990, John Hopkins University Press.

Turlington L, Moldin SO: Assessing the demand for psychiatric genetic counseling, *Am J Hum Genet* 55:A144, 1994.

Vogel F, Motulsky AG: *Human genetics: problems and approaches,* New York, 1986, Springer-Verlag.

Wang V, Marsh FH: Ethical principles and cultural integrity in health care delivery: Asian ethnocultural perspectives in genetic services. *Genet Couns* 1:81-92, 1992.

Weissman M et al: *Affective disorders.* In Robins LN, Regier DA, editors: *Psychiatric disorders in America: the epidemiologic catchment area study,* New York, N.Y., 1991, Free Press.

Young ID: *Introduction to risk calculation in genetic counseling,* New York, N.Y., 1991, Oxford University Press.

Chapter 24

Ambrosini PJ et al: Antidepressant treatments in children and adolescents. I. Affective Disorders, *J Am Acad Child Adolesc Psychiatry* 32:1-6, 1993.

Barkley RA et al: The adolescent outcome of hyperactive children diagnosed by research criteria. I. An 8-year prospective follow-up study, *J Am Acad Child Adolesc Psychiatry* 26:317-325, 1990.

Brent DA et al: Psychiatric risk factors for adolescent suicide: a case-control study, *J Am Acad Child Adolesc Psychiatry* 32:521-529, 1993.

Cicchetti D, Toth SL: A developmental psychopathology perspective on child abuse and neglect, *J Am Acad Child Adolesc Psychiatry* 34:541-565, 1995.

Costello EJ et al: Psychopathology in pediatric primary care: the new hidden morbidity, *Pediatrics* 82:415-424, 1988.

Costello EJ et al: How can epidemiology improve mental health services for children and adolescents? *J Am Acad Child Adolesc Psychiatry* 32:1106-1113, 1993.

Dulcan MK: Using psychostimulants to treat behavioral disorders of children and adolescents, *J Child Adolesc Psychopharmacol* 1:7-20, 1990.

Green WH: Nonstimulant drugs in the treatment of attention-deficit hyperactivity disorder, *Child Adolesc Psychiatr Clin North Am* 1:449-465, 1992.

Ialongo NS et al: The effects of multimodal intervention with attention-deficit hyperactivity disorder children: a 9-month follow-up, *J Am Acad Child Adolesc Psychiatry* 32:182-189, 1993.

Jellinek MS et al: Pediatric symptom checklist: screening school-age children for psychosocial dysfunction, *J Pediatr* 112:201-209, 1988.

Jones MB, Offord DR: Reduction in antisocial behavior in poor children by nonschool skill-development, *J Child Psychol Psychiatry* 30:737-750, 1989.

Kazdin AE, editor: *Conduct disorders in childhood and adolescence,* Newbury Park, Calif., 1987, Sage.

Kazdin AE: Adolescent mental health: prevention and treatment programs, *Am Psychol* 48:127-141, 1993.

Kovacs M, Ho V, Pollock MH: Criterion and predictive validity of the diagnosis of adjustment disorder: a prospective study of youths with new-onset insulin-dependent diabetes mellitus, *Am J Psychiatry* 152:523-528, 1995.

Kovacs et al: Depressive disorders in childhood, *Arch Gen Psychiatry* 41:229-237, 1984.

Leonard HL, editor: Anxiety disorders, *Child Adolesc Psychiatr Clin North Am* 2:563-838, 1993.

Lewis DO: From abuse to violence: psychophysiological consequences of maltreatment, *J Am Acad Child Adolesc Psychiatry* 31:383-391, 1992.

McConaughy SH: Evaluating behavioral and emotional disorders with the CBCL, TRF, and YSR cross-informant scales, *J Emotion Behav Disord* 1:40-52, 1993.

Mannuzza S et al: Adult outcome of hyperactive boys: educational achievement, occupational rank, and psychiatric status, *Arch Gen Psychiatry* 50:565-576, 1993.

Offer D, Schonert-Reich KA: Debunking the myths of adolescence: findings from recent research, *J Am Acad Child Adolesc Psychiatry* 31:1003-1014, 1992.

Rao U et al: Unipolar depression in adolescents: clinical outcome in adulthood, *J Am Acad Child Adolesc Psychiatry* 34:566-578, 1995.

Rotheram-Borus MJ et al: Brief cognitive-behavioral treatment for adolescent suicide attempters and their families, *J Am Acad Child Adolesc Psychiatry* 33:508-517, 1994.

Shaffer D et al: Preventing teenager suicide: a critical review, *J Am Acad Child Adolesc Psychiatry* 27:675-687, 1988.

Sturm R, Wells KB: How can care of depression become more cost-effective? *JAMA* 273:51-58, 1995.

Wilson MD, Joffe A: Adolescent medicine, *JAMA* 273:1657-1659.

Chapter 25

Abernethy DR: *Psychotropic drugs and the aging process: pharmacokinetic and pharmacodynamics.* In Salzman C, editor: *Clinical geriatric psychopharmacology,* ed 2, Baltimore, 1992, Williams and Wilkins.

Barraclough BM: Suicide in the elderly, *Br J Psychiatry* (Special supplement 6):87-97, 1971.

Belitsky R, McGlashan T: The manifestations of schizophrenia in late life: a dirth of data, *Schizophr Bull* 19:683-685, 1993.

Blazer DG, Bachar JR, Manton KG: Suicide in late life: review and commentary, *J Am Geriatr Soc* 34:519-525, 1986.

Blumenthal SJ, Kupfer DJ, editors: *Suicide over the life cycle: risk factors, assessment, and treatment of suicidal patients,* Washington, D.C., 1990, American Psychiatric Press.

Conwell Y, Caine ED: Rational suicide and the right to die: reality and myth, *N Engl J Med* 325:1100-1103, 1991.

Copeland AR: Suicide among the elderly: The Metro-Dade County experience, 1981-83, *Med Sci Law* 27:32-36, 1987.

Cummings JL: Depression and Parkinson's disease: a review, *Am J Psychiatry* 149:443-454, 1992.

Davidson M et al: Severity of symptoms in chronically institutionalized geriatric schizophrenic patients, *Am J Psychiatry* 152:197-207, 1995.

Drevets WC, Rubin EH: Psychotic symptoms and the longitudinal course of senile dementia of the Alzheimer type, *Biol Psychiatry* 25:39-48, 1989.

Drevets WC et al: A functional anatomical study of unipolar depression, *J Neurosci* 12:3628-3641, 1992.

Folstein MF, Folstein SE, McHugh PR: Mini-Mental State: a practical method for grading the cognitive state of patients for the clinician, *J Psychiatr Res* 12:189-198, 1975.

Foster JR: *Normal aging: biological aspects.* In Lazarus LW, editor: *Essentials of geriatric psychiatry: a guide for health professionals,* New York, 1988, Springer Publishing Company.

Frasure-Smith N, Lesperance F, Talajic M: Depression following myocardial infarction, *JAMA* 270:1819-1825, 1993.

Frierson RL: Suicide attempts by the old and the very old, *Arch Intern Med* 151:141-144, 1991.

Gold DD: Late age of onset schizophrenia: present but unaccounted for, *Compr Psychiatry* 25:225-237, 1984.

Goldberg TE et al: Course of schizophrenia: neuropsychological evidence for a static encephalopathy, *Schizophr Bull* 19:797-804, 1993.

Greenblatt D: Basic pharmacokinetic principles and their application to psychotropic drugs, *J Clin Psychiatry* 54(suppl):8-13, 1993.

Hing E, Bloom B: Long-term care for the functionally dependent elderly, *Vital Health Stat* 13:104, 1990, National Center for Health Statistics.

Hirano A, Llena J: *Structure of neurons in the aging nervous system.* In Calne D, editor: *Neurodegenerative diseases,* Philadelphia, 1994, W.B. Saunders.

Holden NL: Late paraphrenia or the paraphrenias? A descriptive study with a 10-year follow-up, *Br J Psychiatry* 150:635-639, 1987.

Jeste DV et al: Treatment of late-life schizophrenia with neuroleptics, *Schizophr Bull* 19:817-830, 1993.

Katzman R et al: Validation of a short orientation-memory-concentration test of cognitive impairment, *Am J Psychiatry* 140:734-739, 1542, 1983.

Kay DWK et al: The differentiation of paranoid from affective psychoses by patient's premorbid characteristics, *Br J Psychiatry* 129:207-215, 1976.

Koller WM, Megaffin B: *Parkinson's disease and parkinsonism.* In Coffey CE, Cummings JL, editors: *Textbook of geriatric neuropsychiatry,* Washington, D.C., 1994, American Psychiatric Press.

Lesser IM et al: Brain imaging in late-life schizophrenia and related psychoses, *Schizophr Bull* 19:773-782, 1993.

Levanthal EA: *Biological aspects.* In Sadavoy J, Lazarus LW, Jarvik LF, editors: *Comprehensive review of geriatric psychiatry,* Washington, D.C., 1991, American Psychiatric Press.

Lustman PJ et al: Depression in adults with diabetes, *Diabetes Care* 15:1631-1639, 1992.

Malmgren R: *Epidemiology of aging.* In Coffey CE, Cummings JL, editors: *Textbook of geriatric neuropsychiatry,* Washington, D.C., 1994, American Psychiatric Press.

McConnell H, Duffy J: *Neuropsychiatric aspects of medical therapies.* In Coffey CE, Cummings JL, editors: *Textbook of geriatric neuropsychiatry,* Washington, D.C., 1994, American Psychiatric Press.

McIntosh JL: Epidemiology of suicide in the elderly, *Suicide Life Threat Behav* 22:15-35, 1992.

Miller M: *Suicide after sixty: the final alternative,* New York, 1979, Springer Publishing Company.

Morris PLP et al: Association of depression with 10-year post stroke mortality, *Am J Psychiatry* 150:124-129, 1993.

Pearlson GD, Petty RG: *Late-life onset psychoses.* In Coffey CE, Cummings JL, editors: *Textbook of geriatric neuropsychiatry,* Washington, D.C., 1994, American Psychiatric Press.

Poon LW, Siegler IC: *Psychological aspects of normal aging.* In Sadavoy J, Lazarus LW, Jarvik LF, editors: *Comprehensive review of geriatric psychiatry,* Washington, D.C., 1991, American Psychiatric Press.

Powers RE: *Neurobiology of aging.* In Coffey CE, Cummings JL, editors: *Textbook of geriatric neuropsychiatry,* Washington, D.C., 1994, American Psychiatric Press.

Preskorn S: Pharmacokinetics of antidepressants: why and how they are relevant to treatment, *J Clin Psychiatry* 54(suppl):14-33, 1993.

Ratcliff G, Saxton J: *Age-associated memory impairment.* In Coffey CE, Cummings JL, editors: *Textbook of geriatric neuropsychiatry,* Washington, D.C., 1994, American Psychiatric Press.

Robins E: *The final months,* New York, 1981, Oxford University Press.

Rubin EH: *Depression and dementia.* In Morris J, editor: *Handbook of dementing illnesses,* New York, 1994, Marcel Dekker.

Rubin EH, Kinscherf DA: Psychopathology of very mild dementia of the Alzheimer type, *Am J Psychiatry* 146:1017-1021, 1989.

Rubin EH, Zorumski CF, Burke WJ: Overlapping symptoms of geriatric depression and Alzheimer-type dementia, *Hosp Commun Psychiatry* 39:1074-1079, 1988.

Rubin EH et al: The influence of major depression on clinical and psychometric assessment of senile dementia of the Alzheimer type, *Am J Psychiatry* 148:1164-1171, 1991.

Schneider EL, Guralnik JM: The aging of America, *JAMA* 263:2335-2340, 1990.

Shulman K: Suicide and parasuicide in old age: a review, *Age Ageing* 7:201-209, 1978.

U.S. Bureau of Census, *Statistical abstract of the United States,* ed 114, Washington, D.C., 1994, author.

Yesavage JA, Brink TL: Development and validation of a geriatric depression screening scale: a preliminary report, *J Psychiatr Res* 17:37-49, 1983.

Warheit GJ, Longino CF, Bradsher JE: *Sociocultural aspects.* In Sadavoy J, Lazarus LW, Jarvik LF, editors: *Comprehensive review of geriatric psychiatry,* Washington, D.C., 1991, American Psychiatric Press.

Chapter 26

Altschuler LL: Pharmacologic management of psychiatric illness during pregnancy: dilemmas and guidelines, *Am J Psychiatry* 153:592-606, 1996.

Atkinson JH, Grant I: Natural history of neuropsychiatric manifestations of HIV disease, *Psychiatr Clin North Am* 17:17-33, 1994.

Black KJ: Diagnosing depression after stroke, *South Med J* 88:699-708, 1995.

Bright DA: Postpartum mental disorders, *Am Fam Physician* 50:595-598, 1994.

Brockington IF, Meakin CJ: Clinical clues to the aetiology of puerperal psychosis, *Prog Neuropsychopharmacol Biol Psychiatry* 18:417-429, 1994.

Carney RM, Freedland KE, Jaffe AS: Insomnia and depression prior to myocardial infarction, *Psychosom Med* 52:603-609, 1990.

Carney RM et al: Major depressive disorder in coronary artery disease, *Am J Cardiol* 60:1273-1275, 1987.

Carney RM et al: Major depressive disorder predicts cardiac events in patients with coronary artery disease, *Psychosom Med* 50:627-633, 1988.

Carney RM et al: Ventricular techycardia and psychiatric depression in patients with coronary artery disease, *Am J Med* 95:23-28, 1993.

Clouse RE: Anxiety and gastrointestinal illness, *Psychiatr Clin North Am* 11:399-417, 1988.

Clouse RE, Lustman PJ: Gastrointestinal symptoms in diabetic patients: lack of association with neuropathy, *Am J Gastroenterol* 84:868-872, 1989.

Craven JL, Rodin GM, Littlefield C: The Beck Depression Inventory as a screening device for major depression in renal dialysis patients, *Int J Psychiatry* 18:365-374, 1988.

Craven JL et al: The diagnosis of depression in renal dialysis patients, *Psychosom Med* 49:482-492, 1987.

Cummings JL: Depression and Parkinson's disease: a review, *Am J Psychiatry* 149:443-454, 1992.

Cummings JL, Trimble MR: *Concise guide to neuropsychiatry and behavioral neurology,* Washington, D.C., 1995, American Psychiatric Press.

DeVane CL: Pharmacogenetics and drug metabolism of newer antidepressant agents, *J Clin Psychiatry* 55(12 suppl):38-47, 1994.

Figiel GS et al: ECT-induced delirium in depressed patients with Parkinson's disease, *J Neuropsychiatry Clin Neurosci* 3:405-411, 1991.

Folstein SE: *Huntington's disease: a disorder of families*, Baltimore, 1989, Johns Hopkins University Press.

Freedland KE et al: Underdiagnosis of depression in patients with coronary artery disease: the role of nonspecific symptoms, *Int J Psychiatry Med* 22:221-229, 1992.

Gavard JA, Lustman PJ, Clouse RE: Prevalence of depression in adults with diabetes, *Diabetes Care* 16:1167-1178, 1993.

Goldberg RJ: Diagnostic dilemmas presented by patients with anxiety and depression, *Am J Med* 98:278-284, 1995.

Goodnick PJ, Henry JH, Buki VMV: Treatment of depression in patients with diabetes mellitus, *J Clin Psychiatry* 56:128-136, 1995.

Gorelick PB, Ross ED: The aprosodias: further functional-anatomical evidence for the organisation of affective language in the right hemisphere, *J Neurol Neurosurg Psychiatry* 50:553-560, 1987.

Guengerich FP: Catalytic selectivity of human cytochrome P450 enzymes: relevance to drug metabolism and toxicity, *Toxicol Lett* 70:133-138, 1994.

Henrickson GA et al: Depression in hemodialysis patients, *Psychosomatics* 30:284-285, 1989.

Jorge RE et al: Depression and anxiety following traumatic brain injury, *J Neuropsychiatry Clin Neurosci* 5:369-374, 1993.

Kendler KS et al: Stressful life events, genetic liability, and onset of an episode of major depression in women, *Am J Psychiatry* 152:833-842, 1995.

Kennedy SH, Craven JL, Roin GM: Major depression in renal dialysis patients: an open trial of antidepressant therapy, *J Clin Psychiatry* 50:60-63, 1989.

Lane EA: Renal function and the disposition of antidepressants and their metabolites, *Psychopharmacol Bull* 27:533-540, 1991.

Leigh H, Kramer SI: *The psychiatric manifestations of endocrine disease.* In Stollerman GH, editor: *Advances in internal medicine,* Chicago, 1984, Mosby.

Lishman WA: *Organic psychiatry: the psychological consequences of cerebral disorder,* ed 2, Boston, 1987, Blackwell Scientific Publications.

Lloyd GG, Cawley RH: Distress or illness? A study of psychological symptoms after myocardial infarction, *Br J Psychiatry* 142:120-125, 1983.

Lustman PJ: Anxiety disorders in adults with diabetes mellitus, *Psychiatr Clin North Am* 11:419-432, 1988.

Lustman PJ, Griffith LS, Clouse RE: Depression in adults with diabetes: results of 5-yr follow-up study, *Diabetes Care* 11:605-612, 1988.

Lustman PJ et al: Depression in adults with diabetes, *Diabetes Care* 15:1631-1639, 1992.

Lustman PJ et al: Effects of nortriptyline on depression and glycemic control in diabetes: results of a double-blind, placebo-controlled trial, *Psychosom Med* submitted for publication, 1996.

McDaniel JS et al: Depression in patients with cancer, *Arch Gen Psychiatry* 52:89-99, 1995.

Mayberg HS: Frontal lobe dysfunction in secondary depression, *J Neuropsychiatry Clin Neurosci* 6:428-442, 1994.

Migliorelli R et al: Prevalence and correlates of dysthymia and major depression among patients with Alzheimer's disease, *Am J Psychiatry* 152:37-44, 1995.

Minden SL, Schiffer RB: Affective disorders in multiple sclerosis: review and recommendations for clinical research, *Arch Neurol* 47:98-104, 1990.

Platz C, Kendell RE: A matched-control follow-up and family study of 'puerperal psychoses,' *Br J Psychiatry* 153:90-94, 1988.

Pons G, Rey E, Matheson I: Excretion of psychoactive drugs into breast milk, *Clin Pharmacokinet* 27:270-289, 1994.

Preskorn SH: Antidepressant drug selection: criteria and options, *J Clin Psychiatry* 55(9 Suppl A):6-22, 1994.

Price JS: Chronic depressive illness, *Br Med J* 1:1200-1201, 1978.

Rifkin A: Depression in physically ill patients, *Postgrad Med* 92:147-154, 1992.

Ross ED: The aprosodias: functional-anatomic organization of the affective components of language in the right hemisphere, *Arch Neurol* 38:561-569, 1981.

Ross ED, Rush AJ: Diagnosis and neuroanatomical correlates of depression in brain-damaged patients: implications for a neurology of depression, *Arch Gen Psychiatry* 38:1344-1354, 1981.

Schleifer SJ et al: The nature and course of depression following myocardial infarction, *Arch Intern Med* 149:1785-1789, 1989.

Smith MD, Hong BA, Robson AM: Diagnosis of depression in patients with end-stage renal disease, *Am J Med* 79:160-166, 1985.

Starkstein SE, Preziosi TJ, Robinson RG: Sleep disorders, pain, and depression in Parkinson's disease, *Eur Neurol* 31:352-355, 1991.

Starkstein SE, Robinson RG, editors: *Depression in neurologic disease,* Baltimore, 1993, Johns Hopkins University Press.

Turkington RW: Depression masquerading as diabetic neuropathy, *JAMA* 243:1147-1150, 1980.

Videbech P, Gouliaev G: First admission with puerperal psychosis: 7-14 years of follow-up, *Acta Psychiatr Scand* 91:167-173, 1995.

Chapter 27

Allgulander C: Suicide and mortality patterns in anxiety neurosis and depressive neurosis, *Arch Gen Psychiatry* 51:708-712, 1994.

Arató M et al: Retrospective psychiatric assessment of 200 suicides in Budapest, *Acta Psychiatr Scand* 77:454-456, 1988.

Åsgård U: A psychiatric study of suicide among urban Swedish women, *Acta Psychiatr Scand* 82:115-124, 1990.

Barraclough B et al: A hundred cases of suicide: clinical aspects, *Br J Psychiatry* 125:355-373, 1974.

Beskow J: Suicide and mental disorder in Swedish men, *Acta Psychiatr Scand* 277(suppl):1-138, 1979.

Blackburn IM et al: The efficacy of cognitive therapy in depression: a treatment trial using cognitive therapy and pharmacotherapy, each alone and in combination, *Br J Psychiatry* 139:181-189, 1981.

Bowers WA: Treatment of depressed in-patients: cognitive therapy plus medication, relaxation plus medication, and medication alone, *Br J Psychiatry* 156:73-78, 1990.

Caldwell CB, Gottesman II: Schizophrenics kill themselves too: a review of risk factors for suicide, *Schizophrenia Bull* 16:571-589, 1990.

Cheng ATA: Mental illness and suicide: a case-control study in Taiwan, *Arch Gen Psychiatry* 52:594-603, 1995.

Chynoweth R, Tonge JI, Armstrong J: Suicide in Brisbane: a retrospective psychosocial study, *Austr N Z J Psychiatry* 14:37-45, 1980.

Clendenin WW, Murphy GE: Wrist cutting: new epidemiological findings, *Arch Gen Psychiatry* 25:465-469, 1971.

Coryell W, Noyes R, Clancy J: Excess mortality in panic disorder: a comparison with primary unipolar depression, *Arch Gen Psychiatry* 39:701-703, 1982.

Davidson KM: Diagnosis of depression in alcohol dependence: changes in prevalence with drinking status, *Br J Psychiatry* 166:199-204, 1995.

Delong WB, Robins E: The communication of suicidal intent prior to psychiatric hospitalization: a study of 87 patients, *Am J Psychiatry* 117:695-705, 1961.

Dorpat TL, Ripley HS: A study of suicide in the Seattle area, *Compr Psychiatry* 1:349-359, 1960.

Elkin I et al: National Institute of Mental Health Treatment of Depression Collaborative Research Program: general effectiveness of treatments, *Arch Gen Psychiatry* 46:971-982, 1989.

Fawcett J: Suicidal depression and physical illness, *JAMA* 219:1303-1306, 1972.

Goldacre M, Seagroatt V, Hawton K: Suicide after discharge from psychiatric care, *Lancet* 342:283-286, 1993.

Hagnell O, Rorsman B: Suicide in the Lundby study: a comparative investigation of clinical aspects, *Neuropsychobiology* 5:61-73, 1979.

Henriksson MM et al: Mental disorders and comorbidity in suicide, *Am J Psychiatry* 150:935-940, 1993.

Isacsson G, Boëthius G, Bergman U: Low level of antidepressant prescription for people who later commit suicide: 15 years of experience from a population-based drug database in Sweden, *Acta Psychiatr Scand* 85:444-448, 1992.

Isometsaa ET et al: Suicide in major depression, *Am J Psychiatry* 151:530-536, 1994.

Kapamadžija B, Biro M, Sovljanski M: Socio-psihijatrijska i patomorfoloska analiza, 100 izvrsenih samoubistava, *Soc Psihijat* 10:35-56, 1982.

Keller MB: Depression: a long-term illness, *Br J Psychiatry* 165(suppl 26):9-15, 1994.

Mann JJ, Kapur S: The emergence of suicidal ideation and behavior during antidepressant pharmacotherapy, *Arch Gen Psychiatry* 48:1027-1033, 1991.

Marzuk PM et al: Increased risk of suicide in persons with AIDS, *JAMA* 259:1333-1337, 1988.

Mitterauer B: Mehrdimensionale Diagnostik von 121 Suiziden im Bundesland Salzburg im Jahre 1978, *Wien Med Wochenschr* 9:229-234, 1981.

Murphy GE: The physician's responsibility for suicide. II. Errors of omission, *Ann Intern Med* 82:305-309, 1975.

Murphy GE, Robins E: Social factors in suicide, *JAMA* 199:303-308, 1967.

Murphy GE et al: Suicide and alcoholism: interpersonal loss confirmed as a predictor, *Arch Gen Psychiatry* 36:65-69, 1979.

Murphy GE et al: Cognitive therapy and pharmacotherapy: singly and together in the treatment of depression, *Arch Gen Psychiatry* 41:33-41, 1984.

Murphy GE et al: Multiple risk factors predict suicide in alcoholism, *Arch Gen Psychiatry* 49:459-463, 1992.

Noyes RN: Suicide and panic disorder: a review, *J Affective Disord* 22:1-11, 1991.

Rich CL, Runeson BS: Similarities in diagnostic comorbidity between suicide among young people in Sweden and the United States, *Acta Psychiatr Scand* 86:335-339, 1992.

Rich CL, Young D, Fowler RC: San Diego suicide study. I. Young vs. old subjects, *Arch Gen Psychiatry* 43:577-582, 1986.

Rich CL et al: San Diego suicide study. III. Relationships between diagnoses and stressors, *Arch Gen Psychiatry* 45:589-592, 1988.

Robins LN, Locke BZ, Regier DA: *Psychiatric disorders in America,* New York, 1991, The Free Press.

Robins E et al: Some clinical considerations in the prevention of suicide based on a study of 134 successful suicides, *Am J Public Health* 49:888-899, 1959.

Runeson B: Mental disorder in youth suicide: DSM-III-R axes I and II, *Acta Psychiatr Scand* 79:490-497, 1989.

Teicher MH, Glod C, Cole Jo: Emergence of intense suicidal preoccupation during fluoxetine treatment, *Am J Psychiatry* 147:207-210, 1990.

United States Department of Health and Human Services: Annual medical examiner data, (from the Drug Abuse Warning Network) Series I, Number 13-B, Rockville, 1995, DHHS Publication No. (SMA)95-3019.

Vollrath M, Angst J: Outcome of panic and depression in a seven year follow-up: results of the Zurich study, *Acta Psychiatr Scand* 80:591-596, 1989.

Chapter 28

Appelbaum PS, Gutheil TG: *The clinical handbook of psychiatry and the law,* ed 2, Baltimore, 1991, Williams and Wilkins.

Developments in the law: civil commitment of the mentally ill, *87 Harv L Rev,* 1974.

Grisso T: *Evaluating competencies: forensic assessments and instruments,* vol 7, *Perspectives in law and psychology,* Sales BD, series editor, New York, 1986, Plenum Press.

Gutheil TG: *Legal issues in psychiatry.* In Kaplan HI, Sadock BJ, editors: *Comprehensive textbook of psychiatry,* ed 6, vol 2, Baltimore, 1995, Williams and Wilkins.

Melton GB et al: *Psychological evaluations for the courts,* New York, 1987, Guilford Press.

Missouri Revised Statutes §475.010.

Prosser WL: *Handbook of the law of torts,* ed 4, St. Paul, Minn., 1971, West Publishing Company.

Simon RI: *Clinical psychiatry and the law,* Washington, D.C., 1987, American Psychiatric Press.

Chapter 29

Appelbaum PS, Roth LS: Competency to consent to research, *Arch Gen Psychiatry* 39:951-958, 1982.

Beresford T: *Alcohol abuse and liver transplantation.* In Craven J, Rodin GM, editors: *Psychiatric aspects of organ transplantation,* New York, 1992, Oxford University Press.

Brody BA: Assessing empirical research in bioethics, *Theor Med* 14:211-219, 1993.

Bursztain HJ et al: Beyond cognition: the role of disordered affective states in impairing competence to consent to treatment, *Bull Am Acad Psychiatry Law* 19:383-388, 1991.

Cohen C, Benjamin M: Alcoholics and liver transplantation, *JAMA* 265:1299-1301, 1991.

Dinwiddie SH: Physician-assisted suicide: epistemological problems, *Int J Med Law* 11:345-352, 1992.

Emanuel EJ, Emanuel LL: Four models of the physician-patient relationship, *JAMA* 267:2221-2226, 1992.

Freeman A et al: *Assessment of transplant candidates and prediction of outcome.* In Craven J, Rodin GM, editors: *Psychiatric aspects of organ transplantation,* New York, 1992, Oxford University Press.

Goldman MJ, Gutheil TG: The misperceived duty to report patients' past crimes, *Bull Am Acad Psychiatry Law* 22:407-410, 1994.

Goodwin JS: Mercy killing: mercy for whom? *JAMA* 265:326, 1991.

Guze SB: The need for toughmindedness in psychiatric thinking, *South Med J* 63:662-671, 1970.

Guze SB: *Why psychiatry is a branch of medicine,* New York, 1992, Oxford University Press.

Humber JM, Almeder RF, Kasting GA, editors: *Physician-assisted death,* Totowa, N.J., 1993, Humana Press.

Levenson JLL, Olbrisch ME: Psychosocial evaluation of organ transplant candidates: a comparative study of process, criteria, and outcomes in heart, liver, and kidney transplantation, *Psychosomatics* 34:314-323, 1993.

Meier DE: *Doctors' attitudes and experiences with physician-assisted death: a review of the literature.* In Humber JM, Almeder RF, Kasting GA, editors: *Physician-assisted death,* Totowa N.J., 1993, Humana Press.

Moss AH, Siegler M: Should alcoholics compete equally for liver transplantation? *JAMA* 265:1295-1298, 1991.

Ortenlicher D: Physician participation in assisted suicide, *JAMA* 262:1844-1845, 1989.

Pellegrino ED, Thomasma DC: *For the patient's good,* Oxford, England, 1988, Oxford University Press.

Rosenblum VG, Forsythe CD: The right to assisted suicide: protection of autonomy or an open door to social killing? *Issues Law Med* 6:4-31, 1990.

Thomasma DC: *The ethics of physician-assisted suicide,* In Humber JM, Almeder RF, Kasting GA, editors: *Physician-assisted death,* Totowa N.J., 1993, Humana Press.

Webb WL, Rothschild BS, Monroe L: *Ethics and psychiatry.* In Hales RE, Yudofsky SC, Talbott JA, editors: *Textbook of psychiatry,* ed 2, Washington, D.C., 1994, American Psychiatric Press.

Index

E

I

W

Y

Z